Eye Pathology

An Atlas and Text

SECOND EDITION

To Michael with my best regards ...

Eye Pathology

An Atlas and Text

SECOND EDITION

RALPH C. EAGLE, JR., MD

Director, Department of Pathology
Wills Eye Institute
The Noel T. and Sara L. Simmonds Professor of Ophthalmic Pathology
Wills Eye Institute
Professor of Ophthalmology and Pathology
Jefferson Medical College of Thomas Jefferson University
Philadelphia, Pennsylvania

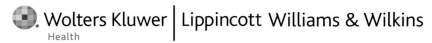

Wolters Kluwer | Lippincott Williams & Wilkins
Health

Philadelphia · Baltimore · New York · London
Buenos Aires · Hong Kong · Sydney · Tokyo

Senior Executive Editor: Jonathan W. Pine, Jr.
Senior Product Manager: Emilie Moyer
Senior Manufacturing Manager: Benjamin Rivera
Marketing Manager: Lisa Lawrence
Senior Designer: Stephen Druding
Production Service: SPi Global

Second Edition

© 2011 by LIPPINCOTT WILLIAMS & WILKINS, a WOLTERS KLUWER business

Two Commerce Square
2001 Market Street
Philadelphia, PA 19103 USA
LWW.com

First Edition © 1999 by W.B. Saunders

Printed in China

Library of Congress Cataloging-in-Publication Data
Eagle, Ralph C., Jr., author.
  Eye pathology : an atlas and text / Ralph C. Eagle, Jr., MD, Director, Department of Pathology, Wills Eye Institute, The Noel T. and Sara L. Simmonds Professor of Ophthalmic Pathology, Wills Eye Institute, Professor of Ophthalmology and Pathology, Jefferson Medical College of Thomas Jefferson University, Philadelphia, Pennsylvania. — Second edition.
       p. ; cm.
  Includes bibliographical references and index.
  ISBN 978-1-60831-788-2 (hardback)
  1. Eye—Pathophysiology. 2. Eye—Pathophysiology—Atlases. I. Title.
  [DNLM: 1. Eye Diseases—pathology—Atlases. WW 17]
  RE67.E24 2010
  617.7—dc22
                                                                              2010046343

Care has been taken to confirm the accuracy of the information presented and to describe generally accepted practices. However, the authors, editors, and publisher are not responsible for errors or omissions or for any consequences from application of the information in this book and make no warranty, expressed or implied, with respect to the currency, completeness, or accuracy of the contents of the publication. Application of the information in a particular situation remains the professional responsibility of the practitioner.

The authors, editors, and publisher have exerted every effort to ensure that drug selection and dosage set forth in this text are in accordance with current recommendations and practice at the time of publication. However, in view of ongoing research, changes in government regulations, and the constant flow of information relating to drug therapy and drug reactions, the reader is urged to check the package insert for each drug for any change in indications and dosage and for added warnings and precautions. This is particularly important when the recommended agent is a new or infrequently employed drug.

Some drugs and medical devices presented in the publication have Food and Drug Administration (FDA) clearance for limited use in restricted research settings. It is the responsibility of the health care provider to ascertain the FDA status of each drug or device planned for use in their clinical practice.

To purchase additional copies of this book, call our customer service department at (800) 638-3030 or fax orders to (301) 223-2320. International customers should call (301) 223-2300.

Visit Lippincott Williams & Wilkins on the Internet: at LWW.com. Lippincott Williams & Wilkins customer service representatives are available from 8:30 am to 6 pm, EST.

In memory of Ewa

This book is also dedicated to my teachers Myron Yanoff and Ramon L. Font and to my former chief William S. Tasman for his friendship and strong and unwavering support of ophthalmic pathology during his long and distinguished tenure as Ophthalmologist-in-Chief at the Wills Eye Institute.

PREFACE

During the past three decades, I have taught ophthalmic pathology to medical students, interns, and ophthalmologists-in-training at the Wills Eye Institute, the Lancaster Course in Ophthalmology, the Armed Forces Institute of Pathology (AFIP) Ophthalmic Pathology course, the Wills Review of Ophthalmology, and eye hospitals and academic institutions on four continents. In the past, students expressed a need for a basic eye pathology text that was fairly comprehensive, yet concise enough to be read and mastered in a relatively short time. The first edition of *Eye Pathology: An Atlas and Basic Text* sought to fulfill that need. Positive feedback received from students and colleagues suggests that I was successful in achieving that goal.

The second edition of my textbook incorporates changes that are designed to make it even better. The second edition has been printed in standard "portrait" format. All of the figures have been reprocessed and they are now incorporated in the text. The text has been updated and lengthened a bit, incorporating new advances and developments in ophthalmology and genetics. A short introductory chapter on ocular anatomy and histology has been included, and some areas that were covered too superficially in the first edition were expanded. These include intraocular tumors in adults, corneal dystrophies, melanocytic lesions of the conjunctiva, ocular and adnexal lymphomas, and the use of immunohistochemistry in diagnosis.

Finally, a substantial review quiz comprising more than 400 multiple-choice questions has been added to help the reader review and reinforce learning of the material. The online quiz includes more than 100 questions based on photos.

The second edition of *Eye Pathology: An Atlas and Text* is designed to serve as a basic introduction to eye pathology that can be read and mastered during an ophthalmic pathology elective. In addition, it is a well-illustrated resource for residents who are studying for the Ophthalmic Knowledge Assessment Program (OKAP) examinations or Board certification in ophthalmology. To fulfill the latter goal, the text is relatively short, succinct, and factually-rich (almost a précis); there are many large color figures and photomontages; and the figure legends intentionally highlight important facts and "buzz words" that students are expected to know. The book should also benefit surgical pathologists who wish to learn more about eye pathology, and need a short, well–illustrated reference by the gross dissection bench or microscope.

Why study ophthalmic pathology, anyway? Most would agree that an understanding of ocular disease and pathologic mechanisms that lead to blindness is a prerequisite for quality ophthalmic practice. A physician cannot diagnose a disease that he or she has never heard of.

In 1984, Dr. Frederick A. Jakobiec eloquently addressed this issue in his introduction to a special issue of the Journal Ophthalmology dedicated to basic science and ophthalmology:

"Unless one knows the natural course of a disease, it is not possible to decide whether an intervention has been efficacious or not. At a time when we are witnessing the progressive commercialization of ophthalmology and the slackening of traditional standards of professional behavior, one of the few remaining constraints that might prevent us from becoming high-tech mountebanks, peddling star wars' nostrums that are expensive and potentially meretricious, is our well-founded and ethically enhancing knowledge of ocular disease."

Dr. Jakobiec's words still ring true today.

Ralph C. Eagle, Jr., MD
Director, Department of Pathology, Wills Eye Institute
November 2010

CONTENTS

1 An Introduction to Ocular Anatomy and Histology

A paired, hollow, spherical organ, the human eye is slightly less than an inch in diameter (Fig. 1-1A). Internally, it is divided into anterior and posterior chambers and a much larger vitreous cavity, which comprises most of its posterior segment. The anterior chamber is bounded anteriorly by the cornea and posteriorly by the anterior surfaces of the iris and lens (Fig. 1-1B). The posterior chamber is bounded anteriorly by the iris pigment epithelium (IPE), laterally by the ciliary processes that form the pars plicata of the ciliary body, and posteriorly by the "face" or anterior surface of the vitreous humor. Both anterior and posterior chambers are filled with watery aqueous humor, which is secreted by the ciliary epithelium on the ciliary processes.

The vitreous humor fills most of the posterior segment. The most delicate connective tissue in the body, the vitreous humor is a transparent gel composed of hyaluronic acid and a framework of delicate fibrils of type II collagen. Centrally, the anterior face of the vitreous abuts the posterior surface of the lens, which is located directly behind the iris in the posterior chamber, and is supported by a suspensory ligament of zonular fibers. The concavity in the anterior face of the vitreous that holds the lens is called the patellar fossa, and the retrolental space of Berger is interposed between the lens and the vitreous. Posteriorly, the vitreous lines the inner surface of the retina. Anteriorly, it is firmly adherent to the vitreous base, which straddles the ora serrata, the junction between the peripheral retina and the pars plana of the ciliary body. The vitreous also has relatively firm attachments to the margin of the optic disc and major retinal vessels. A curved channel called Cloquet canal runs through the center of the vitreous from the lens to the optic nerve. Overlying the optic nerve head, the posterior part of Cloquet canal widens to form a space resembling an inverted funnel called the area Martegiani.

The eye wall is composed of three concentric coats that vary markedly in their cellularity and composition (Fig. 1-1C,D). The three layers are readily separated during gross dissection. The outer coat includes the white sclera that merges with the transparent cornea at the corneoscleral limbus. Paucicellular and composed largely of dense collagenous connective tissue, the outer layer constitutes the eye's tough fibrous exoskeleton that confines and protects its contents of fluid and delicate neural tissues. The collagenous lamellae of the sclera are larger and more irregular than that of the cornea.

The eye's innermost coat is composed of neuroectodermal tissues derived from the optic cup. Highly cellular and largely devoid of connective tissue, these structures include the neurosensory retina, the retinal pigment epithelium (RPE), the ciliary epithelium, and the IPE. Embryologically, this inner layer of neuroectodermal tissues is derived from an outpouching of the forebrain called the optic vesicle. The neuroectoderm is a polarized layer of epithelial cells with characteristic apical and basal features. Microvilli and cilia typically are found on the apical surface of the cells, which are joined near their apices by intercellular connections called terminal bars. The bases of the cells rest on a basement membrane or basal lamina. The basal lamina serves as the attachment for extracellular matrix material.

The optic vesicle is lined externally by a basement membrane, and the apical surface of its neuroectodermal cells projects into its lumen. Later, as the optic vesicle invaginates to form the optic cup on day 27 of gestation, the apical surfaces of the inner and outer layer of cells become approximated. This "apex to apex" orientation continues throughout life. The inner layer of the optic cup goes on to form the posterior layer of IPE, the inner nonpigmented layer of ciliary epithelium, and the neurosensory retina. Its outer layer forms the anterior half of the IPE, which includes the dilator muscle, the outer pigmented layer of ciliary epithelium, and the RPE.

The two layers of cells that compose the iris and ciliary epithelia retain "apex to apex" orientation found in the optic cup with basal laminae on their external surfaces. Both layers are firmly fused together. Both layers are pigmented in the IPE. The ciliary epithelium is a half-pigmented bilayer; its outer layer is pigmented and its inner layer is nonpigmented (see Fig. 1-5D). During microscopy, this "two-toned" bilayer of cells readily serves to identify ciliary body tissue. At the ora serrata, the outer layer of pigmented ciliary epithelium continues posteriorly as the RPE, and the inner layer of nonpigmented ciliary epithelium abruptly thickens to form the neurosensory retina, with its complex lamellar architecture. Posterior to the ora serrata, the layers derived from the inner and outer layers of the optic cup are not fused. A potential space called the subretinal space is present between the retina and the RPE. The apical surfaces of both tissues project into the subretinal space and interdigitate. Retinal detachment or separation is marked by the accumulation of fluid in this potential space.

In routine microscopic sections, the IPE appears to be a single layer, since its two layers of cells are obscured by heavy pigmentation (Fig. 1-2D). Both layers are apparent in bleached sections, however. The iris dilator muscle appears as an eosinophilic band on the anterior surface of the IPE. The dilator is not a separate structure. Rather, it is composed of cellular processes arising from the basal surface of the anterior layer of cells, which are nonpigmented and have smooth muscle differentiation. The sphincter muscle

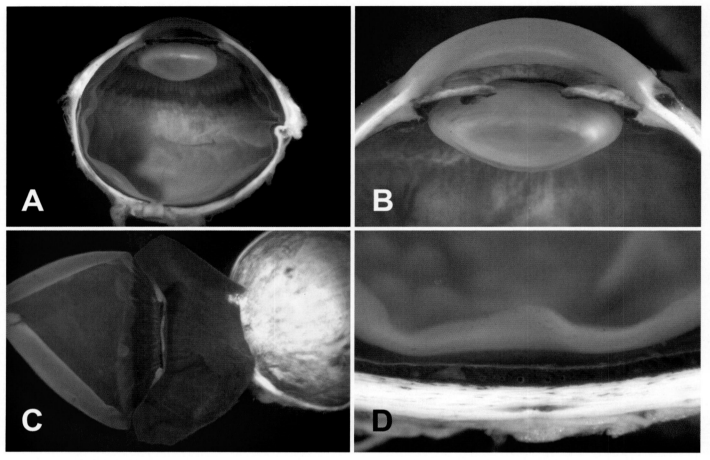

Fig. 1-1. A. Slightly less than an inch in diameter, the eye is composed of an anterior chamber and a much larger posterior vitreous cavity. **B.** The anterior chamber is bounded anteriorly by the cornea and posteriorly by the iris and lens. The lens is situated in the posterior chamber behind the pupil. **C.** The eye is composed of three concentric coats that are easily separated during dissection. **D.** Posteriorly, the three coats are evident as the sclera, pigmented choroid, and the retina.

of the iris, which encircles and constricts the pupil, is also derived from the IPE but separates from it during development, forming a distinct structure. Continuity of the sphincter muscle with the IPE can be observed microscopically in fetal eyes. The sphincter is about 1 mm in width and is separated from the IPE by a layer of connective tissue that becomes more prominent with increasing age.

Clinically, the IPE is visible at the edge of the pupil as the pigment ruff or frill, which corresponds to the margin of the optic cup (Fig. 1-2C). This is the only neuroectodermal tissue of the eye that can be seen with the slit lamp biomicroscope without supplementary lenses. The granules of neuroepithelial melanin in the iris pigment epithelial cells are large and spherical in shape in contrast to RPE granules, which typically are ellipsoidal. Granules of neuroectodermal melanin are always larger than the dustlike melanosomes found in uveal stromal cells. The IPE is maximally pigmented in all eyes.

A peripheral colony of brainlike tissue, the neurosensory retina is a complex, highly cellular tissue composed of cells that are arranged in regular layers (Fig. 1-3A). Ten retinal layers including the RPE are identified. It is relatively easy

to remember the microscopic anatomy of the retina if one recalls that the retina is a three-neuron system composed of three layers of cells: photoreceptors and first- and second-order neurons. Regarding orientation, the term *inner* refers to the layers of cells that are located closest to the vitreous cavity or the center of the eye. *Outer* denotes layers that are located nearer to the sclera. The nuclei of retinal cells are arranged in distinct bands called nuclear layers. The nuclei of the photoreceptors and first-order neurons (bipolar cells) form the outer nuclear layer (ONL) and inner nuclear layer (INL), respectively. The retinal ganglion cells (the second-order neurons) comprise the innermost layer of nuclei in the retina. The ganglion cell layer (GCL) varies markedly in thickness. Surrounding the fovea, the GCL is five or more cells thick. Multilamination of the GCL is an excellent histologic marker for the macula or perifoveal part of the retina. The GCL is thin in the peripheral retina. Peripheral to the vascular arcades formed by the superior and inferior temporal retinal arterioles, the ganglion cells form a discontinuous monolayer.

The plexiform layers of the retina are composed of axons and dendrites. The outer plexiform layer (OPL) is

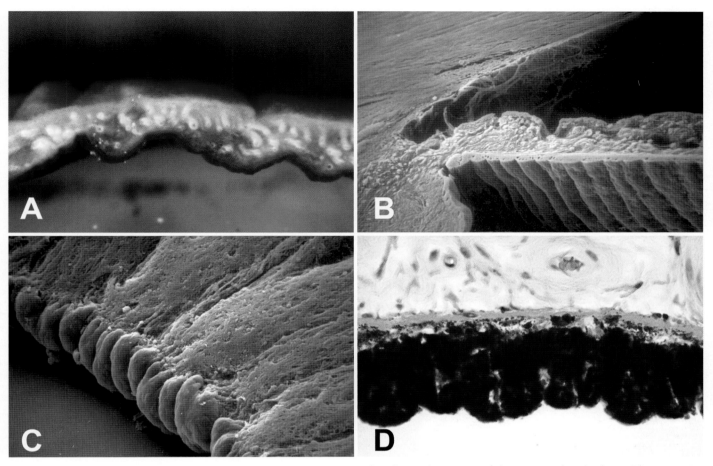

Fig. 1-2. The iris. A. The pigment in this brown iris is concentrated in the melanocytes of the anterior border layer. The posterior IPE is maximally pigmented. Cuffs of collagen highlight iris stromal vessels. **B.** SEM shows circumferential ridges on posterior surface of the neuroectodermal IPE. Iris stroma is derived from the neural crest. **C.** Termination of the IPE at pupillary margin forms beaded pigment ruff. **D.** The two layers comprising the IPE are fused and maximally pigmented. The dilator muscle is evident as an eosinophilic band on its stromal surface. It is composed of cellular processes with smooth muscle differentiation. (**B.** SEM ×40, **C.** SEM ×320, **D.** H&E ×250)

interposed between the ONL and INL, and the inner plexiform layer separates the INL from the GCL. The inner plexiform layer is truly plexiform: its whole breadth is comprised of an intricately interweaving tangle of ramifying neuronal processes. In contrast, only the narrow inner band of the OPL is truly plexiform. Its wider outer part contains an orderly parallel array of photoreceptor axons called Henle fibers. Although Henle fibers occur throughout the retina, the eponym generally is applied to the radially oriented photoreceptor axons surrounding the fovea. A line of synaptic connections comprising cone pedicles, rod spherules, and the dendrites of bipolar cells delimits the outer margin of the truly plexiform part of the OPL (Fig. 1-3B). This linear row of synapses is called the middle limiting membrane (MLM). Like the retina's external limiting membrane (XLM), the MLM is not a basement membrane (the only true basement membrane of the retina is the internal limiting membrane or ILM). The MLM delimits the vascularized inner part of the retina; capillaries from the central retinal artery penetrate no deeper than the MLM. External to the

MLM, the retina is avascular and depends on the choroidal circulation for oxygen and nutrients. The OPL is a watershed zone between the dual vascular supplies of the retina. This factor contributes to the localization of edema fluid and hard exudates in OPL.

The INL contains the nuclei of bipolar, amacrine, horizontal, and Mueller cells. Bipolar cells predominate. The horizontal cell nuclei are found in the outer part, and the amacrine cell nuclei in the inner part of the INL. The nuclei of the Mueller cells can lie at any level of the INL. Accessory glial cells including fibrous and protoplasmic astrocytes and oligodendrocyte-like cells are confined to the nerve fiber, ganglion cell, and inner plexiform layers of the retina. Hence, gliosis does not occur after central retinal artery occlusion because these cells are killed.

As we have seen, the orientation of cells in the optic vesicle and cup persists in the adult eye. The internal limiting membrane (ILM) of the retina corresponds to the basal lamina on the inner layer of the optic cup. A true basement membrane, the ILM is synthesized by the basal

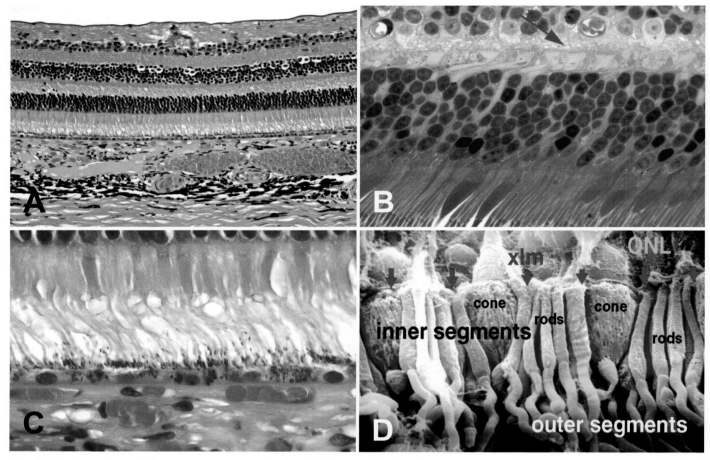

Fig. 1-3. The retina. A. The retina is composed of orderly layers of cell nuclei (nuclear layers) and plexiform layers composed of axons and dendrites. The photoreceptors rest on the RPE on the inner surface of the choroid. **B.** The MLM (**arrow**) is a linear band of synapses connecting photoreceptor cell axons and bipolar cell dendrites in the anterior part of the OPL. **C.** The inner and outer segments of the photoreceptors project through the fenestrated XLM into the subretinal space. The tips of the outer segments interdigitate with pigmented processes on the apical surface of the RPE. **D.** False colorized SEM highlights inner and outer segments of rods and cones. Cones are distinguished by the conical configuration of their inner segments. Photoreceptor nuclei comprise ONL. (**A.** H&E ×50, **B.** Toluidine blue ×250, H&E ×250, SEM ×2,500)

foot processes of the giant glial cells of Mueller, which span the entire thickness of the retina. The ILM serves as an attachment point for the fine fibrils of type II collagen that comprise the fibrillar component of the vitreous humor. Intricately interweaving processes of the Mueller cells totally fill the interstices between the retinal neurons and serve to segregate their receptive surfaces. There is little or no extracellular space in the retina.

The Mueller cells are polarized. Electron microscopy discloses microvilli on their apical surfaces, which project into the subretinal space between the photoreceptors. A belt desmosome of intercellular junctions called the XLM is found in the outer or apical part of the neurosensory retina. Not a true basement membrane, the XLM is composed of permeable adherent junctions (zonulae adherentes) that join the apices of the Mueller cells and the rod and cone cells. The XLM is permeable and does not form a barrier to fluid or macromolecules. The XLM has been called the fenestrated membrane of Verhoeff. The inner and outer segments of the rods and cones project through this fenestrated membrane into the subretinal space where they are surrounded by extracellular matrix material rich in hyaluronidase-resistant acid mucopolysaccharide (Fig. 1-3C). Cone cell nuclei are located next to the XLM in the ONL.

Rods and cones are distinguished light microscopically by the shape of their inner segments (Fig. 1-3D). The inner segments of rods are slender rodlike cylinders, while extrafoveal cones are conical in shape. Highly specialized cones that resemble rods are densely packed in the cone-rich fovea. The photoreceptor inner segments are packed with mitochondria that provide energy for the photochemistry of vision, which occurs in the photoreceptor outer segments. Photoreceptor inner and outer segments are joined by a connecting cilium that has the characteristic 9 + 0 pattern of microtubular doublets found in central nervous system cilia. Photoreceptors probably are derived from modified cilia, which are found on the apical surface of cells.

The outer segments of the photoreceptors contain stacks of thin discs composed of cellular membranes. The arrangement of the membranous discs has been likened to a stack of coins or potato chips packaged in cylindrical containers. Visual pigments such as rhodopsin are incorporated as transmembrane proteins in the disc membranes. Separate, free-floating discs occur in rods. The discs in cone outer segments are not separate structures; they comprise a continuous, sinuously folded structure formed by invaginations of the outer cell membrane.

Photoreceptor outer segments project from the apical surface of the retina into the subretinal space where they are enveloped by the microvillous processes on the apical surface of the RPE, the polarized monolayer of pigmented cells derived from the outer layer of the optic cup. The RPE cells are firmly joined near their apices by a girdle of intercellular connections called *zonulae occludentes*. These tight junctions form a barrier to the passage of molecules and constitute the outer part of the blood–retinal barrier. Large ellipsoidal granules of melanin pigment measuring approximately 1 μm in diameter are found in the apical cytoplasm of the RPE cells. Granules of lipofuscin pigment fill the basal cytoplasm. This "wear and tear" pigment is derived from the incomplete digestion of photoreceptor outer segments by the RPE's phagolysosomal system and gradually accumulates with age. The lipofuscin is relatively inapparent in routine Hematoxylin and eosin (H&E) sections, but the pigment is autofluorescent and is vividly disclosed by UV fluorescent microscopy (Fig. 1-4D). The nuclei of the RPE cells are located in the basal cytoplasm near Bruch membrane.

An intact layer of RPE is vital to the health and function of the adjacent neurosensory retina (Fig. 1-4). In flat preparations, the cells comprising this pigmented monolayer are hexagonal in shape, resembling the familiar pattern of the bathroom tile (Fig. 1-4B). The pigment in the RPE is largely responsible for the reddish brown color of the fundus seen grossly or ophthalmoscopically (Fig. 1-4A). This is readily demonstrated in the laboratory by focally denuding Bruch membrane with a cotton swab. Removal

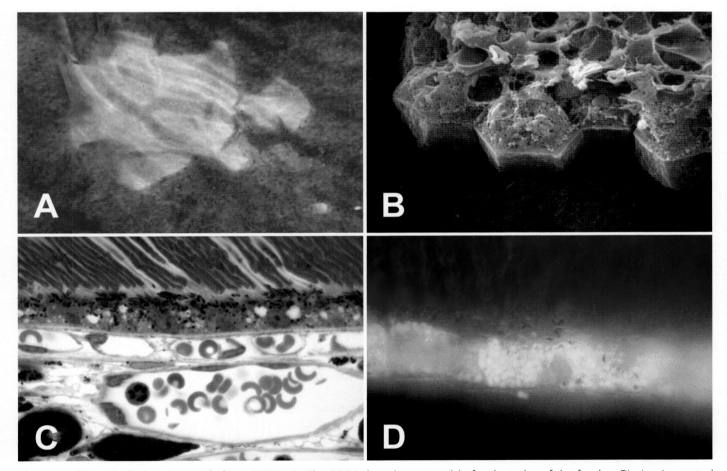

Fig. 1-4. The retinal pigment epithelium (RPE). A. The RPE is largely responsible for the color of the fundus. Rip in pigmented layer discloses large vessels in underlying choroid separated by uveal pigment. **B.** SEM shows hexagonal monolayer of RPE cells covering the inner surface of Bruch membrane. **C.** Photomicrograph shows elliptical granules of RPE melanin in apical cytoplasm of RPE cells. The choriocapillaris abuts the outer surface of Bruch membrane. **D.** Fluorescent microscopy discloses yellow granules of autofluorescent lipofuscin pigment in the basal cytoplasm of the RPE cells. (**B.** SEM ×1,250, **C.** Toluidine blue ×250, UV fluorescent microscopy ×400)

of the RPE discloses the larger choroidal vessels, which are visible through Bruch membrane, which is semitransparent. Melanin pigment within choroidal melanocytes between the vessels serves to highlight the latter. In heavily pigmented people, the density of pigmentation between the vessels may impart a tigroid or tiger-striped appearance to the fundus.

The RPE rests on a specialized layer of connective tissue called Bruch membrane, which rests on, and delimits the inner surface of the choroid (Fig. 1-4C). Bruch membrane is a sandwichlike structure composed of extracellular matrix material. Its inner and outermost layers are the basement membranes of the RPE cells and the endothelial cells of the choriocapillaris, respectively. The basement membrane of the RPE corresponds to the basement membrane on the outer surface of the optic cup. Bruch membrane is largely composed of type I collagen and has a central core of elastic tissue. As we age, Bruch membrane gradually thickens and becomes increasingly periodic acid-Schiff (PAS)-positive. Basophilic foci of calcification are often found in the posterior parts of Bruch membrane in the elderly. Transmission electron microscopy demonstrates that the thickening of Bruch membrane is caused by the gradual accumulation of linear and vesicular structures.

The choroid is the posterior and largest part of the uveal tract, the eye's central coat, which is interposed between the outer sclera and the innermost layer of neuroectodermal tissue (Fig. 1-1D). Intermediate in cellularity, the uveal tract is pigmented and richly vascular. The term uveal reflects the fanciful resemblance of this coat to a black-purple grape (uva = grape in Latin) noted when early anatomists removed the sclera. Derived from the neural crest, the uvea comprises the iris stroma, the stroma of the ciliary body, and the choroid.

The highly vascular choroid contains three layers of blood vessels that increase in size as they near the sclera (Fig. 1-3A). An interconnected layer of leaky, fenestrated capillaries called the choriocapillaris rests directly beneath the Bruch membrane (Fig. 1-4C). A second layer of medium-sized vessels called Sattler layer and an outer layer of larger vessels called Haller layer also are present. The choroidal stroma contains connective tissue and dendritic melanocytes that vary in their pigment content depending on the patient's race and eye color. An equivalent number of melanocytes is present in all races, but darkly pigmented individuals have larger cells filled with larger melanin granules. The melanin granules found in uveal melanocytes are quite small and dustlike. They are readily distinguished from the large ellipsoidal granules of melanin found in the apical cytoplasm of the RPE cells.

The middle part of the uveal tract called the ciliary body is interposed between the iris and the choroid (Fig. 1-5). The ciliary body has two major components, the pars plicata (also called the "corona ciliaris") and the pars plana (Fig. 1-5B). The anterior pars plicata is composed of a ring of 70 to 80 ciliary processes. The ciliary processes project into and encircle the posterior chamber, and their nonpigmented epithelial cells secrete the watery aqueous humor that fills the cavity and the anterior chamber. The aqueous humor flows through the pupil toward specialized "drains" located in the anterior chamber "angle" formed by the junction of the iris and cornea. Small white nodules occasionally are observed incidentally on individual ciliary processes during gross dissection, particularly in the eyes of older individuals. These represent small foci of pseudoadenomatous proliferations of the nonpigmented ciliary epithelium called Fuchs (or coronary) adenomas. They undoubtedly represent the smallest eponymic "neoplasms" in the human body.

The ciliary processes of infants are smooth and pigmented. With age, the processes become increasingly thickened, convoluted, and hyalinized as collagenous connective tissue accumulates around the vessels in their cores (Fig. 1-5C,D). The hyalinized ciliary processes in older patients appear white. With experience, one can roughly estimate a patient's age from the degree of hyalinization evident grossly or microscopically. The pars plana or flat part of the ciliary body is located posterior to the pars plicata and forms a circular band that extends to the ora serrata. The term ora serrata, which means "toothed mouth," is derived from the serrated appearance of this junction caused by the presence of anteriorly projecting dentate processes of peripheral retina separated by concavities called oral bays (Fig. 1-5B). Dentate processes and oral bays are prominent in the nasal ora serrata, while the temporal ora is relatively smooth. This finding can serve as anatomic landmark to orient the eye during gross examination. In some eyes, elongated dentate processes of peripheral retinal tissue called meridional processes deeply invade, or even bridge, the pars plana. Posterior to the ora, the peripheral retina often has a moth-eaten pattern of darker spaces reflecting the almost ubiquitous presence of peripheral microcystoid degeneration (see retinal chapter below).

The bilayer of half pigmented ciliary epithelium that forms part of the eye's inner neuroectodermal layer (Fig. 1-5D) is discussed above. The stroma of the ciliary body is composed largely of smooth muscle. In routine histologic sections, the ciliary muscle appears as an elongated triangle, but in actuality, the structure is a circular sphincter. The ciliary muscle has longitudinal, radial, and circular parts. The longitudinal ciliary muscle of Brücke attaches to the sclera spur, a ridge of connective tissue that is located directly behind trabecular meshwork and the Canal of Schlemm. The scleral spur is the only spot where the ciliary body is firmly attached to the sclera. The ciliary muscle's primary function is focusing or accommodation, which is discussed in the lens section below.

The iris is the anterior, visible part of the uveal tract (Fig. 1-2). The structure is named after Iris, the Greek goddess of the rainbow, an appellation that undoubtedly reflects the range of eye colors found in different peoples. The iris has two components, the posterior IPE derived from neuroectoderm (see above) and the iris stroma, derived from the neural crest. Its major component, the iris stroma is a loosely arranged tissue that contains pigmented

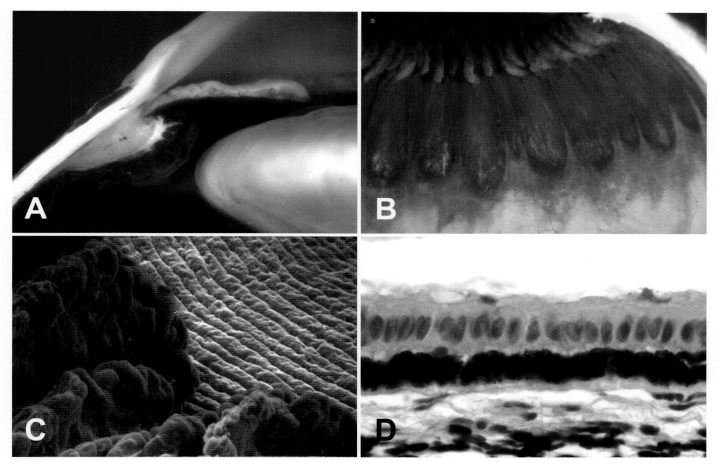

Fig. 1-5. Ciliary body. A. The pars plicata of the ciliary body is composed of ciliary processes, which project into the posterior chamber directly behind the iris. **B.** The flat pars plana is interposed between the ring of ciliary processes comprising the pars plicata and the retina. The ora serrata is the junction between the pars plana and the retina. The nasal ora serrata, shown here, has prominent dentate processes and concave oral bays. **C.** Scanning electron micrograph shows convoluted surface of ciliary processes and circumferential folds on posterior surface of the IPE. **D.** The ciliary epithelium, shown here on the pars plana, is a half pigmented bilayer. Its nonpigmented inner layer is continuous with the retina at the ora serrata. (**C.** SEM ×50, **D.** H&E ×250)

and nonpigmented cells set in an abundant extracellular matrix containing bundles of type I collagen fibrils and hyaluronidase-sensitive glycosaminoglycans. The cells include melanocytes and fibroblasts. The greatest concentration of iris melanocytes is found in the avascular anterior border layer deep to an inconspicuous discontinuous sheet of fibroblasts (Fig. 1-2A). The iris vessels have an undulating radial orientation. Ensheathed by a thick mantle of collagen fibers, these "thick-walled" vessels have a characteristic histologic appearance that is not encountered elsewhere in the body. The characteristic histologic appearance of its vessels serves to distinguish iris from choroidal tissue in evisceration specimens. Most iris vessels are located in the middle layers of the iris stroma. In blue irides, radiating iris vessels are visible clinically because the melanocytes comprising the anterior border layer lack pigment and are transparent. The melanocytes in darker irides are opacified by pigment, obscuring the vessels. In general, the number and size of melanin granules within iris melanosomes increase in darker irides.

The anterior surface of the iris has an irregular contour. The pupillary portion of the iris, which is located central to the roughly stellate collarette, is thinner. Embryologically, this thinning results from atrophy of the anterior stromal caused by resorption of the pupillary membrane. The anterior surface of broader, thicker peripheral ciliary zone is grooved by contraction furrows. Defects in the anterior stroma called the crypts of Fuchs are evident clinically. The iris muscles are discussed above. Heavily pigmented, rounded clump cells of Koganei are often found in the stroma near the sphincter muscle. These can be melanophages or displaced neuroepithelial cells.

The crystalline lens is situated in the posterior chamber behind the iris (Fig. 1-6). The lens is the only large transparent cellular tissue in the body and is the only intraocular structure that is derived embryologically from the surface ectoderm. Early in gestation, the surface ectoderm overlying the optic vesicle thickens to form the lens placode, which subsequently invaginates to form the lens vesicle, as the neuroectodermal optic vesicle invaginates to form the optic cup. The

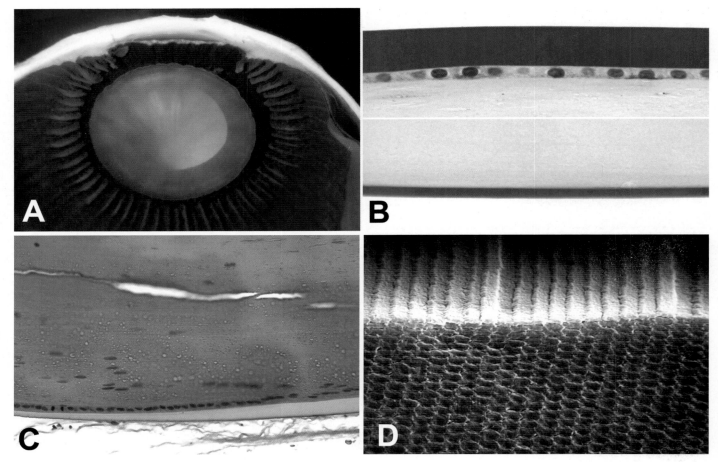

Fig. 1-6. The lens. A. The lens is situated in the posterior chamber behind the iris. The lens is composed of highly differentiated epithelial cells called lens fibers. **B.** A monolayer of cuboidal lens epithelial cells is present beneath the anterior lens capsule. The posterior capsule is much thinner. **C.** The epithelial monolayer terminates at the equatorial lens bow, where the cells elongate to form the secondary lens fibers. **D.** SEM shows that the lens fibers are tightly packed in a paracrystalline fashion. (**B.** H&E ×100, **B. top and bottom,** PAS ×250, **D.** SEM ×160)

epithelial cells of the posterior part of the vesicle elongate anteriorly forming the primary lens fibers that fill the cavity of the optic vesicle. These fibers persist as the central embryonic nucleus in the adult lens. An anterior monolayer of cuboidal cells persists as the anterior lens epithelium throughout life (Fig. 1-6C). Secondary lens fibers are formed by division of lens epithelial cells near the equator of the lens. Seven to eight millimeters in length, these long, straplike cells extend from the anterior to the posterior pole of the lens, totally enveloping the nucleus. The formation of secondary lens fibers continues throughout life; new fibers are laid down in concentric lamellae peripherally in an onionlike fashion. The nuclei of the newly formed peripheral lens fibers form a curved bow near the equator (Fig. 1-6B). These highly specialized epithelial cells lose their nuclei shortly after formation. Tightly packed in a nearly paracrystalline fashion (Fig. 1-6D), the lens fibers are joined together by ball and socket joints that minimize extracellular space. The lens has no vessels or nerves and is almost totally devoid of connective tissue, except for its thick enveloping capsule

of basement membrane (Fig. 1-6C). The anterior capsule is much thicker than the posterior capsule, whose caliber is less than the diameter of an erythrocyte. Like other basement membranes, the lens capsule stains intensely with the PAS stain. The lens epithelial cells retain the ability to synthesize collagen and may do so under pathologic conditions.

The primary optical function of the lens is focusing or accommodation. Divergent light rays from near objects must be bent or refracted more to sharply focus them on the retina. When a near object (e.g., this page) is examined, the ciliary muscle contracts, relaxing the tension on the zonular fibers that form the suspensory ligament of the lens (Fig. 1-7). The ciliary muscle is a circular or sphincter muscle. Its central aperture becomes smaller when it contracts. When distant objects are examined and the eye is at rest, the zonular fibers pull on the lens and flatten it. Relaxation of the zonular fibers during accommodation allows the lens to assume a more spherical configuration, which has a shorter radius of curvature and greater refractive power. Refractive power is inversely proportional to the radius of curvature of a lens.

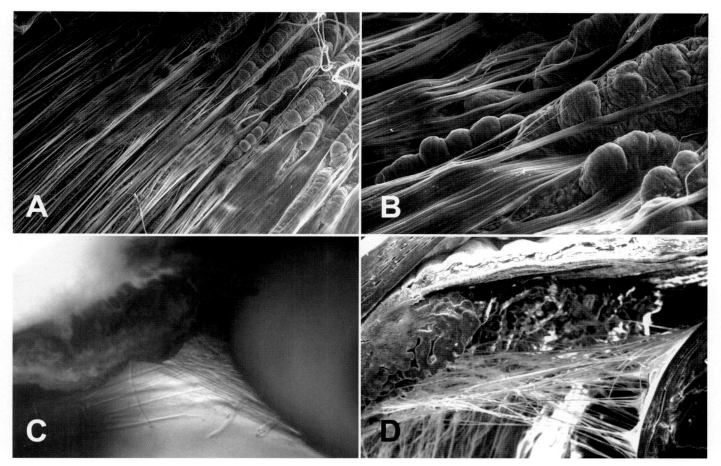

Fig. 1-7. The suspensory ligament of the lens. A. SEM discloses zonular fibers traversing the pars plana. **B.** Bundles of zonular fibers pass through valleys between ciliary processes. **C.** Two groups of zonular fibers are disclosed by retroillumination in macrophoto. **D.** Anterior and posterior groups of zonular fibers delimit triangular canal of Hanover at the lens equator. (**A.** SEM ×10, **B.** SEM ×80, **D.** SEM ×20)

The cornea (Fig. 1-8) is the eye's major refractive element with an optical power of approximately 45 diopters. It is the anterior, transparent part of the eye's tough outer fibrous coat and is continuous with the sclera at the limbus. The bulk of the cornea is composed of interweaving lamellae of type I collagen fibers, which are spaced in an exquisitely regular fashion. Artifactitious clefts separate the stromal lamella in routine histologic sections (Fig. 1-8A). The stroma contains flattened dendriform fibroblast-like cells called keratocytes. A nonkeratinized epithelium five cells in thickness covers the anterior surface of the cornea (Fig. 1-8B). This is composed of basal cells, wing cells, and flattened surface squamous cells. The epithelium normally has an inconspicuous basement membrane and rests on a feltwork of modified stroma called Bowman membrane or layer that appears as a homogeneous, hyaline band. A delicate monolayer of flattened endothelial cells, derived embryologically from the neural crest, lines the posterior surface of the cornea (Fig. 1-8C,D). The endothelium secretes a thick basement membrane called Descemet membrane, which stains intensely with the PAS stain (Fig. 1-8C).

Anvil-shaped, hyaline excrescences called Hassall-Henle warts stud the inner surface of the peripheral part of Descemet membrane in older patients. They resemble the guttae that occur in the central cornea in Fuchs endothelial dystrophy.

The intraocular pressure is governed by a delicate balance between the production of aqueous humor by the nonpigmented ciliary epithelial cells and its egress or outflow from the eye. Most aqueous humor exits via the traditional aqueous outflow pathway that consists of the trabecular meshwork and the canal of Schlemm, which are located in the peripheral anterior chamber in the anterior or corneoscleral part of the angle formed by the cornea and peripheral iris (Fig. 1-9). Smaller amounts of aqueous exit through nontraditional pathways that include iris vessels and posterior uveoscleral outflow via the ciliary body and the vortex veins.

The trabecular meshwork is a sievelike structure that is nestled in the anterior crotch of the scleral spur (Fig. 1-9B–D). The scleral spur serves as an important anatomic landmark in both clinical and pathologic

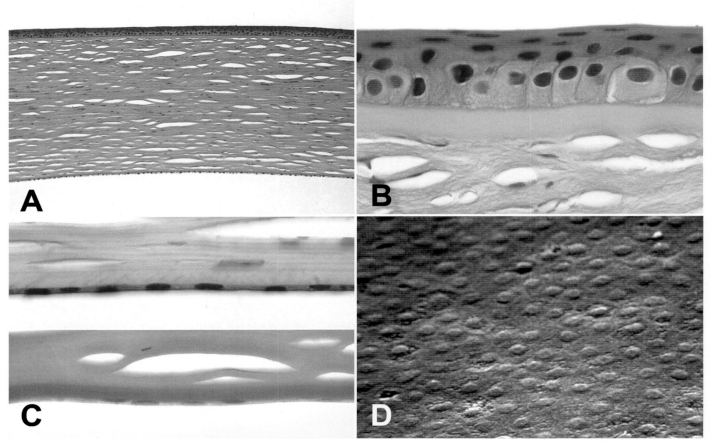

Fig. 1-8. **The cornea. A.** Most of the cornea is composed of collagenous stroma with keratocytes and lamellae separated by arti-factitious clefts. **B.** The corneal epithelium rests on the anterior surface of Bowman layer, a hyaline band of modified stroma. The epithelium is typically five cells in thickness. **C.** A flattened monolayer of corneal endothelial cells rests on the posterior surface of the Descemet membrane, which is PAS-positive (**below**). **D.** SEM discloses a regular mosaic of endothelial cells. (**A.** H&E ×50, **B.** H&E ×250, **C. top**, H&E ×250, **bottom**, PAS ×250, **D.** SEM ×160)

practice. The longitudinal fibers of the ciliary muscle are firmly attached to the posterior aspect of the scleral spur (Fig. 1-9D). During microscopy, the spur is found by following the ciliary muscle fibers to their insertion. The trabecular meshwork is composed of an interconnected network of small beams or trabeculae (Fig. 1-9B). The beams are made of collagen with a central core of elastic tissue and are encompassed by trabecular endothelial cells and a thin layer of endothelial basement membrane. The inner, corneoscleral part of the meshwork is composed of concentrically oriented plates of connective tissue containing pores, which are out of register. The interstices of the meshwork do not communicate directly with the lumen of the canal of Schlemm but are separated by a thin layer of extracellular matrix material called the juxtacanalicular connective tissue. Schlemm canal is a modified vein that is lined by a continuous layer of endothelial cells. Schlemm canal runs circumferentially around the chamber angle, giving off branches or collector channels that traverse the sclera and discharge their contents into the epibulbar veins via the aqueous veins of Ascher.

The anterior surface of the eyeball and the posterior surface of eyelids are covered by a delicate transparent mucous membrane called the conjunctiva. The term conjunctiva is derived from the Latin meaning "to bind together." It connects the eye with the eyelids.

The conjunctiva consists of a nonkeratinized stratified columnar epithelium that rests on a connective tissue stroma or substantia propria (see Fig. 5-1). The conjunctival epithelium is two to five cells in thickness and contains mucous glands called goblet cells whose contents appear clear or bluish in routine H&E sections and are vividly PAS-positive. Goblet cells are more numerous nasally, especially in the semilunar fold (plica semilunaris).

Topographically, the conjunctiva is divided into bulbar, forniceal, and tarsal (or palpebral) parts. The bulbar conjunctiva covers the anterior surface of the eyeball and is freely movable. The stroma or substantia propria of the bulbar conjunctiva is composed of loose, areolar connective tissue and is easily ballooned up by edema fluid (chemosis) or injected anesthetic. In contrast, the palpebral conjunctiva is firmly adherent to the tarsal plate and

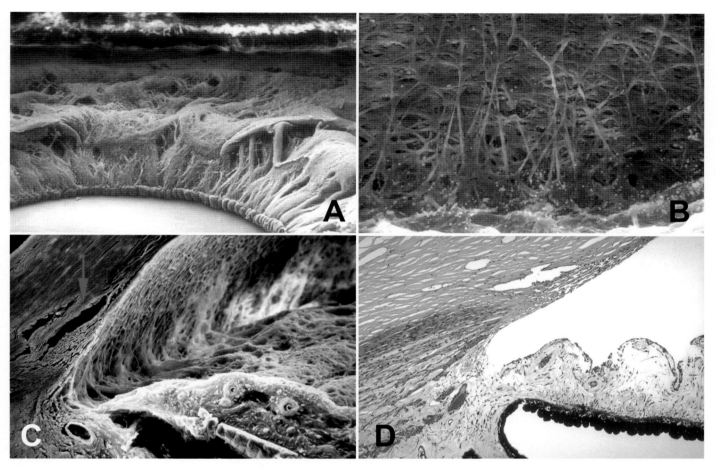

Fig. 1-9. The iridocorneal angle and aqueous outflow pathways. A. Electronic charging artifact highlights the trabecular mesh-work in the periphery of the anterior chamber in this SEM. **B.** Thin trabecular beams comprising the inner part of the trabecular meshwork are evident in SEM. **C.** *Arrow* in SEM points to the canal of Schlemm in the outer wall of the iridocorneal angle external to the trabecular meshwork. **D.** The trabecular meshwork and canal of Schlemm are nestled in the anterior crotch of the scleral spur. The longitudinal ciliary muscle inserts onto the posterior aspect of the spur. (**A.** SEM ×20, **B.** SEM ×80, **C.** SEM ×60, **D.** H&E ×50)

does not move freely. Multiple epithelial invaginations or crypts called the pseudoglands of Henle usually occur in the palpebral conjunctiva. The forniceal conjunctiva that arches around the superior and inferior culs-de-sac is redundant and folded to facilitate eye movements. Several small accessory lacrimal glands of Krause are found beneath the forniceal conjunctiva, and accessory glands of Wolfring occur at the upper and lower margins of the tarsal plates. Lymphocytes and plasma cells normally are found in the conjunctival stroma and constitute part of the eye's normal defense mechanisms.

The caruncle is a small fleshy nodule located on the nasal surface of the eye medial to the semilunar fold. The term caruncle means "a little piece of flesh." An island of skin surrounded by conjunctiva, the caruncle is covered by keratined squamous epithelium with fine hairs. In addition to pilosebaceous units, the stroma contains fat and lobules of accessory lacrimal gland tissue (the glands of Popoff).

The eyelids are flaps of modified skin with highly modi-fied epidermal appendages that cover and protect the eye (Fig. 13-1A–F). The anterior surface of the eyelid is covered

by skin, and its posterior surface is lined by a mucous mem-brane, the palpebral conjunctiva, which is closely applied to the tarsal plate. The tarsal plate is a curved plate of dense connective tissue that serves as the lid's internal skeleton. Striated fibers of the orbicularis muscle are found between the skin and the anterior surface of the tarsus. The orbic-ularis muscle encircles the eyelid fissure forming a large sphincter that functions during eyelid closure. The bundles of the orbicularis are sectioned transversely in standard his-tologic sections. A mucocutaneous junction between the eyelid skin and conjunctiva occurs near the eyelid margin. Here, the epidermis is mildly thickened and has small rete ridges. Just anterior to the lid margin, slit lamp biomicros-copy discloses a line of tiny meibomian gland orifices. The meibomian glands are large sebaceous glands that occupy almost the entire length of the tarsal plate and are oriented perpendicular to the lid margin. The oily secretion of the meibomian glands helps to retard evaporation of the tear film. About 25 meibomian glands are present in the upper lid and 20 in the lower lid. The meibomian glands in the upper lid are much longer, reflecting the greater length of the upper tarsal plate (11 mm). The upper lid is identified grossly and in tissue sections by the length of the tarsal plate and the lid's roughly rectangular shape. The shape of the lower lid is roughly triangular. The greater mass of meibomian gland tissue in the upper tarsus probably explains why sebaceous carcinoma occurs most often in the upper lid. The eyelid fissure is encircled by a protective ring of cilia (eyelashes). The hair bulbs of the cilia are located deep within the lid next to the tarsal plate. Malignant tumors such as sebaceous gland carcinoma that arise deep in the substance of the lid often produce loss of lashes (madarosis).

Other eyelid glands bear eponyms. The sebaceous glands of the eyelashes are the glands of Zeis. Sebaceous glands are holocrine glands. The glandular secretion called sebum is composed of entire cells (*holos*—whole). Cellular division occurs in the peripheral germinative layer of sebaceous gland lobules. As new cells form, the older cells are pushed toward the center of the glandular lobule. The cells degenerate as they mature. Their nuclei become karyorrhectic and pyknotic, and the cytoplasm becomes intensely lipidized and foamy.

The glands of Moll are apocrine sweat glands. Their dilated lumina are lined by tall, eosinophilic cells capped with the "apical snouts" that characterize apocrine decapitation secretion. Eccrine sweat glands, which bear no eponym, also are found. Glandular epithelial cells remain intact during eccrine secretion. The glands of Wolfring or Ciaccio are small accessory lacrimal glands that are located at the proximal margins of the tarsal plates. There are two to five glands of Wolfring at the upper margin of the superior tarsal plate and two glands at the lower margin of the lower tarsus. Other accessory lacrimal glands called the glands of Krause are found near the conjunctival fornix. The accessory lacrimal glands are responsible for baseline tear secretion. The main lacrimal gland releases copious amounts of watery secretion (endogenous irrigating fluid) in response to emotional stimuli or severe ocular irritation.

The eye is contained in a protective pear-shaped cavity in the skull called the orbit, which contains about 30 mL of highly specialized tissue (see Fig. 14-1). Other orbital contents include the optic nerve, which is a specialized tract of the central nervous system; the cartilaginous

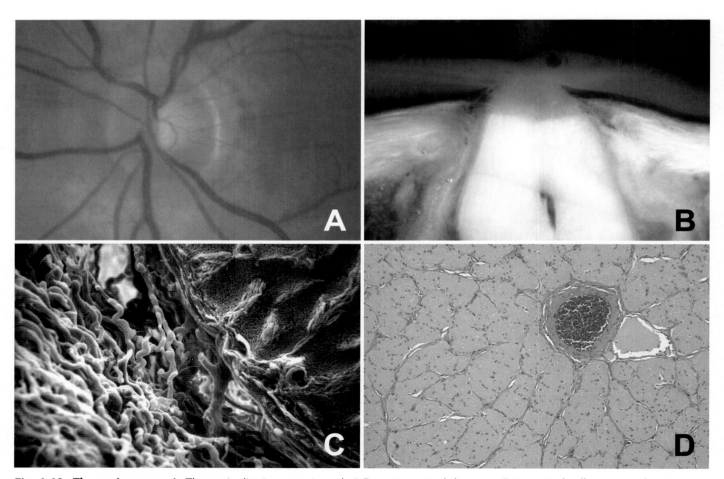

Fig. 1-10. The optic nerve. A. The optic disc is approximately 1.5 mm in vertical diameter. **B.** Longitudinally sectioned optic nerve shows abrupt termination of creamy myelin at the posterior margin of the lamina cribrosa. **C.** SEM of optic nerve meninges shows spidery arachnoidal processes bridging cleft between the optic nerve (**at right**) and the dura (**at left**). Septa of pia matter extend into the substance of the nerve, compartmentalizing its axons. **D.** Pial septa and central retinal vessels are seen in photomicrograph of transversely sectioned nerve. (**C.** SEM ×160, **D.** H&E ×100)

trochlea, smooth and striated muscle; vessels; nerves; fatty and fibrous connective tissue; and the lacrimal gland, a minor salivary gland. The orbit communicates with the intracranial cavity through several fissures and foramina, and several of its bony walls contain paranasal sinuses. The eye and the remainder of the orbital contents, which are delimited anteriorly by a septum of fibrous tissue, are protected by the eyelids, retractable flaps of skin equipped with highly specialized epidermal appendages. The epithelial-lined components of the nasolacrimal drainage system are located in the inferonasal part of the orbit.

The optic nerve is a tract of the central nervous system that connects the eye and the brain (Fig. 1-10). The nerve has intraorbital, intracanalicular, and intracranial portions and is about 50 mm in total length. It is composed of the axons of the retinal ganglion cells, interstitial cells including oligodendrocytes, astrocytes, and microglia, and fibrovascular septa of the pia mater. The retinal nerve fibers exit the eye through the lamina cribrosa in the posterior sclera and extend to the optic chiasm, and then to the lateral geniculate body via the optic tracts. Behind the lamina cribrosa, the axons are myelinated. Here, the nerve measures about 3 mm in diameter. In contrast, the diameter of the optic disc is only 1.5 mm. Dense collagenous dura, the spidery trabeculated arachnoid and the vascularized pia mater comprise the meninges of the optic nerve. The optic nerve is encompassed by firmly adherent pia mater, and its substance is compartmentalized by septa of pial connective tissue.

BIBLIOGRAPHY

Fine BS, Yanoff M. *Ocular Histology: A Text and Atlas*, 2nd ed. Hagerstown, MD: Harper & Row, 1979.

Hogan MJ, Alvarado JA, Weddell JE. *Histology of the Human Eye*. Philadelphia, PA: W.B. Saunders, 1971.

Jakobiec FA. *Ocular Anatomy, Embryology, and Teratology*. Philadelphia, PA: Harper & Row, 1982.

Snell RS, Lemp MA. *Clinical Anatomy of the Eye*, 2nd ed. Boston, MA: Blackwell Scientific Publications, 1998.

2 Congenital and Developmental Anomalies

INTRODUCTION

Congenital anomalies are developmental disorders that are present at birth. Congenital malformations are caused by chromosomal abnormalities, mutant genes, and major environmental factors such as infections, drugs and toxins, or radiation. In many instances, the cause is unknown. Heritable disorders are genetically determined and may or may not affect the phenotype. Heritable traits may be manifest at birth, or they may become obvious later in life.

Etiologic factors that act early during embryogenesis (conception to 2 weeks) or the initial stages of ocular organogenesis (2 weeks to 3 months) tend to have profound effects on ocular development. The development of the eye commences about 24 days after fertilization when the optic pits form in the anterior part of the embryo's neuroectodermal plate. The pits subsequently evaginate to form the optic vesicles, which invaginate to form the optic cups 4 days later. The neuroectoderm comprising the inner layer of the optic cup is destined to form the neurosensory retina, the nonpigmented ciliary epithelium, and the posterior layer of iris epithelium, while the outer layer of the optic cup gives rise to the retinal pigment epithelium (RPE), the pigmented ciliary epithelium, and the anterior layer of iris pigment epithelium, which includes the dilator muscle. The optic vesicles induce the formation of the lens placodes in the overlying surface ectoderm. The lens placodes invaginate to form the lens vesicles as the optic cups form. Transitory fissures develop in the outer wall of the optic cups on day 29. These embryonic fissures give the hyaloid arteries access to the interior of the developing eye. The fissures subsequently are obliterated by fusion, which usually is complete by the 6th week of gestation. Abnormalities affecting each of these events can become manifest as severe developmental anomalies.

Primary **anophthalmos** is a rare anomaly caused by failure of optic vesicle evagination. Primary anophthalmos usually is bilateral and occurs sporadically in otherwise healthy individuals. Secondary anophthalmos is caused by suppression of the entire anterior part of the neural tube, which is lethal. In consecutive anophthalmos, the optic vesicle evaginates and then undergoes degeneration. Histologic examination of the orbit usually discloses rudimentary neuroectodermal structures, which are absent in primary anophthalmos.

SYNOPHTHALMIA/CYCLOPIA

Synophthalmia/cyclopia is a striking anomaly caused by a failure of formation or induction of the anterior neural tube including the eye fields (Fig. 2-1A,B). Although it is often called a fusion anomaly, synophthalmia/cyclopia actually reflects a failure of complete bicentricity to emerge. The disorder is a continuum of anomalies that involves the brain, nose, orbits, and bones in addition to the eyes. Bicentricity fails to emerge at an early stage; cells that are induced as eye tissue complete all stages of development with a high degree of fidelity. The greatest degree of ocular differentiation occurs anteriorly and laterally; there is duplication of anterior ocular structures and fusion posteriorly with a single optic nerve. A rudimentary nose or nasal proboscis is present above the single midline orbit (Fig. 2-1A). The proboscis is caused by faulty migration of the frontonasal processes. Failure of bicentricity also involves the forebrain, invariably producing a malformation called holoprosencephaly, which is marked by failure of the brain to divide into right and left hemispheres. Most cases of this clinical spectrum have synophthalmia; true cyclopia is exceedingly rare. The lethal malformation usually is sporadic, but it may be a manifestation of trisomy 13. Dominantly and recessively inherited familial cases have been reported. Holoprosencephaly has been linked to mutations in a number of genes including the human sonic hedgehog gene on chromosome 7q36 and the SIX3 sine oculo hemeobox gene on chromosome 2p21. Pregnant ewes who ingest toxic alkaloids from the false hellebore plant *Veratrum californicum* on the 14th or 15th day of gestation give birth to cyclopic lambs.

Congenital cystic eye is a very rare anomaly caused by complete failure of optic vesicle invagination. Partial arrest in vesicle invagination probably causes extreme microphthalmos, which may simulate anophthalmos clinically. Congenital nonattachment of the retina is caused by faulty invagination of the optic cup and failure of its inner and outer layers to meet posteriorly.

Uveal colobomas are developmental anomalies caused by faulty closure of the embryonic fissure. Derived from the Greek word for "mutilation," coloboma is defined as "a condition where a portion of the structure of the eye is lacking." Colobomas typically are located inferonasally in the territory of the fissure. They can involve the iris, ciliary body, choroid, or any combination of the three, and also may affect the optic nerve. Because the primary defect in a typical coloboma is in the neuroectoderm, absence of the mesectodermal uveal stroma is a secondary phenomenon. Occasionally, the uveal tissue undergoes dysplasia or metaplasia forming cartilage, muscle or fat. An absolute scotoma is present in the region of the coloboma because the overlying retina is absent or dysplastic.

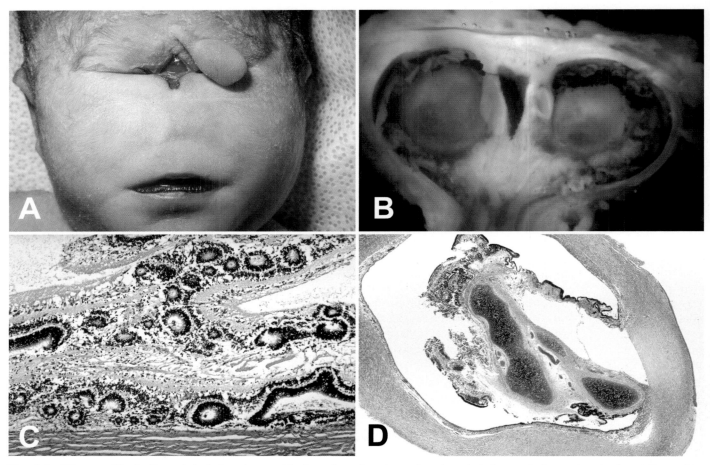

Fig. 2-1. Trisomy 13. A. Synophthalmia, trisomy 13. A pedunculated nasal proboscis is located above the single midline orbit.
B. Synophthalmia, trisomy 13. Small, synophthalmic eye from infant shown in Figure 2-1A has two lenses and a single optic nerve.
Septum between lenses contains two foci of hyaline cartilage. Mass of dysplastic retina fills vitreous cavity. **C.** Coloboma and retinal
dysplasia, trisomy 13. Mass of disorderly dysplastic retina containing large multilayered rosettes adheres directly to the sclera within
the coloboma. The choroid is absent. **D.** Intraocular cartilage, trisomy 13. Mesenchymal tissue filling coloboma surrounds a focus of
hyaline cartilage in severely microphthalmic eye. (**C.** Hematoxylin-eosin (H&E), ×25, **D.** H&E, ×10)

Although most colobomas are sporadic, they occasionally
are inherited as isolated ocular defects, usually in an autosomal dominant fashion with incomplete penetrance.
Colobomas occur in infants with CHARGE syndrome and the
Cat Eye, Kabuki, Wolf-Hirschhorn (4p–), and 13q deletions
syndromes as well. In addition to colobomas, infants with
CHARGE syndrome have congenital heart defects, choanal
atresia, mental retardation, and genital and ear anomalies.
CHARGE syndrome is associated with mutations or complete
deletion of the CHD7 (helicase DNA-binding protein-7)
gene on chromosome 8q12. Colobomas also are characteristic findings in several syndromes caused by the duplication
or deletion of chromosomes or chromosomal fragments
including trisomy 13. Colobomas in severely microphthalmic
(<10 mm) eyes from infants with trisomy 13 often contain
foci of hyaline cartilage and dysplastic retina (Fig. 2-1C,D).

Coloboma with cyst is a severe form of embryonic fissure anomaly characterized by a cystic outpouching of
ectatic sclera that communicates with the interior of the

eye through a posterior coloboma (Fig. 2-2). The intraocular
contents protrude outward through the fissure, and the cyst
is lined by a layer of atrophic or dysplastic neuroectodermal tissue. The cyst may become much larger than the eye
(microphthalmos with cyst).

Atypical colobomas are not related to closure of the
embryonic fissure and can occur anywhere. Macular colobomas probably result from intrauterine infections such as
congenital toxoplasmosis. Colobomas of the eyelid occur
in Goldenhar syndrome.

Optic nerve aplasia usually is unilateral and occurs sporadically in individuals who have no systemic abnormalities. The optic nerve is absent and the retina is avascular
and lacks ganglion cells and axons.

Malformations that are localized to a single ocular
structure usually are related to damage that occurs during
the fetal period of ocular development (3rd to 9th month).
Most are discussed in the chapters on individual ocular
structures that follow.

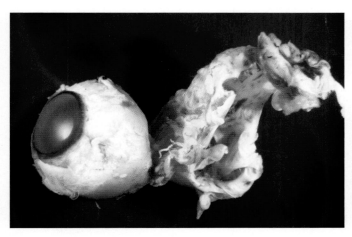

Fig. 2-2. Microphthalmos with cyst. Cystic outpouching of ectatic sclera is larger than microphthalmic eye. The lumen of the cyst was lined by atrophic neuroectodermal tissue and it communicated with the interior of the eye through an optic nerve coloboma. The cyst ruptured intraoperatively.

CHROMOSOMAL ANOMALIES

Ocular malformations occur in a number of chromosomal duplication or deletion syndromes. **Down syndrome (trisomy 21)** is the most common chromosomal syndrome and the most common cause of mental retardation. The "mongoloid" appearance of patients with Down syndrome is caused by an upward and outward slanting of their palpebral fissures, which are almond shaped. Other ocular findings include epicanthal folds, significant refractive errors, especially high myopia, cataract, and strabismus, usually esotropia, which occurs in approximately 40%. Congenital ectropion, iris hypoplasia, keratoconus with acute hydrops, and an increased number of retinal vessels crossing the optic disc margin also occur.

Brushfield spots appear as a concentric ring of white or yellowish spots on the anterior surface of the iris in 85% of blue- or hazel-eyed patients with Down syndrome (Fig. 2-3). Brushfield spots are focal condensations of stromal collagen that are visible through the transparent anterior border layer of the blue iris, and tend to be accentuated by concurrent iris atrophy. Discrete stromal condensations that resemble Brushfield spots called Kruckmann-Wolfflin bodies occur in some normal persons with blue or hazel eyes.

Severe ocular malformations including anophthalmos, synophthalmia/cyclopia, microphthalmia, PHPV, retinal dysplasia, colobomas, and intraocular cartilage occur in infants with **trisomy 13 (Patau syndrome)** (Fig. 2-1A–D). Affected infants have cleft lips and palates, cardiac and pulmonary defects, arrhinencephaly and holoprosencephaly. Few survive the first year of life.

Epicanthal folds, ptosis, blepharophimosis, microphthalmos, corneal opacities, and congenital glaucoma are found in trisomy 18 (Edwards syndrome), the second most common autosomal trisomy.

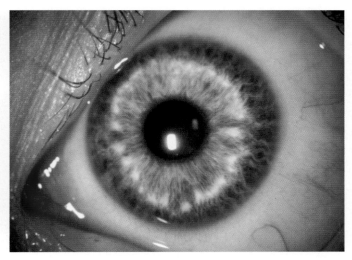

Fig. 2-3. Brushfield spots, trisomy 21. Focal stromal condensations form a ring of white spots in the middle third of the iris in a blue-eyed patient with Down Syndrome. (Photo courtesy of Dr. Edward A. Jaeger, from Eagle RC Jr. Congenital, developmental and degenerative disorders of the iris and ciliary body. In: Albert DM, Jakobiec FA, eds. *Principles and Practice of Ophthalmology. Clinical Practice*, vol. 1. Philadelphia, PA: Saunders, 1993:367–389.)

Retinoblastoma occurs in the 13q– syndrome if the deletion includes the q1-4 band. The 22q+ syndrome includes microphthalmia, the posterior ulcer of von Hippel, and severe retinal dysplasia. Ocular abnormalities have been reported in the 18p–, 18q–, 18 ring chromosome, 5p– (cri-du-chat), and the 4p– (Wolf-Hirschhorn) syndromes.

HERITABLE DISORDERS WITH OCULAR MANIFESTATIONS

A variety of heritable disorders caused by genetic mutations have ocular manifestations.

Most cases of **aniridia** are caused by mutations in the PAX6 gene on the short arm of chromosome 11. The term aniridia is a misnomer; most cases have severely hypoplastic irides that are hidden clinically by opaque limbal tissues (Fig. 2-4). Aniridia is a spectrum of ocular disease that also includes foveal and optic nerve hypoplasia, cataract, secondary glaucoma, and corneal opacification. Eighty-five percent of aniridic patients have autosomal dominant familial aniridia, which is an isolated ocular defect. The association of sporadic aniridia and Wilms tumor or nephroblastoma is called Miller syndrome and accounts for about 13% of cases. Miller syndrome is caused by deletions in the short arm of chromosome 11 that include both the PAX6 gene and another closely linked tumor suppressor gene (WT1) involved in the pathogenesis of Wilms tumor. The PAX6 gene plays a central role in ocular development throughout the animal kingdom. PAX6 mutations have been identified in patients with other anterior segment

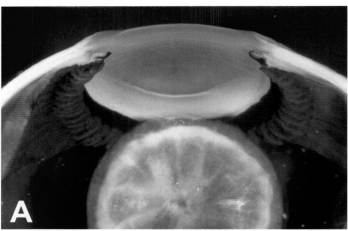
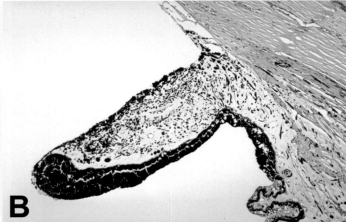

Fig. 2-4. Aniridia. A. Overhang of opaque limbal tissue hides skirt of hypoplastic iris in peripheral anterior chamber. The lens dislocated during sectioning of eye obtained postmortem from adult with familial aniridia. **B.** Stubby hypoplastic iris leaflet from eye seen grossly in (**A**) has thickened pigment epithelium and lacks sphincter and dilator muscles. (H&E, ×25)

malformations including Peters anomaly and autosomal dominant keratitis.

A number of heritable ocular diseases are caused by mutations in genes on the X chromosome and show X-linked recessive inheritance. They include color blindness (Daltonism), juvenile x-linked retinoschisis, some cases of retinitis pigmentosa, the Nettleship-Falls type of ocular albinism, Fabry disease, Hunter disease, Norrie disease, and Lowe syndrome. Incontinentia pigmenti (Bloch-Sulzberger) shows X-linked dominant inheritance. It occurs only in girls and boys with Klinefelter syndrome and is lethal in normal males.

Other ocular disorders occur predominantly in men because they are caused by mutations in maternally transmitted mitochondrial DNA. These include Leber hereditary optic neuropathy and the Kearns-Sayre, MERRF, and MELAS syndromes.

Autosomal recessively inherited disorders with prominent ocular manifestations include several types of albinism (foveal hypoplasia), systemic mucopolysaccharidoses including Hurler, Scheie, and Maroteaux-Lamy syndromes (corneal clouding), the lysosomal storage diseases Tay-Sachs disease and Niemann-Pick disease (macular cherry-red spot), Wilson disease (Kayser-Fleischer ring), the sickle hemoglobinopathies (neovascular sea fans), myotonic dystrophy (presenile cataract), alkaptonuria (sclera pigmentation), osteogenesis imperfecta (blue sclera), homocystinuria (ectopia lentis), and ocular-scoliotic Ehlers-Danlos syndrome (corneal and scleral rupture).

PHAKOMATOSES (FAMILIAL TUMOR SYNDROMES)

The term phakomatosis is applied to several heritable disorders that have important systemic and ocular findings. The primary phakomatoses include von Recklinghausen neurofibromatosis (NF-1), tuberous sclerosis complex (TSC), and von Hippel-Lindau (VHL) disease, which are autosomal dominant disorders, as well as Sturge-Weber syndrome (SWS), which is sporadic. Recent advances in molecular genetics have made the basic concept of phakomatosis outdated. Mutations in recessive tumor suppressor genes have been identified in all three of the classic dominantly inherited phakomatoses. The WHO classification of tumors of the central nervous system (CNS) no longer includes the term phakomatosis. NF-1, TSC, and VHL are included as familial tumor syndromes.

VON RECKLINGHAUSEN NEUROFIBROMATOSIS (NF-1)

Von Recklinghausen neurofibromatosis (NF-1) is one of the most common hereditary diseases, because the NF-1 gene, which is located on chromosome 17, is quite large and is subject to mutation. Neurofibromin, the protein product of the NF-1 gene, (17q11.2) normally interacts with the protein product of the ras oncogene to dampen growth stimulatory signals. NF-1 is characterized by tumors composed of Schwann cells, which typically occur on the skin as multiple fibroma molluscum. Deforming elephantiasis neuromatosa is caused by diffuse neurofibromatous infiltration (Fig. 2-5). The presence of more than six cutaneous café au lait spots >1.5 cm in diameter is a diagnostic criterion.

Ocular findings in NF-1 are numerous and include plexiform neurofibromas of the eyelid and orbit; an "S"-shaped lid fissure; congenital glaucoma, particularly if the upper lid is involved by neurofibromatous tissue; Lisch nodules on the iris, hamartomatous infiltration of the uvea with tactile corpuscle-like ovoid bodies (Fig. 2-6); retinal and optic nerve gliomas; dysplasia of the sphenoid bone (Orphan Annie sign); pulsating exophthalmos; and a slight

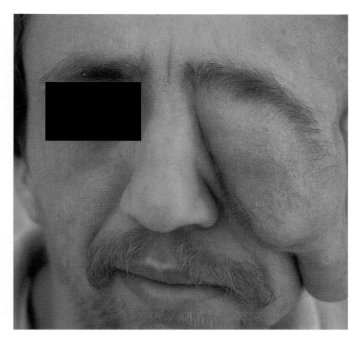

Fig. 2-5. Elephantiasis neuromatosa, Von Recklinghausen neurofibromatosis (NF-1). Pendulous mass of hamartomatous tissue involves left upper lid and forehead. (Courtesy of Dr. Dario Savino-Zari, Caracas, Venezuela.)

increased risk for uveal melanoma. Lisch nodules (Fig. 2-7) are the most common ocular manifestation of NF-1. These melanocytic hamartomas are a useful diagnostic criterion for NF-1 because they are found on the anterior surface of the iris in nearly all affected adults, and develop before cutaneous neurofibromas. Plexiform neurofibromas are composed of a plexus composed of markedly enlarged nerves that are swollen by a disorderly proliferation of Schwann cells and endoneural fibroblasts in a mucinous matrix (Fig. 2-8).

Neurofibromatosis type 2 (NF-2) is a totally separate disease caused by mutations in the merlin gene on chromosome 22 (22q12.2). Bilateral schwannomas of the 8th cranial nerve are the disorder's classic manifestation. Ocular findings include presenile posterior subcapsular cataracts, epiretinal membranes, combined hamartoma of the RPE and retina, and optic nerve sheath meningiomas.

TUBEROUS SCLEROSIS COMPLEX

The TSC is caused by mutations in either of two genes, TSC1 located on chromosome 9q34 and TSC2 on chromosome 16p13, which encode for the proteins hamartin and tuberin, respectively. Hamartin and tuberin form a complex that normally suppresses mTOR signaling. The classic clinical triad of TSC includes epilepsy, mental retardation, and facial lesions called adenoma sebaceum, which actually are angiofibromas. Astrocytic hamartomas and astrocytomas occur in the retina in about half of patients with tuberous sclerosis. Astrocytomas overlying the optic disc have been called giant drusen of the optic nerve. Retinal astrocytomas may be confused clinically with retinoblastoma. More mature lesions typically contain calcospherites and have been called mulberry nodules. The astrocytic hamartomas of the retina are typically nonprogressive. Larger retinal giant cell astrocytomas are encountered rarely. These resemble subependymal giant cell astrocytomas of the CNS histopathologically and often grow, causing total retinal detachment and lost eyes (Fig. 2-9). Large astrocytomas in the brain typically have a tuberlike appearance and may calcify forming "brain stones." Visceral tumors in TSC include renal angiomyolipomas and cardiac rhabdomyomas. Pleural cysts can predispose to spontaneous pneumothorax. Other skin lesions include subungual fibromas, shagreen patches, and ash leaf lesions.

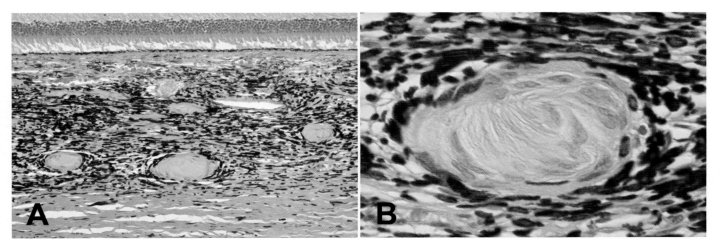

Fig. 2-6. Von Recklinghausen neurofibromatosis (NF-1) Choroidal infiltrate, NF-1. A. The choroid is massively thickened by a hamartomatous infiltrate that contains an increased number of melanocytes and nonpigmented ovoid bodies that resemble tactile corpuscles. **B.** Ovoid body in choroidal infiltrate, NF-1. Delicately laminated appearance of ovoid body reflects the presence of concentric Schwann cell processes. (**A.** H&E, ×50, **B.** H&E, ×250)

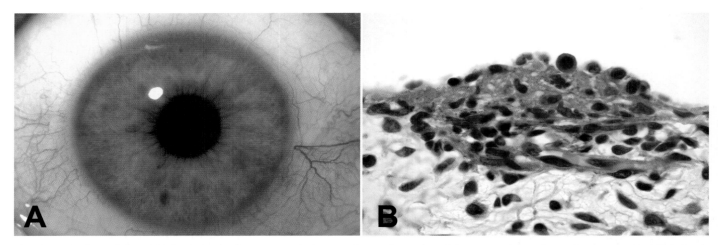

Fig. 2-7. Lisch nodules, NF-1. A. Multiple tan or pale brown dome-shaped nodules on surface of iris of patient with NF-1. Lisch nodules occur in nearly all affected adults with NF-1 and are a useful diagnostic criterion. **B.** Focus of partially pigmented cells rests on anterior iridic surface. Lisch nodules are melanocytic hamartomas. (**B.** H&E, ×250)

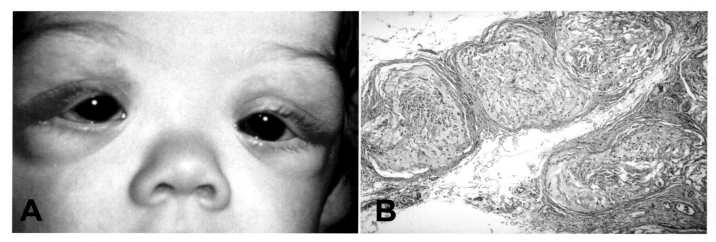

Fig. 2-8. Plexiform neurofibroma, NF-1. A. Infant with NF-1 has bilateral plexiform neurofibromas of upper eyelids and enlarged corneas indicative of secondary buphthalmos. **B.** Markedly enlarged nerves forming plexiform neurofibroma are swollen by a disorderly proliferation of Schwann cells and endoneural fibroblasts in a mucinous matrix. (**B.** H&E, ×25)

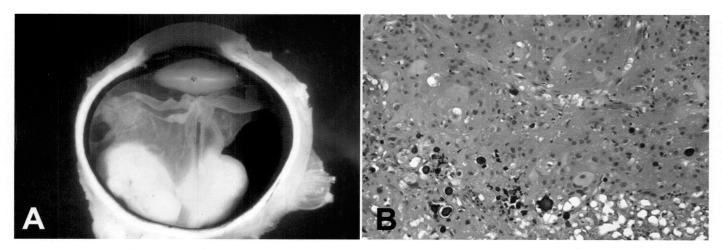

Fig. 2-9. A. TSC, retinal giant cell astrocytoma. Large bilobed astrocytoma caused retinal detachment in young girl with well-documented tuberous sclerosis. The macroscopic appearance of the tumor resembles retinoblastoma. **B.** Photomicrograph of retinal giant cell astrocytoma in (**A**) shows large astrocytes with copious amounts of eosinophilic cytoplasm. A few basophilic spherules of calcium (calcospherites) are seen below. Other parts of the tumor were extensively necrotic. (**B.** H&E, ×50)

VON HIPPEL-LINDAU DISEASE (ANGIOMATOSIS RETINAE)

VHL disease (angiomatosis retinae) is a dominantly inherited familial cancer syndrome caused by germline mutations in the VHL tumor suppressor gene located on chromosome 3p25. VHL protein is part of a complex that normally targets proteins for degradation including hypoxia-inducible factor 1a (HIF1a), an important transcription factor that stimulates tumors by inducing abnormal cellular growth and angiogenesis.

Cherrylike retinal "angiomas" with large feeding and draining vessels are the characteristic ocular manifestation of the syndrome (Fig. 2-10). These retinal lesions should be called retinal hemangioblastomas because they are identical histologically to hemangioblastomas that occur in the cerebellum of many affected patients. The retinal hemangioblastomas are bilateral in 50% of cases, can arise from the retina in an exophytic or endophytic fashion, may involve the optic disc or nerve, and often produce a Coats-like exudative maculopathy. Histopathologically, the hemangioblastomas are composed of capillaries within a matrix of foamy, lipidized stromal cells (Fig. 2-11). Molecular genetic studies demonstrating loss of heterozygosity within the stromal cells indicates that they are the primary constituent of the neoplasm. The capillaries are a secondary response to upregulation of vascular endothelial growth factor (VEGF) by the stromal cells.

Patients are also at risk for pheochromocytoma and renal cell carcinoma. Endolymphatic sac tumors cause hearing loss or tinnitus in about 10% of patients with VHL.

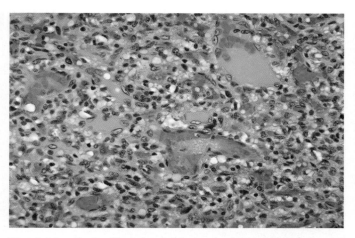

Fig. 2-11. Retinal hemangioblastoma, VHL disease. Retinal tumor is composed of capillaries and lipidized stromal cells. Histology of retinal tumor is identical to CNS hemangioblastoma. (H&E, ×100)

STURGE-WEBER SYNDROME (ENCEPHALOTRIGEMINAL ANGIOMATOSIS)

SWS (encephalotrigeminal angiomatosis) is a nonheritable congenital syndrome characterized by a facial port wine stain or nevus flammeus, an ipsilateral hemangioma of the meninges and brain, and "train track" intracranial calcification. Ocular findings include ipsilateral glaucoma and a diffuse cavernous hemangioma of the ipsilateral choroid (Fig. 2-12). It has been suggested that SWS may be caused by mosaicism for a lethal gene.

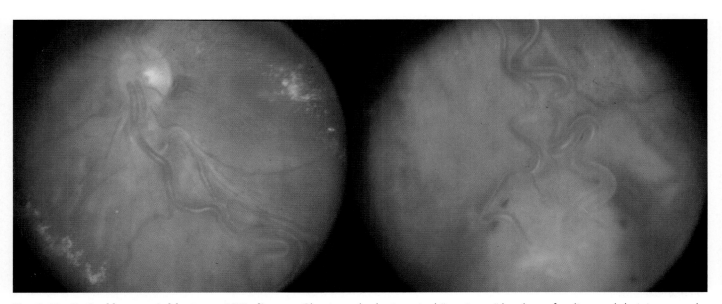

Fig. 2-10. Retinal hemangioblastoma, VHL disease. Classic endophytic retinal "angioma" has large feeding and draining vessels. Lipid exudate is present in posterior fundus **at left.**

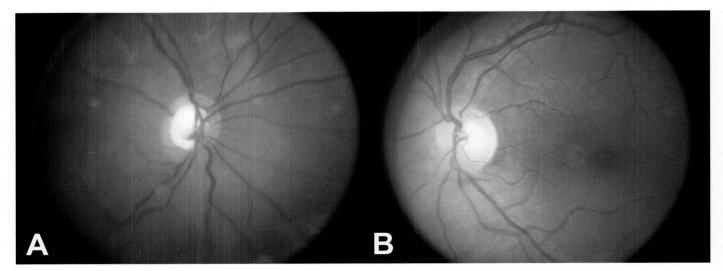

Fig. 2-12. Sturge Weber syndrome. A. Diffuse hemangioma obscures normal details of choroid and imparts "tomato ketchup" appearance to right fundus. Severe glaucomatous cupping of the right optic disc is present. **B.** The left eye is normal. The patient had a right facial nevus flammeus that involved the upper eyelid.

Other disorders that have been included with the phakomatoses include **cavernous hemangioma of the retina**, the **Wyburn-Mason syndrome**, the **organoid nevus (nevus sebaceus of Jadassohn) syndrome,** and **ataxia telangiectasia**. Large, nonleaking retinal arteriovenous malformations (AVMs) occur in the nonhereditary syndrome of Wyburn and Mason. Twenty to thirty percent of patients have associated midbrain AVMs. The organoid nevus syndrome is characterized by cutaneous sebaceous nevi that may spawn basal cell carcinomas, seizures, epibulbar complex choristomas, and yellow fundus lesions that may represent intrascleral cartilage or bone. Ataxia-telangiectasia (A-T) is a pleiotropic autosomal recessive disorder characterized by cerebellar ataxia, immunodeficiency, specific developmental defects, profound predisposition to cancer, and acute radiosensitivity. Ocular findings include telangiectatic conjunctival vessels and oculomotor apraxia. The ATM gene normally is involved in DNA and cellular repair mechanisms.

Infections that occur during pregnancy and other harmful factors in the maternal environment such as drugs, toxins and radiation can have devastating effects on the fetus. The most severe complications are associated with events that occur early in the first trimester. Maternal infections with ocular complications include rubella, toxoplasmosis, syphilis, cytomegalic inclusion disease, herpes simplex virus, and AIDS. Drugs that cause congenital ocular anomalies include thalidomide, retinoic acid, LSD, cocaine, and ethanol (fetal alcohol syndrome).

BIBLIOGRAPHY

General References
Duke-Elder S. The Iris. *Congenital Deformities*, vol. 3, part 2. London, UK: Henry Kimpton, 1964:256.

Glaser T, Jepeal L, Edwards JG, et al. PAX6 gene dosage effect in a family with congenital cataracts, aniridia, anophthalmia and central nervous system defects. *Nat Genet* 1994;7:463–471.
Mann I. *The Development of the Human Eye*. New York, NY: Grune & Stratton, 1950.
Mann I. *Developmental Abnormalities of the Eye*. Philadephia, PA: JB Lippincott, 1957.
Pagon RA. Ocular coloboma. *Surv Ophthalmol* 1981;25:223–223.
Pagon RA, Graham JM, Zonana J, et al. Coloboma, congenital heart disease, and choanal atresia with multiple anomalies: CHARGE association. *J Pediatr* 1981;99:223–227.
Rosias PR, Sijstermans JM, Theunissen PM, et al. Phenotypic variability of the cat eye syndrome. Case report and review of the literature. *Genet Couns* 2001;12:273–282.
Schubert HD. Schisis-like rhegmatogenous retinal detachment associated with choroidal colobomas. *Graefes Arch Clin Exp Ophthalmol* 1995;233:74–79.
Schubert HD. Structural organization of choroidal colobomas of young and adult patients and mechanism of retinal detachment. *Trans Am Ophthalmol Soc* 2005;103:457–472.
Torczynski E, Jacobiec FA, Johnston MC, et al. Synophthalmia and cyclopia: a histopathologic, radiographic, and organogenetic analysis. *Doc Ophthalmol* 1977;44:311–378.
Waardenburg P, Franceschetti A, Klein D. *Genetics and Ophthalmology*. Springfield, IL: Charles C Thomas, 1961.

Chromosomal Anomalies
Brushfield T. Mongolism. *Brit J Child Dis* 1924;21:241.
Donaldson D. The significance of spotting of the iris in mongols. Brushfield's spots. *Arch Ophthalmol* 1961;65:26–31.
Hoepner J, Yanoff M. Ocular anomalies in trisomy 13–15: an analysis of 13 eyes with two new findings. *Am J Ophthalmol* 1972;74:729–737.
Howard RO. Classification of chromosomal eye syndromes. *Int Ophthalmol* 1981;4:77–91.
Jaeger E. Ocular findings in Down's syndrome. *Trans Am Ophthalmol Soc* 1980;78:808–845.
Wilcox LJ, Bercovitch L, Howard R. Ophthalmic features of chromosome deletion 4p- (Wolf-Hirschhorn syndrome). *Am J Ophthalmol* 1978;86:834–839.

Aniridia and Other Iris Anomalies

Davis A, Cowell JK. Mutations in the PAX6 gene in patients with hereditary aniridia. *Hum Mol Genet* 1993;2:2093–2097.

Duke-Elder S. *Persistent Pupillary Membrane. Congenital Deformities*, vol. 3, part 2, London, UK: Henry Kimpton, 1964:775.

Edward D, Al Rajhi A, Lewis RA, et al. Molecular basis of Peters anomaly in Saudi Arabia. *Ophthalmic Genet* 2004;25:257–270.

Elsas F, Maumenee I, Kenyon K, et al. Familial aniridia with preserved ocular function. *Am J Ophthalmol* 1977;83:718–724.

Glaser T, Walton DS, Maas RL. Genomic structure, evolutionary conservation and aniridia mutations in the human PAX6 gene. *Nat Genet* 1992;2:232–239.

Graw J. Genetic aspects of embryonic eye development in vertebrates. *Devel Genet* 1996;18:181–197.

Grindley JC, Davidson DR, Hill RE. The role of Pax-6 in eye and nasal development. *Development* 1995;121:1433–1442.

Hanson IM, Fletcher JM, Jordan T, et al. Mutations at the PAX6 locus are found in heterogeneous anterior segment malformations including Peters' anomaly. *Nat Genet* 1994;6:168–173.

Hingorani M, Williamson KA, Moore AT, et al. Detailed ophthalmologic evaluation of 43 individuals with PAX6 mutations. *Invest Ophthalmol Vis Sci* 2009;50:2581–2590.

Lee H, Khan R, O'Keefe M. Aniridia: current pathology and management. *Acta Ophthalmol* 2008;86:708–715.

Mackman G, Brightbell F, Opitz J. Corneal changes in aniridia. *Am J Ophthalmol* 1979;87:497–502.

Margo CE. Congenital aniridia: a histopathologic study of the anterior segment in children. *J Paed Ophthalmol Strab* 1983;20:192–198.

Miller R, Fraumeni JJ, Manning M. Association of Wilms' tumor with aniridia, hemihypertrophy, and other congenital malformations. *N Engl J Med* 1964;270:922–927.

Mirzayans F, Pearce WG, MacDonald IM, et al. Mutation of the PAX6 gene in patients with autosomal dominant keratitis. *Am J Hum Genet* 1995;57:539–548.

Nelson LB, Spaeth GL, Nowinski T, et al. Aniridia: a review. *Surv Ophthalmol* 1984;28:621–642.

Ramaesh K, Ramaesh T, Dutton GN, et al. Evolving concepts on the pathogenic mechanisms of aniridia related keratopathy. *Int J Biochem Cell Biol* 2005;37:547–557.

Warburg M, Mikkelsen M, Andersen SR, et al. Aniridia and interstitial deletion of the short arm of chromosome 11. *Metab Pediatr Ophthalmol* 1980;4:97–102.

Neurofibromatosis

Anonymous. Neurofibromatosis. Conference Statement. National Institutes of Health Consensus Development Conference. *Arch Neurol* 1988;45:575–578.

Huson SM, Compston DA, Harper PS. A genetic study of von Recklinghausen neurofibromatosis in south east Wales. II. Guidelines for genetic counselling. *J Med Genet* 1989;26:712–721.

Lewis RA, Riccardi VM. Von Recklinghausen neurofibromatosis. Incidence of iris hamartomata. *Ophthalmology* 1981;88:348–354.

Lisch K. Ueber Beteiligung der Augen, insbesondere das Vorkommen von Irisknotchen bei der Neurofibromatose (Recklinghausen). *Zeitschrift fur Augenheilkunde* 1937;93:137–143.

Mindel JS, Rubenstein AE, Wallace S, et al. Congenital Horner's syndrome does not alter Lisch nodule formation. *Ann Neurol* 1994;35:123–124.

Perry H, Font R. Iris nodules in von Recklinghausen neurofibromatosis. Electron microscopic confirmation of their melanocytic origin. *Arch Ophthalmol* 1982;100:1635–1640.

Ragge NK, Falk RE, Cohen WE, et al. Images of Lisch nodules across the spectrum. *Eye* 1993;7:95–101.

Ragge NK, Traboulsi EI. The phakomatoses. In: Traboulsi EI, ed. *Genetic Diseases of the Eye*. New York, NY: Oxford University Press, 1998:733–775.

Sakurai T. Multiple neurofibroma patient showing multiple flecks on the anterior surface of the iris. *Acta Soc Ophthalmol Jpn* 1935;39:87–93.

Traboulsi EI. *A Compendium of Inherited Disorders and the Eye*. New York, NY: Oxford University Press, 2005.

Williamson TH, Garner A, Moore AT. Structure of Lisch nodules in neurofibromatosis type 1. *Ophthalmic Paediatr Genet* 1991;12:11–17.

Tuberous Sclerosis

Alper JC, Holmes LB. The incidence and significance of birthmarks in a cohort of 4,641 newborns. *Pediatr Dermatol* 1983;1:58–68.

Au KS, Pollom GJ, Roach ES, et al. TSC1 and TSC2 gene mutations: detection and genotype/phenotype correlation. *Am J Hum Genet* 1998;63S:350.

Au KS, Williams AT, Gambello MJ, et al. Molecular genetic basis of tuberous sclerosis complex: from bench to bedside. *J Child Neurol* 2004;19:699–709.

Davies DM, Johnson SR, Tattersfield AE, et al. Sirolimus therapy in tuberous sclerosis or sporadic lymphangioleiomyomatosis. *N Engl J Med* 2008;358:200–203.

Eagle RC Jr, Shields JA, Shields CL, et al. Hamartomas of the iris and ciliary epithelium in tuberous sclerosis complex. *Arch Ophthalmol* 2000;118:711–715.

El-Hashemite N, Zhang H, Henske EP, et al. Mutation in TSC2 and activation of mammalian target of rapamycin signalling pathway in renal angiomyolipoma. *Lancet* 2003;361:1348–1349.

European Chromosome 16 Tuberous Sclerosis Consortium. Identification and characterization of the tuberous sclerosis gene on chromosome 16. *Cell* 1993;75:1305–1315.

Gunduz K, Eagle RC Jr, Shields CL, et al. Invasive giant cell astrocytoma of the retina in a patient with tuberous sclerosis. *Ophthalmology* 1999;106:639–642.

Margo CE, Barletta JP, Staman JA. Giant cell astrocytoma of the retina in tuberous sclerosis. *Retina* 1993;13:155–159.

Robertson DM. Ophthalmic manifestations of tuberous sclerosis. *Ann N Y Acad Sci* 1991;615:17–25.

Shields JA, Eagle RC Jr, Shields CL, et al. Aggressive retinal astrocytomas in four patients with tuberous sclerosis complex. *Trans Am Ophthalmol Soc* 2004;102:139–147.

Ulbright TM, Fulling KH, Helveston EM. Astrocytic tumors of the retina. Differentiation of sporadic tumors from phakomatosis-associated tumors. *Arch Pathol Lab Med* 1984;108:160–163.

Weiner DM, Ewalt DH, Roach ES, et al. The tuberous sclerosis complex: a comprehensive review. *J Am Coll Surg* 1998;187:548–561.

Yeung RS. Multiple roles of the tuberous sclerosis complex genes. *Genes Chromosomes Cancer* 2003;38:368–375.

Von Hippel-Lindau Syndrome

Chan CC, Collins AB, Chew EY, et al. Molecular pathology of eyes with von Hippel-Lindau (VHL) disease: a review. *Retina* 2007;27:1–7.

Chew EY. Ocular manifestations of von Hippel-Lindau disease: clinical and genetic investigations. *Trans Am Ophthalmol Soc* 2005;103:495–511.

Couch V, Lindor NM, Karnes PS, et al. von Hippel-Lindau disease. *Mayo Clin Proc* 2000;75:265–272.

Decker HJ, Weidt EJ, Brieger J. The von Hippel-Lindau tumor suppressor gene. A rare and intriguing disease opening new insight into basic mechanisms of carcinogenesis. *Cancer Genet Cytogenet* 1997;93:74–83.

Friedrich CA. Von Hippel-Lindau syndrome. A pleomorphic condition. *Cancer* 1999;86(11 Suppl):2478–2482.

Grossniklaus HE, Thomas JW, Vigneswaran N, et al. Retinal hemangioblastoma. A histologic, immunohistochemical, and ultrastructural evaluation. *Ophthalmology* 1992;99:140–145.

Jakobiec FA, Font RL, Johnson FB. Angiomatosis retinae: an ultrastructural study and lipid analysis. *Cancer* 1976;38: 2042–2056.

Kim HJ, Butman JA, Brewer C, et al. Tumors of the endolymphatic sac in patients with von Hippel-Lindau disease: Implications for their natural history, diagnosis, and treatment. *J Neurosurg* 2005;102:503–512.

Lonser RR, Kim HJ, Butman JA, et al. Tumors of the endolymphatic sac in von Hippel-Lindau disease. *N Engl J Med* 2004;350:2481–2486.

Singh A, Shields J, Shields C. Solitary retinal capillary hemangioma: Hereditary (von Hippel-Lindau disease) or nonhereditary? *Arch Ophthalmol* 2001;119:232–234.

Singh AD, Nouri M, Shields CL, et al: Retinal capillary hemangioma: a comparison of sporadic cases and cases associated with von Hippel-Lindau disease. *Ophthalmology* 2001;108: 1907–1911.

Sturge-Weber Syndrome

Goldberg RE, Pheasant TR, Shields JA. Cavernous hemangioma of the retina: a four-generation pedigree with neurocutaneous manifestations and an example of bilateral retinal involvement. *Arch Ophthalmol* 1979;97:2321–2232.

Hamm H. Cutaneous mosaicism of lethal mutations. *Am J Med Genet* 1999;85(4):342–345.

Happle R. Lethal genes surviving by mosaicism: a possible explanation for sporadic birth defects involving the skin. *J Am Acad Dermatol* 1987;16:899–906. *Am Acad Ophthalmol Otolaryngol* 1978;85:276–286.

Messmer E, Font RL, Laqua H, et al. Cavernous hemangioma of the retina. Immunohistochemical and ultrastructural observations. *Arch Ophthalmol* 1984;102:413–418.

Phelps CD. The pathogenesis of glaucoma in Sturge-Weber syndrome. *Trans Am Acad Ophthalmol Otolaryngol* 1978;85: 276–286.

3 Inflammation

INTRODUCTION

During the evolutionary struggle for survival, a complex series of defense mechanisms (that we in its totality call inflammation) has evolved. The inflammatory response involves a variety of specialized effector cells and a bewilderingly complex interplay of cells, mediators, and biochemical reactions that serves to protect the body against microorganisms and cancer. In addition, the inflammatory process includes mechanisms to repair and restore tissues that have been damaged by foreign invaders, trauma, or chemical and physical agents. The wide spectrum of opportunistic infections and tumors that afflict patients who have the acquired immunodeficiency syndrome (AIDS) underscores generally how effective the intact immune system, the cornerstone of the inflammatory process, is in protecting us from potential invaders.

Fantone and Ward defined inflammation as "a reaction of the microcirculation characterized by movement of fluid and white blood cells from the blood into the extravascular tissues. This is frequently an expression of the host's attempt to localize and eliminate metabolically altered cells, foreign particles, microorganisms, or antigens." The inflammatory cells and the biochemical mediators of inflammation largely reside within the lumina of blood vessels. In contrast, the majority of the body's cells are located in the extravascular compartment, where invasion by microorganisms also generally begins. Hence, inflammatory cells and macromolecules such as antibodies and components of the complement system must leave the vessels and enter the tissues if they are to combat microbial invaders or dispose of dead or damaged cells or other materials. Vasoactive inflammatory mediators such as histamine, serotonin, kinins, prostaglandins, and platelet activating factor cause vasodilation and increase vascular permeability, allowing cells and antibodies access to the tissues. A second heterogenous group of nonimmunoglobulin protein mediators called cytokines recruit and stimulate inflammatory cells. Cytokines are synthesized and secreted by inflammatory cells and include the interleukins, interferons, and colony stimulating factors. Other cell adhesion molecules including selectins, integrins, and cadherins are involved in cellular homing, adhesion, and cell-to-cell interactions. The details of this complex series of interactions are beyond the scope of this introductory chapter.

Vasodilation and increased vascular permeability are responsible for several of the cardinal manifestations of inflammation including *tumor* or swelling, *calor* or heat, and *rubor* or redness (Fig. 3-1). Heat and redness reflect increased blood flow and swelling, the collection of serum and other blood components in the extracellular space. Some inflammatory mediators (e.g., some of the prostaglandins) cause pain and stimulate the contraction of smooth muscle. Spasm of the ciliary muscle and sphincter muscle of the iris contributes to the pain of anterior uveitis, which usually is ameliorated by strong cycloplegic drugs such as atropine. Pain, pupillary miosis, and photophobia are helpful clinical markers that serve to differentiate iridocyclitis from conjunctivitis.

The increased vascular permeability that occurs in inflammation is readily evident to the ophthalmologist during slit lamp biomicroscopy. Aqueous humor normally is almost totally devoid of protein. The protein content rises when inflammation disrupts the blood–ocular barrier. A focused beam of light illuminating the anterior chamber becomes visible, just as a projector beam is visible in a smoky room. This phenomenon, which is termed aqueous "flare" or "ray," is caused by the Tyndall effect. The intensity of the aqueous flare correlates fairly well with the severity of the inflammation and may be roughly quantified and noted in the clinical record. Individual inflammatory cells also are evident on slit lamp examination as motes of light. The quantity of cells is also roughly estimated and recorded. The cells normally move with the convection currents in the aqueous. (They sink anteriorly where the aqueous is cooled by the cornea and rise posteriorly where the aqueous is heated by the iris.) Absence of cellular convection currents may indicate clotting of fibrin-rich aqueous in a case with severe vascular permeability. Adhesions readily form in the fibrin-rich milieu of ocular inflammation. Adhesions between the iris and the lens called posterior synechiae can block the flow of aqueous humor through the pupil from the posterior chamber. The pupil is said to be secluded if its entire circumference

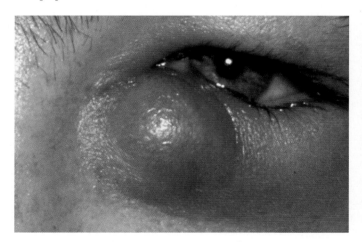

Fig. 3-1. Acute dacryocystitis. Signs of acute inflammation including swelling and erythema are evident in the region of infected lacrimal sac and lower lid.

is bound down by posterior synechiae (seclusio pupillae). Secondary closed-angle glaucoma can develop if the synechiae are not broken. Cycloplegic/mydriatic drugs help to prevent these adhesions by dilating the pupil. Aggregates of inflammatory cells called keratic precipitates or KPs form on the posterior surface of the cornea. The KPs may be small or large and lardaceous. The latter, which are often called "mutton-fat" keratin precipitates, typically occur in eyes that have chronic granulomatous inflammation.

Functio laesa or loss of function is the final cardinal manifestation of inflammation. Although many common ocular inflammations such as conjunctivitis or chalazion are short-lived incapacitations or annoyances, severe inflammations or infections, particularly those that affect the interior of the eye, can cause blindness. Stereotyped inflammatory responses that are designed to protect the body against external invaders can totally destroy the delicate tissues of the eye. A small bacterial infection may be inconsequential in the skin, but it can totally destroy an eye. Even if an intraocular bacterial infection is expediently sterilized, the normal processes of regeneration and repair often cause blindness. A delicate membrane of connective tissue <1 mm long can profoundly affect visual acuity if it forms in an inopportune location. Likewise, minor alterations in the structure of the transparent ocular media (cornea, lens, or vitreous) can markedly degrade their optical properties. One must also remember that the eye's neurosensory components are incapable of regeneration or repair like central nervous system tissue. Blindness caused by retinal damage or destruction is irrevocable and untreatable.

THE CLASSIFICATION OF INFLAMMATION

Histopathologically, inflammation is categorized into acute and chronic categories based on the type of inflammatory cells that are found in the tissue or exudate. **Acute inflammation** usually is characterized by the presence of polymorphonuclear leukocytes or "polys." Lymphocytes and plasma cells are found in chronic nongranulomatous inflammation, and their presence generally denotes involvement of the immune system. Activated macrophages or epithelioid histiocytes and inflammatory giant cells characterize chronic granulomatous inflammation.

POLYMORPHONUCLEAR LEUKOCYTES

The polymorphonuclear leukocyte, neutrophil, or poly is the primary cell found in acute inflammation (Fig. 3-2A). The polymorphonuclear leukocyte is the body's first line of cellular defense. These cells phagocytize bacteria and other foreign material, and their cytoplasm contains many primary and secondary granules that harbor a wide variety of digestive enzymes that they use to kill and digest microorganisms. Polys have pink cytoplasm and a multilobed (typically trilobed) nucleus in routine sections stained with hematoxylin and eosin (H&E). Degenerated polys with round karyorrhectic nuclei frequently are observed in focal collection of polys called abscesses. The term suppurative inflammation refers to the presence of an exudate called pus, which is composed of numerous polys and tissue destruction. Polymorphonuclear leukocytes do not proliferate at the site of inflammation. They are produced in the bone marrow and delivered via the blood stream to the site of inflammation, where they die. They are attracted to the site of injury by chemotactic gradients, adhere to receptors or adhesion molecules on the vascular endothelial cells (margination), and pass through the capillary wall into the tissue (diapedesis). The cell walls of polys have receptors for the Fc component of immunoglobulin. These Fc receptors aid in the phagocytosis of bacteria that have been bound to antibodies in a process called opsonization.

Clinically, acute inflammation is characterized by the presence of pus. Copious quantities of purulent exudate occur in patients who have hyperacute conjunctivitis such as that caused by gonococcus. A layered collection of polys called a hypopyon accumulates in the inferior part of the anterior chamber in eyes with acute keratitis or endophthalmitis. Vitreous abscesses form in acute purulent endophthalmitis. The polys in the vitreous abscess occasionally are arranged in a linear fashion, reflecting the orientation of the type II collagen fibrils that constitute the framework of the vitreous humor.

EOSINOPHILS

Eosinophilic leukocytes or eosinophils are recognized by their intensely eosinophilic, orange, granular cytoplasm and their bilobed nuclei (Fig. 3-2B). Eosinophils are about the same size as polys. Their cytoplasmic granules have a characteristic rhomboid crystalloid configuration disclosed by electron microscopy. The eosinophil granules are rich in acid phosphatase and other lysosomal enzymes and also contain a unique eosinophilic major basic protein that is toxic to certain parasites and normal host cells. Eosinophils are involved in the phagocytosis of antigen antibody complexes and are known to modulate inflammatory reactions mediated by mast cells. The presence of numerous eosinophils in tissue sections is highly suggestive of either an allergic reaction or a parasitic infestation.

LYMPHOCYTES

Lymphocytes are mononuclear cells that are 7 to 8 μm in diameter. Lymphocytes appear as blue spheres in smears and tissue sections; their nuclei are round and intensely

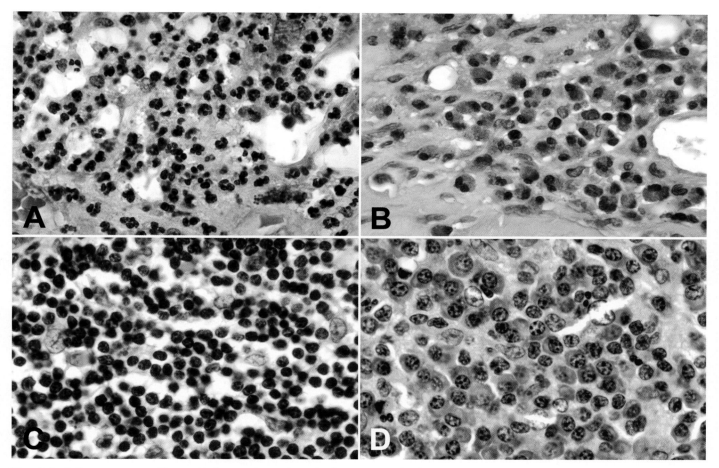

Fig. 3-2. Inflammatory cells. A. Polymorphonuclear leukocytes. Polys have multilobed nuclei and eosinophilic cytoplasm. The polys in this field are well preserved. A few mononuclear histiocytes also are present in the acute inflammatory infiltrate. **B. Eosinophils.** The cytoplasm of eosinophils contains intensely eosinophilic granules. The nuclei are bilobed. The presence of eosinophils usually suggests the presence of allergy or a parasite. **C. Lymphocytes.** Lymphocytes have round, intensely basophilic nuclei and scanty cytoplasm that usually is inapparent in routine light microscopic sections. Many subtypes of lymphocytes can be identified with special immunohistochemical stains. **D. Plasma cells.** Plasma cells have round, eccentrically located nuclei with a cartwheel or clock-face pattern of chromatin clumping. The cytoplasm is basophilic because it contains large quantities of ribosomal RNA used in antibody synthesis. The Golgi apparatus is evident light microscopically as a perinuclear "hof." **(A–D.** H&E ×250)

basophilic, and the cytoplasm is so scanty that it is often inapparent (Fig. 3-2C). Lymphocytes play a dominant role in chronic inflammation and in both humoral and cell-mediated immunity. Multiple subtypes of lymphocytes have been characterized. B lymphocytes are formed in the bone marrow and are involved in humoral immunity. B lymphocytes differentiate into plasma cells, the chief antibody-producing cells of the body. T lymphocytes, which originate in the thymus, include effector and regulatory subtypes. Effector T cells participate in delayed hypersensitivity and mixed lymphocyte reactions and are a prominent constituent of benign reactive lymphoid infiltrates. Regulator T cells (T-helper/amplifier [T4] and suppressor/cytotoxic [T8] cells) modulate the immune response. T4 cells, which are responsible for initiating the immune response, are preferentially infected and killed by human immunodeficiency virus (HIV), which binds to the CD4 receptor. Other lymphocyte subtypes include killer, natural killer, and null cells.

PLASMA CELLS

Plasma cells are activated B lymphocytes. Plasma cells are the body's primary source of circulating antibodies. These antibody factories have a characteristic appearance (Fig. 3-2D). Round and eccentrically located, the nucleus has dense clumps of chromatin that adhere to the inner surface of its membrane in a pattern that has been likened to a cart wheel or clock face. Unlike lymphocytes, plasma cells have an abundant quantity of cytoplasm, which is largely occupied by rough endoplasmic reticulum (RER) used to synthesize immunoglobulin. In routine sections stained with H&E, the cytoplasm of plasma cells has a distinctly basophilic or purple hue caused by the affinity of the basic dye hematoxylin for ribosomal RNA in the RER. The Golgi apparatus of plasma cell is apparent light microscopically as a lighter staining crescent next to the nucleus called the perinuclear "hof"

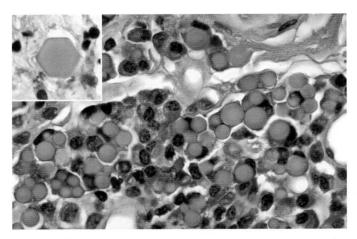

Fig. 3-3. Russell bodies. The uniformly eosinophilic spherules in this chronic inflammatory infiltrate are crystalloids of immuno-globulin called Russell bodies. A rare hexagonal Russell body is seen in the **inset**. (**Both figures**, H&E ×250)

(German, "courtyard"). The cytoplasm of plasma cells may become eosinophilic as the cells produce large quantities of immunoglobulin. Eosinophilic crystals of immunoglobulin called Russell bodies occasionally form in the cytoplasm of plasma cells (Fig. 3-3). Usually round, but occasionally square or even hexagonal, Russell bodies reflect the "terminal con-stipation" plasma cells by immunoglobulin. They generally denote an inflammatory process of some chronicity and may be found intracellularly or free in the tissue. Dutcher bodies are similar smaller crystalline inclusions of antibody mol-ecules that appear to be intranuclear but actually reside in an intranuclear cytoplasmic inclusion. Positive staining with the periodic acid-Schiff (PAS) stain indicates that Russell or Dutcher bodies are composed either of IgA or IgM molecules. A cell that contains multiple small intracytoplasmic Russell bodies is called a morula cell of Mott.

An inflammatory infiltrate composed of lymphocytes and varying numbers of plasma cells characterizes **chronic nongranulomatous inflammation**. Although lymphocytes and plasma cells occasionally constitute an acute inflam-matory response to certain viral infections, the presence of these cells usually indicates that the immune system has been activated (Fig. 3-4). Special stains for microorganism generally are nonrevealing in chronic nongranulomatous inflammation.

MAST CELLS

Mast cells are often called tissue basophils, although there is evidence that they are derived from different precursor cells in the bone marrow. Mast cells play an extremely important role in acute anaphylaxis (Type I hypersensitivity reaction). IgE antibody molecules made by allergic individuals bind to Fc receptors on the plasma membrane of mast cells. Subsequent interaction between the appropriate antigen and two IgE molecules causes mast cell degranulation and the release of potent vaso-active substances including histamine, serotonin, and heparin, which have an immediate effect on vascular permeability. Severe itching and the acute onset of con-junctival edema or chemosis are clinical symptoms and signs of acute allergic conjunctivitis of the anaphylactic type (Fig. 3-5B).

Mast cells vaguely resemble plasma cells in tissue sec-tions but have a centrally placed nucleus (Fig. 3-5A). In routine H&E sections, they lack the prominent array of basophilic granules disclosed by Wright stain. The cyto-plasm of mast cells is PAS-positive, and its constituent granules are stained intensely blue by the acid-fast stain. Mast cells are found in the conjunctival substantia propria

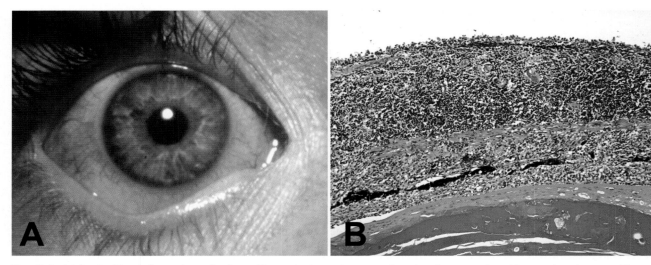

Fig. 3-4. Iritis. A. The inflamed eye had pupillary miosis and an anterior chamber reaction. No exudate is seen. The patient had pain and photophobia. **B.** Histopathology exam of another case shows massive thickening of the iris stroma by an infiltrate of lymphocytes and plasma cells. The disrupted iris pigment epithelium adheres to the anterior surface of the cataractous lens. No microorganisms were detected. (**B.** H&E ×50)

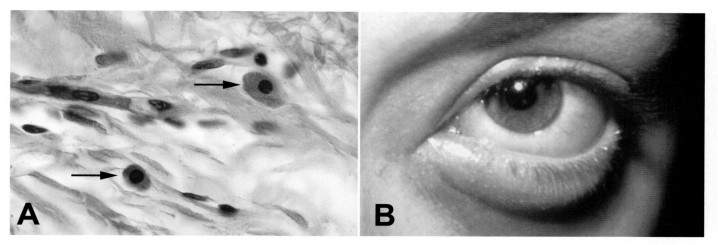

Fig. 3-5. A. Mast cells. Mast cells (*arrows*) in tissue sections have round, centrally located nuclei. The cytoplasm is mildly basophilic in routine sections stained with H&E and stains intensely with PAS. **B. Acute allergic conjunctivitis.** Conjunctival chemosis is evident in the photo of a laboratory worker with acute anaphylactic conjunctivitis. The patient was allergic to animal dander and experienced the sudden onset of severe itching. (**A.** H&E ×250)

in allergic disorders such as vernal conjunctivitis and giant papillary conjunctivitis. They are also common in some neoplasms such as neurofibromas.

MACROPHAGES

Macrophages or histiocytes are the body's second line of cellular defense and its chief phagocytic cell. Macrophages are derived from circulating monocytes. They are relatively large mononuclear cells (larger than polys) that have an eccentric reniform or kidney-shaped nucleus. Macrophages have a great capacity to phagocytize material, but unlike polys they cause little tissue damage. Prior to phagocytosis, newly formed macrophages have a modest amount of eosinophilic cytoplasm. In ophthalmic pathology, macrophages generally are characterized by the substances that

they have phagocytized. They include macrophages that have ingested blood breakdown products such as hemosiderin and erythrocyte ghost cells, lipid material seen as foamy vacuoles, and other materials such as degenerated lens protein or melanin (Fig. 3-6).

Macrophages play an important role as antigen-presenting cells in the initial stages of the immune response. They phagocytize and process antigenic material and present appropriate epitopes to helper T cells in conjunction with class II major histocompatibility molecules (called HLA-DR in humans), which are located in their cell membranes. During activation, macrophages produce a lymphokine called interleukin-1 (IL-1) that produces fever and is thought to induce the production of a second cellular messenger interleukin-2 by the T cells. They also secrete a wide variety of powerful biologic molecules called monokines that are important, even pivotal, participants in the inflammatory response.

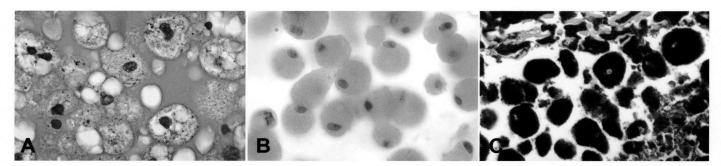

Fig. 3-6. Macrophages. A. Lipid-laden macrophages, subretinal fluid. The frothy vacuolated cytoplasm is filled with lipid vacuoles and scattered elliptical granules of RPE melanin. The surrounding subretinal fluid is protein-rich and intensely eosinophilic. The patient had radiation retinopathy. **B. Lens-laden macrophages, phacolytic glaucoma.** These macrophages have copious quantities of eosinophilic cytoplasm that reflects the ingestion of degenerated lens protein released from an advanced cortical cataract. **C. Melanophages, melanocytomalytic glaucoma.** Macrophages have ingested melanin pigment released from necrotic iris melanocytoma. (**A–C.** H&E, original magnification ×250)

EPITHELIOID HISTIOCYTES AND INFLAMMATORY GIANT CELLS

Under certain circumstances macrophages or histiocytes transform into more metabolically active forms called epithelioid cells or epithelioid histiocytes (see Fig. 3-9A, later in this chapter). Activation typically occurs when the histiocytes encounter large quantities of antigenic material that is relatively insoluble or indigestible. Some microorganisms, particularly those that proliferate intracellularly, stimulate the formation of epithelioid histiocytes. Classic examples include the mycobacteria that cause tuberculosis and leprosy, fungi, and parasites such as schistosomes.

Epithelioid histiocytes are termed "epithelioid" (-oid, resembling; epithelioid, like epithelium) because these cells have abundant eosinophilic cytoplasm and superficially resemble simple epithelial cells. If epithelioid histiocytes are observed histopathologically in a chronic inflammatory infiltrate, the inflammation is termed granulomatous. Epithelioid histiocytes are required for the diagnosis of chronic granulomatous inflammation. Inflammatory giant cells are another characteristic feature of chronic granulomatous inflammation (Figs. 3-7 and 3-8). Inflammatory giant cells are a multinucleated syncytium formed by the fusion of epithelioid histiocytes.

Several kinds of inflammatory giant cells are recognized histopathologically. The **Langhans giant cell,** which typically is seen in tuberculosis, has a peripheral rim of nuclei and homogenous cytoplasm (Fig. 3-7A). **Foreign body giant cells** have nuclei, which are randomly dispersed or are centrally located, and their cytoplasm contains particulates of foreign material in large vacuoles (Fig. 3-8). When an extremely large foreign body is encountered, numerous foreign body giant cells adhere to its outer surface, forming an encompassing cytoplasmic barrier that "insulates" the foreign material from the rest of the body. The **Touton giant cell** occurs in chronic xanthogranulomatous inflammation (Fig. 3-7B). The classic Touton giant cell is shaped like a target. The "bulls-eye" is a central zone of eosinophilic cytoplasm, which is encircled by a ring of nuclei, which in turn is surrounded by a peripheral wreath of foamy lipidized cytoplasm. Although Touton giant cells classically are associated with juvenile xanthogranuloma (JXG), they also are found in other xanthogranulomatous disorders that affect the ocular adnexa including Erdheim-Chester disease, necrobiotic xanthogranuloma with paraproteinemia, and orbital xanthogranuloma with adult-onset asthma.

GRANULOMATOUS INFLAMMATION

By definition, to be classified as *chronic granulomatous,* an inflammatory infiltrate must contain epithelioid histiocytes and/or inflammatory giant cells. Clinically, the term granulomatous is applied to ocular inflammation when large lardaceous "mutton-fat" KPs are observed. Mutton-fat KPs are miniature granulomas composed of aggregated epithelioid histiocytes. If granulomatous inflammation is noted clinically or histopathologically, a causative organism or specific etiologic agent should be sought. If granulomatous inflammation is encountered in tissue sections, it is imperative that stains for acid-fast organisms, fungi, and bacteria (and occasionally silver stains for spirochetes) be performed. The specimen should also be examined with polarization microscopy to rule out the presence of foreign material that can be inconspicuous. **Sarcoidosis** is a relatively common cause of granulomatous ocular inflammation (Figs. 3-9 and 3-10A). A diagnosis of exclusion, sarcoidosis should be suspected when a characteristic pattern of discrete noncaseating granulomas is found and special stains for microorganisms are negative. Granulomatous

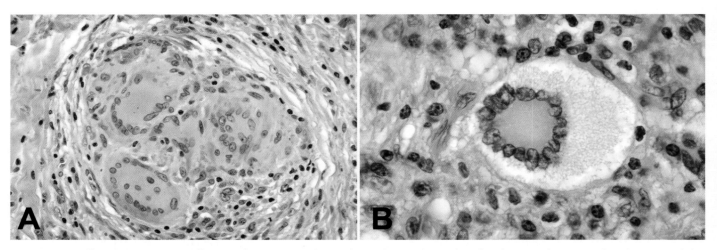

Fig. 3-7. A. Inflammatory giant cells, Langhans type. The nuclei are located peripherally. The cytoplasm is uniformly eosinophilic. Langhans giant cells are found in tuberculosis and other granulomatous diseases. **B. Touton giant cells, juvenile xanthogranuloma.** Fully developed Touton giant cells have a target configuration. A peripheral rim of frothy lipidized cytoplasm surrounds a ring of nuclei which in turn encompasses a central bull's eye of eosinophilic cytoplasm. Touton giant cells are found in JXG and other xanthogranulomatous diseases. (**A.** H&E ×100, **B.** H&E ×250)

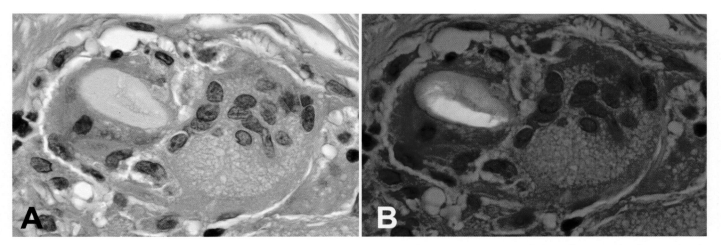

Fig. 3-8. Foreign body giant cell. A. The cytoplasm of the giant cell at left contains an oval cellulose fiber. **B.** The foreign body shows vivid birefringence during polarization microscopy. The nuclei of foreign body giant cells are arranged haphazardly. (**A.** H&E ×250, **B.** H&E with crossed polarizers ×250)

inflammation occasionally is a response to endogenous material. Examples include the response to lipid in chalazia and the thick layer of giant cells bordering keratin in the lumen of dermoid cysts with discontinuous epithelial linings.

PATTERNS OF CHRONIC GRANULOMATOUS INFLAMMATION

The arrangement of the epithelioid histiocytes and other inflammatory cells differs in various chronic granulomatous disorders. These histologic patterns are often helpful in the diagnostic assessment of ocular specimens. Diffuse, discrete and zonal patterns of granulomatous inflammation occur in ocular tissues.

The **diffuse pattern** of chronic granulomatous inflammation characteristically occurs in sympathetic uveitis

(ophthalmia) (Fig. 4-5) and other diseases such as lepromatous leprosy. The epithelioid histiocytes and inflammatory giant cells are diffusely scattered amongst a background infiltrate composed of lymphocytes and plasma cells. The arrangement of the cellular elements has been likened to salt and pepper; the eosinophilic epithelioid histiocytes with their abundant cytoplasm comprise the "salt" that is diffusely dispersed within a "peppery" background of basophilic lymphocytes.

Discrete, well-circumscribed aggregates of epithelioid histiocytes characteristically occur in sarcoidosis (Fig. 3-9 and 3-10A). Hence, the **discrete pattern** of chronic granulomatous inflammation is often called the sarcoidal pattern. The tubercles of epithelioid histiocytes and giant cells in sarcoidosis are sharply delimited from the surrounding infiltrate of round cells, which is comprised largely of helper T lymphocytes. The discrete granulomas in sarcoidosis are noncaseating and they typically lack the cheesy

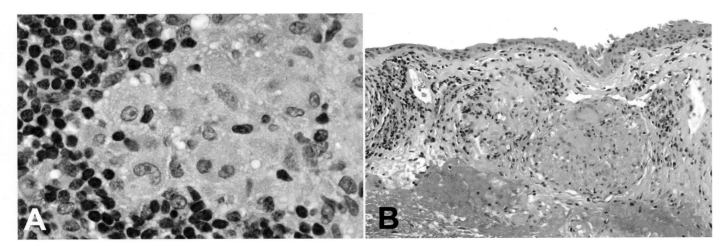

Fig. 3-9. A. Epithelioid histiocytes, sarcoidosis. The epithelioid histiocytes comprising the discrete granuloma have abundant quantities of eosinophilic cytoplasm and vesicular nuclei with nucleoli. **B. Positive conjunctival biopsy, sarcoidosis.** Substantia propria contains several discrete granulomas consistent with sarcoidosis. (**A.** H&E ×250, **B.** H&E ×100)

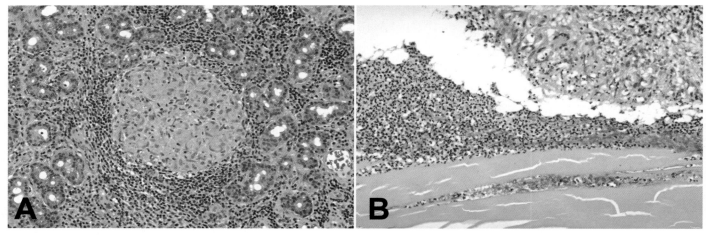

Fig 3-10. Patterns of granulomatous inflammation. A. Discrete granuloma, chronic dacryoadenitis, sarcoidosis. An infiltrate of lymphocytes, rich in helper T cells, surrounds a discrete noncaseating granuloma composed of epithelioid histiocytes and inflammatory giant cells. Scattered acini and ducts persist. **B. Zonal granulomatous reaction, phacoantigenic uveitis (phacoanaphylaxis).** Polymorphonuclear leukocytes infiltrating substance of ruptured lens (below) constitute the first zone of inflammatory cells. A second zone of epithelioid histiocytes surrounds the polys. The clear space separating the two zones of cells is a sectioning artifact. A third zone of nongranulomatous inflammation occurs peripherally. (**A.** H&E ×50, **B.** H&E ×100)

or caseous central necrosis that is a characteristic feature of tuberculosis. Sarcoidosis is a diagnosis of exclusion, however, and special stains for microorganisms should always be performed. Discrete granulomas do occur in other diseases such as miliary tuberculosis and tuberculoid leprosy. In addition, polarization microscopy should be done to exclude particles of foreign material. Silica and beryllium can incite granulomatous inflammation that can mimic sarcoidosis.

Concentric zones of inflammatory cells surround a central nidus of antigenic material in the **zonal pattern** of chronic granulomatous inflammation. The classic example in general pathology is the palisading granuloma that surrounds a nidus of devitalized collagen in rheumatoid arthritis. The classic examples of zonal granulomatous inflammation in the eye are rheumatoid scleritis (see Fig. 6-31) and the rare autoimmune disorder, phacoanaphylactic endophthalmitis (phacoantigenic uveitis).

Phacoanaphylactic endophthalmitis (phacoanaphylaxis) or phacoantigenic uveitis is a severe zonal granulomatous inflammatory reaction that envelops the lens and follows trauma (Fig. 3-10B). In the past, the avascular encapsulated lens was thought to be an immune-sequestered structure, and phacoanaphylaxis, in turn, was considered the body's attempt to reject this "foreign tissue" after its antigens were exposed by injury. These classic concepts are now known to be erroneous. The lens *is not* an immune-sequestered structure; lens proteins or crystallins are expressed elsewhere in the body and antilens antibodies have been found in the sera of normal individuals using modern sensitive assay techniques. Furthermore, if the immune sequestration theory were valid, phacoantigenic uveitis should be an extremely common disease in the current era

of early extracapsular surgery. Residual undenatured lens material almost always remains in the capsular bag after planned extracapsular surgery. Despite this, phacoanaphylactic endophthalmitis remains an extremely rare disease, and very few cases have been documented after extracapsular surgery and intraocular lens implantation.

Phacoanaphylaxis is currently thought to be an immune complex disease (Type III hypersensitivity reaction) involving loss of immune tolerance. Histopathologically, the zonal inflammatory reaction is centered around a lens whose capsule is ruptured or fragments of lens substance (Fig. 3-10B). The central zone of inflammatory cells that infiltrates the substance of the lens is composed of polymorphonuclear leukocytes (first line of cellular defense). The polys are attracted by chemotactic molecules such as C5a that are generated when complement is activated by the formation of immune complexes of antilens antibodies and lens antigens. A second zone of granulomatous inflammation composed of epithelioid histiocytes (activated macrophages, the second line of cellular defense) and giant cells surrounds the inner collection of polys. A third zone of nongranulomatous inflammation containing granulation tissue and lymphocytes and plasma cells occurs peripherally.

Granulation tissue forms during the reparative phase of inflammation and plays an important role in wound healing. Granulation tissue is composed of proliferating capillaries, activated fibroblasts with contractile properties called myofibroblasts, and a mixture of inflammatory cells including polys, lymphocytes, plasma cells, macrophages, and eosinophils (Fig. 3-11). The myofibroblasts are involved in scar contraction. A "pyogenic granuloma" is an inappropriate, exuberant proliferation of granulation tissue that typically arises after minor trauma (Fig. 5-13).

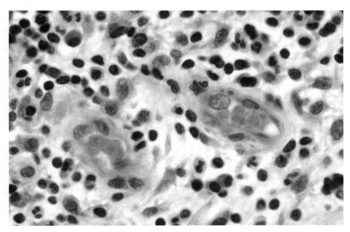

Fig. 3-11. Granulation tissue. A mixed inflammatory infiltrate comprised of lymphocytes, plasma cells, polys, and macrophages surrounds proliferating capillaries and spindle-shaped myofibroblasts. (H&E ×250)

ENDOPHTHALMITIS AND PANOPHTHALMITIS

Endophthalmitis is defined as inflammation, usually acute and infectious in cause, that involves one or more of the ocular coats and adjacent intraocular cavities. Clinically, the term usually denotes an infection that involves the vitreous. As the name implies, panophthalmitis is a more extensive ocular infection that has spread to involve all of the ocular coats including the sclera and occasionally the orbit as well.

Endophthalmitis and panophthalmitis usually are caused by bacteria and less often by yeast and filamentous fungi. The ocular contents, especially the vitreous humor, are an excellent culture medium that will support the growth of relatively avirulent organisms including saprophytes. These intraocular infections usually are suppurative; that is, they are acute and are characterized by the presence of myriad polymorphonuclear leukocytes (polys) that accumulate in the vitreous cavity as a vitreous abscess. Tissue destruction, a hallmark of suppurative inflammation, is caused by the release of digestive enzymes by degenerating polys. The visual prognosis in endophthalmitis is often poor because the retina and other structures bordering the abscess may be destroyed.

Bacterial endophthalmitis usually presents 1 to 2 days postoperatively with severe pain, turbid media, and a hypopyon. Eyes with acute purulent bacterial endophthalmitis typically contain a large solitary vitreous abscess (Fig. 3-12A). Histopathology shows extensive necrosis and dissolution of uveal and retinal tissues and occasionally intraocular hemorrhage (Fig. 3-12B). In contrast to the infiltrate of polys in the vitreous, the choroid often contains lymphocytes and plasma cells because Bruch membrane acts as a natural barrier that confines the acute inflammation. In chronic cases, an ingrowth of granulation tissue from the uvea breaches the neuroepithelium and invades and organizes the vitreous abscess. Bacterial colonies may be conspicuous in some cases, but extensive dispersion of ocular pigment can make identification of bacteria difficult. The clinical course of fungal endophthalmitis usually is more indolent than bacterial endophthalmitis. Multiple vitreous microabscesses are a characteristic finding in **fungal endophthalmitis** (Fig. 3-13).

Endophthalmitis is called exogenous when the eye is invaded by organisms from the external environment. **Exogenous endophthalmitis** usually is caused by bacteria or fungi introduced during ocular surgery or penetrating trauma (Fig. 3-12A). Other avenues of exogenous infection

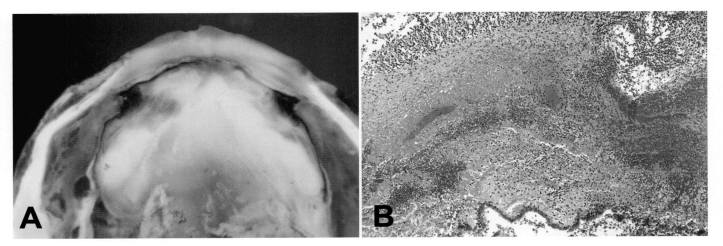

Fig. 3-12. A. Acute endophthalmitis, secondary to *Bacillus cereus*. A large abscess comprised of polymorphonuclear leukocytes fills the vitreous cavity. The exogenous infection developed rapidly after organisms were introduced through a corneal laceration. The anterior chamber is flat and the choroid is detached. The retina was totally necrotic. **B. Retinal necrosis, acute bacterial endophthalmitis.** Polys fill the vitreous (above). The retina is almost totally necrotic and shows loss of its normal lamellar architecture. Focal hemorrhage is present. (**B.** H&E ×50)

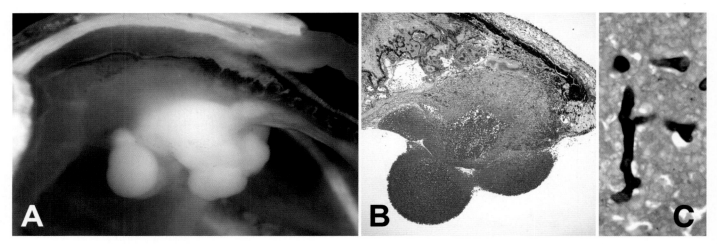

Fig. 3-13. Fungal endophthalmitis. A. Multiple small vitreous microabscesses are present. Vitreous microabscesses are a characteristic finding in fungal endophthalmitis. **B.** Photomicrograph shows characteristic microabscesses in posterior chamber. **C.** GMS fungal stain discloses fungal hyphae within a microabscess. (**B.** H&E ×10, **C.** Gomori methenamine silver ×250)

are infected corneal ulcers that perforate or infected filtering blebs in patients who have undergone fistulization surgery for glaucoma. Staphylococci, streptococci, Gram-negative rods, and fungi are common causes of exogenous endophthalmitis. The term **localized endophthalmitis** refers to infection by relatively avirulent organisms such as *Propionibacterium acnes* or *Candida parapsilosis*, which are sequestered within the lens capsular bag after extracapsular cataract extraction with intraocular lens implantation (Fig. 3-14). Such infections tend to be chronic and smoldering and often incite a granulomatous response.

Endogenous endophthalmitis usually is caused by the hematogenous dissemination of organisms to the eye. Endogenous endophthalmitis can complicate septicemia, subacute bacterial endocarditis, meningococcemia, and systemic fungal infections such as candidiasis, aspergillosis, or nocardiosis in immunocompromised patients

(Fig. 3-15). The posterior segment usually harbors the bulk of the inflammatory process in an endogenous infection. Other important endogenous infections are the necrotizing retinitis caused by the herpesviruses cytomegalovirus (CMV), varicella-zoster virus (VZV), and herpes simplex virus (HSV), and the protozoan parasite *Toxoplasma gondii*.

VIRAL RETINITIS

Cytomegalovirus retinitis (Fig. 3-16) is the most common opportunistic intraocular infection in patients who have the acquired immunodeficiency syndrome (AIDS) and can also affect patients who are immunosuppressed following transplant surgery or cancer chemotherapy. Before the institution of HAART therapy, nearly one third of AIDS patients developed CMV retinitis. CMV retinitis is a devastating

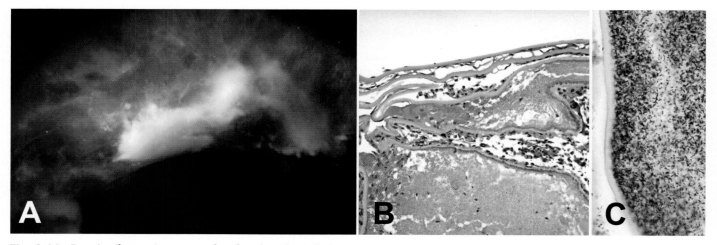

Fig. 3-14. *Propionibacterium acnes* localized endophthalmitis. A. Large intracapsular colony of bacteria forms whitish plaque within the excised lens capsular bag. Chronic granulomatous uveitis developed months after extracapsular cataract extraction. **B.** Large colony of sequestered diphtheroids forms basophilic granular deposit within the explanted lens capsular bag. **C.** Bacterial colony beneath anterior lens capsule is composed of pleomorphic Gram-positive bacteria. (**B.** H&E ×50, **C.** Tissue Gram stain ×250)

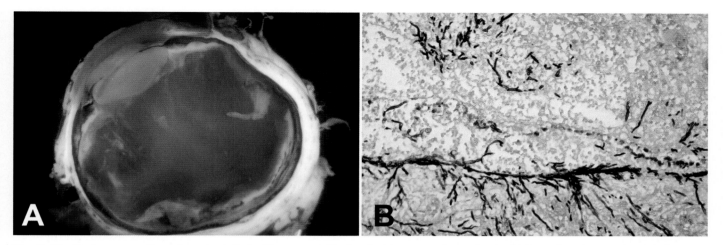

Fig. 3-15. Endogenous fungal endophthalmitis, aspergillosis. A. The posterior retina is thickened and necrotic and the posterior choroid is thickened. Inflammatory cells partially opacify the vitreous. **B.** Fungal stain discloses characteristic linear array of fungal hyphae on the inner surface of Bruch membrane. Branching septate hyphae also infiltrate the retina and choroidal stroma. (**B.** Gomori methenamine silver, ×50)

ocular complication of AIDS because it causes total retinal destruction and blindness if untreated.

Ophthalmoscopically, acute CMV infection causes coagulative necrosis and opacification of the retina, which appears yellowish white. Posterior retinal infections usually begin along vessels and often are marked by heavy infiltration and hemorrhage, which are responsible for an ophthalmoscopic appearance that has been likened to "crumbled cheese and ketchup." Peripheral lesions have a granular appearance and little or no hemorrhage.

The term cytomegalovirus is derived from the cellular enlargement, which is a characteristic cytopathic effect of the virus (Fig. 3-16). In this regard, CMV differs from the other herpesviruses that cause necrotizing retinitis. All retinal herpesvirus infections are characterized histopathologically

by the presence of Cowdry type A intranuclear inclusions comprised of virions. The intranuclear inclusions found in cells infected by CMV are often called "owl's eye" inclusions because they typically are quite large and are surrounded by a clear halo. Multiple intracytoplasmic inclusions also occur in cells infected with CMV.

Light microscopy discloses markedly enlarged abnormal retinal cells containing "owl's eye" inclusions in the necrotic retina (Fig. 3-16C). Areas that are opaque clinically typically show full-thickness retinal destruction. The transition between healthy and totally necrotic retina is often abrupt. The underlying choroid contains acute and chronic inflammatory cells. CMV can also infect the retinal pigment epithelium (RPE). The vitreous in CMV retinitis is often relatively clear in contrast to the intense vitritis seen in ocular toxoplasmosis.

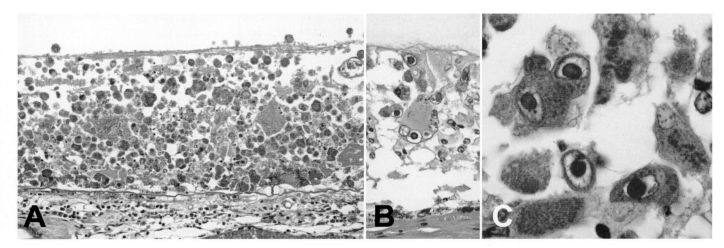

Fig. 3-16. Cytomegalovirus retinitis. A. Full-thickness destruction of the retina and RPE are present. The infected retina contains enlarged cells. The patient had received chemotherapy for lymphoma. **B.** The infected retina contains a multinucleated giant cell with viral inclusions. **C.** Clear haloes surrounding large Cowdry type A intranuclear inclusions of CMV impart an "owl's eye" appearance to infected nuclei. Smaller cytoplasmic inclusions also are present. (**A.** Hematoxylin-eosin ×100, **B.** Hematoxylin-eosin ×120, **C.** Hematoxylin-eosin ×400)

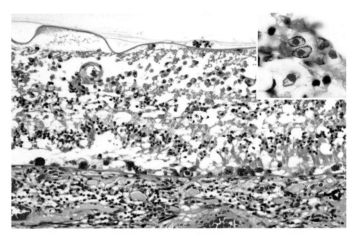

Fig. 3-17. Progressive Outer Retinal Necrosis (PORN) syndrome. Necrosis involves all retinal layers including RPE. Cowdry type A intranuclear inclusions of VZV are seen in inset. The patient had AIDS. (**Main figure**, H&E ×100; **inset**, H&E ×250) (Case presented by Dr. Curtis Margo at the 1994 meeting of the Verhoeff Society, Rochester, Minnesota.)

Necrotizing retinitis caused by *Herpes simplex* or *varicella-zoster virus* occurs in the **acute retinal necrosis** (ARN) or **bilateral acute retinal necrosis** (BARN) syndromes. Classic ARN syndrome occurs in presumably healthy patients who are not immunosuppressed. A similar ocular infection can occur in immunosuppressed patients, however. The Cowdry type A intranuclear inclusions are smaller than the "owl's eye" inclusions of CMV and cytomegaly is not observed. The visual prognosis in patients who have ARN is often poor because severe postinfectious retinal atrophy predisposes to retinal holes and detachment. VZV infection of the retina in AIDS patients causes the **progressive outer retinal necrosis** (PORN) syndrome, which begins with deep multifocal retinal opacification and rapidly progresses to total retinal necrosis (Fig. 3-17).

Eosinophilic viral inclusions are found postmortem in retinal neurons and glial cells in children who have **subacute sclerosing panencephalitis (SSPE),** a slow virus infection of the CNS by the measles virus. SSPE can present with visual loss from a macular neuroretinitis (measles maculopathy). The average age at onset is 7 years, and boys are predominantly affected (3:1). As mental deterioration progresses toward decerebration, patients develop seizures and myoclonic jerks with distinctive EEG changes.

TOXOPLASMA RETINOCHOROIDITIS

Ocular toxoplasmosis is an infestation by the obligatory intracellular protozoan parasite *Toxoplasma gondii,* whose definitive host is the cat. Toxoplasmosis is a retinochoroiditis; the neurotropic parasite infests the retina and the central nervous system primarily. The multiplicative activity of the organisms themselves causes coagulative necrosis of retinal tissue; toxoplasma proliferate in the cytoplasm of the parasitized retinal cells until the cells rupture. Infected portions of the retina are totally destroyed, and the area of primary retinal infection is usually sharply demarcated (Fig. 3-18A). The primary retinitis is associated with a secondary chronic choroiditis that may spread to involve the sclera producing a focal or segmental panophthalmitis. An example of a zonal granulomatous inflammatory reaction modified by anatomy, the inflammatory infiltrate is confined to the choroid by the structural barrier of Bruch membrane and usually contains epithelioid histiocytes.

The name *Toxoplasma* (toxon = bow) is derived from the crescentic shape of the tachyzoites, which are the rapidly multiplying free form of the parasite (Fig. 3-18B). Tachyzoites occasionally are identified in the infected retina, but the diagnosis usually is confirmed by the identification of toxoplasma cysts in sections stained with PAS (Fig. 3-18C). Toxoplasma cysts are filled with hundreds of slowly proliferating bradyzoites, which are released when the cyst walls rupture. Reactivation of infection in adults is caused by the release of organisms that have remained encysted and dormant in the margins of old congenital chorioretinal scars.

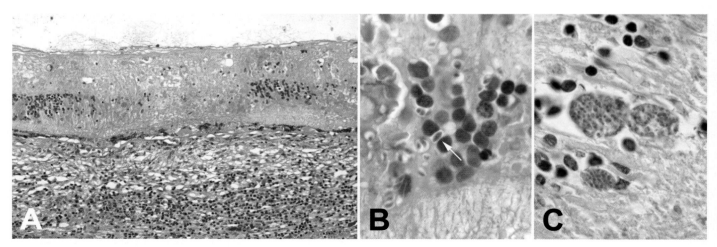

Fig. 3-18. Toxoplasma retinochoroiditis. A. The infected retina is almost totally necrotic. The choroid is thickened by chronic granulomatous inflammation. **B.** The *arrow* denotes toxoplasma tachyzoite in largely necrotic retina. **C.** Three intraretinal toxoplasma cysts filled with bradyzoites are present. (**A.** H&E ×50, **B.** H&E ×250, **C.** H&E ×250)

In the past it was thought that most cases of ocular toxoplasmosis in the United States were acquired *in utero* by transplacental transmission of the parasite from a newly infected mother to her fetus. Acquired toxoplasmosis is more common than previously thought, however, and acquired disease related to dietary habits and poor hygiene is relatively common in some parts of the world.

Congenital retinochoroiditis produces atrophic and pigmented craterlike chorioretinal scars, which typically are located in the macula and were once called atypical colobomas. The macular region is affected primarily because it is profusely vascularized and the parasite is disseminated hematogenously. The old scars of ocular toxoplasmosis appear white because the sclera has been bared by full-thickness choroidal destruction. Intensely pigmented clumps of hyperplastic RPE also typically are found. Active infection causes focal retinal opacification and necrosis and an intense inflammatory infiltrate in the vitreous composed of histiocytes and lymphocytes. The intense vitritis markedly reduces visual acuity and may partially obscure the underlying focus of white infected retina. This latter appearance has been likened to a "headlight in a fog." Toxoplasmosis is one of the opportunistic infections that can occur in patients with AIDS.

UVEITIS

Uveitis refers to inflammation of the uveal tract, the middle pigmented and heavily vascularized coat of the eye that includes the iris, ciliary body, and choroid. Endogenous chronic nongranulomatous iridocyclitis, a poorly understood immunological disorder, is encountered most frequently in clinical practice. Uveitis is often idiopathic, but it may be associated with systemic disorders including juvenile rheumatoid arthritis, ankylosing spondylitis, Reiter syndrome, ulcerative colitis, regional enteritis, or Behçet disease. Microscopy discloses an infiltrate of lymphocytes and plasma cells in the uveal stroma in eyes with nongranulomatous uveitis (Fig. 3-4). Russell bodies and morula cells may be quite common in chronic cases.

Clinical or pathological evaluation may disclose a specific cause in patients who have chronic granulomatous uveitis. **Sarcoidosis** is the most common cause of granulomatous uveitis. Approximately 38% of patients with systemic sarcoidosis will have ocular involvement at some point in their disease. Granulomatous intraocular inflammation can also be caused by tuberculosis, leprosy, syphilis, parasites, and fungal infections including candidiasis, coccidioidomycosis, histoplasmosis, blastomycosis, and sporotrichosis. Granulomatous inflammation is also found in sympathetic uveitis and Vogt-Koyanagi-Harada disease.

Behçet disease is a systemic immune complex disease that causes occlusive vasculitis. Genital and oral aphthous ulcers and recurrent nongranulomatous iridocyclitis with hypopyon are characteristic manifestations and diagnostic criteria. Ocular involvement also is marked by retinal vasculitis, which leads to hemorrhagic retinal infarction and retinal detachment. Especially common in the Middle and Far East, Behçet disease is associated with HLA phenotypes HLA-B5 and its subtype HLA-Bw51. Patients who have ocular Behçet disease usually become blind if they are not treated with immunosuppressive drugs.

THE SEQUELAE OF OCULAR INFLAMMATION

The sequelae of ocular inflammation include corneal scarring and vascularization, band keratopathy, cataract, and secondary glaucoma. The latter is often closed angle in type and is caused by inflammatory posterior synechiae between the iris and lens. Intraocular fibrosis and membranes are caused by the organization of inflammatory debris. A **cyclitic membrane** is a fibrous membrane that bridges the anterior part of the vitreous cavity behind the lens from ciliary body to ciliary body (Fig. 3-19). Cyclitic membranes are caused by fibrous organization of the anterior

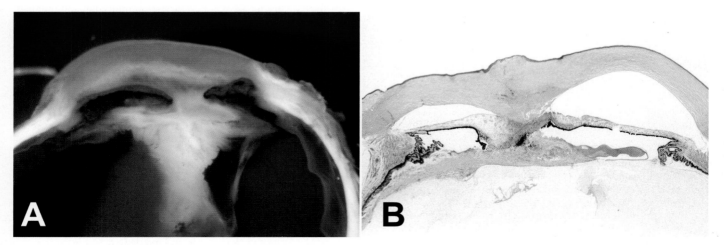

Fig. 3-19. Cyclitic membrane. A. The chronically detached retina adheres anteriorly to the white mass of fibrous connective tissue filling the posterior chamber. Cyclitic membranes are caused by fibrous organization of the vitreous. **B.** Cyclitic membrane incorporates lens remnants. The iris is incarcerated in the central corneal wound. (**B.** H&E ×5)

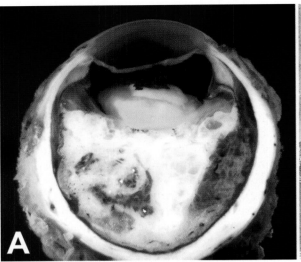
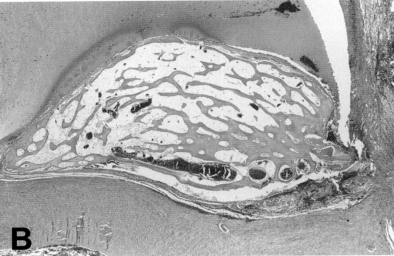

Fig. 3-20. A. Pathological phthisis bulbi (atrophia bulbi with shrinkage and disorganization). Mass of totally detached gliotic retina and metaplastic bone fills disorganized interior of chronically blind and painful eye. The angle is closed by peripheral anterior synechiae. The pupil adheres to the lens at the site of a white anterior subcapsular cataract. **B. Osseous metaplasia of the RPE.** A Large focus of metaplastic bone containing fatty marrow rests on the inner surface of juxtapapillary choroid. Intraocular bone is often found in phthisical eyes with long-standing retinal detachments. **(B.** H&E ×10)

vitreous. Contraction of inflammatory membranes causes tractional detachment of the ciliary body or retina. Ocular hypotony and shrinkage frequently result from the disorganization and destruction of intraocular structures. Clinically, the term phthisical is applied to blind hypotonus eyes that are soft, partially collapsed, and have a vaguely cuboid shape caused by rectus muscle traction. The pathologic diagnosis **phthisis bulbi (atrophia bulbi with shrinkage and disorganization)** is reserved for eyes that are markedly atrophic and disorganized and have thickened folded sclera (Fig. 3-20A). The interior of such phthisical eyes usually is filled with scar tissue, and intraocular structures are unrecognizable. The term **atrophia bulbi with shrinkage** is used if intraocular structures can be identified. Intraocular ossification (**osseous metaplasia of the RPE**) is commonly observed in phthisical and atrophic eyes that have chronic retinal detachments (Fig. 3-20B).

BIBLIOGRAPHY

General References

Chensue SW, Ward PA. Inflammation. In: Damjanov I, Linder J, eds. *Anderson's Pathology*, 10th ed. St. Louis, MO: CV Mosby, 1996:387–415.

Cotran RS, Kumar V, Robbins SL. Inflammation and repair. In: Cotran RS, Kumar V, Robbins SL, eds. *Pathologic Basis of Disease*, 5th ed. Philadelphia, PA: WB Saunders, 1994:51–92.

Fantone JC, Ward PA. Inflammation. In: Rubin E, Farber JL, eds. *Pathology*. Philadelphia, PA: JB Lippincott, 1994:32–67.

Gallin JI, Goldstein IM, Snyderman R, eds. *Inflammation: Basic Principles and Clinical Correlates*. New York, NY: Raven Press, 1988.

Green WR. Inflammatory diseases and conditions of the eye. In: Spencer W, ed. *Ophthalmic Pathology: An Atlas and Textbook*, vol. 3, Philadelphia, PA: WB Saunders, 1996:1864–2110.

Howes EL, Rao NA. Basic mechanisms in pathology, Chapter 13. In: Spencer W, ed. *Ophthalmic Pathology: An Atlas and Textbook*, vol. 4. Philadelphia, PA: WB Saunders, 1996:2935–3044.

Naumann GOH, Naumann LR. Intraocular inflammations. In: Naumann GOH, Apple DJ, eds. *Pathology of the Eye*. New York, NY: Springer-Verlag, 1986:99–184.

Ormerod LD, Margo CE. Changing patterns of ocular infectious disease. In: Grossniklaus HE, Margo CE, eds. *Advances in Ophthalmic Pathology. Ophthalmol Clin North Am* 1995;8:109–124.

Pepose JS, Holland GN, Wilhelmus KR, eds. *Ocular Infection and Immunity*. St. Louis, MO: CV Mosby, 1996.

Proia AD. Inflammation. In: Garner A, Klintworth GK, eds. *Pathobiology of Ocular Disease. A Dynamic Approach*. New York, NY: Marcel Dekker, 1994:63–100.

Roitt I, ed. *Essential Immunology*. Oxford, UK: Blackwell Scientific Publications, 1988.

Inflammatory Mediators

Albelda SM, Buck CA. Integrins and other cell adhesion molecules. *FASEB J* 1990;4:2868–2880.

Albelda SM, Smith CW, Ward PA. Adhesion molecules and inflammatory injury. *FASEB J* 1994;8:504–512.

Arai KI, Lee F, Miyajima A, et al. Cytokines: coordinators of immune and inflammatory responses. *Annu Rev Biochem* 1990;59:783–836.

Cochrane CG, Gimbrone MA Jr, eds. *Cellular and Molecular Mechanisms of Inflammation. Vascular Adhesion Molecules*. San Diego, CA: Academic Press, 1991:1–181.

Cochrane CG, Gimbrone MA Jr, eds. *Cellular and Molecular Mechanisms of Inflammation. Signal Transduction in Inflammatory Cells, Part A*. San Diego, CA: Academic Press, 1992:1–195.

Dinarello CA. Biology of interleukin 1. *FASEB J* 1988;2:108–115.

Harlan JM, Liu DY, eds. *Adhesion. Its Role in Inflammatory Disease*. New York, NY: WH Freeman & Company, 1992:1–202.

Kunkel SL, Remick DG, eds. *Cytokines in Health and Disease*. New York, NY: Marcel Dekker, 1992:1–568.

Le J, Vilcek J. Tumor necrosis factor and interleukin 1: cytokines with multiple overlapping biological activities. *Lab Invest* 1987;56:234–248.

Movat HZ. Tumor necrosis factor and interleukin-1: role in acute inflammation and microvascular injury. *J Lab Clin Med* 1987;110:668–681.

Inflammatory Cells

Adams DO, Hamilton TA. The activated macrophage and granulomatous inflammation. *Curr Top Pathol* 1989;79:151–167.

Becker EL. Leukocyte stimulation: receptor, membrane, and metabolic events. Introduction and summary. *Fed Proc* 1986;45:2148–2150.

Cochrane CG. Mechanisms coupling stimulation and function in leukocytes. Introduction. *Fed Proc* 1984;43:2729–2731.

Elsbach P, Weiss J. Oxygen-dependent and oxygen-independent mechanisms of microbicidal activity of neutrophils. *Immunol Lett* 1985;11:159–163.

Fantone JC, Ward PA. Role of oxygen-derived free radicals and metabolites in leukocyte-dependent inflammatory reactions. *Am J Pathol* 1982;107:395–418.

Johnston RB Jr. Current concepts: immunology. Monocytes and macrophages. *N Engl J Med* 1988;318:747–752.

Kay AB. The eosinophilic leukocyte. In: Dale MM, Foreman JC, eds. *Textbook of Immunopharmacology*. Oxford, UK: Blackwell Scientific Publications, 1989:68–76.

Lewis CE, McGee GOD, eds. *The Natural Immune System. The Macrophage*. Oxford, UK: IRL Press at Oxford University Press, 1992.

Thomas R, Lipsky PE. Monocytes and macrophages. In: Kelley WN, Harris ED Jr, Ruddy S, et al., eds. *Textbook of Rheumatology*, 4th ed. Philadelphia, PA: WB Saunders, 1993:286–303.

van Furth R. Development and distribution of mononuclear phagocytes. In: Gallin JI, Goldstein IM, Snyderman R, eds. *Inflammation. Basic Principles and Clinical Correlates*. New York, NY: Raven Press, 1992:325–340.

Weiss SJ, LoBuglio AF. Phagocyte-generated oxygen metabolites and cellular injury. *Lab Invest* 1982;47:5–18.

Weller PF. The immunobiology of eosinophils. *N Engl J Med* 1991;374:1110–1118.

Granulomatous Inflammation

Boros DL. Granulomatous inflammation. In: Zembala M, Asherson GL, eds. *Human Monocytes*. San Diego, CA: Academic Press, 1989:313–381.

Ferry AP. The histopathology of rheumatoid episcleral nodules: an extra-articular manifestation of rheumatoid arthritis. *Arch Ophthalmol* 1969;82:77–88.

Font RL, Fine BS, Messmer E, et al. Light and electron microscopic study of Dalen-Fuchs nodules in sympathetic ophthalmia. *Ophthalmology* 1982;90:66–75.

Jakobiec FA, Marboe CC, Knowles DM II, et al. Human Sympathetic ophthalmia. An analysis of the inflammatory infiltrate by hybridoma-monoclonal antibodies, immunochemistry, and correlative electron microscopy. *Ophthalmology* 1983;90:76–95.

Lubin JR, Albert DM, Weinstein M. Sixty-five years of sympathetic ophthalmia. A clinicopathologic review of 105 cases (1913–1978). *Ophthalmology* 1980;87:109–121.

Marak GE. Phacoanaphylactic Endophthalmitis. *Surv Ophthalmol* 1992;36:325–329.

Obenauf CD, Shaw HE, Wyndor CF, et al. Sarcoidosis and its ocular manifestations. *Am J Ophthalmol* 1978;86:648–655.

Rao NA, Marak GE, Hidayat AA. Necrotizing scleritis. A clinicopathologic study of 41 cases. *Ophthalmology* 1985;92:1542–1549.

To KW, Jakobiec FA, Zimmerman LE. Sympathetic uveitis. In: Albert DM, Jakobiec FA, eds. *Principles and Practice of Ophthalmology: Clinical Practice*, vol. 1. Philadelphia, PA: WB Saunders, 1994:496–503.

Bacterial Endophthalmitis

Allen HF, Mangiaracine AB. Bacterial endophthalmitis after cataract surgery. *Arch Ophthalmol* 1974;91:3–7.

Jensen AD, Naidoff MA. Bilateral meningococcal endophthalmitis. *Arch Ophthalmol* 1973;90:396–398.

Meisler DM, Mandelbaum S. Propionibacterium-associated endophthalmitis after extracapsular cataract extraction: review of reported cases. *Ophthalmology* 1989;96:54–61.

Meisler DM, Palestine AG, Vastein DW, et al. Chronic Propionibacterium endophthalmitis after extracapsular cataract extraction and intraocular lens implantation. *Am J Ophthalmol* 1986;102:733–739.

O'Brien TP, Green WR. Endophthalmitis. In: Mandell GL, Douglas RG Jr, Bennett JE, eds. *Principles and Practice of Infectious Diseases*, 4th ed. New York, NY: Churchill Livingstone, 1993.

Piest KL, Kincaid MC, Tetz MR, et al. Localized endophthalmitis: A newly described cause of the so-called toxic lens syndrome. *J Cataract Refract Surg* 1987;13:498–510.

Shammas HF. Endogenous E. coli endophthalmitis. *Surv Ophthalmol* 1977;21:428–435.

Fungal Endophthalmitis

Abbott RL, Forster RK, Rebell G. Listeria monocytogenes endophthalmitis with a black hypopyon. *Am J Ophthalmol* 1978;86:715–719.

Brod RD, Clarkson JG, Flynn HM Jr, et al. Endogenous fungal endophthalmitis. In: Tasman W, Jaeger EA, eds. *Duane's Clinical Ophthalmology*. New York, NY: Harper & Row, 1990:1–39.

Caya JG, Farmer SG, Williams GA, et al. Bilateral *Pseudallescheria boydii* endophthalmitis in an immunocompromised patient. *Wis Med J* 1988;87:11–14.

Chen CJ. Nocardia asteroides endophthalmitis. *Ophthalmic Surg* 1983;14:502–505.

Demicco DD, Reichman RC, Violette EJ, et al. Disseminated aspergillosis presenting with endophthalmitis. A case report and a review of the literature. *Cancer* 1984;53:1995–2001.

Edwards JE Jr, Foos RY, Montgomerie JA, et al. Ocular manifestations of Candida septicemia: review of 76 cases of hematogenous *Candida endophthalmitis*. *Medicine* 1974;53:47–75.

Ferry AP, Font RL, Weinberg RS, et al. Nocardial endophthalmitis: report of two cases studied histopathologically. *Br J Ophthalmol* 1988;72:55–61.

Fine BS, Zimmerman LE. Exogenous intraocular fungus infections with particular reference to complications of intraocular surgery. *Am J Ophthalmol* 1959;48:151–165.

Gregor RJ, Chong CA, Augsburger JJ, et al. Endogenous *Nocardia asteroides* subretinal abcess diagnosed by transvitreal fine-needle aspiration biopsy. *Retina* 1989;9:118–121.

Ho PC, Tolentino FI, Baker AS. Successful treatment of exogenous *Aspergillus endophthalmitis*: a case report. *Br J Ophthalmol* 1984;68:412–415.

McGuire TW, Bullock JD, Bullock JD Jr, et al. Fungal endophthalmitis. An experimental study with a review of 17 human ocular cases. *Arch Ophthalmol* 1991;109:1289–1296.

Michelson PE, Stark WJ, Reeser F, et al. Endogenous *Candida endophthalmitis*. Report of 13 cases and 16 from the literature. *Int Ophthalmol Clin* 1971;11:125–147.

O'Brien TP, Green WR. Fungus infections of the eye and periocular tissues. In: Garner A, Klintworth GK, eds. *Pathology of Ocular Disease. A Dynamic Approach*, 2nd ed. New York, NY: Marcel Dekker, 1993.

Weishaar PD, Flynn HW Jr, Murray TG, et al. Endogenous aspergillus endophthalmitis. Clinical features and treatment outcomes. *Ophthalmology* 1998;105:57–65.

Wong KW, Tasman W, Eagle RC Jr, et al. Bilateral *Candida parapsilosis* endophthalmitis. *Arch Ophthalmol* 1997;115:670–672.

HIV/AIDS

Pepose JS, Holland GN, Nestor MS, et al. Acquired immune deficiency syndrome: pathogenic mechanisms of ocular disease. *Ophthalmology* 1985;92:472–484.

Rajeev B, Rao NA. Advances in ocular pathology in AIDS. In: Grossniklaus HE, Margo CE, eds. *Advances in Ophthalmic Pathology*. *Ophthalmol Clin North Am* 1995;8:125–141.

Rao NA, Zimmerman PL, Boyer D, et al. A clinical, histopathologic, and electron microscopic study of *Pneumocystis carinii* choroiditis. *Am J Ophthalmol* 1989;107:218–228.

Viral Retinitis

Culbertson WW, Blumenkranz MS, Haines H, et al. The acute retinal necrosis syndrome. 2. Histopathology and etiology. *Ophthalmology* 1982;89:1317–1325.

Duker JS, Blumenkranz MS. Diagnosis and management of the acute retinal necrosis (ARN) syndrome. *Surv Ophthalmol* 1991;35:327–343.

Fisher JP, Lewis ML, Blumenkranz M, et al. The acute retinal necrosis syndrome. 1. Clinical manifestations. *Ophthalmology* 1982;89:1309–1316.

Font RL, Jenis EH, Tuck KO. Measles maculopathy associated with subacute sclerosing panencephalitis. *Arch Pathol* 1973;96:168–174.

Holland GN. The progressive outer retinal necrosis syndrome. *Int Ophthalmol* 1994;18:163–165.

Murray HW, Knox DL, Green WR, et al. Cytomegalovirus retinitis in adults: a manifestation of disseminated viral infection. *Am J Med* 1977;63: 574–584.

Pavesio CE, Mitchell SM, Barton K, et al. Progressive outer retinal necrosis (PORN) in AIDS patients: a different appearance of varicella-zoster retinitis. *Eye* 1995;9:271–276.

Pepose JS, Holland GN. Cytomegalovirus infections of the retina. In: Ryan S, ed. *Retina*, 2nd ed., vol. 2. St. Louis, MO: Mosby, 1994:1559–1570.

Uveitis

Bell R, Font RL. Granulomatous anterior uveitis caused by Coccidioides immitis. *Am J Ophthalmol* 1972;74:93–98.

Inomata H, Kohno T, Rao NA, et al. Vasculitis and intraocular neovascularization in Behçet's disease: histopathology of the early and advanced late stages. In: Dernouchamps JP, Verougstraete C, Caspers-Velu L, et al., eds. *Proceedings of the Third International Symposium on Uveitis. Brussels, Belgium, May 24–27, 1992*. New York, NY: Kugler Publications, 1993:349–355.

Knox DL. Uveitis associated with systemic disease. In: Albert DM, Jakobiec FA, eds. *Principles and Practice of Ophthalmology: Clinical Practice*, vol. 1. Philadelphia, PA: WB Saunders, 1994:465–474.

Mullaney J, Collum LM. Ocular vasculitis in Behçet's disease. A pathological and immunohistochemical study. *Int Ophthalmol* 1985;7:183–191.

O'Brien JM, Albert DM, Foster CS. Anterior uveitis. In: Albert DM, Jakobiec FA, eds. *Principles and Practice of Ophthalmology: Clinical Practice*, vol. 3. Philadelphia, PA: WB Saunders, 1994:1745–1770.

Park SS, To KW, Friedman AH, et al. Infectious causes of posterior uveitis. In: Albert DM, Jakobiec FA, eds. *Principles and Practice of Ophthalmology: Clinical Practice*, vol. 1. Philadelphia, PA: WB Saunders, 1994:450–464.

Parasitic Infection

Anderson J, Font RL. Ocular onchocerciasis. In: Binford CH, Connor DH, eds. *Pathology of Tropical and Extraordinary Diseases*, vol. II. Washington, DC: Armed Forces Institute of Pathology, 1976:360.

Gagliuso DJ, Teich SA, Freidman AH, et al. Ocular toxoplasmosis in AIDS patients. *Trans Am Ophthalmol Soc* 1990;88:63–86.

Naumann G, Gunders AE. Pathogenesis of the posterior segment lesion of ocular onchocerciasis. *Am J Ophthalmol* 1973;75:82–89.

O'Connor GR. Manifestations and management of ocular toxoplasmosis. *Bull NY Acad Sci* 1970;174:192–210.

Perkins ES. Ocular toxoplasmosis. *Br J Ophthalmol* 1973;57:1–17.

4 Ocular Trauma

Many eyes that are enucleated have a past history of nonsurgical or surgical trauma. The eye can be totally destroyed by severe injuries that violate the integrity of its protective coats and scatter its contents. Less devastating injuries cause blindness by disrupting the normal anatomical and functional relationships between the eye's highly specialized tissues. Retinal detachment, retinal avulsion anteriorly from the ora serrata or posteriorly from the optic nerve, avulsion of the optic nerve from the globe, iridodialysis or cyclodialysis, lens dislocation, and choroidal rupture are examples. By disrupting pristine anatomical relationships, trauma also exposes new surfaces that cells can proliferate on. These include the inner and outer surfaces of the retina after retinal detachment, the posterior face of the vitreous exposed by vitreous detachment, or anterior chamber structures made accessible to surface epithelium by poorly apposed wounds in the cornea. Cellular proliferation on these newly exposed surfaces leads to permanent adhesions between structures, membrane formation, fibrosis, traction, retinal detachment, and glaucoma. Hemorrhage commonly complicates trauma. The blood opacifies transparent ocular media such as the vitreous and may cause secondary glaucoma by occluding aqueous outflow pathways. In addition, intraocular hemorrhage causes expulsion and irrevocable loss of vital intraocular structures when it accumulates in the suprauveal space and fills the interior of the eye (expulsive choroidal hemorrhage). Blindness also can result when the body's normal mechanisms of regeneration and repair cause scarring that affects highly differentiated transparent tissues or when fibrous membranes exert traction on vital structures. For example, the fibrous organization of tracts of hemorrhage in the vitreous left by perforating missiles ultimately can cause tractional retinal detachment. Trauma also predisposes to infection by destroying the eye's normal protective barriers. Infection is always a danger after ocular trauma, even minor injuries such as corneal abrasions. Organisms introduced by penetrating injuries or contaminated intraocular foreign bodies of metallic, vegetable, or even endogenous animal (e.g., hair, skin) composition can cause exogenous endophthalmitis.

The terms penetrating and perforating are commonly applied to ocular injuries that produce defects in the integrity of the ocular coats. A penetrating injury partially cuts or tears a structure. A perforation is a through-and-through injury that completely cuts or tears through a structure (Fig. 4-1). To use these terms properly, one must specify the structure that is involved. For example, a corneal laceration is both a perforating injury of the cornea and a penetrating injury of the globe. Most corneal foreign bodies produce a small penetrating injury in the anterior stroma

that is filled by the corneal epithelium forming an epithelial facette (Fig. 4-2A).

The ophthalmic pathology laboratory frequently processes eyes that have been ruptured by severe blunt trauma, have severe corneoscleral lacerations caused by sharp objects, or have been perforated by missiles such as BBs (Fig. 4-3). Pathologic examination of some severely traumatized eyes reveals a disrupted scleral shell filled with blood and scant remnants of intraocular tissue. Most cases show intraocular hemorrhage and loss or incarceration of intraocular structures. Massive intraocular hemorrhage typically involves the vitreous, and subretinal and suprauveal spaces. Loss of intraocular contents is caused by the space-occupying effect of expanding suprauveal hemorrhage and compression of the eye by the surrounding orbital tissue and forceful eyelid closure. Both mechanisms elevate the intraocular pressure (IOP) and expel the intraocular tissues through the open wound. Tissues that frequently are lost or incarcerated in the wound include the iris, lens, ciliary body, vitreous, and

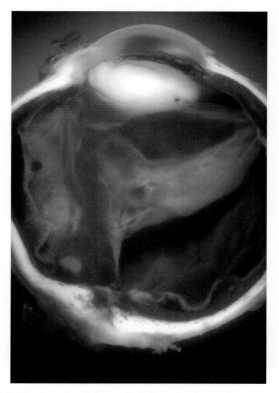

Fig. 4-1. Perforating injury of globe. Ocular perforation caused by BB gun is a through-and-through injury with entrance and exit wounds in limbus and sclera, respectively. The track of the BB is marked by fresh blood. Posteriorly detached vitreous also contains ochre-colored degenerated blood.

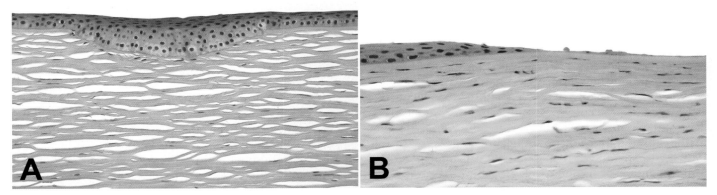

Fig. 4-2. A. Epithelial facette, cornea. The epithelium fills crater in Bowman membrane and anterior stroma caused by corneal foreign body. **B. Corneal abrasion.** The sliding epithelium healing the corneal abrasion has tapering margin. (**A.** Hematoxylin-eosin [H&E] ×100, **B.** H&E ×100.)

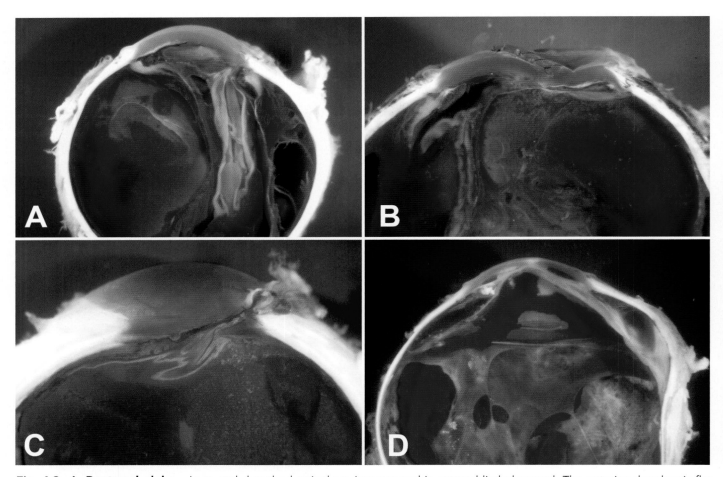

Fig. 4-3. A. Ruptured globe. Lens and detached retinal are incarcerated in sutured limbal wound. The anterior chamber is flat and part of the iris is absent. A massive suprauveal hemorrhage fills half of the posterior segment. **B. Corneal laceration.** A sutured laceration is present in the central cornea. The lens and half of the iris are absent, and the detached retina is drawn toward the wound. Most of the blood filling the interior of the eye is located in the suprauveal space. **C. Uveal and retinal incarceration in limbal wound.** Pigmented uveal tissue and orange band of detached retina extend extraocularly through scleral wound. Degenerated blood fills the interior of the globe. **D. Old ruptured globe.** Organized vitreous is incarcerated in the central corneal scar. Anterior uvea and lens are absent.

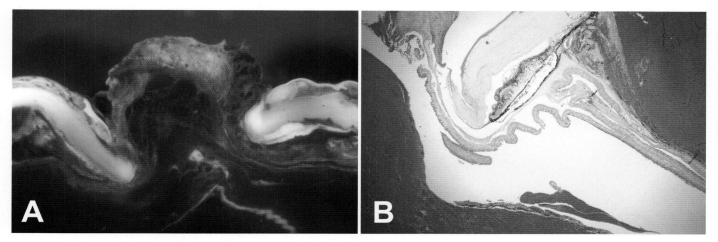

Fig. 4-4. Spontaneous expulsive hemorrhage. **A.** A knuckle of uveal tissue is expelled extraocularly through lips of gaping perforation in the infected cornea by massive suprauveal hemorrhage. A hypopyon fills the residual anterior chamber. **B.** Detached retina and hemorrhagic detachment of choroid extend extraocularly through perforation in infected cornea. Blood detaches the ciliary body at right. Neovascular glaucoma predisposed to acute keratitis and corneal perforation. (H&E ×5.)

occasionally the retina and choroid. Prolapsed intraocular tissue excised during the repair of corneoscleral lacerations should always be submitted for pathologic examination. If retina is found, the prognosis is poor.

Expulsive choroidal hemorrhage caused by an expanding suprauveal hematoma is a dreaded complication of ocular surgery. Intraoperative rupture of a sclerotic arteriole caused by the sudden hypotony of surgery causes the expanding hemorrhage in the suprachoroidal space. Spontaneous expulsive choroidal hemorrhage can also complicate corneal perforation in glaucomatous eyes (Fig. 4-4).

SYMPATHETIC UVEITIS (SYMPATHETIC OPHTHALMIA)

Expedient enucleation of eyes that are severely traumatized and hopelessly blind is strongly advised as prophylaxis against a rare autoimmune disorder called sympathetic uveitis, which affects and potentially can blind *both* eyes after unilateral trauma. Sympathetic uveitis (ophthalmia) is a severe bilateral granulomatous inflammation of the uveal tract that follows unilateral trauma or surgery, which usually is complicated by the incarceration of uveal tissue in the wound (Fig. 4-5). Blurred vision, photophobia, and signs of granulomatous inflammation develop in the uninjured or *sympathizing* eye simultaneous with exacerbation of signs and symptoms in the injured or *exciting* eye.

Sympathetic uveitis is thought to be a T-cell–mediated autoimmune response to uveal or retinal antigens released by the injury. Uveal pigment, retinal S antigen, and interphotoreceptor retinoid–binding protein could be possible antigens. Sympathetic uveitis occurs between 2 weeks and 1 year postinjury in about 90% of cases, most cases occurring during the 3-week to 3-month interval. Sympathetic uveitis generally will not develop if the injured eye is enucleated within 1 week of the injury. If enucleation of the

injured eye is delayed, the noninjured eye still remains at risk. There is some evidence that enucleation of the inciting eye decreases the severity of the inflammation in the sympathizing eye after bilateral uveitis develops. Rare cases of sympathetic uveitis have been reported after ocular evisceration. These probably are related to antigenic material left behind in scleral emissarial canals, which typically are involved by granulomatous inflammation.

Sympathetic uveitis is a clinicopathologic diagnosis. There must be a history of unilateral trauma followed by bilateral uveitis. Four characteristic features are found on histopathologic examination. The uvea is thickened by a diffuse granulomatous infiltrate composed of epithelioid histiocytes, inflammatory giant cells, and lymphocytes of the T-suppressor/cytotoxic subtype (Fig. 4-5A). The choriocapillaris is not destroyed by the inflammation (sparing of the choriocapillaris) (Fig. 4-5B). The epithelioid histiocytes and giant cells usually contain granules of phagocytized uveal pigment (Fig. 4-5D). Nodular aggregates of epithelioid cells, which focally detach the retinal pigment epithelium (RPE), are found on the inner surface of Bruch membrane (Fig. 4-5C). These Dalen-Fuchs nodules are not pathognomonic for sympathetic uveitis because they also occur in sarcoidosis and Vogt-Koyanagi-Harada disease. The uveal infiltrate rarely contains plasma cells. Eosinophilia may be found in deeply pigmented patients, in whom the inflammation typically is more severe. Sympathetic uveitis usually spares the retina. One should consider another diagnosis if retinal involvement is found distant from the site of injury. Although their immunopathogenic mechanisms differ, both sympathetic ophthalmia and phacoantigenic uveitis may occur concurrently in the same traumatized eye. Atypical histopathologic features occur in some cases, generally are associated with severe choroidal inflammation, and may be a response to high doses of antigenic material. Progressive subretinal fibrosis with multifocal granulomatous chorioretinitis is thought to be a variant of sympathetic ophthalmia.

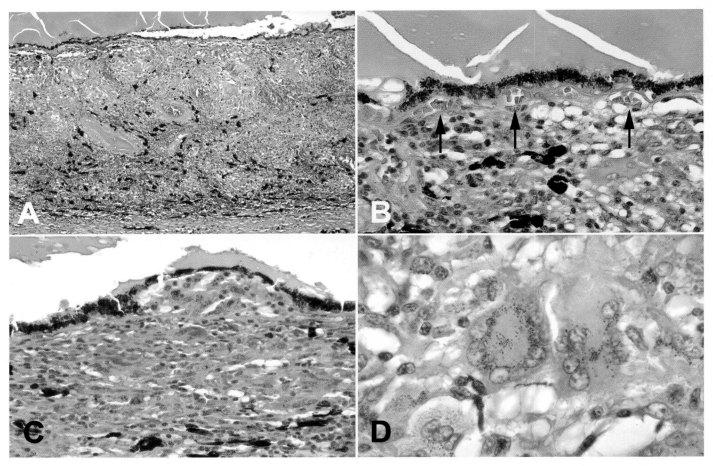

Fig. 4-5. Sympathetic uveitis. A. The choroid is massively thickened by a diffuse granulomatous infiltrate of epithelioid histiocytes, giant cells, and lymphocytes. **B.** Sparing of the choriocapillaris. *Arrows* denote persistent choriocapillaris beneath Bruch membrane and the RPE. **C. Dalen-Fuchs nodule, sympathetic uveitis.** Aggregate of epithelioid histiocytes on the inner surface of Bruch membrane focally detaches RPE. Underlying choroid contains diffuse granulomatous inflammatory infiltrate rich in epithelioid histiocytes. **D.** Giant cells in choroidal infiltrate contain granules of melanin pigment. (**A.** H&E ×25, **B.** H&E ×100, **C.** H&E ×100, **D.** H&E ×250.)

CONTUSION INJURIES

Minor contusion injuries often cause abrasions of the corneal epithelium that rapidly heal by epithelial sliding (Fig. 4-2B). Severe contusion injuries can rupture the cornea and/or sclera. A rupture caused by blunt trauma can occur directly at the site of impact. In other instances, the thinnest parts of the globe such as the limbus, or the scleral behind the insertion of the rectus muscles or adjacent to the optic nerve, are involved indirectly by force vectors transmitted by the essentially incompressible globe.

Contusion injuries need not disrupt the integrity of the cornea or sclera to wreak severe intraocular havoc. Ocular contusion injuries can rupture Descemet membrane, the lens, or choroid; detach or avulse the retina from its attachments to the ora serrata (Fig. 4-6) or optic nerve; or fracture photoreceptor outer segments causing Berlin edema or commotio retinae. Late cystoid macular degeneration or macular holes are common sequelae. Other anterior segment complications include lens dislocation, contusion rosette cataract (Fig. 4-7A), postcontusion angle recession, iridodialysis, cyclodialysis, and hyphema.

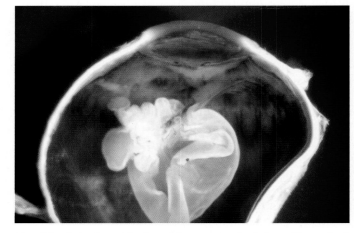

Fig. 4-6. Anterior retinal avulsion, contusion injury. The retina's attachments to the ora serrata have been disrupted. A hyphema fills the anterior chamber.

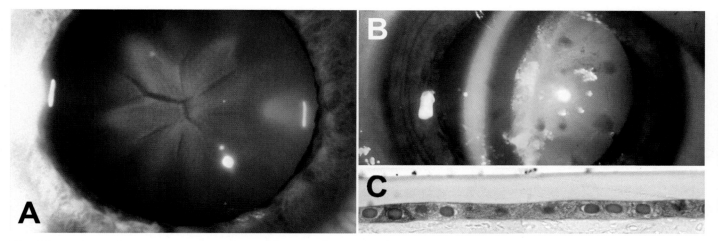

Fig. 4-7. A. Contusion rosette cataract. Petalliform configuration of traumatic cataract reflects damage to superficial lens fibers. This type of cataract serves as a clinical marker for ocular contusion injury. **B. Siderotic cataract.** Iron from intraocular foreign body has formed rusty deposits beneath the anterior capsule of cataractous lens. **C.** Prussian blue reaction highlights iron in the lens epithelium. (**C.** Iron stain ×100.)

Blood staining of the corneal stroma is a potential complication of chronic hyphema (Fig. 4-8). Whether corneal blood staining develops or not depends on the health of the corneal endothelium, the IOP, and the duration of the hyphema. Blood staining may occur within 48 hours if the IOP is high. The corneal stroma contains small particles of hemoglobin, not intact erythrocytes. Golden-brown granules of hemosiderin are found in the cytoplasm of the keratocytes.

During a contusion injury of the anterior segment, the lens and iris act together as a ball valve that confines the aqueous humor to the anterior chamber. The incompressible aqueous humor conveys the force of the blow to the weakest parts of the anatomy, which are subject to damage (Fig. 4-9). The iris may be ripped from the ciliary body at its root where it is very thin (iridodialysis). In other cases, the tenuous attachment of the ciliary muscle to the scleral spur is disrupted, causing detachment of the ciliary body or **cyclodialysis** (Fig. 4-9D).

Tears into the anterior face of the ciliary body cause **postcontusion angle recession** (Fig. 4-9A–C). The tear usually extends between the external longitudinal fibers of the ciliary muscle and its radial and circumferential fibers, which are located centrally (Fig. 4-9A). The injury usually detaches the inner uveal part of the trabecular meshwork and disrupts the greater arterial circle of the iris causing anterior chamber hemorrhage (hyphema). The root of the iris is displaced posteriorly by the tear. Afterwards, gonioscopy discloses widening of the ciliary body band. Microscopic examination of acutely traumatized eyes often reveals ischemic necrosis of the iris and ciliary body. In chronic cases, the residual ciliary muscle typically has a fusiform configuration reflecting ischemic atrophy of its inner parts.

Postcontusion angle recession can cause late-onset unilateral open-angle glaucoma. When they are stable, patients who have had hyphemas always should be gonioscoped to exclude traumatic angle recession. Less than 10% of patients who have postcontusion angle recession actually develop glaucoma. Microscopic examination of blind glaucomatous eyes with recessed angles that are enucleated typically reveals a new layer of Descemet membrane on the inner surface of the damaged trabecular meshwork.

INTRAOCULAR FOREIGN BODIES

Fragments of foreign material often are left inside the eye during perforating injuries (Fig. 4-10). How well the eye tolerates an intraocular foreign body depends on the chemical composition of the foreign material and whether it is sterile or contaminated with microorganisms. Foreign bodies composed of vegetable matter are often contaminated with fungi and typically cause a violent inflammatory response.

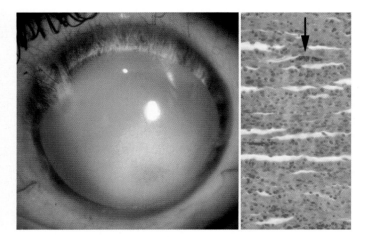

Fig. 4-8. Corneal blood staining. Central cornea is opacified by ochre deposit. Histopathology of corneal stroma discloses small particles of hemoglobin that are much smaller than intact erythrocytes. One of the keratocytes contains granules of golden-brown hemosiderin pigment (*arrow*). (**Right panel,** H&E ×250.)

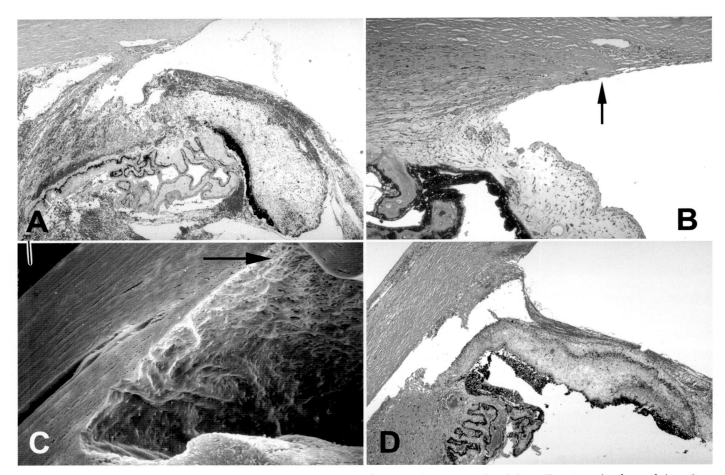

Fig. 4-9. Contusion injuries, anterior segment. A. Acute angle recession, contusion injury. Tear into the face of the ciliary body is located internal to the longitudinal part of the ciliary muscle, which remains attached to the scleral spur. A layer of blood rests on the anterior surface of the iris, which shows early necrosis. **B. Postcontusion angle recession.** The iris root is displaced posteriorly, markedly widening the ciliary body band. *Arrow* points to scleral spur. The ciliary processes are displaced posteriorly and the residual ciliary muscle has a fusiform configuration. Incidental pseudoexfoliation is present. **C. Postcontusion angle recession.** *Arrow* in SEM denotes trabecular meshwork. The iris root is displaced posteriorly, widening the ciliary body band. The ciliary muscle is fusiform in shape. **D. Cyclodialysis, contusion injury.** The ciliary body has been avulsed from its attachment to the scleral spur. The iris shows early necrosis. A hyphema is present. (**A.** H&E ×25, **B.** H&E ×50, **C.** SEM ×40, **D.** H&E ×25.)

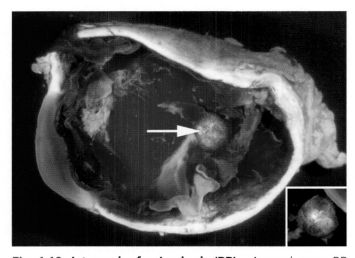

Fig. 4-10. Intraocular foreign body (BB). *Arrow* denotes BB surrounded by blood and disrupted retina and choroid in disorganized interior of the ruptured globe. Pars plana entrance wound is seen at top left. **Inset** shows foreign body.

In contrast, foreign bodies of glass and plastic usually are inert and are well tolerated. Iron foreign bodies, which are relatively common, have a toxic effect on the retina, lens epithelium, and aqueous outflow pathways if they are chronically retained. Ferrous iron is more toxic than ferric iron. Ocular **siderosis** is marked by the deposition of iron in epithelial or neuroectodermal derivatives (epithelia of cornea, lens, and ciliary body, iris musculature, retina, and RPE) (Figs. 4-7B and 4-11). An identical deposition of hematogenous iron (hemosiderosis) can complicate repeated chronic intraocular hemorrhage (Fig. 4-12A). Foreign bodies comprised of >90% copper incite a severe sterile purulent reaction, while retained fragments of brass or bronze that contain 70% to 90% copper cause deposition in Descemet membrane and the lens capsule (**chalcosis**) (Fig. 4-12B). An analogous deposition of copper occurs in these thick basement membranes in Wilson hepatolenticular degeneration and is responsible for the characteristic Kayser-Fleischer ring and sunflower cataract.

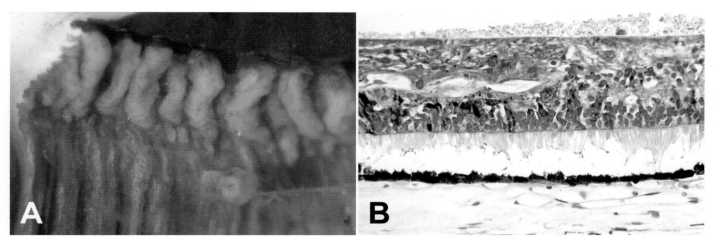

Fig. 4-11. Siderosis. A. Ciliary processes in the eye with chronically retained intraocular iron foreign body show rusty discoloration. **B.** Intense Prussian blue reaction discloses iron in neurosensory retina and RPE. **(B.** Iron Stain ×100.)

CHEMICAL INJURIES

Chemical injuries by strong acid and alkali usually involve the anterior part of the eye. The severity of the injury usually depends on the nature and strength of the agent and the duration of contact. Acid burns are nonprogressive and generally are less severe than alkali burns because penetration is limited by a buffering action of the tissues. Histology usually shows superficial coagulative necrosis of the conjunctival and/or corneal epithelium. In contrast, alkali penetrates deeply causing denaturation of protein, saponification of fat, and necrosis of intraocular structures (Fig. 4-13). Alkali injuries usually are progressive because the alkali is difficult to neutralize and the necrosis of stromal fibroblasts precludes replacement or repair of denatured corneal collagen. In addition, vascular occlusion caused by necrosis of the vascular endothelium produces tissue ischemia. A white porcelain appearance of the conjunctiva after an alkali burn is a clinical sign of severe ischemia and an indicator of poor prognosis. Collagenase made by polymorphonuclear leukocytes infiltrating the necrotic stroma contributes to corneal dissolution and ulceration.

WOUND HEALING

Many complications that occur after ocular surgery are related to poor wound healing. Ocular wounds heal by the formation of scar tissue. The mechanisms involved in wound healing differ depending on what ocular tissue is involved.

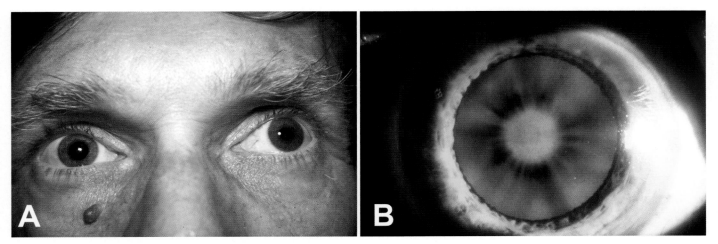

Fig. 4-12. A. Heterochromia iridum, hemosiderosis. Iris of blind, exotropic left eye shows *greenish* discoloration caused by iron deposition. Chronic vitreous hemorrhage caused ocular hemosiderosis. **B. Chalcosis lentis.** Sunflower cataract caused by copper deposition in lens capsule developed in eye with intraocular foreign body composed of copper alloy. The central disc of the "sunflower" corresponds to the diameter of the undilated pupil and the petals to radial ridges in the iris pigment epithelium. (Courtesy of Prof. Dr. med. Wolfgang Lieb, University of Würzburg, from Eagle RC Jr. Congenital, developmental and degenerative disorders of the iris and ciliary body. In: Albert DM, Jakobiec FA, eds. *Principles and Practice of Ophthalmology. Clinical Practice.* vol. 1. Philadelphia, PA: Saunders, 1993:367–389.)

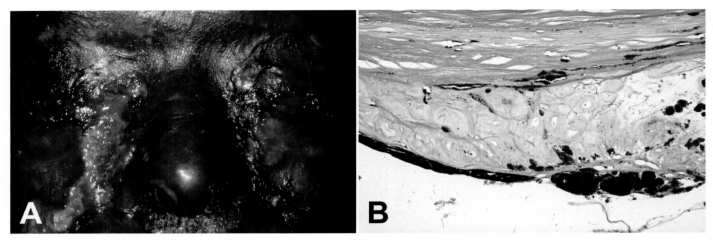

Fig. 4-13. Alkali injury. A. The patient was blinded by strong alkali drain cleaner poured on his eyes while asleep. **B.** Alkali has penetrated deep into the eye causing total necrosis of the iris, which adheres to the posterior surface of the cornea. Necrotic iris and cornea appear acellular. (**B.** H&E ×50.)

The healing of limbal wounds involves a proliferation of granulation tissue derived from the episclera and the substantia propria of the conjunctiva. Epithelial migration and an early proliferation of granulation tissue rapidly seal the superficial aspect of well-apposed wounds, and a plug of fibrin, which polymerizes on the exposed collagen in the wound, prevents the leakage of aqueous humor. The posterior wound gapes slightly and elastic Descemet membrane curves inwardly. Granulation tissue enters the external part of the wound at about 8 days and has extended the full length of the wound by 2 weeks. By this time, migrating endothelial cells have covered the posterior wound. These cells eventually will synthesize a new layer of Descemet membrane. The fibroblastic component of the granulation tissue produces collagen, which is initially randomly arranged. As the scar matures and becomes less vascularized, collagen is progressively produced, and the fibers mature and undergo reorientation.

Unlike the limbus, the central cornea is an avascular site. Hence, granulation tissue is not involved in the healing of central corneal wounds (Fig. 4-14). Initially, the lips of the wound swell, functionally sealing the wound, which gapes anteriorly and posteriorly. A fibrin plug forms and Descemet membrane retracts and curves inwardly. Neighboring corneal endothelial cells are lost. The anterior surface of the wound is reepithelialized by surface epithelial sliding, which enters the gaping anterior part of the wound and fills it with an epithelial plug. The anterior surface of the wound usually is reepithelialized by 12 hours. Three or four days following an injury, stromal fibroblasts enter

Fig. 4-14. Scar of corneal laceration. Periodic acid-Schiff (PAS) stain **(at right)** highlights gap in Descemet membrane in scar of well-healed and fairly well-approximated corneal laceration. (**A.** H&E ×50; **B.** PAS, ×50.)

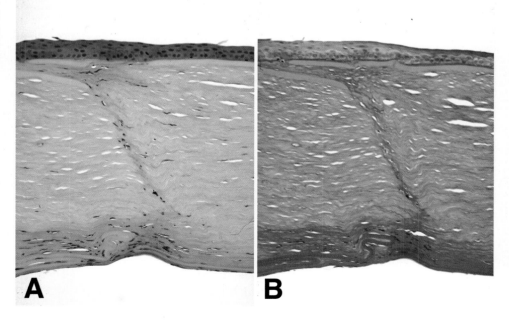

the wound and begin to elaborate collagen. The plug of surface epithelium regresses as stromal wound healing proceeds, and regression generally is complete by 2 weeks. By that time, the sliding endothelium has extended across the posterior defect and has begun to lay down a new layer of Descemet membrane. During the next 6 months, the cellularity of the scarred area gradually decreases and the character and orientation of the collagen becomes more regular.

Unsutured wounds of the iris do not heal. Iridectomies remain patent unless they are closed by pigment epithelial migration. Most wounds in the lens lead to cataract formation. Small rents in the capsule may be closed by posterior synechiae and be repaired by fibrous metaplasia of lens epithelium and capsular reformation. The sclera itself does not participate in the healing of defects. Full-thickness scleral wounds heal by an ingrowth of granulation tissue from both the episclera and the superficial choroid.

Retinal cells do not regenerate. Retinal scars are produced by glial cells, not fibroblasts. The internal limiting membrane and Bruch membrane provide architectural planes for glial scarring. RPE cells may contribute to the retinal scars.

SURGICAL COMPLICATIONS

Poorly apposed or poorly healed limbal surgical wounds cause a variety of postoperative complications. Leaky wounds cause hypotony, serous choroidal detachments, and loss and flattening of the anterior chamber, which can lead to secondary angle closure or corneal endothelial damage as a result of lens corneal touch. Poorly healed wounds also allow microorganisms to enter the interior of the eye and can provide an avenue for surface epithelial invasion of the anterior chamber. Incarceration of uvea or vitreous in wounds can contribute to permanent fistula formation

(vitreous wick) and increase the chance of postoperative infection or epithelial downgrowth.

Epithelial downgrowth (ingrowth) is a devastating complication of surgical or nonsurgical trauma in which corneal or conjunctival epithelium gains access to the anterior chamber and proliferates on the back of the cornea, the trabecular meshwork, the anterior surface of the iris, and even more posteriorly located structures (Fig. 4-15A). Most cases occur after cataract surgery or penetrating keratoplasty. Patients typically present with a translucent sheet of epithelial cells that slowly grows down the back surface of the cornea. In occasional instances where posterior corneal epithelization is not obvious, epithelial downgrowth may present several months postoperatively with pain, glaucoma, and intensifying inflammatory signs. Several mechanisms can obstruct aqueous outflow in eyes with epithelial downgrowth. These include sheets of epithelium covering the trabecular meshwork, peripheral anterior synechia formation, and blockage of the trabecular meshwork by desquamated epithelial cells.

Histopathologically, the intraocular epithelium may approximate the normal surface epithelium in thickness, or it may be markedly attenuated. The advancing edge of the epithelial sheet on the posterior corneal surface typically is prominent. Epithelium growing on vascularized structures such as the iris often is thicker than that on the cornea. The anterior surface of the iris usually is flattened by the epithelial sheet. Occasionally, the epithelium extends through the pupil onto the iris pigment epithelium and ciliary body, and rarely, it may extend onto the inner surface of the peripheral retina causing a tractional retinal detachment.

Clinically, the presence of epithelium on the iris can be confirmed by laser photocoagulation, which causes blanching of the transparent cells. The prognosis of epithelial downgrowth usually is poor. Although some cases can be cured by extensive *en bloc* resection of ocular tissue,

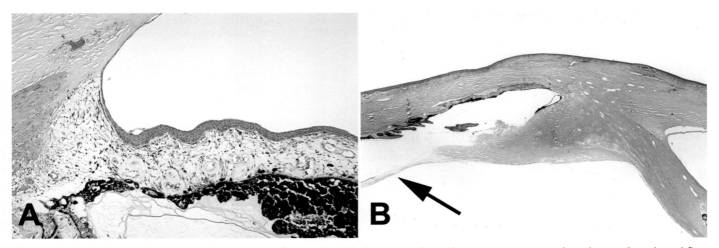

Fig. 4-15. A. Epithelial downgrowth. A sheet of corneal epithelium introduced by trauma covers trabecular meshwork and flattens the anterior iridic surface. **B. Fibrous ingrowth.** Thick membranes of dense collagenous connective tissue have formed on scaffold of vitreous incarcerated in central corneal wound. An extensive anterior synechia is seen at top left. *Arrow* denotes anterior vitreous face. (**A.** H&E ×50, **B.** H&E ×5.)

the intraocular epithelial proliferation is often diffuse, extensive, and impossible to totally eradicate. Experimental studies suggest that a healthy population of corneal endothelial cells tends to retard epithelial migration by means of cellular contact inhibition.

Fibrous ingrowth also complicates poor wound closure, particularly when there has been intraoperative vitreous loss (Fig. 4-15B). Incarcerated vitreous serves as a growth scaffold for fibroblasts, which invade the interior of the eye, produce collagen, and transform the vitreous into a mass of dense fibrous scar tissue.

Fibrous metaplasia of the RPE is another major source of intraocular scarring. RPE hyperplasia and metaplasia typically occur after retinal detachment, which abolishes the outer retina's normal inhibitory effect on RPE proliferation. Papillary proliferation, the formation of large drusen-like structures, and pseudoadenomatous proliferation of the RPE ensue. The RPE synthesizes large quantities of extracellular matrix material, including granular drusenoid material, collagen, and ultimately bone. Massive fibrous and **osseous metaplasia of the RPE** are commonly found in chronically blind phthisical eyes, which often must be decalcified before they can be dissected. The bone always is found on the inner surface of Bruch membrane. The bone is a mature lamellar bone and may contain fatty marrow (Fig. 3-20B).

The term **phthisis bulbi** is applied clinically to blind hypotonous eyes that are soft, shrunken, and partially collapsed and have a vaguely cuboid configuration caused by traction of the four rectus muscles. Pathologically, the diagnosis of phthisis bulbi (atrophia bulbi with shrinkage and disorganization) is reserved for profoundly atrophic globes that have markedly thickened and folded sclera and generally unrecognizable intraocular structures. If the intraocular structures can be identified, the term atrophia bulbi with shrinkage is used.

Superficial absorption of ultraviolet light causes punctate keratopathy (welder's flash, snow blindness). Relatively low doses of ionizing radiation can cause cataract. Radiation-induced occlusion of the retinal capillary bed is the cause of radiation retinopathy.

BIBLIOGRAPHY

Surgical Trauma

Apple DJ, Mamilis N, Loftfield K, et al. Complications of intraocular lenses: a historical and histochemical review. *Surv Ophthalmol* 1984;29:1–54.

Apple DJ, Mamalis N, Olson RJ, et al. *Intraocular Lenses: Evolution, Designs, Complications and Pathology.* Baltimore, MD: Williams & Wilkins, 1989.

Bettman JW Jr. Pathology of complications of intraocular surgery. *Am J Ophthalmol* 1969;68:1037–1050.

Cerasoli JR, Kasner D. A follow-up of vitreous loss during cataract surgery managed by anterior vitrectomy. *Am J Ophthalmol* 1971;71:1040–1043.

Friedman AH, Henkind P. Corneal stromal overgrowth after cataract extraction. *Br J Ophthalmol* 1970;54:528–534.

Gass JDM, Norton EWD. Cystoid macular edema and papilledema following cataract extraction. *Arch Ophthalmol* 1966;76:646–661.

Kohnen T, Koch DD, Font RL. Lensification of the posterior corneal surface. An unusual proliferation of lens epithelial cells. *Ophthalmology* 1997;104:1343–1347.

Kuchle M, Green WR. Epithelial ingrowth: a study of 207 histopathologically proven cases. *Ger J Ophthalmol* 1996;5:211–223.

Magnante DO, Bullock JD, Green WR. Ocular explosion after peribulbar anesthesia: case report and experimental study. *Ophthalmology* 1997;104:608–615.

McDonnel PJ, Patel A, Green WR. Comparison of intracapsular and extracapsular cataract surgery: histopathologic study of eyes obtained postmortem. *Ophthalmology* 1985;92:1208–1225.

Sassani JW, John T, Cameron JD, et al. Electron microscopic study of corneal epithelial endothelial interactions in organ culture. *Ophthalmology* 1984;91:553–557.

Swan KC. Fibroblastic ingrowth following cataract surgery. *Arch Ophthalmol* 1973;89:445–449.

Von Domarius D, Naumann GOH. Accidental and surgical trauma and wound healing of the eye. In: Naumann GOH, Apple DJ, eds. *Pathology of the Eye.* New York, NY: Springer-Verlag, 1986:185–248.

Wiener MJ, Trentacoste J, Pon DM, et al. Epithelial downgrowth: a 30-year clinicopathological review. *Brit J Ophthalmol* 1989;73:6–11.

Williams DK, Rentiers PK. Spontaneous expulsive choroidal hemorrhage. A clinicopathologic report of two cases. *Arch Ophthalmol* 1970;83:191–194.

Winslow RL, Stevenson W III, Yanoff M. Spontaneous expulsive hemorrhage. *Arch Ophthalmol* 1974;92:33–36.

Wolter JR. Expulsive hemorrhage: a study of histopathological details. *Graefes Arch Clin Exp Ophthalmol* 1982;219:155–158.

Nonsurgical Trauma

Barr CC, Mitchell D. Penetrating ocular injury caused by nylon cord fragment from electric lawn trimmer. *Ophthalmic Surg* 1983;14:741–743.

Blanton FM. Anterior chamber angle recession and secondary glaucoma. *Arch Ophthalmol* 1964;72:39–43.

Broderick JD. Corneal blood staining after hyphema. *Br J Ophthalmol* 1972;56:589–593.

Cox MS, Schepens CL, Freeman HM. Retinal detachment due to ocular contusion. *Arch Ophthalmol* 1966;76:678–685.

Dunn ES, Jaeger EA, Jeffers JB, et al. The epidemiology of ruptured globes. *Ann Ophthalmol* 1992;24:405–410.

Esmaeli B, Elner SG, Schork MA, et al. Visual outcome and ocular survival after penetrating trauma. A clinicopathologic study. *Ophthalmology* 1995;102:393–400.

Gregor Z, Ryan SJ. Combined posterior contusion and penetrating injury in the pig eye. I. A natural history study. *Br J Ophthalmol* 1982;66:793–798.

Gregor Z, Ryan SJ. Combined posterior contusion and penetrating injury in the pig eye. II. Histologic features. *Br J Ophthalmol* 1982;66:799–804.

Hagler WS, North AW. Retinal dialysis and retinal detachment. *Arch Ophthalmol* 1968;79:376–388.

Helveston EM. Eye trauma in childhood. *Pediatr Clin North Am* 1975;22:501–511.

Honig MA, Barraquer J, Perry HD, et al. Forceps and vacuum injuries to the cornea: histopathologic features of twelve cases and review of the literature. *Cornea* 1996;15:463–472.

Kempster RC, Green WR, Finkelstein D. Choroidal rupture. Clinicopathologic correlation of an unusual case. *Retina* 1996;16:57–63.

Manche EE, Goldberg RA, Mondino BJ. Air bag-related ocular injuries. *Ophthalmic Surg Lasers Imaging* 1997;28:246–250.

Martin DF, Awh CC, McCuen BW, et al. Treatment and pathogenesis of traumatic chorioretinal rupture (sclopetaria). *Am J Ophthalmol* 1994;117:190–200.

Meredith TA, Gordon PA. Pars plana vitrectomy for severe penetrating injury with posterior segment involvement. *Am J Ophthalmol* 1987;103:549–554.

Messmer EP, Gottsch J, Font RL. Blood staining of the cornea: a histopathologic analysis of 16 cases. *Cornea* 1984;3:205–212.

Pearlstein ES, Agapitos PJ, Cantrill HL, et al. Ruptured globe after radial keratotomy. *Am J Ophthalmol* 1988;106:755–756.

Rudd JC, Jaeger EA, Freitag SK, et al. Traumatically ruptured globes in children. *J Pediatr Ophthalmol Strabismus* 1994;31:307–311.

Russell SR, Olsen KR, Folk JC. Predictors of scleral rupture and the role of vitrectomy in severe blunt ocular trauma. *Am J Ophthalmol* 1988;105:253–257.

Ryan SJ. Penetrating ocular trauma and pars plana vitrectomy. *Trans New Orleans Acad Ophthalmol* 1983;31:129–136.

Schein OD, Hibberd PL, Shingleton BJ, et al. The spectrum and burden of ocular injury. *Ophthalmology* 1988;95:300–305.

Smiddy WE, Green WR. Retinal dialysis: pathology and pathogenesis. *Retina* 1982;2:94–116.

Spalding SC, Sternberg P Jr. Controversies in the management of posterior segment ocular trauma. *Retina* 1990;10:76–82.

Sternberg P Jr, de Juan E Jr, Green WR, et al. Ocular BB injuries. *Ophthalmology* 1984;91:1269–1277.

Winthrop SR, Cleary PE, Minckler DS, et al. Penetrating eye injuries: a histopathological review. *Br J Ophthalmol* 1980;64:809–817.

Wolff SM, Zimmerman LE. Chronic secondary glaucoma associated with retrodisplacement of the iris root and deepening of the anterior chamber secondary to contusion. *Am J Ophthalmol* 1962;54:547–562.

Sympathetic Uveitis

Auw-Haedrich C, Loeffler KU, Witschel H. Sympathetic ophthalmia: an immunohistochemistry study of four cases. *Ger J Ophthalmol* 1996;5:98–103.

Croxatto JO, Galentine P, Cupples HP, et al. Sympathetic ophthalmia after pars plana vitrectomy-lensectomy for endogenous bacterial endophthalmitis. *Am J Ophthalmol* 1981;91:342–346.

Font RL, Fine BS, Messmer E, et al. Light and electron microscopic study of Dalen-Fuchs nodules in sympathetic ophthalmia. *Ophthalmology* 1982;90:66–75.

Gass JD. Sympathetic ophthalmia following vitrectomy. *Am J Ophthalmol* 1982;93:552–558.

Green WR, Maumenee AE, Sanders TE, et al. Sympathetic uveitis following evisceration. *Trans Am Acad Ophthalmol Otolaryngol* 1972;76:625–644.

Jakobiec FA, Marboe CC, Knowles DM II, et al. Human Sympathetic ophthalmia. An analysis of the inflammatory infiltrate by hybridoma-monoclonal antibodies, immunochemistry, and correlative electron microscopy. *Ophthalmology* 1983;90:76–95.

Lubin JR, Albert DM, Weinstein M. Sixty-five years of sympathetic ophthalmia. A clinicopathologic review of 105 cases (1913–1978). *Ophthalmology* 1980;87:109–121.

Marak GE. Phacoanaphylactic endophthalmitis. *Surv Ophthalmol* 1992;36:325–329.

Morse PH, Duke JR. Sympathetic ophthalmitis. Report of a case, proven pathologically, eight years after original injury. *Am J Ophthalmol* 1969;68:508–512.

To KW, Jakobiec FA, Zimmerman LE. Sympathetic uveitis. In: Albert DM, Jakobiec FA, eds. *Principles and Practice of Ophthalmology: Clinical Practice*, vol. 1. Philadelphia, PA: WB Saunders, 1994:496–503.

Wilson MW, Grossniklaus HE, Heathcote JG. Focal posttraumatic choroidal granulomatous inflammation. *Am J Ophthalmol* 1996;121:397–404.

Intraocular Foreign Bodies

Hanna C, Fraunfelder FT. Lens capsule change after intraocular copper. *Ann Ophthalmol* 1973;5:9–12.

Masciulli L, Andersen DR, Charles S. Experimental ocular siderosis in the squirrel monkey. *Am J Ophthalmol* 1972;74:638–661.

Rosenthal AR, Appleton B, Hopkins JL. Intraocular copper foreign bodies. *Am J Ophthalmol* 1974;78:671–678.

Seland JH. The nature of capsular inclusions in lenticular chalcosis. Report of a case. *Acta Ophthalmol Copenh* 1976;54:99–108.

Talamo JH, Topping TM, Maumenee AE, et al. Ultrastructural studies of cornea, iris and lens in a case of siderosis bulbi. *Ophthalmology* 1985;92:1675–1680.

Chemical Burns

Brown SI, Weller CA, Akiya S. Pathogenesis of ulcers of the alkali-burned cornea. *Arch Ophthalmol* 1970;83:205–208.

Hirst LW, Fogle JA, Kenyon KR, et al. Corneal epithelial regeneration and adhesions following acid burns in the rhesus monkey. *Invest Ophthalmol Vis Sci* 1982;23:764–773.

Radiation Injuries

Bagan SM, Hollenhorst RW. Radiation retinopathy after irradiation of intracranial lesions. *Am J Ophthalmol* 1979;88:694–697.

Brown GC, Shields JA, Sanborn G, et al. Radiation optic neuropathy. *Ophthalmology* 1982;89:1489–1493.

Brown GC, Shields JA, Sanborn G, et al. Radiation retinopathy. *Ophthalmology* 1982;89:1494–1501.

Buschke W, Friedenwald JS, Moses SG. Effect of ultraviolet irradiation on corneal epithelium: mitosis, nuclear fragmentation, post-traumatic cell movements, loss of tissue cohesion. *J Cell Comp Physiol* 1945;26:147–164.

Cogan DG, Donaldson DD. Experimental radiation cataracts. I. Cataracts in the rabbit following single x-ray exposure. *Arch Ophthalmol* 1951;45:508–522.

Noble KG, Kupersmith MJ. Retinal vascular remodelling in radiation retinopathy. *Br J Ophthalmol* 1984;68:475–478.

5 Conjunctiva

The conjunctiva is a delicate mucous membrane that covers the anterior surface of the eyeball and the posterior surface of eyelids. The term conjunctiva is derived from the Latin meaning "to bind together."

The nonkeratinized stratified columnar epithelium of the conjunctiva is two to five cells in thickness and contains mucous glands called goblet cells whose contents appear clear or bluish in routine H&E sections and are vividly periodic acid-Schiff (PAS)-positive (Fig. 5-1). Goblet cells are more numerous nasally, especially in the semilunar fold (plica semilunaris).

Topographically, the conjunctiva is divided into bulbar, forniceal, and tarsal (or palpebral) parts. The bulbar conjunctiva covers the surface of the eyeball and is freely movable. The stroma or substantia propria of the bulbar conjunctiva is composed of loose, areolar connective tissue and is easily ballooned-up by edema fluid (chemosis) or injected anesthetic. In contrast, the palpebral conjunctiva adheres firmly to the tarsal plate and does not move freely. Multiple glandlike epithelial invaginations or crypts called pseudoglands of Henle usually occur in the palpebral conjunctiva. The forniceal conjunctiva that arches around the superior and inferior cul-de-sacs is redundant and folded to facilitate eye movements. Several small accessory lacrimal glands of Krause are found beneath the forniceal conjunctiva, and accessory glands of Wolfring occur at the upper and lower margins of the tarsal plates. Lymphocytes and plasma cells normally are found in the conjunctival stroma and constitute part of the eye's normal defense mechanisms.

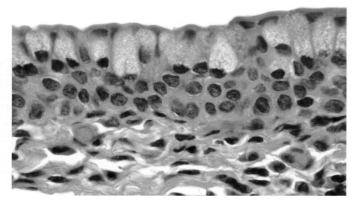

Fig. 5-1. Conjunctival epithelium. The stratified squamous epithelium of the conjunctiva is nonkeratinized and contains mucin-producing goblet cells that are most numerous in the nasal bulbar conjunctiva. Chronic inflammatory cells normally are present in the substantia propria. (Hematoxylin-eosin [H&E] ×250)

DEVELOPMENTAL LESIONS

Congenital **epibulbar dermoids** are choristomatous masses that usually occur at the limbus temporally. They are composed of coarse, interweaving bundles of collagenous connective tissue and are covered by conjunctival or corneal epithelium or skinlike epithelium with epidermal appendages (Fig. 5-2A). **Dermolipomas (lipodermoids)** are solid dermoids comprised largely of adipose tissue (Fig. 5-2B). These yellowish tan, soft fusiform tumors usually are located in the superotemporal quadrant. Bilateral epibulbar dermoids and dermolipomas occur in two thirds of patients with Goldenhar syndrome, which also includes vertebral anomalies, preauricular appendages, and aural fistulas. Epibulbar dermoids that contain cartilage and/or ectopic lacrimal gland tissue are called **complex choristomas** (Fig. 5-2C). (A choristoma is a congenital tumor composed of tissue that is not normally found in an area.) Epibulbar dermoids also occur in the organoid nevus syndrome (Nevus sebaceus of Jadassohn). Solid epibulbar dermoids should not be confused with dermoid cysts, which usually occur in the superotemporal orbit, or so-called conjunctival dermoids, which are a rare variant of cystic dermoid that occurs in the nasal orbit and is lined by conjunctival epithelium. Other congenital lesions of the conjunctiva include **ectopic lacrimal gland** and **episcleral osseous choristoma**. Episcleral osseous choristomas are plaques of mature lamellar bone that are located in the superotemporal quadrant (Fig. 5-2D).

CONJUNCTIVITIS

Most inflammatory diseases of the conjunctiva are treated medically and are rarely seen in the ophthalmic pathologic laboratory, except as scrapings or smears.

Conjunctivitis can be acute or chronic and can be caused by numerous infectious or noninfectious agents including bacteria, viruses, fungi, and protozoans. Allergy is another important cause of conjunctivitis.

The clinical manifestations of acute conjunctivitis include redness (conjunctival injection or hyperemia), chemosis (conjunctival edema), and exudation. The exudate in acute purulent bacterial conjunctivitis contains numerous polymorphonuclear leukocytes (Fig. 5-3). Histologic sections (obtained incidentally) show edema and infiltration of the conjunctival epithelium and substantia propria by polys and an exudate composed of a mixture of polys, fibrin, mucous, and necrotic cellular debris. Clinically, the presence of copious quantities of pus

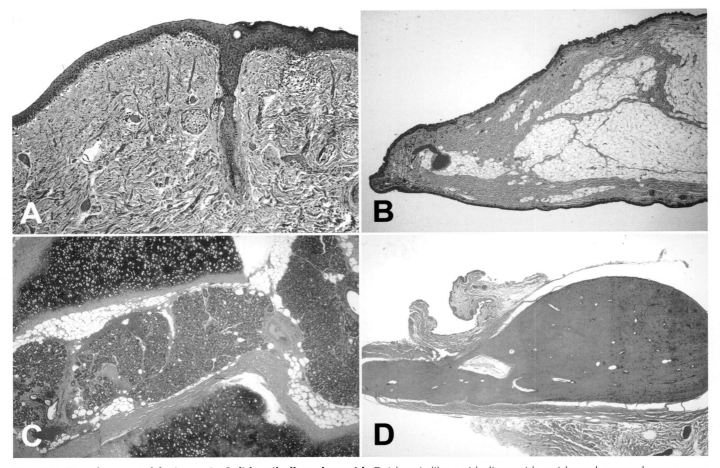

Fig. 5-2. Developmental lesions. A. Solid epibulbar dermoid. Epidermis-like epithelium with epidermal appendages covers the apex of epibulbar choristoma and merges with nonkeratinized ocular surface epithelium on its sloping margin. The stroma is composed of coarse interweaving bundles of collagen. **B. Dermolipoma (lipodermoid).** A dermolipoma is a solid epibulbar dermoid comprised largely of adipose tissue. Most dermolipomas occur on the superotemporal surface of the globe. **C. Complex choristoma, organoid nevus syndrome.** This epibulbar complex choristoma contains hyaline cartilage, ectopic lacrimal gland, and fat. The surface of the choristoma was lined by skinlike epithelium with epidermal appendages. A choristoma is a congenital tumor composed of tissue that is not normally found in an area. **D. Osseous choristoma, conjunctiva.** This rare type of epibulbar choristoma is composed of a plaque of mature lamellar bone. Most occur in the superotemporal quadrant. (**A.** H&E ×50, **B.** H&E ×10, **C.** H&E ×10, **D.** H&E, ×10)

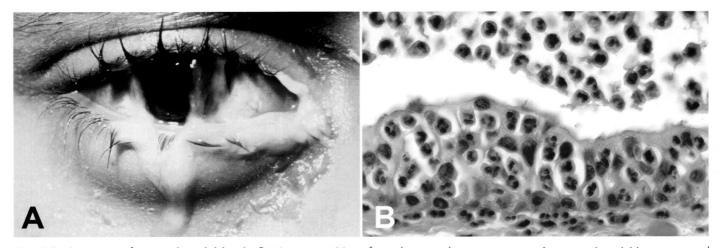

Fig. 5-3. Acute purulent conjunctivitis. A. Copious quantities of purulent exudate are present. Acute conjunctivitis was caused by *Haemophilus influenzae*. **B.** Polys infiltrate the edematous conjunctival epithelium and are the major cellular constituent of the purulent exudate. The focus of acute conjunctivitis was found incidentally in a tumor resection specimen. (**B.** H&E ×250)

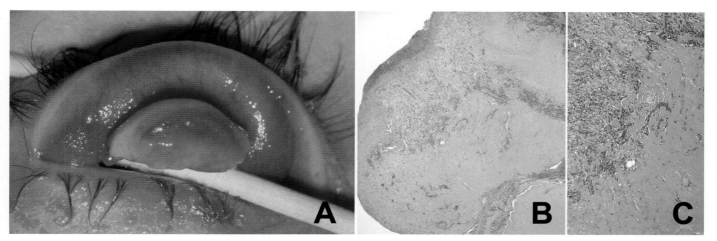

Fig. 5-4. Ligneous conjunctivitis. A. Inflammatory mass on upper palpebral conjunctiva had a firm, woody consistency. It recurred several times and was composed largely of fibrin. **B.** Ligneous conjunctivitis is composed of granulation tissue and sheets of intensely eosinophilic acellular amorphous fibrin, seen at higher magnification in (**C**). **C.** Ligneous conjunctivitis has been linked to mutations in the plasminogen gene. (**A.** Photo courtesy of Dr. Joseph Calhoun, Wills Eye Institute.) (**B.** H&E ×25, **C.** H&E ×50)

(hyperacute conjunctivitis) should suggest the possibility of gonococcal infection.

Inflammatory membranes or pseudomembranes can develop in severely inflamed eyes. These adhere to the conjunctiva and are composed of fibrin and inflammatory cells. True membranes occur in Stevens-Johnson syndrome or bacterial infections by β-hemolytic *Streptococcus, Neisseria gonorrhea*, or *Corynebacterium diphtheriae*. True conjunctival membranes are firmly adherent to the epithelium and bleeding occurs when removal is attempted.

Conjunctival pseudomembranes are less adherent and can be peeled without bleeding. Pseudomembranes may complicate infection by adenovirus 8 (epidemic keratoconjunctivitis or EKC) and adenovirus 3 (pharyngoconjunctival fever or PCF). They also form in patients with certain severe bacterial infections (*Staphylococcus, Streptococcus, N. meningitidis, Pseudomonas*, or coliforms), or complicate chemical burns, foreign bodies, benign mucous membrane pemphigoid, or ligneous conjunctivitis.

Ligneous conjunctivitis is a rare form of chronic pseudomembranous conjunctivitis that is marked by a massive accumulation of fibrin (Fig. 5-4). The term ligneous refers to the firm, woody consistency of the large masses of fibrin that comprise the pseudomembranes. Ligneous conjunctivitis typically occurs in children but may recur in adults. Treatment is often challenging because the inflammation is persistent and the pseudomembranes often recur rapidly after excision. Histopathology shows two components: granulation tissue and sheets of intensely eosinophilic acellular amorphous material, which has been shown to be composed predominantly of fibrin by immunohistochemical stains (Fig. 5-4B,C). The mass of fibrin also incorporates other serum components such as immunoglobulin. The granulation tissue component (like all granulation tissue) is rich in acid mucopolysaccharide ground substance. Lesions that resemble those found in the

conjunctiva can affect other mucous membranes including the larynx, vagina, and ear. Ligneous conjunctivitis is an autosomal recessive trait caused by mutations in the gene for plasminogen on chromosome 6q26.

Acute anaphylactic conjunctivitis is marked by the abrupt onset of severe conjunctival edema (chemosis), mild injection, and itching. The latter is an important clinical symptom of ocular allergy (Fig. 3-5). The release of inflammatory mediators such as histamine and serotonin by mast cells in the substantia propria causes the signs and symptoms in persons who are sensitized to antigens such as ragweed pollen or animal dander. Such atopic individuals produce IgE that is incorporated into the cell membranes of the mast cells. Mast cell degranulation occurs when the appropriate antigen is reencountered. The release of vasoactive substances markedly increases the permeability of conjunctival vessels, which leads to an outpouring of fluid that fills the areolar substantia propria of the bulbar conjunctiva causing chemosis. Contact hypersensitivity to topical medications can cause severe ocular injection, itching, and eyelid erythema in postoperative patients.

CHRONIC CONJUNCTIVITIS

Chronic follicular conjunctivitis and chronic papillary conjunctivitis are the conjunctiva's two basic patterns of response to chronic inflammatory stimuli. **Chronic follicular conjunctivitis** represents a reactive follicular hyperplasia of the population of lymphocytes that normally resides in the substantia propria. This lymphoid hyperplasia can be a reaction to a variety of stimuli. Conjunctival follicles are evident clinically as gray-white, round to oval elevations with an avascular center (Fig. 5-5). Microscopically, the substantia propria contains an intense basophilic infiltrate of benign lymphocytes and plasma cells that often contains

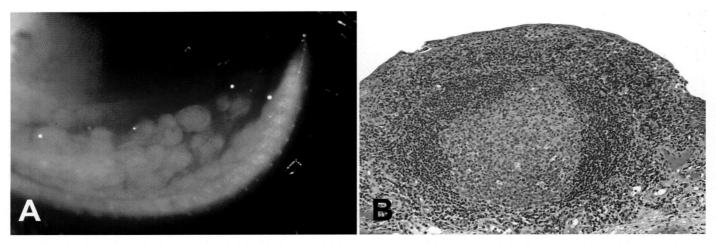

Fig. 5-5. A. Chronic follicular conjunctivitis. Conjunctival follicles are caused by reactive follicular hyperplasia of the tissue's normal resident population of lymphocytes. The round to oval, gray-white elevations are avascular centrally. **B. Conjunctival follicle.** The follicle is composed of an avascular sheet of basophilic lymphocytes. A germinal center is present. The overlying epithelium is thinned. (**B.** H&E ×25)

follicular centers. The conjunctival epithelium overlying the lymphoid follicles is often thinned.

Conjunctival follicles occur in some types of acute viral conjunctivitis. They are typically observed in acute adenovirus infections such as EKC and PCF, herpes simplex virus (HSV) conjunctivitis, swimming pool conjunctivitis (Newcastle virus), and the acute hemorrhagic conjunctivitis caused by enterovirus 70.

Infectious causes of chronic follicular conjunctivitis include trachoma, psittacosis, moraxella, and infectious mononucleosis. *Chlamydiae*, which are small obligate intracellular parasites that are sensitive to antibiotics, cause trachoma, inclusion conjunctivitis, psittacosis, and lymphogranuloma venereum.

Trachoma is the most important infectious cause of blindness in the world. Trachoma is caused by serotypes A, B, and C of *Chlamydia trachomatis*. In endemic areas, trachoma is spread by direct contact with infected ocular secretions. Poor hygiene and insect vectors such as flies contribute to the spread of the disease.

Trachoma is marked by bilateral keratoconjunctivitis, which may be asymmetric. The initial infection involves the conjunctival epithelial cells and stimulates epithelial hyperplasia. Conjunctival smears stained with the Giemsa stain show a mixed inflammatory exudate, which contains both lymphocytes and polys as well as large macrophages laden with phagocytized cellular debris called Leber cells. The conjunctival epithelial cells contain diagnostic basophilic intracytoplasmic inclusions of Halberstaedter and Prowazek (Fig. 5-6). More specific direct immunofluorescent tests and a dipstick immunoassay designed for field testing also are available.

An intense infiltration of the substantia propria by chronic inflammatory cells follows the initial epithelial infection. Numerous lymphoid follicles occur on the upper tarsus. In florid cases, the follicles develop central areas of necrosis that

can extend superficially forming small ulcerations. Follicles also occur in the fornix and at the limbus. In the latter stages of the disease, the remnants of follicles may be evident at the limbus as saucerlike depressions called Herbert pits. As the disease progresses, papillary hypertrophy of the conjunctiva supplants the follicular response. Pannus formation is another characteristic feature of trachoma. The inflammatory pannus of trachoma is marked by a downgrowth of subepithelial vessels from the superior limbus that destroys Bowman membrane. Scarring occurs in the late stages of trachoma. A linear scar called Arlt line, which extends across the upper tarsus parallel to the lid margin, is one of the diagnostic criteria for trachoma listed by the World Health Organization. (Other diagnostic criteria include lymphoid follicles on the upper tarsus, a vascular pannus, and active limbal follicles or Herbert pits. Two are diagnostic.)

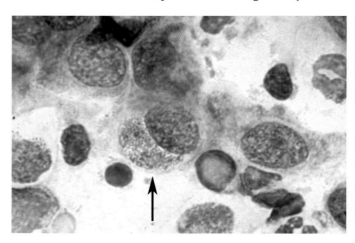

Fig. 5-6. Trachoma, conjunctival smear. The *arrow* denotes large basophilic intracytoplasmic inclusion of Halberstaedter and Prowazek in epithelial cell in Giemsa-stained smear. The inflammatory exudate includes both polys and lymphocytes. (Giemsa, ×250)

Blindness in trachoma typically results from sequelae that develop in the cicatricial stage. Severe conjunctival drying and epidermalization result from the loss of epithelial goblet cells and obstruction of the ducts of the main and accessory lacrimal glands. Lid scarring also causes entropion and trichiasis that predispose to severe corneal scarring as well as corneal ulceration and secondary bacterial infection.

Serotypes D through K of *Chlamydia trachomatis* cause inclusion conjunctivitis or paratrachoma in developed countries. Inclusion blennorrhea, an infantile form of inclusion conjunctivitis, is an important cause of acute purulent conjunctivitis or ophthalmia neonatorum in the newborn. (Other causes include *N. gonorrhoeae* and a chemical conjunctivitis caused by Credé silver nitrate prophylaxis against gonococcal infection.) Infants acquire the disease from an infected mother during passage through the birth canal. Inclusion conjunctivitis is a venereal disease in adults. In contrast to the superior conjunctival involvement found in trachoma, which has superior tarsal involvement, the follicles in inclusion conjunctivitis occur in the lower fornix.

Chronic follicular conjunctivitis can also be a response to cosmetics; topical medications such as atropine, eserine, or IDU; viral particles shed by a molluscum contagiosum on the eyelid margin; or the feces of crab lice infesting the lashes (phthiriasis palpebrarum). The lids and lashes should always be carefully (and expeditiously) examined when unilateral follicles are encountered during clinical exam.

Papillary hypertrophy is the second relatively non-specific reaction that occurs in some patients with chronic conjunctivitis (Fig. 5-7). Papillary hypertrophy typically develops on the tarsal conjunctiva and is marked by proliferation of the conjunctival epithelium and hyperplasia of the substantia propria. Pale avascular valleys that contain deep infoldings of conjunctival epithelium separate

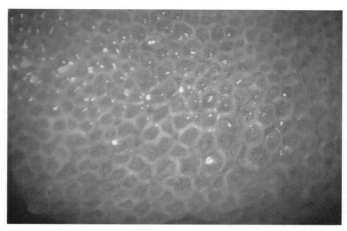

Fig. 5-7. Conjunctival papillae. Avascular valleys separate papillae on superior tarsal conjunctiva. Fine vessels are seen in the center of the papillae. (Photo courtesy of Dr. Dario Savino-Zari, Caracas, Venezuela.)

individual papillae, which have a richly vascular stroma and a central tuft of blood vessels (Fig. 5-8B). This contrasts with lymphoid follicles, which typically are avascular. Papillae contain a moderately intense infiltrate composed of a variety of inflammatory cells. Eosinophils and mast cells usually are present, and the sheets of lymphocytes and follicular centers found in chronic follicular conjunctivitis are absent.

Giant papillae, which have been likened to cobblestones, occur on the superior tarsus in **vernal conjunctivitis**, a bilateral chronic recurrent disease that typically afflicts adolescent males who have a history of atopy (Fig. 5-8). The term vernal reflects the characteristic exacerbation of signs and symptoms that occurs in the spring. Itching is a characteristic symptom. Patients have a thick, ropy chewing gum–like mucus rich in eosinophils and Charcot-Leyden granules. The latter is termed the

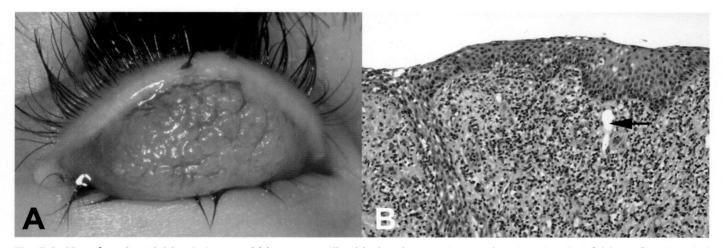

Fig. 5-8. Vernal conjunctivitis. A. Large cobblestone papillae blanket the superior tarsal conjunctiva. **B.** Infolding of conjunctival epithelium (**at left**) extends into the valley separating two large "cobblestone" papillae. The *arrow* points to the central vessel in the papilla. Moderately intense inflammatory infiltrate includes chronic inflammatory cells and eosinophils. (**B.** H&E, ×50)

Maxwell-Lyons sign. Conjunctival smears contain eosinophils and eosinophilic granules. The large "cobblestone" papillae may abrade the cornea producing painful shield-like ulcerations of the superior corneal epithelium. A limbal variant of vernal conjunctivitis marked by papillae at the superior limbus also occurs. "Limbal vernal" is said to be more common in black patients. Horner-Trantas dots, which are intraepithelial and subepithelial collections of eosinophils and cellular debris, occasionally occur near the limbus. Histopathologically, vernal conjunctivitis is characterized by papillary hypertrophy of the conjunctiva. The edematous fibrovascular core of the papillae contains an infiltrate of lymphocytes and plasma cells and numerous eosinophils.

Giant papillary conjunctivitis occurs in long-term wearers of hard and soft contact lenses and even ocular prostheses. Probably a cell-mediated hypersensitivity reaction stimulated by the accumulation of immunogenic material on the surface of foreign material, giant papillary conjunctivitis shares similarities with vernal conjunctivitis, but usually has fewer eosinophils.

Phlyctenular keratoconjunctivitis is thought to be a hypersensitivity reaction to bacterial proteins. In the past, it classically was associated with tuberculosis, but now most cases probably are related to staphylococcal blepharitis. Phlyctenular conjunctivitis is marked clinically by the presence of 2- to 3-mm whitish inflammatory nodules on the bulbar conjunctiva. A zone of dilated vessels surrounds the nodules and the overlying epithelium is ulcerated. Microscopically the nodules are composed of acute and chronic inflammatory cells.

CHRONIC GRANULOMATOUS CONJUNCTIVITIS

A chronic inflammatory infiltrate that includes epithelioid histiocytes and inflammatory giant cells occurs in several conjunctival diseases. Discrete noncaseating granulomas are found in biopsies from patients with sarcoidosis (Fig. 3-9B). The granulomas may be evident clinically as small yellowish tan nodules in the inferior fornix. Extensive subepithelial infiltration by sarcoidosis can stimulate symblepharon formation. The conjunctiva can be biopsied when sarcoidosis is suspected clinically and a tissue diagnosis is required. Bilateral blind conjunctival biopsy will be positive in about 50% of patients with sarcoidosis, despite the absence of obvious nodules or ocular inflammation clinically.

Granulomatous conjunctivitis with associated regional lymphadenopathy, usually a preauricular node, constitutes **Parinaud oculoglandular syndrome**. The differential diagnosis of Parinaud oculoglandular syndrome is rather extensive and includes a number of relatively rare infectious disorders caused by variety of microorganisms including bacteria, spirochetes, chlamydiae, rickettsia, fungi, and viruses.

Cat scratch fever is a relatively common cause of Parinaud oculoglandular syndrome (Fig. 5-9). The disease is caused by *Bartonella henselae*, a bacterium that usually is inconspicuous in routine Gram stains because it is only faintly Gram negative. The infected conjunctiva contains an intense infiltrate of histiocytes with foci of necrosis. The Warthin-Starry silver stain often reveals masses of bacteria in the necrotic areas. There usually is a history of a cat scratch that typically does not involve the eye or face. Conjunctival involvement results from a bacteremia. A focal angiomatous response to *Bartonella*, called bacillary angiomatosis, has been reported in the conjunctiva of immunosuppressed patients. Granulomatous conjunctivitis in response to the irritating hairs or setae of certain species of caterpillars is called ophthalmia nodosa. The setae occasionally migrate into the anterior chamber causing severe intraocular inflammation.

Synthetic fiber granuloma is a foreign body giant cell reaction to a "fuzz ball" of synthetic fabric fibers lodged in the inferior conjunctival fornix (Fig. 5-10). Most cases have occurred in infants and young children. Synthetic fiber granuloma has been confused with ophthalmia nodosa histopathologically. Particulates of inorganic delustering agent incorporated into the fibers and knife chatter marks on the ends of sectioned fibers serve to differentiate the synthetic fabric fibers from caterpillar setae. The condition is also called teddy bear granuloma after the source of the fibers in some patients.

Allergic conjunctival granuloma is a bilateral condition marked by the presence of yellowish nodules on the ocular surface, which is thought to be a response to parasitic infestation, probably by nematodes. Histopathology discloses granulomatous inflammation and eosinophilia centered around intensely eosinophilic deposits of antigen-antibody complexes called the Splendore-Hoeppli

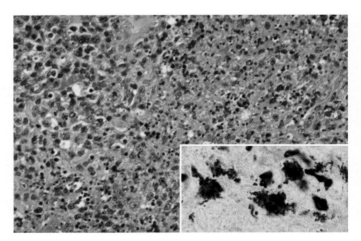

Fig. 5-9. Cat scratch disease, conjunctiva. The intense chronic inflammatory infiltrate contains a focus of necrotic karyorrhectic cells. Silver stain discloses masses of bacteria (*Bartonella henselae*) in **inset**. The patient developed unilateral granulomatous conjunctivitis and a preauricular node after being scratched by a cat. (**Main figure**, H&E ×100; **inset**, Warthin-Starry ×250)

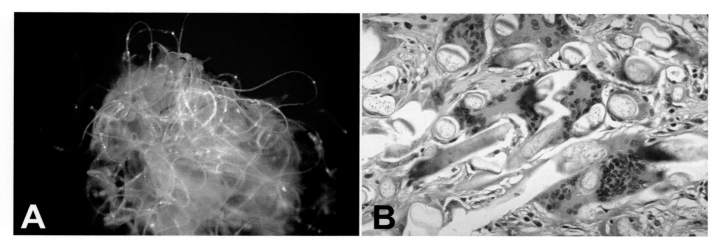

Fig. 5-10. Synthetic fiber granuloma. A. "Fuzz ball" of synthetic fabric fibers that stimulated chronic granulomatous inflammatory response in inferior fornix. **B.** Foreign body giant cells encompass yellow synthetic fabric fibers that contain dark particulates of delustering agent added to opacify the plastic. (**B.** H&E ×100)

phenomenon. Nematode fragments are identified histologically in less than one fifth of cases.

Parasitic and mycotic infections of the conjunctiva are rare in the United States. Adult *Loa loa* worms that have migrated to the subconjunctival space occasionally are found in visitors from West and Central Africa (Fig. 11A). These worms cause itching, pain, and the disconcerting sensation of a mobile foreign body. Systemic infestation with *Trichinella spiralis* (trichinosis) causes fever, eosinophilia, periorbital swelling, edema of the eyelids, and conjunctiva and subconjunctival hemorrhages and petechiae. *Rhinosporidium seeberi*, an unusual fungus with a pathognomonic histologic appearance, causes strawberry-like papillary conjunctival granulomas that are studded with white microabscesses. Although rhinosporidiosis has been

reported in the United States, most cases occur in India and Southeast Asia. Microsporidia and *Pneumocystis carinii* can cause conjunctivitis in patients with HIV/AIDS (Fig. 5-11B).

Ocular cicatricial pemphigoid (OCP) is a systemic autoimmune disease with ocular and systemic manifestations. A type II hypersensitivity reaction, OCP is thought to occur when environmental factors, probably viruses, stimulate genetically susceptible individuals to make autoantibodies (IgG) directed against epithelial basement membrane zone components including the beta-4 subunit of alpha-6-beta-4 integrin and laminin 5/epiligrin (Fig. 5-12). Similar diseases also occur in some patients receiving topical medication or as a paraneoplastic effect of nonocular cancer. Antibody deposition and complement activation cause chronic inflammation and stimulate fibroblasts to

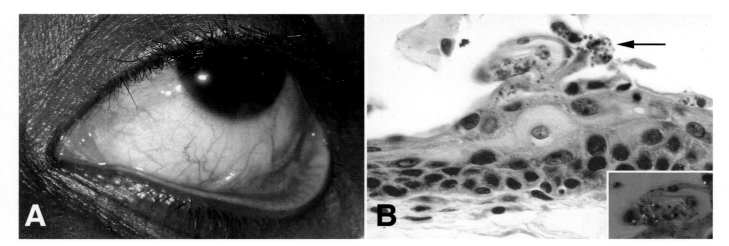

Fig. 5-11. A. Loiasis. Nematode is seen beneath inferior bulbar conjunctival in the eye of a West African student who presented to the Wills Eye Institute ER with a severe foreign body sensation. (Photo courtesy of Michael A. DellaVechia, MD, PhD, Director of Emergency Room Services, Wills Eye Institute.) **B. Microsporidial keratoconjunctivitis**. The *arrow* points to minute microsporidial parasites (*Encephalitozoon hellem*) in the conjunctival epithelium from an AIDS patient with chronic keratoconjunctivitis. Polarization microscopy discloses birefringent polar bodies in inset. (**Main figure**, H&E ×250; **inset**, H&E, polarization ×250. [Case presented by Dr. Ramon L. Font at the 1992 meeting of Eastern Ophthalmic Pathology Society, Jekyll Island, Georgia.])

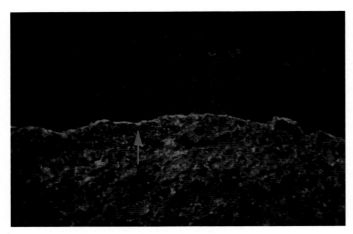

Fig. 5-12. Ocular cicatricial pemphigoid. Immunofluorescent microscopy discloses deposition of IgA in conjunctival basement membrane (*arrow*). (Immunofluorescence, ×250. [Courtesy of Dr. C. Stephen Foster, Boston, Massachusetts.])

produce collagen causing abnormal conjunctival scarring. Conjunctival bullae rarely form in OCP. Progressive cicatrization causes foreshortening of the conjunctival fornices, symblepharon formation, and drying due to compromise of lacrimal gland and meibomian gland ductules. The end stage of the disease is marked by epidermalization of the cornea and conjunctival epithelium and adherence of the lids to the globe. Routine conjunctival biopsies are nondiagnostic; specialized immunohistochemical procedures are required to show immunoglobulin or complement deposition in the epithelial basement membrane. These must be performed on fresh frozen sectioned tissue.

Severe subepithelial fibrosis, symblepharon formation, severe ocular drying, and trichiasis complicate Stevens-Johnson syndrome (erythema multiforme), which is thought to be a type III hypersensitivity reaction to microbes or drugs characterized by circulating IgA containing immune complexes and lymphocytic vasculitis. Conjunctival involvement by pemphigus vulgaris is marked by intraepithelial bulla formation; therefore, subepithelial scarring and symblepharon formation do not occur. In pemphigus vulgaris, autoantibodies are directed against desmoglein 3, a protein component of desmosomes joining epithelial cells.

The normal reparative phase of the inflammatory response is marked by the production of granulation tissue, which plays an important role in wound healing. An inappropriate, **exuberant proliferation of granulation tissue** may develop on the surface of the globe or conjunctiva after surgery or trauma. Ophthalmologists apply the thoroughly ingrained term **pyogenic granuloma** to these relatively common inflammatory tumors. Ophthalmic pathologists diagnose these lesions as "exuberant granulation tissue (pyogenic granuloma)" to distinguish them from an acquired type of capillary hemangioma called pyogenic granuloma by dermatopathologists. (The latter lesions usually are relatively devoid of inflammatory cells and rarely occur on the conjunctiva or eyelid.) The richly vascular mass of exuberant granulation tissue typically has a smooth, rounded surface and is red or pink in color (Fig. 5-13A). A paler hue may reflect superficial necrosis or adherent exudate. These lesions often arise quite rapidly, which serves to differentiate them from true neoplasms.

The mass of granulation tissue is composed of proliferating capillaries, activated fibroblasts with contractile properties called myofibroblasts, and a spectrum of acute and chronic inflammatory cells including polymorphonuclear leukocytes, lymphocytes, plasma cells, histiocytes, and occasional eosinophils and mast cells (Fig. 5-13B). The inflammatory infiltrate usually lacks epithelioid histiocytes and inflammatory giant cells unless it harbors residual lipogranulomatous inflammation from a previously drained chalazion. The vessels in pyogenic granuloma usually radiate from the base or stalk of the lesion. This

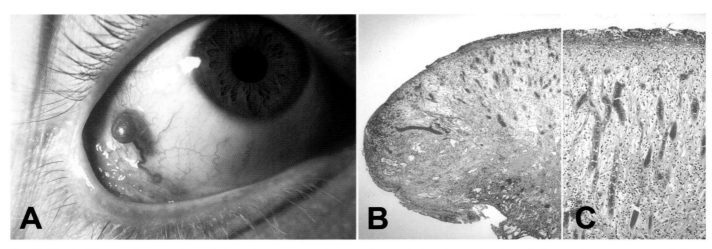

Fig. 5-13. A. "Pyogenic granuloma." Round, smooth, red mass of granulation tissue developed after strabismus surgery. **B.** Exuberant proliferation of granulation tissue forms smooth-surfaced pedunculated mass. **C.** Radially oriented vessels and inflammatory cells are seen at higher magnification. (**B.** H&E ×10, **C.** H&E ×25)

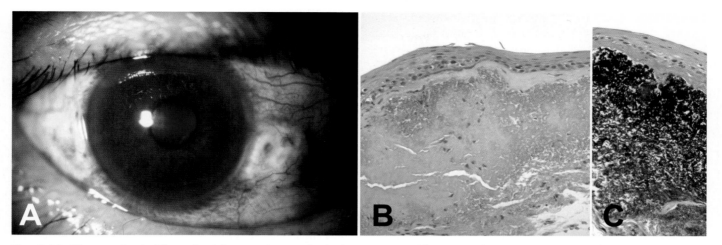

Fig. 5-14. Pinguecula. A. The yellowish mounds near the limbus are caused by actinic damage to conjunctival stromal connective tissue. **B.** The grayish deposit of elastotic degeneration elevates limbal epithelium. The deposit has granular and hyalinized areas. **C.** Material shows intense positive staining for elastic tissue that is not quenched by pretreatment with elastase. (**B.** H&E ×100, **C.** Verhoeff–van Gieson ×125)

radial vascular pattern and the prominent inflammatory cell component differentiate pyogenic granuloma from hemangioma on histopathologic examination.

DEGENERATIONS

Chronic light exposure damages the stromal connective tissue of the bulbar conjunctiva exposed in the interpalpebral fissure. This actinic damage is evident clinically as a yellowish white or gray-white opacification of the subepithelial tissue. In advanced cases, a raised yellowish mound called a **pinguecula** forms near the limbus (Fig. 5-14A). Microscopy discloses an acellular grayish granular deposit of extracellular matrix material beneath the limbal epithelium, which usually is elevated and thinned (Fig. 5-14B). Some

pinguecula contain thickened vermiform fibrils of degenerated collagen; others contain deposits of hyaline material such as those found in chronic actinic keratopathy. The damaged matrix material stains positively (black) with the Verhoeff–van Gieson stain for elastic tissue (Fig. 14C). Pretreatment with the enzyme elastase does not abolish positive staining for elastic tissue. Hence, the term elastoid is applied. The degenerative process actually may involve the production of abnormal elastic tissue components by light damaged fibroblasts. Similar foci of elastotic degeneration often are found in pterygia.

Conjunctival amyloidosis usually is a localized phenomenon that occurs in healthy adults who do not have systemic amyloidosis (Fig. 5-15). The degeneration can involve any part of the conjunctiva. The subepithelial amyloid can form circumscribed polypoid, yellowish, waxy nodules on

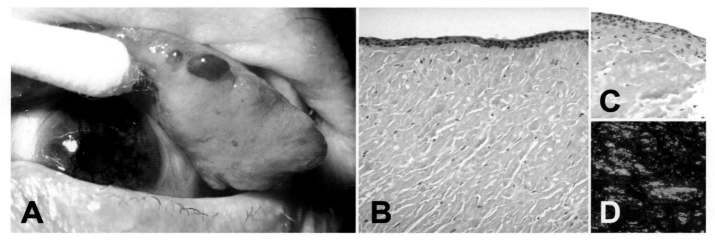

Fig. 5-15. Conjunctival amyloidosis. A. Large amyloid deposit forms yellowish mass on the tarsal surface of the upper lid. Sebaceous carcinoma was suspected clinically. **B.** Substantia propria contains extensive eosinophilic deposit of acellular amorphous amyloid. Amyloid shows positive (*orange*) staining with *Congo red* (**C**) and *apple green* birefringence with polarization microscopy (**D**). (**B.** H&E ×25; **C.** Congo red ×50, **D.** Congo red with crossed polarizers, ×50)

the epibulbar surface or may diffusely infiltrate the substantia propria. Intralesional hemorrhage is often found. Light microscopy discloses relatively acellular amorphous deposits of eosinophilic hyaline material (Fig. 5-15B). Special stains, usually Congo red, and polarization microscopy are used to confirm the diagnosis (Fig. 15C,D). Conjunctival amyloidosis is often composed of immunoglobulin light chains.

CONJUNCTIVAL CYSTS

Conjunctiva cysts occur congenitally or may develop secondarily when surface epithelium is entrapped or implanted in the stroma during surgery or trauma. Conjunctival inclusion cysts are lined by conjunctival epithelium, which may be attenuated. The lumen appears empty or it may be filled with mucinous material and/or proteinaceous fluid. Cysts also form when conjunctival crypts or pseudoglands of Henle become occluded and dilate. The proteinaceous luminal contents of such cysts occasionally undergo inspissation and even calcification, forming irritating concretions that literally feel like "grains of sand" in the eye. Another type of conjunctival cyst is caused by the blockage of an accessory lacrimal gland duct. Such cysts are analogous to sweat ductal cysts of the eyelid skin. They have a clear empty lumen and are lined by a dual layer of ductal epithelium.

CONJUNCTIVAL TUMORS

There are three basic categories of conjunctival tumors. The great majority of benign and malignant neoplasms of the conjunctiva arise from the squamous epithelium, associated melanocytes, or the lymphoid cells that normally reside in the substantia propria.

SQUAMOUS EPITHELIAL LESIONS

Squamous epithelial lesions of the conjunctiva include benign papillomas, actinic keratoses, and the spectrum of ocular surface squamous neoplasia (OSSN) that begins as intraepithelial neoplasia and can progress to invasive squamous cell carcinoma. Rare keratoacanthomas of the conjunctiva have been reported. Bilateral benign leukoplakic lesions occur on the conjunctiva and other mucous membranes in hereditary benign intraepithelial dyskeratosis.

Most **conjunctival papillomas** of the conjunctiva are composed of multiple fronds or fingerlike projections of conjunctival epithelium that enclose cores of vascularized connective tissue (Fig. 5-16). The vessels in the fronds of the papilloma are visible through the transparent epithelium as multiple "hair pin" vascular loops. Conjunctival papillomas in children may be multiple, and they tend to recur after excision. Many are caused by infection with human papilloma virus (HPV) 6 or 11. Benign papillomas occasionally contain foci of dysplastic epithelium. Such areas are marked by thickening of the epithelium, absence of goblet cells, cytologic atypia, and mitotic figures that are not confined to the basal cell layer.

The term papilloma signifies a growth pattern. Although conjunctival papillomas typically are benign, malignant tumors of the squamous epithelium occasionally grow in a papillomatous fashion. In malignant lesions, the epithelium comprising the papillomatous growth is thickened and replaced totally or in part by atypical cells. The former is termed papillary squamous cell carcinoma *in situ*.

Squamous cell lesions of the conjunctiva tend to occur in the sun-exposed part of the conjunctiva near the limbus, where there is a population of proliferating stem cells. Clinically, it is often impossible to distinguish between actinic keratoses, which recur infrequently after excision, and the spectrum of conjunctival intraepithelial neoplasia

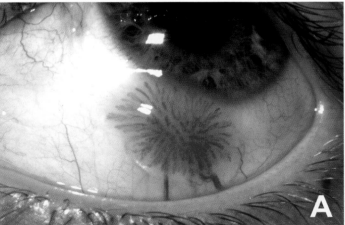
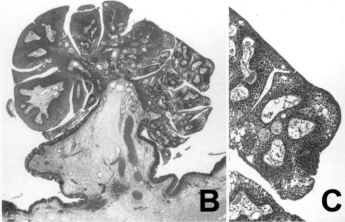

Fig. 5-16. Conjunctival papilloma. A. Vessels in fibrovascular cores of epithelial fronds are visible as hair pin vascular loops through transparent conjunctival epithelium. This benign epithelial tumor occurred in a child. **B.** Benign pedunculated tumor is composed of multiple fronds of conjunctival epithelium that surround cores of fibrovascular tissue. **C.** Fronds are seen at higher magnification. (**B.** H&E ×10, **C.** H&E ×50)

(CIN—see below), which tends to recur, and includes cases of *in situ* and invasive squamous cell carcinoma.

Most **actinic keratoses** are focal leukoplakic lesions that occur on the surface of pinguecula or pterygia (Fig. 5-17). Histopathology discloses irregular focal acanthosis of the epithelium by atypical epidermoid cells, a surface plaque of parakeratosis, and actinic elastosis in the substantia propria. Excisional biopsy usually is curative.

Conjunctival intraepithelial neoplasia (CIN) is a spectrum of squamous epithelial disease, in which part or all of the conjunctival epithelium is replaced by the proliferation of a new clone of neoplastic cells spawned by a mutation in the basal germinative layer. Intraepithelial neoplasia is often called conjunctival dysplasia. The newer term CIN is derived from the terminology applied to an analogous spectrum of intraepithelial malignancy that involves the uterine cervix. The term Bowen disease should never be applied to the conjunctiva.

Most cases of CIN arise near the limbus in the interpalpebral part of the conjunctiva (Fig. 5-18A,B). The palpebral conjunctiva is rarely affected. Patients usually have a history of extensive sun exposure. In many cases, the abnormal epithelium appears diffusely thickened and has a gelatinous appearance clinically. Leukoplakia may be present, however. Leukoplakia (white plaque) signifies keratin production and is good evidence that a lesion is composed of squamous cells. More advanced lesions form epibulbar tumors that may have a vascularized, papillary configuration. Corneal involvement may be evident as contiguous areas of grayish epithelial thickening. In rare instances, the process may be confined to the cornea.

Microscopic examination typically shows an abrupt transition between the normal conjunctival epithelium and the affected part (Fig. 5-18D). Compared to normal epithelium, the dysplastic epithelium shows increased cellularity, poor maturation, and a disorderly arrangement of its

cells (Fig. 5-18C,D). Part or all of the epithelium is replaced by the new proliferating clone of neoplastic cells. The basal part of the epithelium is replaced first because the mutational event occurs there. The involved epithelium is often massively thickened or acanthotic, sometimes measuring eight to ten times the normal thickness. The abnormal cells may have a spindled configuration with scant cytoplasm or may show epidermoid differentiation with copious quantities of eosinophilic cytoplasm. Varying degrees of atypia are possible. Mitoses are not confined to the basal cell layer where mitotic activity normally takes place and may be found throughout the thickened epithelium. Lesions caused by HPV infection may show koilocytosis. Depending on the amount of surface differentiation that persists, the degree of dysplasia is roughly graded as mild, moderate, or severe. If the entire thickness of the epithelium is replaced and there is no evidence of maturation or surface differentiation, the process is termed carcinoma *in situ* (Fig. 5-18D). The epithelial basement membrane remains intact in carcinoma *in situ*. Carcinoma *in situ* has a good prognosis because the malignant cells have not gained access to the blood vessels and lymphatics in the conjunctival stroma.

Intraepithelial carcinoma can progress to **invasive squamous cell carcinoma** (Fig. 5-19A). This occurs when tumor cells break through the epithelial basement membrane and invade the conjunctival stroma. Invasive squamous cell carcinoma does have a potential for metastatic spread (usually to regional lymph nodes), but the frequency of metastasis fortunately is low. In many cases, the squamous cell carcinoma tends to be papillary in configuration and forms an exophytic mass on the surface of the globe (Fig. 5-19B).

Most conjunctival squamous cell carcinomas remain superficial and rarely invade the eye or orbit. Most are successfully eradicated by local excision. Invasion of the eye

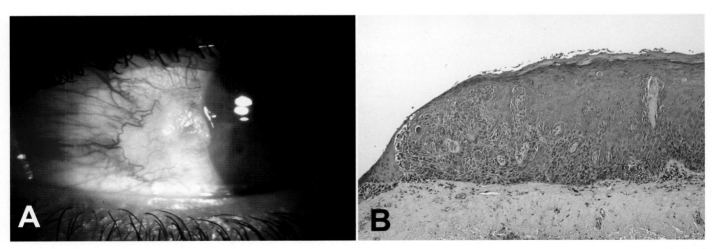

Fig. 5-17. Actinic keratosis, conjunctiva. A. Elevated leukoplakic lesion is located near the limbus in the exposed interpalpebral part of the conjunctiva. Leukoplakia indicates keratin-producing squamous cell lesion. **B.** Hyperkeratosis and parakeratosis is present on the surface of thick plaque of epidermoid cells, which arises abruptly from normal epithelium. The underlying stroma shows actinic elastosis. (**B.** H&E ×50)

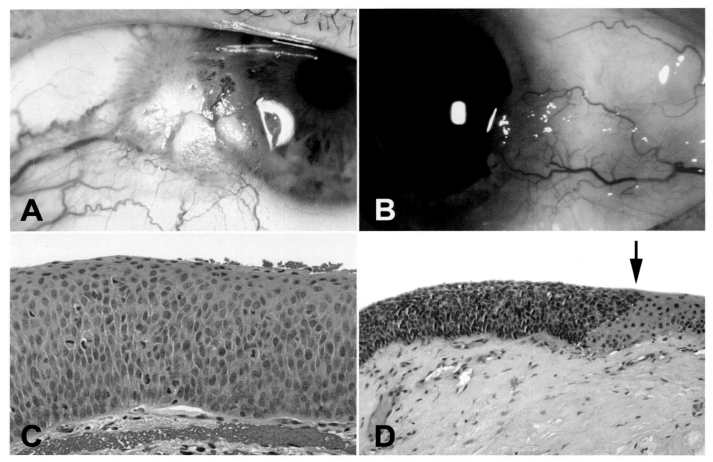

Fig. 5-18. A. Squamous cell carcinoma, conjunctiva. The tumor is located near the limbus in the interpalpebral part of conjunctiva. Limbal tumor is leukoplakic indicating keratin production. Peripheral corneal invasion and prominent feeder vessels are evident. **B. Conjunctival intraepithelial neoplasia.** Gelatinous lesion has arisen from the exposed interpalpebral conjunctiva at limbus. Excisional biopsy is required for definitive diagnosis of conjunctival squamous lesions. **C. Conjunctival intraepithelial neoplasia (severe dysplasia).** The thickened epithelium is largely replaced by atypical cells, but a small amount of surface differentiation persists. The epithelial basement membrane is intact. Mitotic figures are present within the acanthotic epithelium. **D. Conjunctival intraepithelial neoplasia (carcinoma *in situ*).** The epithelium at left has been totally replaced by atypical squamous cells and appears hypercellular and basophilic compared to the segment of normal limbal epithelium at right. The *arrow* denotes transition that is characteristically abrupt. The carcinoma is *in situ* because the epithelial basement membrane is intact. (**C.** H&E ×200, **D.** H&E ×100)

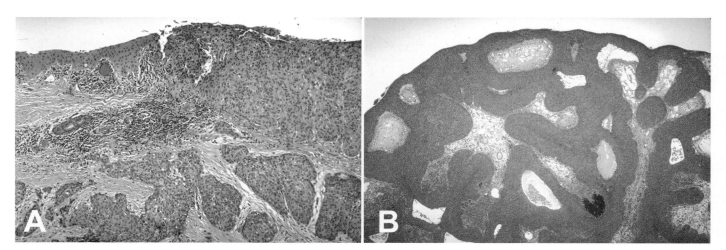

Fig. 5-19. A. Invasive squamous cell carcinoma, conjunctiva. Nests and islands of squamous cell carcinoma invade the substantia at right. The tumor cells have broken through the epithelial basement membrane. A characteristically abrupt junction separates the tumor from a segment of normal limbal conjunctiva at left. **B. Papillary squamous cell carcinoma *in situ*.** The epithelial component of exophytic papillary lesion is totally comprised of highly atypical squamous epithelium consistent with carcinoma *in situ*. (**A.** H&E ×50, **B.** H&E ×10)

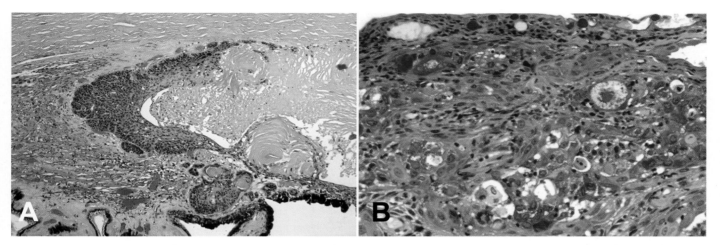

Fig. 5-20. A. **Anterior chamber invasion by conjunctival squamous cell carcinoma**. Tumor lines angle and iris surface and infiltrates iris stroma. Desquamated keratin fills the anterior chamber. B. **Mucoepidermoid carcinoma, conjunctiva.** PAS stain highlights focal mucin production by conjunctival carcinoma. Mucoepidermoid carcinoma of the conjunctiva can behave aggressively. (**A.** H&E ×50, **B.** PAS ×100)

or orbit occurs infrequently, but enucleation and orbital exenteration occasionally are required (Fig. 5-20A). Poorly differentiated spindle cell carcinomas or mucoepidermoid carcinomas of the conjunctiva can behave aggressively, as can tumors in immunosuppressed patients who have HIV/AIDS or have undergone organ transplantation. Mucoepidermoid carcinomas contain pools of mucous and goblet cells (Fig. 5-20B). Positive immunohistochemical stains for cytokeratin may be necessary to differentiate spindle cell carcinoma from other spindle cell tumors. The rare clear cell variant of mucoepidermoid carcinoma can be confused histopathologically with sebaceous carcinoma. **Hereditary benign intraepithelial dyskeratosis** (Witkop–Von Sallmann syndrome) is an autosomal

dominantly inherited trait characterized by keratinized plaques of hyperplastic epithelium that occur bilaterally in the bulbar conjunctiva and are associated with ocular injection (Fig. 5-21A). The disorder can also affect the buccal mucosa. The surface plaque of keratin is composed of round or oval dyskeratotic cells that are found throughout the thickened epithelium (Fig. 5-21B). The condition is always benign. Although cases have been reported elsewhere, most affected patients belong to a triracial isolate called the Haliwa-Saponi Indians from Halifax and Warren Counties in North Carolina. Visual loss occurs rarely when the disease affects the corneal epithelium. Affected patients have a duplication of two alleles in chromosome 4q35.

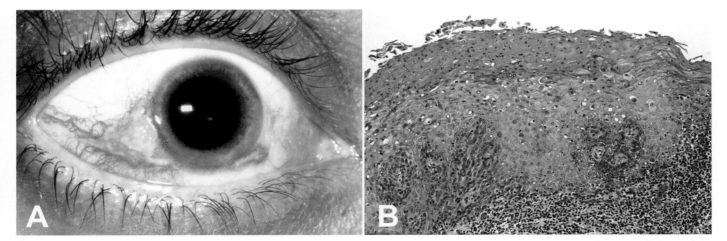

Fig. 5-21. **Hereditary benign intraepithelial dyskeratosis, conjunctiva. A.** Two leukoplakic lesions are present. The other eye and buccal mucosa also were involved. The patient traced her ancestry to Halifax County, North Carolina. (From Shields CL, Shields JS, et al. Hereditary benign intraepithelial dyskeratosis. *Arch Ophthalmol* 1987;105:422–423. Copyright 1987, American Medical Association.) **B. Hereditary benign intraepithelial dyskeratosis, conjunctiva.** Parakeratin plaque composed of plump dyskeratotic cells covers acanthotic epithelium. Single dyskeratotic cells are seen in the deeper part of the benign lesion. The underlying substantia propria contains a heavy infiltrate of lymphocytes. (**B.** H&E ×50)

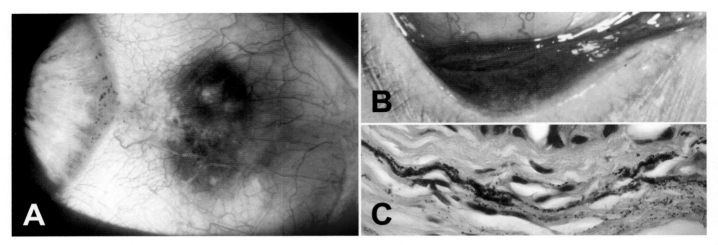

Fig. 5-22. A. Ochronosis. Brownish deposit of homogentisic acid discolors the sclera near the insertion of medial rectus tendon. A few globules of pigment are seen in the peripheral cornea. **B. Argyrosis, conjunctiva.** Chronic administration of silver-containing eye drops has caused grayish discoloration of forniceal conjunctiva. **C.** Photomicrograph shows deposition of silver granules in substantia propria. (**C.** H&E ×250)

PIGMENTED LESIONS OF THE CONJUNCTIVA

Most pigmented lesions of the conjunctiva are composed of melanocytes. Melanocytic lesions of the conjunctiva include racial melanosis, benign freckles and lentigines, several types of nevi, and malignant melanoma and its clinically important precursor primary acquired melanosis (PAM). Conjunctival pigmentation can develop in certain systemic diseases, such as Addison disease and ochronosis (Fig. 5-22A), or may be caused by systemic (phenothiazines, tetracycline) or topical drugs (epinephrine) or the deposition of metals, such as silver (argyrosis) (Fig. 5-22B).

Conjunctival freckles or **ephelides** are flat patches of pigmentation. Histopathology shows increased pigmentation of the epithelial basal cell layer. An identical picture is seen in **racial** or **constitutional melanosis** and in the early stages of PAM (Fig. 5-23).

Conjunctival nevi are benign hamartomatous tumors composed of modified melanocytes called nevus cells, which are derived embryologically from the neural crest (Figs. 5-24 and 5-25). Although nevi are considered to be congenital lesions, they often are detected towards the end of the second decade. Apparent growth and increased pigmentation of conjunctival nevi is often caused by elevated levels of hormones during puberty or pregnancy (Fig. 5-24). Excisional biopsy is usually performed for cosmetic reasons, or when apparent enlargement or the deepening of pigmentation raises concern about possible malignant transformation. Conjunctival nevi are the most common conjunctival tumor in children, comprising 64% of lesions in a large series by Shields. Fewer than 1% evolve into melanoma.

Conjunctival nevi are classified topographically based on the location of the nevus cells in relation to the epithelium. The nevus cells are located at the epithelial-subepithelial

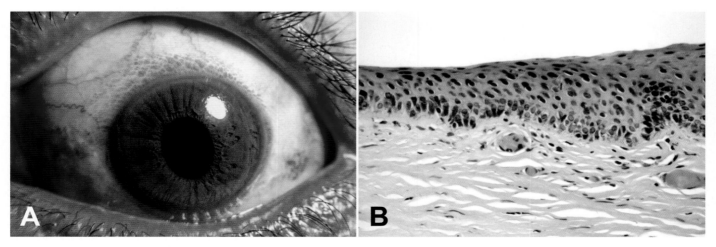

Fig. 5-23. Constitutional melanosis. A. Patchy conjunctival pigmentation occurred in both eyes of a dark-complexioned individual. **B.** Squamous epithelial cells contain melanin pigment. Atypical melanocytic hyperplasia is not present. (**B.** H&E ×100)

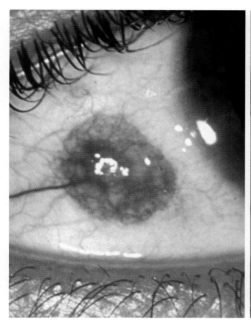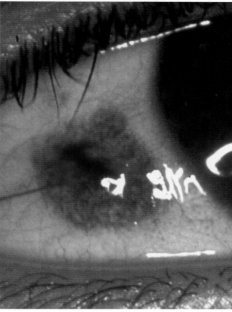

Fig. 5-24. Hormone-induced changes in conjunctival nevus. Compound cystic nevus was photographed at age 11 (**left**) and age 13 (**right**). Cytologically benign lesion appears larger and more intensely pigmented after menarche. The nevus contains multiple cysts.

junction in junctional nevi. Nevus cells are confined to the conjunctival stroma in subepithelial nevi, which are the counterpart of intradermal nevi in the skin. Most conjunctival nevi are compound nevi, which have both junctional and subepithelial components (Fig. 5-25). Junctional activity tends to decrease markedly with age. Junctional nevi are rare in childhood and almost never occur in adults. Hence, any lesion in an adult that appears to be a junctional nevus should be considered to be PAM until proven otherwise. Purely subepithelial nevi generally are found in older adults.

Microscopically, nevus cells often form aggregates called nests. Polarity may be present, that is, more superficial nevus cells tend to be larger, while cells deeper in the stroma tend to be smaller and may have a lymphocytoid appearance reflecting scanty cytoplasm. Bland multinucleated nevoid giant cells are seen in some cases.

Most compound conjunctival nevi are cystic; the nevus contains cystic invaginations and occasionally solid rests of conjunctival epithelium (Fig. 5-25). These intralesional microcysts can be seen with the slit lamp in some cases, an observation that can suggest the diagnosis clinically. The cysts tend to enlarge with age. The pigment content of conjunctival nevi varies markedly. Some nevi are dark brown; others are totally amelanotic and may appear pink if inflamed.

Blue nevi are composed of melanocytes that are located deep to the epithelium in the stroma or epibulbar tissues. Blue nevi are composed of bland dendriform melanocytes. A deep blue nevus that typically involves the deep stroma,

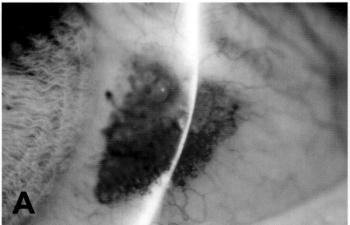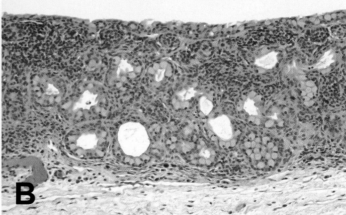

Fig. 5-25. Compound cystic nevus, conjunctiva. A. Slit beam highlights cysts in pigmented conjunctival nevus at the limbus. **B.** Lightly pigmented nevus contains characteristic cystic rests of conjunctival epithelium with goblet cells. Nevus cells are present at the junctional position and in the substantia propria. (**B.** H&E ×50)

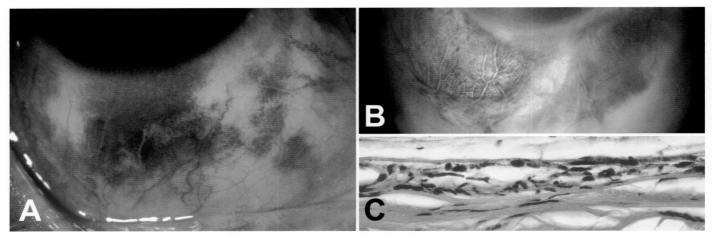

Fig. 5-26. Congenital ocular melanocytosis. A. Patchy, slate gray pigmentation is caused by dendriform melanocytes deep in epibulbar tissues beneath the conjunctiva. (Photograph courtesy of Dr. Jerry A. Shields, Wills Eye Institute.) **B.** Epibulbar pigment on the surface of the globe (above) appears brown where it is exposed by defect in the conjunctiva. Tyndall effect makes pigment beneath intact conjunctiva (**at right**) appear gray. The eye was obtained postmortem from a patient with Nevus of Ota who developed leptomeningeal melanoma. **C.** Photomicrograph shows dendritic melanocytes in epibulbar tissue. (**C.** H&E, ×100)

epibulbar connective tissue, and adnexal skin occurs in congenital oculodermal melanocytosis or the Nevus of Ota (Fig. 5-26). Patients with Ota nevus typically have congenital hyperchromic heterochromia iridum (involved eye darker) caused by a diffuse nevus of the ipsilateral uveal tract (Fig. 5-26A). White patients with oculodermal melanocytosis are at risk for uveal, orbital, and CNS malignant melanoma but not conjunctival melanoma. Blue nevi appear blue or slate gray in color because the longer wavelengths of light are absorbed or scattered as the light passes through the epithelium and connective tissue of the overlying conjunctiva (Fig. 5-26B). The conjunctiva moves freely over the deeply situated pigmented cells. If the conjunctival pigmentation moves, the pigment or pigmented cells are associated with the epithelium.

PRIMARY ACQUIRED MELANOSIS AND CONJUNCTIVAL MELANOMA

Although conjunctival melanomas can arise de novo, or from preexisting nevi, almost three fourths develop from a form of *in situ* atypical melanocytic proliferation called **primary acquired melanosis** or **PAM**. Clinically, PAM appears as patchy acquired unilateral pigmentation of the conjunctiva that usually affects middle-aged or elderly white individuals (Fig. 5-27A). The onset is insidious and the pigmentation may wax and wane. The acquired and unilateral nature of the pigmentation serves to distinguish PAM from racial melanosis that occurs bilaterally in heavily pigmented races. PAM can affect black patients, but this is exceedingly rare. About 20% of conjunctival lesions seen at an ocular oncology service were classified as PAM. Patches of conjunctival pigmentation consistent with PAM were found in more than one third (36%) of 146 white

patients over age 10 examined in a cornea clinic. Although PAM is relatively common, conjunctiva melanoma is rare, suggesting that the risk of malignant transformation has been overestimated in the past. A widely cited study from the Armed Forces Institute of Pathology (AFIP) reported that nearly one third of cases (31.7%) of PAM cases progressed to invasive melanoma. However, the authors cautioned that the incidence probably was skewed by referral bias. A more recent clinical study at the Wills Eye Institute Oncology Service found that only 4% of 311 patients with PAM progressed to melanoma. Malignant transformation occurred in 13% of patients who had histologically confirmed PAM with severe atypia. Multivariant analysis showed that the most significant risk factor for recurrence and progression to melanoma was the extent of the pigmentation in clock hours.

PAM is classified into benign and malignant variants on the basis of histopathological examination. Invasive malignant melanomas usually arise from PAM with severe atypia. PAM is classified as atypical if there is any degree of atypical melanocytic hyperplasia.

In **PAM without atypia**, pigment is confined to the conjunctival epithelial cells and there is no evidence of melanocytic hyperplasia, or an increased number of benign melanocytes is present. A benign lesion, PAM without atypia is indistinguishable histopathologically from racial melanosis or a freckle (Fig. 5-23).

Biopsies classified as PAM with mild atypia have atypical melanocytes that are confined to the basal layer of the epithelium in a single cell lentiginous pattern (Fig. 5-27B). Patients who have PAM with mild atypia are at relatively low risk for progression to invasive melanoma.

Atypia is classified as severe if atypical melanocytes are not confined to the basal cell layer of the epithelium and involve its more superficial layers, or form pagetoid

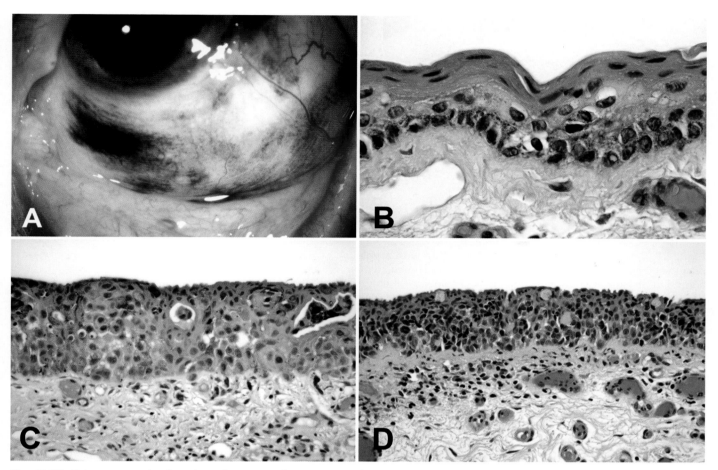

Fig. 5-27. Primary acquired melanosis. A. Patchy conjunctival pigmentation developed slowly in a middle-age white man. The pigment moved with the conjunctiva. PAM is an important precursor of conjunctival melanoma. (Photograph courtesy of Dr. Jerry A. Shields, Wills Eye Institute.) **B. PAM with mild-moderate atypia.** Atypical melanocytes are largely confined to basal part of epithelium. **C. PAM with severe atypia.** The thickened conjunctival epithelium is almost totally replaced by nests of atypical pigmented melanocytes that include epithelioid cells. Some would call this "melanoma *in situ*." **D. PAM with severe atypia, sine pigmento.** There is extensive replacement of the epithelium by atypical melanocytes. Little pigment is present. (**B.** H&E ×250, **C.** H&E ×100, **D.** H&E, ×50)

nests (Fig. 5-27C,D). Pagetoid involvement of the epithelium was associated with a 95% incidence of progression to melanoma in Folberg series from the AFIP. Epithelioid melanocytes are another criterion for **PAM with severe atypia**. Folberg reported that melanoma developed in 75% of cases with epithelioid cells. The term melanoma *in situ* has been proposed for extensive or full-thickness replacement of the epithelium.

Conjunctival melanocytic intraepithelial neoplasia (C-MIN) with or without atypia is a newly proposed alternate term for this disease spectrum. Analogous to the terminology CIN used for squamous lesions of the conjunctiva, C-MIN emphasizes that the atypical melanocytes are confined to the conjunctival epithelium by an intact basement membrane. The author believes that M-CIN might be a more appropriate term.

Invasive melanoma develops when the epithelial basement membrane is violated and a vertical growth phase into the substantia propria ensues. When the pathologist evaluates a biopsy of clinically pigmented conjunctiva, he or she must decide if the pigment is contained within squamous epithelial cells (which occurs in racial melanosis, freckles, and PAM without atypia) or whether an increased number of atypical melanocytes is present (atypical melanocytic hyperplasia). This distinction can be difficult using routine histopathology alone. Immunohistochemistry using melanocytic markers S-100 protein, Melan-A/MART-1, microphthalmia transcription factor (MITF), and melanoma-specific antigen HMB-45 serve as helpful diagnostic aids. Proliferation marker KI-67 can help to distinguish conjunctival nevi from melanoma by highlighting cycling cells.

Patients with PAM should be followed closely with photographic documentation and detailed clinical drawings. Periodic observation is recommended for lesions of the bulbar conjunctiva less than 1 clock hour in extent. Areas of conjunctiva that become thickened and are presumed to be melanoma should be carefully excised using

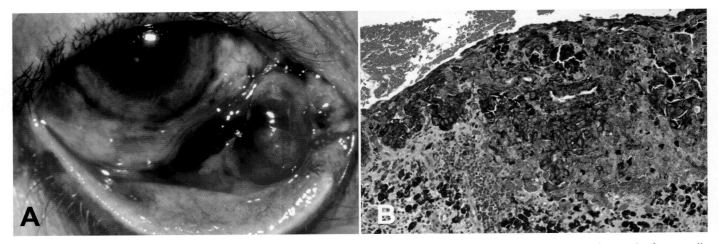

Fig. 5-28. Malignant melanoma arising from PAM with atypia. A. Several nodules of recurrent tumor are located inferonasally near the caruncle. Extensive PAM is present. The patient had a prior incisional biopsy elsewhere. (Photograph courtesy of Drs. Jerry and Carol Shields, Wills Eye Institute.) **B.** The conjunctival epithelium at left is totally replaced by atypical melanocytes. The cells have broken through the epithelial basement membrane forming an invasive malignant melanoma. About 75% of conjunctival melanomas appear to arise from PAM with atypia. (**B.** H&E ×50)

a no-touch technique. Multiple mapping biopsies to determine the extent of the disease have been recommended. Therapy is often challenging. Besides local excision of nodules, extensive cryotherapy and topical chemotherapy with agents such as mitomycin c have been advocated. Rarely, PAM may be totally amelanotic and inapparent clinically. A nodule of invasive melanoma usually is the presenting sign of PAM sine pigmento (Fig. 5-27D).

Conjunctival melanomas are relatively rare tumors (Fig. 5-28). There are about ten uveal melanomas for every conjunctival melanoma in the Registry of Ophthalmic Pathology at the AFIP. Although its behavior is unpredictable, conjunctival melanoma has a better prognosis than uveal melanoma of the ciliary body or choroid. The overall mortality is about 26%. Most (75%) conjunctival melanomas appear to arise from PAM with atypia. Some patients do have a history of an antecedent presumed or biopsy-confirmed conjunctival nevus. Remnants of a nevus are found histopathologically in about one fourth of cases. Some conjunctival melanomas arise de novo.

Conjunctival melanomas do not behave like uveal tumors. Although they do contain spindle and epithelioid cells, the Callender classification for uveal melanoma is not applicable to them. In contrast to uveal melanoma that metastasizes hematogenously to the liver, conjunctival melanomas initially spread to regional lymph nodes, usually the preauricular or intraparotid nodes. The tumor cells then gain access to blood vessels via anastomoses between vessels and lymphatics in the nodes. Factors associated with poorer prognosis include extralimbal tumor location, nasal location, caruncular involvement, involvement of surgical margins, and de novo melanomas without PAM. Several studies have found that inadequate initial surgical management including incisional biopsy and incomplete excision increases risks of local recurrence and metastatic death.

Wide microsurgical excisional biopsy using the "no-touch" technique and supplemental alcohol corneal epitheliectomy and conjunctival cryotherapy is advised. Orbital exenteration is required in 15% to 20% of cases when recurrent malignant melanoma invades the orbit. Such radical surgical therapy probably does not improve prognosis for life but may be necessary to debulk the tumor and relieve local symptoms. Sentinel lymph node biopsy has been recommended for patients with conjunctival melanoma, but its effect on survival is uncertain.

LYMPHOID TUMORS

A spectrum of lymphoid tumors that includes reactive follicular hyperplasias, atypical lymphoid hyperplasias, and malignant lymphomas occurs in the conjunctiva (Fig. 5-29). Many of the lymphomas are low-grade non-Hodgkin B cell tumors of the MALT (mucosa-associated lymphoid tissue) type.

Conjunctival lymphoid tumors typically present as a salmon-colored patch or infiltrate in the fornix or on the epibulbar surface of the globe (Fig. 5-29A,C). The salmon pink color reflects the lesion's fine vascularity. Conjunctival lymphoid tumors cause few symptoms because they lack a connective tissue stroma, are soft and elastic, and mold to the surrounding tissues. They typically are covered by an intact layer of conjunctival epithelium. In MALT lymphoma, the epithelium often contains an infiltrate of lymphocytes (lymphoepithelial lesion.

Lymphoid infiltrates can diffusely involve the substantia propria, or the surface of lesions may be pebbly and multinodular (Fig. 5-29A). The latter pattern typically is seen in follicular hyperplasia or rare cases of follicular lymphoma. In some instances, a conjunctival salmon patch actually may be on the anterior tip of an orbital lymphoid tumor.

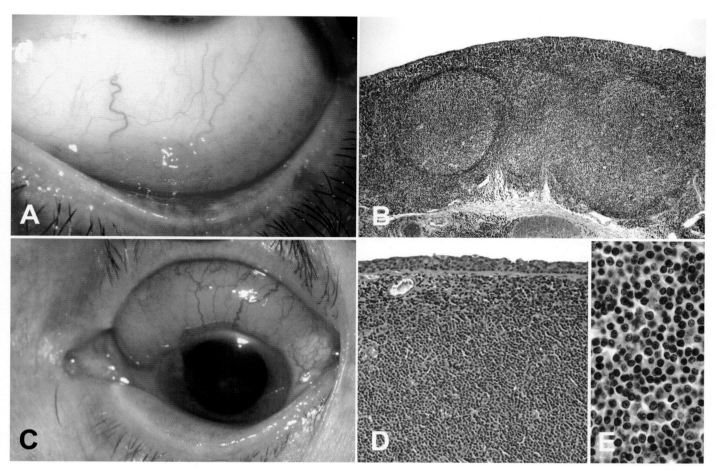

Fig. 5-29. Lymphoid lesions. A. Follicular lymphoid hyperplasia, conjunctiva. Infiltrate in inferior fornix has pebbly surface and salmon color. **B.** Intense stromal infiltrate of benign lymphoid cells comprising follicular hyperplasia contains germinal centers. **C. Malignant lymphoma.** Diffuse "salmon patch" covers the superior part of the globe. **D. Low-grade MALT lymphoma, conjunctiva.** Substantia propria contains diffuse infiltrate of well-differentiated lymphocytes, seen at higher magnification in figure **E**. Flow cytometric analysis disclosed a monoclonal proliferation of B lymphocytes that were expressed CD20 and were negative for CD5 and CD10. Many conjunctival lymphomas are low-grade non-Hodgkin B-cell tumors of the MALT (mucosa-associated lymphoid tissue) type. (**B.** H&E ×25, **D.** H&E ×50, **E.** H&E ×250)

Orbital involvement should be excluded with imaging if it is unclear whether a lesion is purely conjunctival, because orbital lesions have a higher incidence of associated systemic disease.

Histopathologically, **follicular lymphoid hyperplasia** (often called benign reactive lymphoid hyperplasia) is a polymorphous infiltrate composed of mature well-differentiated lymphocytes, often admixed with plasma cells, that contains benign reactive lymphoid follicles or germinal centers (Fig. 5-29B). The reactive follicles are composed of large, pale, mitotically active immunoblasts and harbor tingible body macrophages that contain basophilic bodies of apoptotic nuclear debris. These macrophages process antigens and present it to helper T cells to initiate the immune response. Immunohistochemical stains disclose CD20-positive B lymphocytes in the follicular centers and the surrounding mantle zone. Antiapoptotic Bcl-2 protein normally is absent in the reactive follicles. CD3 positive T cells predominate in the interfollicular zone between the germinal centers.

Most lymphomas of the ocular adnexa are diffuse non-Hodgkin B-cell lymphomas composed largely of a single clone of B lymphocytes that express either kappa or lamda light chains. Clonality is best assessed by flow cytometric analysis of fresh tissue because light chains are labile and usually are destroyed during routine tissue processing. If lymphoma is suspected clinically and a sufficient quantity of fresh, unfixed tissue is available, part should be submitted for flow cytometry. If this is impossible, immunohistochemistry performed on routine paraffin sections usually can establish the diagnosis of lymphoma and classify it as to type. A relatively small panel of antibodies directed against lymphocytic markers CD3, CD5, CD10, CD20, and CD23 often suffices. This occasionally is supplemented with CD43, bcl-2, and cyclin D1. In some cases, gene rearrangement studies are necessary.

B-cell lymphoma cells express immunohistochemical B-cell marker CD20. Demonstration that a lymphoid infiltrated is composed largely of CD20-positive B lymphocytes

Fig. 5-30. Oncocytoma, caruncle. A. Benign cystadenomatous tumor deep in the caruncle is composed of tall bland epithelial cells with copious eosinophilic cytoplasm seen at higher magnification in inset (**B**). The association of conjunctival epithelium with pilosebaceous units identifies the area as the caruncle. (**Main**, H&E ×25, **inset**, H&E ×250)

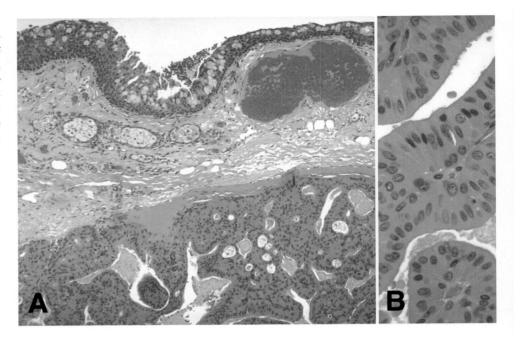

provides circumstantial evidence that it is a lymphoma because chronic inflammatory infiltrates are composed largely of T lymphocytes that stain with T-cell markers such as CD3 and CD5.

Most conjunctival lymphomas are low-grade **extranodal marginal zone lymphomas (EMZL) of mucosa-associated lymphoid tissue** (often called MALT lymphomas) (Fig. 5-29D,E). EMZL comprised more than half (51.6%) of lymphomas in a recent large series of ocular adnexal lymphoid lesions. The cells of MALT lymphomas are CD20 positive but are negative for CD3, CD5, CD10, and CD23. Less often, the conjunctiva is involved by follicular, mantle zone and diffuse large B-cell lymphomas and chronic lymphocytic leukemia/small lymphocytic lymphoma. The latter can be distinguished by morphologic features and characteristic patterns of immunoreactivity.

Conjunctival lymphoma generally has an excellent prognosis. Systematized lymphoma rarely presents in the conjunctiva; most cases are stage IE on presentation. Lymphoma confined to the conjunctiva is associated with systemic lymphoma (prior, concurrent, or subsequent) in about 20% of cases. The 31% incidence of associated systemic disease in 117 cases of conjunctival lymphoid lesions in a recent study probably reflects the inclusion of a significant number (18%) of cases that had concurrent involvement of the orbit or eyelid in addition to a conjunctival salmon patch. In that study, systemic lymphoma was more likely if both conjunctivae were involved or if the tumor involved an extralimbal location.

Treatment depends on whether the disease is localized to the conjunctiva or if systemic lymphoma is present. If a patient has systemic lymphoma, the conjunctival lesion generally responds to systemic chemotherapy. Most patients with localized conjunctival disease are treated with low-dose external beam radiotherapy. Recently, intralesional interferon and systemic rituximab, which avoid the complications of radiotherapy, have been used to treat low-grade primary conjunctival lesions with some success. The role of *Helicobacter pylori* and *Chlamydia psittaci* in conjunctival MALT lymphoma remains controversial.

CARUNCULAR LESIONS

The caruncle is a small nodular island of skin surrounded by conjunctiva near the medial canthus. It is covered by keratinized epithelium and contains sweat glands, fat, accessory lacrimal glands, and pilosebaceous units with delicate hairs. Caruncular masses include nevi, papillomas, senile sebaceous gland hyperplasia, inclusion cysts, and **oncocytomas**. The latter are composed of modified glandular epithelial cells with copious amounts of eosinophilic cytoplasm replete with mitochondria (Fig. 5-30). Rare cases of sebaceous carcinoma arise from the glands of the pilosebaceous units in the caruncle.

BIBLIOGRAPHY

Developmental Lesions

Cunha RP, Cunha MC, Shields JA. Epibulbar tumors in children: a survey of 282 biopsies. *J Pediatr Ophthalmol Strabismus* 1987;24:249–254.

Dreizen NG, Schachat AP, Shields JA, et al. Epibulbar osseous choristoma. *J Pediatr Ophthalmol Strabismus* 1983;20:247–249.

Eijpe AA, Koornneef L, Bras J, et al. Dermolipoma: characteristic CT appearance. *Doc Ophthalmol* 1990;74:321–328.

Elsas FJ, Green WR. Epibulbar tumors in childhood. *Am J Ophthalmol* 1975;79:1001–1007.

Gonnering RS, Fuerste FH, Lemke BN, et al. Epibulbar osseous choristomas with scleral involvement. *Ophthal Plast Reconstr Surg* 1988;4:63–66.

Lucarelli MJ, Ceisler EJ, Talamo JH, et al. Complex choristoma. *Arch Ophthalmol* 1996;114:498–499.

Melki TS, Zimmerman LE, Chavis RM, et al. A unique epibulbar osseous choristoma. *J Pediatr Ophthalmol Strabismus* 1990;27: 252–254.

Oakman JH Jr, Lambert SR, Grossniklaus HE. Corneal dermoid: case report and review of classification. *J Pediatr Ophthalmol Strabismus* 1993;30:388–391.

Pittke EC, Marquardt R, Mohr W. Cartilage choristoma of the eye. *Arch Ophthalmol* 1983;101:1569–1571.

Pokorny KS, Hyman BM, Jakobiec FA, et al. Epibulbar choristomas containing lacrimal tissue. Clinical distinction from dermoids and histologic evidence of an origin from the palpebral lobe. *Ophthalmology* 1987;94:1249–1257.

Roth DB, Shields JA, Shields CL, et al. Lacrimal gland choristoma of the conjunctiva simulating a squamous cell carcinoma. *J Pediatr Ophthalmol Strabismus* 1994;31:62–64.

Shields JA, Eagle RC, Shields CL, et al. Epibulbar osseous choristoma. Computed tomography and clinicopathologic correlation. *Ophthalmic Practice* 1997;15:110–112.

Shields JA, Shields CL, Eagle RC Jr, et al. Ophthalmic features of the organoid nevus syndrome. *Trans Am Ophthalmol Soc* 1996;94:65–86.

Sugar HS. The oculoauriculo-vertebral syndrome of Goldenhar. *Am J Ophthalmol* 1966;62:678–682.

Conjunctivitis

Allansmith MR, Baird RS, Greiner JV. Vernal conjunctivitis and contact lens-associated giant papillary conjunctivitis compared and contrasted. *Am J Ophthalmol* 1979;87:544–555.

Dawson CR, Jones BR, Tarizzo ML. *Guide to Trachoma Control.* Geneva, Switzerland: World Health Organization, 1981:7.

Eagle RC Jr, Brooks SJS, Katowitz JA, et al. Fibrin as a major constituent of ligneous conjunctivitis. (Letter.) *Am J Ophthalmol* 1986;101:493.

Foster CS. The pathophysiology of ocular allergy: current thinking. *Allergy* 1995;50:6–9, discussion 34–38.

Hidayat AA, Riddle PJ. Ligneous conjunctivitis. A clinicopathologic study of 17 cases. *Ophthalmology* 1987;94:949–959.

Leonardi A. Vernal keratoconjunctivitis: pathogenesis and treatment. *Prog Retin Eye Res* 2002;21:319–339.

MacCallan AF. The epidemiology of trachoma. *Br J Ophthalmol* 1931;15:369–411.

Schuster V, Mingers AM, Seidenspinner S, et al. Homozygous mutations in the plasminogen gene of two unrelated girls with ligneous conjunctivitis. *Blood* 1997;90:958–966.

Trocme SD, Kephart GM, Allansmith MR, et al. Conjunctival deposition of eosinophil granule major basic protein in vernal keratoconjunctivitis and contact lens-associated giant papillary conjunctivitis. *Am J Ophthalmol* 1989;108:57–63.

Granulomatous Conjunctivitis

Bergmans AM, Groothedde JW, Schellekens JF, et al. Etiology of cat scratch disease: comparison of polymerase chain reaction detection of *Bartonella* (formerly *Rochalimaea*) and *Afipia felis* DNA with serology and skin tests. *J Infect Dis* 1995;171:916–923.

Lee WR, Chawla JC, Reid R. Bacillary angiomatosis of the conjunctiva. *Am J Ophthalmol* 1994;118:152–157.

Margo CE, Hamed LM. Ocular Syphilis. *Surv Ophthalmol* 1992;37:203–220.

Nichols CW, Eagle RC Jr, Yanoff M, et al. Conjunctival biopsy as an aid in the evaluation of the patient with suspected sarcoidosis. *Ophthalmology* 1980;87:287–291.

Obenauf CD, Shaw HE, Wyndor CF, et al. Sarcoidosis and its ocular manifestations. *Am J Ophthalmol* 1978;86:648–655.

Spektor FE, Eagle RC Jr, Nichols CW. Granulomatous conjunctivitis secondary to *Treponema pallidum*. *Ophthalmology* 1981;88: 863–865.

Wear DJ, Raga HM, Zimmerman LE, et al. Cat scratch disease bacilli in the conjunctiva of patients with Parinaud's oculoglandular syndrome. *Ophthalmology* 1985;92:1282–1287.

Weinberg JC, Eagle RC Jr, Font RL, et al. Conjunctival synthetic fiber granuloma: a lesion that resembles conjunctivitis nodosa. *Ophthalmology* 1984;91:867–872.

Parasitic and Mycotic Infections

Ashton N, Cook C. Allergic granulomatous nodules of the eyelid and conjunctiva. The XXXV Edward Jackson Memorial Lecture. *Am J Ophthalmol* 1978;87:1–28.

Connor DH, Neafie RC, Meyers WM. Loiasis. In: Binford CH, Connor DH, eds. *Pathology of Tropical and Extraordinary Diseases.* Washington, DC: Armed Forces Institute of Pathology, 1976.

Diesenhouse MC, Wilson LA, Corrent GF, et al. Treatment of microsporidial keratoconjunctivitis with topical fumagillin. *Am J Ophthalmol* 1993;115:293–298.

Friedberg DN, Stenson SM, Orenstein JM, et al. Microsporidial keratoconjunctivitis is acquired immunodeficiency syndrome. *Arch Ophthalmol* 1990;108:504–508.

Reidy JJ, Sudesh S, Klafter AB, et al. Infection of the conjunctiva by *Rhinosporidium seeberi*. *Surv Ophthalmol* 1997;41:409–413.

Ruggli GM, Weber R, Messmer EP, et al. *Pneumocystis carinii* infection of the conjunctiva in a patient with acquired immune deficiency syndrome. *Ophthalmology* 1997;104:1853–1856.

Ocular Cicatricial Pemphigoid

Mondino BJ, Ross AN, Rabin BS. Autoimmune phenomena in ocular cicatricial pemphigoid. *Am J Ophthalmol* 1977;83:443–450.

Power WJ, Neves RA, Rodriguez A, et al. Increasing the diagnostic yield of conjunctival biopsy in patients with suspected ocular cicatricial pemphigoid. *Ophthalmology* 1995;102:1158–1163.

Sacks EH, Jakobiec FA, Wieczorek R, et al. Immunophenotypic analysis of the inflammatory infiltrate in ocular cicatricial pemphigoid: further evidence for a T cell-mediated disease. *Ophthalmology* 1989;96:236–243.

Tyagi S, Bhol K, Natarajan K, et al. Ocular cicatricial pemphigoid antigen: partial sequence and biochemical characterization. *Proc Natl Acad Sci U S A* 1996;93:14714–14719.

Amyloidosis

Blodi FC, Apple DJ. Localized conjunctival amyloidosis. *Am J Ophthalmol* 1979;88:346–350.

Demirci H, Shields CL, Eagle RC Jr, et al. Conjunctival amyloidosis: report of six cases and review of the literature. *Surv Ophthalmol* 2006;51:419–33.

Knowles DM, Jakobiec FA, Rosen M, et al. Amyloidosis of the orbit and adnexae. *Surv Ophthalmol* 1975;19:367–384.

O'Donnell B, Wuebbolt G, Collin R. Amyloidosis of the conjunctiva. *Aust N Z J Ophthalmol* 1995;23:207–212.

Conjunctival Tumors

Grossniklaus HE, Green WR, Luckenbach M, et al. Conjunctival lesions in adults. A clinical and histopathologic review. *Cornea* 1987;6:78–116.

McLean IW, Burnier MN, Zimmerman LE, et al. *Tumors of the Eye and Ocular Adnexa, Atlas of Tumor Pathology, Third Series*, Fascicle 12. Washington, DC: Armed Forces Institute of Pathology, 1994.

Seitz B, Fischer M, Holbach LM, et al. Differential diagnosis and prognosis of 112 excised epibulbar epithelial tumors. *Klin Monatsbl Augenheilkd* 1995;207:239–246.

Shields CL, Shields JA. Tumors of the conjunctiva and cornea. *Surv Ophthalmol* 2004;49:3–24.

Shields CL, Demirci H, Karatza E, et al. Clinical survey of 1643 melanocytic and nonmelanocytic conjunctival tumors. *Ophthalmology* 2004;111:1747–1754.

Shields CL, Shields JA. Conjunctival tumors in children. *Curr Opin Ophthalmol* 2007;18:351–360.

Shields JA, Shields CL, De Potter P. Surgical management of conjunctival tumors. The 1994 Lynn B. McMahan Lecture. *Arch Ophthalmol* 1997;115:808–815.

Squamous Epithelial Tumors

Brown HH, Glasgow BJ, Holland GN, et al. Keratinizing corneal intraepithelial neoplasia. *Cornea* 1989;8:220–224.

Cohen B, Green WR, Iliff N, et al. Spindle cell carcinoma of the conjunctiva. *Arch Ophthalmol* 1980;98:1809–1813.

Erie JC, Liesegang TJ, Campbell RJ. Conjunctival and corneal intraepithelial neoplasia: experience at the Mayo Clinic 1920–1983. *Ophthalmology* 1986;93:176–183.

Illif WF, Marbeck R, Green WR. Invasive squamous cell carcinoma of the conjunctiva. *Arch Ophthalmol* 1975;93:119–122.

Kapur R, Sugar J, Edward DP. Conjunctival mucoepidermoid carcinoma: clear cell variant. *Arch Ophthalmol* 2005;123:1265–1268.

Lass JH, Grove AS, Papale JJ, et al. Detection of human papillomavirus DNA sequences in conjunctival papillomas. *Am J Ophthalmol* 1983;95:670–674.

Lee GA, Hirst LW. Ocular surface squamous neoplasia. *Surv Ophthalmol* 1995;39:429–450.

Mauriello JA Jr, Napolitano J, McLean I. Actinic keratosis and dysplasia of the conjunctiva: a clinicopathological study of 45 cases. *Can J Ophthalmol* 1995;30:312–316.

McDonnell JM, McDonnell PJ, Sun YY. Human papillomavirus DNA in tissues and ocular surface swabs of patients with conjunctival epithelial neoplasia. *Invest Ophthalmol Vis Sci* 1992;33:184–189.

Odrich MG, Jakobiec FA, Lancaster WD, et al. A spectrum of bilateral squamous conjunctival tumors associated with human papillomavirus type 16. *Ophthalmology* 1991;98:628–635.

Pizzarello LD, Jakobiec FA. Bowen's disease of the conjunctiva: a misnomer. In: Jakobiec FA, ed. *Ocular and Adnexal Tumors.* Birmingham, AL: Aesculapius, 1978:553–571.

Rao NA, Font RL. Mucoepidermoid carcinoma of the conjunctiva: a clinicopathologic study of five cases. *Cancer* 1976;38:1699–1709.

Schubert HD, Farris RL, Green WR. Spindle cell carcinoma of the conjunctiva. *Graefes Arch Clin Exp Ophthalmol* 1995;233:52–53.

Sjo NC, Heegaard S, Prause JU, et al. Human papillomavirus in conjunctival papilloma. *Br J Ophthalmol* 2001;85:785–787.

Waring GO, Roth AM, Ekins MB. Clinical and pathologic description of 17 cases of corneal intraepithelial neoplasia. *Am J Ophthalmol* 1984;97:547–559.

Melanocytic Lesions

Brownstein S, Jakobiec FA, Wilkinson RD, et al. Cryotherapy for precancerous melanosis (atypical melanocytic hyperplasia) of the conjunctiva. *Arch Ophthalmol* 1981;99:1224–1231.

Busam KJ, Chen YT, Old LJ, et al. Expression of melan-A (MART1) in benign melanocytic nevi and primary cutaneous malignant melanoma. *Am J Surg Pathol* 1998;22:976–982.

Chowers I, Livni N, Solomon A, et al. MIB-1 and PC-10 immunostaining for the assessment of proliferative activity in primary acquired melanosis without and with atypia. *Br J Ophthalmol* 1998;82:1316–1319.

Damato B, Coupland SE. Clinical mapping of conjunctival melanomas. *Br J Ophthalmol* 2008;92:1545–1549.

Damato B, Coupland SE. Conjunctival melanoma and melanosis: a reappraisal of terminology, classification and staging. *Clin Experiment Ophthalmol* 2008;36:786–795.

Damato B, Coupland SE. An audit of conjunctival melanoma treatment in Liverpool. *Eye (Lond)* 2009;23:801–809.

De Potter P, Shields CL, Shields JA, et al. Clinical predictive factors for development of recurrence and metastasis in conjunctival melanoma: a review of 68 cases. *Br J Ophthalmol* 1993;77:624–630.

Dutton JJ, Anderson RL, Schelper RL, et al. Orbital malignant melanoma and oculodermal melanocytosis. Report of two cases and a review of the literature. *Ophthalmology* 1984;91:497–507.

Folberg R, Jakobiec FA, Bernardino VB, et al. Benign conjunctival melanocytic lesions: clinicopathologic features. *Ophthalmology* 1989;96:436–461.

Folberg R, Jakobiec FA, McLean IW, et al. Is primary acquired melanosis of the conjunctiva equivalent to melanoma in situ? *Mod Pathol* 1992;5:2–5, discussion 6–8.

Folberg R, McLean IW, Zimmerman LE. Conjunctival melanosis and melanoma. *Ophthalmology* 1984;91:673–678.

Folberg R, McLean IW, Zimmerman LE. Primary acquired melanosis of the conjunctiva. *Hum Pathol* 1985;16:129–135.

Folberg R, McLean IW, Zimmerman LE. Malignant melanoma of the conjunctiva. *Hum Pathol* 1985;16:136–143.

Jakobiec FA. The ultrastructure of conjunctival melanocytic tumors. *Trans Am Ophthalmol Soc* 1984;82:599–752.

Jakobiec FA, Folberg R, Iwamoto T. Clinicopathologic characteristics of premalignant and malignant melanocytic lesions of the conjunctiva. *Ophthalmology* 1989;96:147–166.

Jakobiec FA, Rini FJ, Fraunfelder FT, et al. Cryotherapy for conjunctival primary acquired melanosis and malignant melanoma. *Opthalmology* 1988;95:1058–1070.

Liesegang TJ. Pigmented conjunctival and scleral lesions. *Mayo Clin Proc* 1994;69:151–161.

Liesegang TJ, Campbell RJ. Mayo Clinic experience with conjunctival melanomas. *Arch Ophthalmol* 1980;98:1385–389.

McDonnell JM, Sun YY, Wagner D. HMB-45 immunohistochemical staining of conjunctival melanocytic lesions. *Ophthalmology* 1991;98:453–458.

Paridaens AD, McCartney AC, Hungerford JL. Multifocal amelanotic conjunctival melanoma and acquired melanosis sine pigmento. *Br J Ophthalmol* 1992;76:163–165.

Paridaens AD, Minassian DC, McCartney AC, et al. Prognostic factors in primary malignant melanoma of the conjunctiva: a clinicopathological study of 256 cases. *Br J Ophthalmol* 1994;78:252–259.

Shields CL, Shields JA. Conjunctival tumors in children. *Curr Opin Ophthalmol* 2007;18:351–360.

Shields JA, Shields CL, Mashayekhi A, et al. Primary acquired melanosis of the conjunctiva: risks for progression to melanoma in 311 eyes: the 2006 Lorenz E. Zimmerman lecture. *Ophthalmology* 2007;115:511–519.

Lymphoid Lesions

Cohen VM, Sweetenham J, Singh AD. Ocular adnexal lymphoma. What is the evidence for an infectious aetiology? *Br J Ophthalmol* 2008;92:446–448.

Coupland SE, Damato B. Lymphomas involving the eye and the ocular adnexa. *Curr Opin Ophthalmol* 2006;17:523–531.

Coupland SE, Krause L, Delecluse HJ, et al. Lymphoproliferative lesions of the ocular adnexa. Analysis of 112 cases. *Ophthalmology* 1998;105:1430–1441.

Ferry JA, Fung CY, Zukerberg L, et al. Lymphoma of the ocular adnexa: a study of 353 cases. *Am J Surg Pathol* 2007;31:170–184.

Jakobiec FA. Ocular adnexal lymphoid tumors: progress in need of clarification. *Am J Ophthalmol* 2008;145:941–950.

Knowles DM, Jakobiec FA, McNally L, et al. Lymphoid hyperplasia and malignant lymphoma occurring in the ocular adnexa (orbit, conjunctiva, and eyelids): a prospective multiparametric analysis of 108 cases during 1977 to 1987. *Hum Pathol* 1990;21:959–973.

Margo CE. Orbital and ocular adnexal lymphoma: evolving concepts. In: Grossniklaus HE, Margo CE, eds. *Advances in Ophthalmic Pathology. Ophthalmol Clin North Am* 1995;8:167–177.

Medeiros LJ, Harris NL. Immunuhistologic analysis of small lymphocytic infiltrates of the orbit and conjunctiva. *Hum Pathol* 1990;21:1126–1131.

Shields CL, Shields JA, Carvalho C, et al. Conjunctival lymphoid tumors: clinical analysis of 117 cases and relationship to systemic lymphoma. *Ophthalmology* 2001;108(5):979–984.

Miscellaneous Lesions

Kiratli H, Shields CL, Shields JA, et al. Metastatic tumours to the conjunctiva: report of 10 cases. *Br J Ophthalmol* 1996;80:5–8.

Margo CE, Grossniklaus HE. Intraepithelial sebaceous neoplasia without underlying invasive carcinoma. *Surv Ophthalmol* 1995;39:293–301.

Tumors of the Caruncle

Chang WJ, Nowinski TS, Eagle RC Jr. A large oncocytoma of the caruncle. *Arch Ophthalmol* 1995;113:382.

Hirsch C, Holz FG, Tetz M, et al. Clinical aspects and histopathology of caruncular tumors. *Klin Monatsbl Augenheilkd* 1997;210: 153–157.

Massry GG, Holds JB, Kincaid MC, et al. Sebaceous gland hyperplasia of the caruncle. *Ophthal Plast Reconstr Surg* 1995;11:32–36.

Rodman RC, Frueh BR, Elner VM. Mucoepidermoid carcinoma of the caruncle. *Am J Ophthalmol* 1997;123:564–565.

Shields CL, Shields JA, White D, et al. Survey of lesions of the caruncle. *Trans Pa Acad Ophthalmol Otolaryngol* 1986;38:528–534.

6 Cornea and Sclera

CORNEAL HISTOLOGY

The cornea is the principal refractive element of the eye. Its anterior surface is covered by a layer of nonkeratinized stratified squamous epithelium five or six cells in thickness. The inconspicuous basement membrane of the epithelium rests on Bowman membrane, a feltwork of modified stroma. The bulk of the cornea is composed of paucicellular collagenous stroma that contains keratocytes and artifactual clefts. The posterior surface of the cornea is lined by the corneal endothelial cells. This delicate monolayer of cells rests on a thick Periodic acid-Schiff (PAS)-positive basement membrane called Descemet membrane, which it secretes (Fig. 1-8).

DEVELOPMENTAL ANOMALIES

The corneal epithelium is derived embryologically from surface ectoderm. The corneal endothelium and stroma are derived from successive waves of migrating neural crest cells.

Developmental anomalies of the cornea include microcornea, defined as <11 mm in greatest diameter, and megalocornea, which is >13 mm. Cornea plana is a bilateral familial trait (autosomal dominant or recessive) characterized by corneal flattening and peripheral opacification. The cornea in sclerocornea resembles sclera. The epithelium is thickened, Bowman membrane is absent, and the

anterior third of the stroma is scarred and vascularized. Solid dermoids and complex choristomas are discussed in Chapter 5.

The **Axenfeld-Reiger syndrome** is a spectrum of developmental anomalies that affects the peripheral cornea, the iris, and the angle and has associated systemic findings. In the past, the terms angle cleavage syndrome and mesodermal dysgenesis were commonly applied to this disorder. Axenfeld-Reiger syndrome is important because about half of affected patients develop glaucoma. Prominence and anterior displacement of Schwalbe line into clear cornea, which is called posterior embryotoxon of Axenfeld, occurs in many patients (Fig. 6-1). Processes of iris stroma often bridge the angle and insert onto the posterior embryotoxon (Axenfeld anomaly). Patients may have iris stromal abnormalities including hypoplasia, and slit, multiple (polycoria), and false pupils (pseudocoria).

Axenfeld-Rieger syndrome is inherited as an autosomal dominant trait. Mutations in the FOXC1, PITX2, and RIEG2 genes have been found in the syndrome. Affected patients can have developmental defects of the face (maxillary hypoplasia) and teeth (anodontia, oligodontia, microdontia, and peg-like incisors) and redundant periumbilical skin. Shields has postulated that the ocular abnormalities in Axenfeld-Rieger syndrome are consistent with a developmental arrest, occurring late in gestation, of certain anterior ocular structures derived from neural crest.

Congenital corneal opacities occur in **Peters anomaly**, a developmental anomaly characterized by a concave

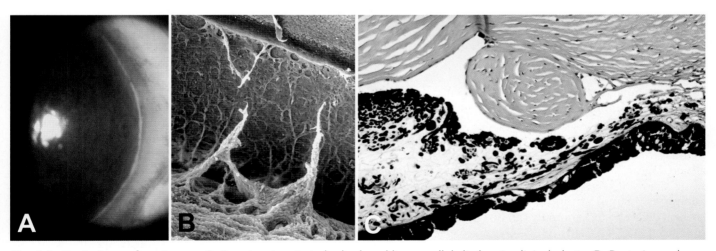

Fig. 6-1. Posterior embryotoxon. A. Prominent, anteriorly displaced line parallels limbus in clinical photo. **B.** Posterior embryotoxon is seen as ridge separating corneal endothelium and trabecular meshwork in scanning electron micrograph of infant eye. Ruptured iris processes bridge angle to embryotoxon. **C.** Large oval mound of connective tissue is interposed between the end of Descemet membrane (Schwalbe line) and the trabecular meshwork. This infant had multiple anterior segment anomalies. (**B.** SEM ×20, **C.** H&E ×50)

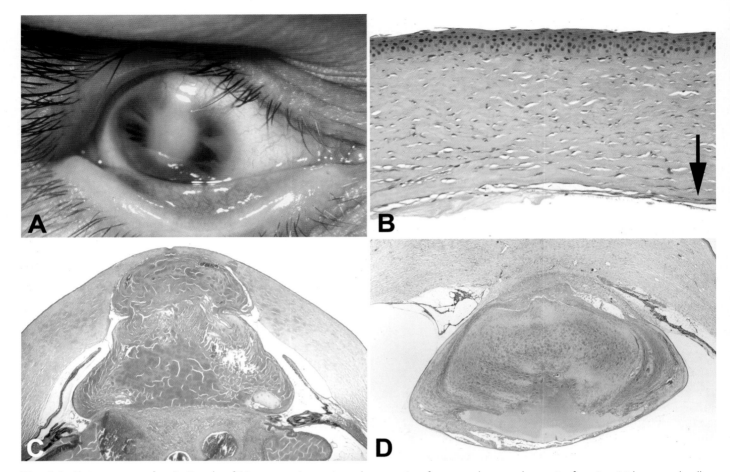

Fig. 6-2. Peters anomaly. A. Bands of iris stroma insert into the margin of a central corneal opacity forming iridocorneal adhesions. The lens was adherent to the posterior cornea centrally. Both eyes were affected. (Photo courtesy of Dr. Irving Raber, Wills Eye Institute.) **B.** The endothelium and Descemet membrane are absent in the region of a central "posterior ulcer." *Arrow* denotes Descemet membrane at margin. The collagenous lamellae of the posterior stroma are thickened and irregular. Bowman membrane is absent and the epithelium is mildly thickened. A central corneal opacity was present clinically. **C.** Keratolenticular adhesion. Lens adheres to large defect in center of cornea. **D.** Peters anomaly with keratolenticular adhesion in child with fetal alcohol syndrome. The cataractous crystalline lens adheres to a posterior ulcer in the central cornea. The iris also attaches to the margin of the ulcer. (Case courtesy of Dr. Nongnart Chan, Philadelphia, Pennsylvania.) (**B.** H&E ×50, **C.** H&E ×10, **D.** H&E ×25)

defect in the central cornea that includes posterior stroma, Descemet membrane, and endothelium (Fig. 6-2). Histopathology shows a central concave defect in the posterior corneal stroma that often contains thickened abnormal lamellae. The endothelium and Descemet membrane are absent within the posterior ulcer, and there is a corresponding area of stromal edema and opacification. Bowman layer may be thickened or absent. The crystalline lens adheres to or is incarcerated within the posterior ulcer in some cases of Peters anomaly, and (Fig. 6-2C,D) iridocorneal adhesions often insert into the periphery of the posterior corneal defect. Peters anomaly can be caused by mutations in PAX6, PITX2, CYP1B1, or FOXC1 genes. Peters anomaly also occurs in fetal alcohol syndrome. This spectrum of developmental anomalies includes the posterior ulcer of von Hippel and posterior keratoconus. The posterior concavity is lined by Descemet membrane and endothelium in posterior keratoconus.

CORNEAL INFLAMMATION

Acute Keratitis and Corneal Ulceration

The anterior surface of the cornea is an interface between the eye and the external environment. Mechanisms that protect the cornea from infection include the corneal epithelium, mucous strands secreted by conjunctival goblet cells that can ensnare microorganisms, and tears that can wash them away. In addition, the tears contain natural antimicrobial substances such as lactoferrin, lysozyme, and antibodies. The latter are made by lymphocytes and plasma cells that are always found in the stroma of the conjunctiva and the parenchyma of the lacrimal gland (Fig. 6-3).

Normally, these mechanisms are remarkably effective. Corneal infection usually develops when these protective mechanisms are compromised, for example, when a contaminated foreign body perforates the epithelium and

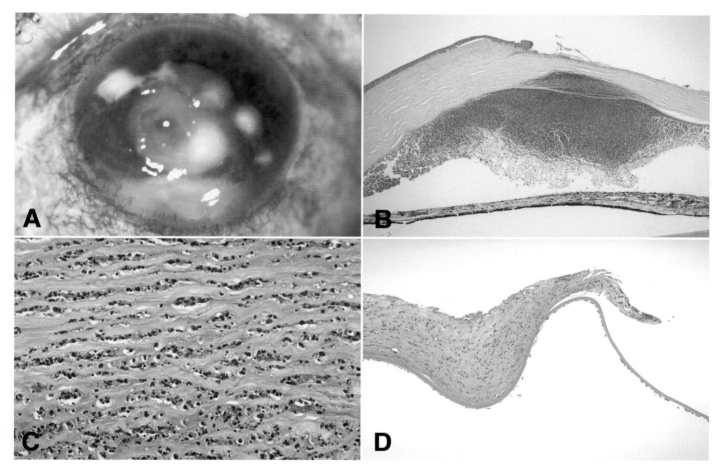

Fig. 6-3. Acute keratitis. A. Clinical photo of acute keratitis with ulceration and hypopyon. **B.** Anterior chamber deep to corneal ulcer contains hypopyon. Iris is flattened by neovascular membrane. **C.** Acute keratitis. Polymorphonuclear leukocytes and inflammatory debris fill clefts between the stromal lamellae. Many polys have pyknotic nuclei and early stromal necrosis is present. **D.** Descemetocele, acute keratitis. An intact layer of Descemet membrane persists in the bed of deep corneal ulcer. The anterior layers of the cornea have been destroyed by inflammation. (**B.** H&E ×25, **C.** H&E ×100, **D.** H&E ×50)

inoculates the corneal stroma, or when the epithelium is abraded or damaged by chronic bullous keratopathy. Finally, a few organisms, most notably *Neisseria gonorrhoeae*, have the ability to invade through an intact epithelium.

Infiltration of the stroma by polymorphonuclear leukocytes occurs in acute bacterial keratitis (Fig. 6-3C). The polys collect in the clefts between adjacent stromal lamellae. Digestive enzymes released by the dying inflammatory cells cause stromal necrosis, which has a smudged basophilic appearance in routine hematoxylin and eosin (H&E) sections. Collagenase made by the corneal epithelium may contribute to dissolution of the stroma. Organisms such as *Pseudomonas* also produce potent enzymes that contribute to corneal destruction. *Pseudomonas keratitis* is characterized by marked stromal edema and dissolution and rapid corneal perforation. The infection can also spread posteriorly into the sclera as a sclerokeratitis (Fig. 6-4).

The epithelium, Bowman membrane, and the anterior stroma are lost in **corneal ulcer**. Corneal perforation results when the infection destroys the full-thickness stroma. Occasionally, a bulging dome of intact, elastic Descemet

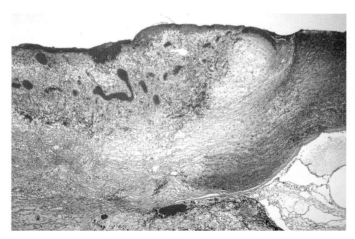

Fig. 6-4. *Pseudomonas* **sclerokeratitis.** *Pseudomonas keratitis* often extends posteriorly as an infectious scleritis. The acutely inflamed cornea (**at right**) appears blue, reflecting necrosis and heavy infiltration by polys. Proteolytic enzymes released by the Gram-negative rods have dissolved the limbal sclera. The angle is closed. (H&E ×20)

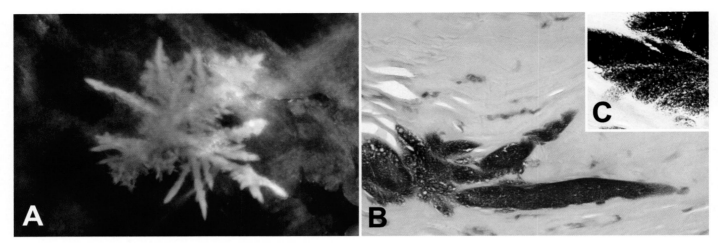

Fig. 6-5. Infectious pseudocrystalline keratopathy. A. Macrophoto shows radiating crystalline appearance of bacterial colony in cornea. **B.** Large basophilic colonies of relatively avirulent streptococci distend interlammelar clefts in relatively noninflamed part of the corneal stroma. **C.** Bacteria are Gram-positive. (**B.** H&E ×100, **C.** Tissue Gram stain ×250)

membrane called a **descemetocele** persists in the floor of the incipient perforation (Fig. 6-3D). Polymorphonuclear leukocytes collect in the lower part of the anterior chamber as a hypopyon, and also typically adhere to the posterior cornea directly beneath the ulcer. The endothelium is often damaged. The tissue Gram stain may disclose myriad microorganisms in the infected cornea or none at all. Bacteria are often found in relatively noninflamed parts of the stroma bordering the inflammatory infiltrate. Perforation or impending perforation of the cornea is an indication for emergent penetrating keratoplasty (corneal transplantation). Cyanoacrylate tissue adhesive often is used to seal corneal perforations. Although the "crazy glue" is lost during processing, its presence is marked by a tell-tale scalloped pattern on the anterior corneal surface.

Infectious pseudocrystalline keratopathy (Fig. 6-5) usually is caused by avirulent strains of streptococci, which proliferate in the relatively noninflamed stroma forming large interlamellar bacterial colonies that have a vaguely crystalline configuration on biomicroscopy. This relatively rare disorder typically occurs in corneal grafts after chronic therapy with corticosteroids. The bacterial colonies are sequestered by a glycocalyx whose formation is stimulated by the steroids.

Fungal keratitis (Fig. 6-6) is rarer than bacterial keratitis, is more prevalent in the South, and often complicates corneal injuries by vegetable matter or steroid therapy in debilitated hosts. Eighty percent of corneal ulcers in the United States are caused by *Aspergillus*, *Candida*, or *Fusarium* species. Clinically, fungal ulcers often have a deep crater with raised edges, and may have smaller satellite lesions. The fungal hyphae readily permeate the stroma and can perforate Descemet membrane and invade the anterior chamber, placing the patient at risk for fungal endophthalmitis (Fig. 6-6D,E).

Fungi may not be detected in superficial smears or scrapings because the hyphae are often found deep in the bed of the ulcer, or in the relatively viable stroma of the ulcer wall (Fig. 6-6C). Hence, corneal biopsy may be required to establish the diagnosis. Fungi and yeast are best shown by the PAS stain or special stains for fungus such as the Gomori methenamine silver (GMS) impregnation stain. The nonspecific fluorochrome calcofluor white binds to cellulose and chitin in cell walls of fungi, pneumocystis, and acanthamoebae. It can be used to detect fungi, but requires an ultraviolet microscope.

M. tuberculosis, *M leprae*, and several strains of atypical mycobacteria such as *M. chelonae* rarely cause corneal infection. Special stains for acid-fast organisms and microbiological cultures are used to diagnose mycobacterial keratitis. The diagnosis is often unsuspected and is frequently delayed. Organisms are often quite numerous in atypical mycobacterial infection.

VIRAL KERATITIS

Herpes simplex (HSV) keratitis (Fig. 6-7) is the most common corneal infection that causes visual loss in the United States and Europe. Most cases of herpetic keratitis are caused by HSV Type I, which causes infection above the waist. The classic clinical manifestation of early ocular herpesvirus infection is dendritic keratitis, a superficial ulcerating infection of the corneal epithelium that has a characteristic branching configuration (Fig. 6-7A). Viral cultures are positive in 75% of cases, and smears show Cowdry type A intranuclear viral inclusions in the infected epithelial cells. The primary epithelial infection tends to be self-limited, lasting 7 to 10 days with complete recovery and disappearance of virus from the primary site of infection. However, recurrences are quite common because the virus remains in a latent state in the trigeminal ganglion where its DNA has been incorporated into the genome of the neurons. Poorly understood trigger mechanisms reactivate the virus, which travels down the sensory nerve to cause overt recurrent disease. One in four

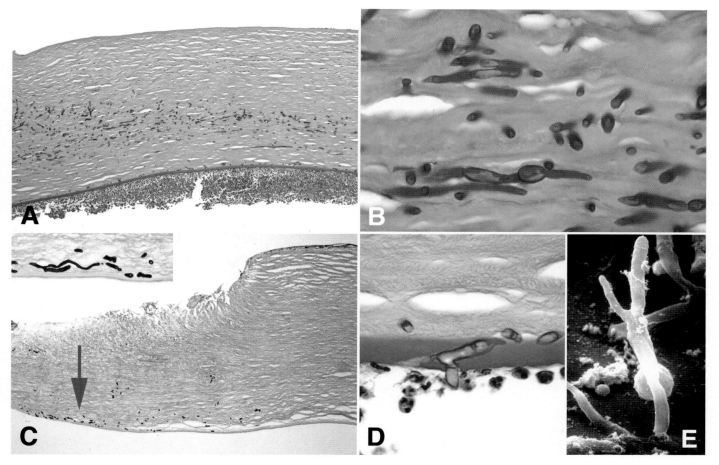

Fig. 6-6. Fungal keratitis. A. Periodic acid-Schiff stain discloses numerous hyphae in mid stroma, seen at higher magnification in **part B**. The corneal epithelium is absent. A hypopyon adheres to the posterior cornea. **C.** Deep hyphae, fungal keratitis. The corneal epithelium and the anterior stroma are absent in the ulcerated area at left. *Arrow* points to GMS-stained hyphae in the deep stroma near Descemet membrane. Hyphae are seen at higher magnification in inset. A superficial scraping of the ulcer bed was negative for fungus. **D.** PAS-positive septate fungal hypha perforates Descemet membrane and invades anterior chamber, which contains poly-morphonuclear leukocytes. **E.** Scanning electron micrographs shows branching fungal hyphae that have invaded anterior chamber. (**A.** PAS ×25, **B.** PAS ×250, **C.** GMS ×50; **Inset**, GMS ×100, **D.** PAS ×250, **E.** SEM ×640)

cases of primary HSV keratitis recur. The recurrence rate rises to 50% after an initial recurrence.

A more serious, potentially blinding form of ocular herpesvirus infection affects the corneal stroma. Although the pathogenesis of **herpes stromal keratitis** is not entirely understood, an immunological response to viral antigens shed from infected corneal epithelial or endothelial cells probably is basis for nonulcerative HSV disciform kerati-tis. The necrotizing form of HSV stromal keratitis actually may involve viral invasion and low-grade replication in the stroma.

Light microscopy of corneal buttons with chronic herpes stromal keratitis typically reveals scarring and vasculariza-tion of the stroma and infiltration by chronic inflammatory cells (Fig. 6-7C). The presence of lymphocytes, plasma cells, and histiocytes in the inflammatory infiltrate in many cases provides evidence for an immunological response. The inflammatory infiltrate frequently includes epithelioid his-tiocytes. These can occur anywhere in the stroma, but they

characteristically coalesce to form giant cells near Descemet membrane (Fig. 6-7D,E). A giant cell reaction to Descemet membrane is not pathognomonic for chronic HSV kerati-tis, but it is highly suggestive. In many cases, there is thin-ning and scarring of the chronically inflamed cornea with loss of Bowman membrane and anterior stroma. Progres-sive stromal loss can lead to corneal perforation in chronic herpetic keratitis. Compensatory hyperplasia of the corneal epithelium is often found in areas of extensive stromal loss (Fig. 6-7F). Viral inclusions are not found light microscopi-cally in the stroma in herpes stromal keratitis. Virions and viral antigens have been detected electron microscopically and immunocytochemically, however.

Varicella zoster virus (VZV), another member of the herpesvirus family, also causes a dendritic keratitis. Zoster dendrites lack the rounded terminal bulbs that typically occur at the end of the branches of HSV dendrites, and are not full-thickness epithelial ulcerations as HSV dendrites are (Fig. 6-7B).

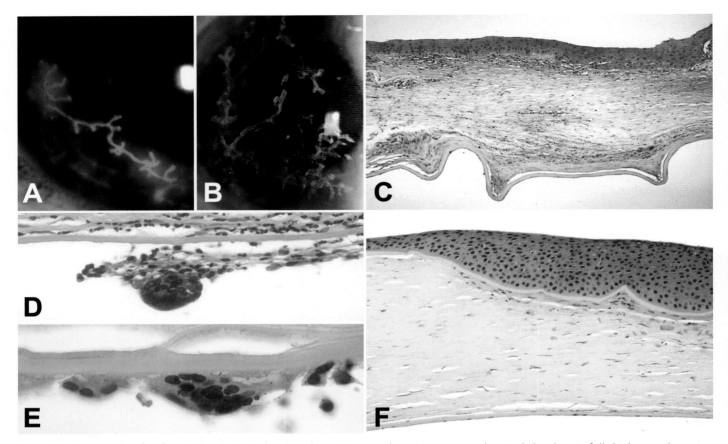

Fig. 6-7. Herpes simplex keratitis. A. HSV dendritic keratitis. Branching Herpes simplex viral dendrite is full-thickness ulceration with terminal bulbs. Dendrite is stained with fluorescein dye. **B.** VZV dendritic keratitis. Dendritiform lesions of varicella-zoster keratitis are composed of heaped-up epithelium. (Both photos courtesy of Dr. Peter Laibson, Wills Eye Institute.) **C.** Chronic herpetic stromal keratitis. The stroma is thin, scarred and chronically inflamed. The inflammatory infiltrate contains lymphocytes, plasma cells and epithelioid histiocytes. Bowman membrane is largely destroyed and the epithelium is irregularly thickened. Descemet membrane is folded. **D, E.** Giant cell reaction to Descemet membrane, Chronic HSV keratitis. Although characteristic, this finding is not pathognomonic for HSV. **F.** Compensatory epithelial hyperplasia, chronic HSV keratitis. The epithelium is markedly thickened overlying an area of stroma loss. Bowman membrane persists in the area of stromal thinning. (**C.** H&E ×50, **D.** H&E ×100, **E.** H&E ×250, **F.** H&E ×50)

Focal subepithelial infiltrates occur in the corneas of patients who have **epidemic keratoconjunctivitis** or EKC, which generally is caused by adenovirus types 8 and 19. The subepithelial infiltrates develop in the later noninfectious stage of the disease and are thought to be composed of lymphocytes attracted by viral antigens. EKC is often a severe, temporarily incapacitating infection, which is highly contagious. Ophthalmologists should take care to avoid infecting themselves and other patients. Patients with EKC usually have preauricular adenopathy.

INTERSTITIAL KERATITIS

In a generic sense, the term interstitial keratitis refers to any nonulcerative inflammation of the corneal stroma. (HSV disciform keratitis is a form of interstitial keratitis.) Other causes of stromal or interstitial keratitis include tuberculosis and leprosy, protozoan parasites such as Acanthamoeba, onchocercal microfilaria, systemic disorders such as sarcoidosis, Hodgkin disease and mycosis fungoides, foreign bodies such as caterpillar setae and plant material, and drugs including gold and arsenic.

In common parlance, however, the term interstitial keratitis generally connotes the severe stromal keratitis that affects patients with congenital syphilis during the first or second decade. Acute luetic interstitial keratitis is marked clinically by a "salmon patch" of intense stromal vascularization and severe photophobia. Lymphocytes infiltrate the edematous stroma. The late sequelae of old syphilitic interstitial keratitis can be relatively subtle: they include a faint diffuse nebulous opacification of the stroma and residual nonperfused ghost vessels located deep in the corneal stroma (Fig. 6-8A). The ghost vessels are best disclosed by the biomicroscopic technique of sclerotic scatter.

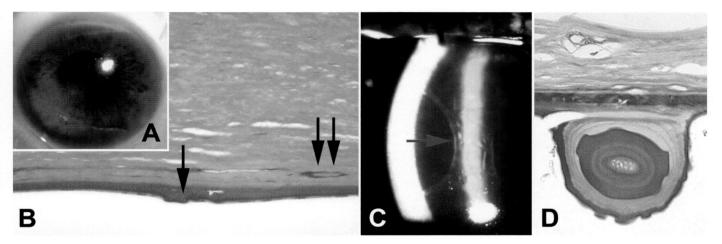

Fig. 6-8. Chronic luetic interstitial keratitis. A. Clinical photo shows faint nebulous opacification of the cornea. **B.** *Double arrow* denotes vessels deep within noninflamed corneal stroma. *Single arrow* points to guttate excrescence on irregularly thickened Descemet membrane. **C.** *Arrow* in clinical photo denotes relucent mass of hypertrophic Descemet membrane material on the posterior cornea. **D.** Photomicrograph shows thick cylinder of PAS-positive basement membrane material studded with guttate excrescences on irregularly thickened Descemet membrane. (**B.** PAS ×100, **C.** Clinical photo courtesy of Dr. Irving Raber, Wills Eye Institute, **D.** PAS ×100)

Histopathologically, Bowman membrane usually is absent. The stroma is free of inflammation, and fine vessels that usually do not contain blood are seen in the posterior third of the stroma, often just anterior to Descemet membrane (Fig. 6-8B). Part of the stroma may have a rarefied vacuolated appearance and will stain intensely for acid mucopolysaccharide. Descemet membrane is often thickened and may be studded with irregular guttate excrescences (Fig. 6-8B). The thickening of Descemet membrane may be massive. Relucent strands and networks of basement membrane material are found on the posterior corneal surface in exceptional cases (Fig. 6-8C,D).

Luetic interstitial keratitis occasionally develops in acquired syphilis, in which corneal involvement is typically unilateral and sectoral. The association of nonluetic interstitial keratitis and vestibuloauditory symptoms is called Cogan syndrome. Cogan syndrome is thought to be an autoimmune disorder.

PARASITIC KERATITIS

Protozoan parasites including microsporidians and the freshwater amebas *Acanthamoeba castellanii* and *A. polyphaga* cause unusual corneal infections. Originally reported in patients with HIV/AIDS, microsporidial keratoconjunctivitis has occurred in immunocompetent individuals as well. The parasite can infect the epithelium of the cornea and conjunctiva or the corneal stroma (Fig. 5-11B).

Acanthamoeba keratitis was initially reported in 1974, and is closely linked to the development and widespread use of soft contact lenses. Acanthamoeba keratitis classically afflicts soft contact lens wearers who use contaminated homemade saline solutions or wear their lenses while swimming or bathing in hot tubs. The keratitis is usually severely painful. Although many cases respond to medical therapy, penetrating keratoplasty (corneal transplantation) may be necessary. The initial stages of acanthamoeba keratitis can be confused with herpetic keratitis if clinical suspicion is low. A ring or annular infiltrate is a characteristic feature of acanthamoeba keratitis, but usually develops in the later stages of the disease (Fig. 6-9A).

Microscopically, acanthamoeba keratitis is often marked by focal detachment or desquamation of the corneal epithelium. In contrast to bacterial or fungal keratitis, the anterior stroma in many cases contains only a relatively sparse infiltrate of inflammatory cells, mainly polys and macrophages (Fig. 6-9B). Stromal necrosis is usually inconspicuous, and stromal vascularization generally is not observed despite a lengthy course that may last months prior to keratoplasty. Amebic cysts in the stroma and epithelium are readily found in sections or smears stained with Giemsa or H&E (Fig. 6-9B–D). The chitinous walls of the acanthamoeba cysts are round or oval, and stain with PAS, GMS, and Giemsa. The cytoplasm typically retracts from the cyst wall in tissue sections. The cysts contain a round nucleus with a distinct nucleolus (Fig. 6-9D). Trophozoites are usually difficult to identify because they resemble macrophages. Intense stromal keratitis with localized abscess formation and palisading granulomatous inflammation can be observed in the late stages of the disease.

Acanthamoeba keratitis can be diagnosed using corneal biopsies, smears, or confocal microscopy. In smears, the organisms are most readily found within sheets of epithelial cells. The nonspecific fluorochrome calcofluor white can disclose cysts during the rapid screening of smears but requires an ultraviolet fluorescent microscope (Fig. 6-9E). Acanthamoebas are cultured on agar

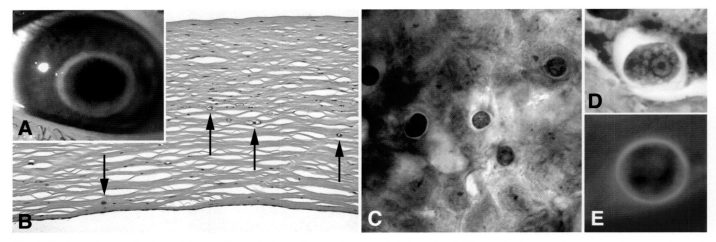

Fig. 6-9. Acanthamoeba keratitis. A. Clinical photo shows characteristic late ring infiltrate. **B.** *Arrows* denote amebic cysts in minimally inflamed corneal stroma. The epithelium is absent. Acanthamoeba cysts are seen in epithelial scraping stained with Giemsa (**C**) and sections stained with H&E (**D**) and calcofluor white (**E**). Cytoplasmic retraction from cyst wall and round nucleus with distinct nucleus are evident in **part D**. (**A.** Clinical photo courtesy of Dr. Elizabeth Cohen, Wills Eye Institute, **B.** H&E ×50, **C.** Giemsa ×100, **D.** H&E ×250, **E.** Calcofluor white ×250)

plates overlain with a layer of *E. coli*. The amebas produce diagnostic linear tracks on the surface of the plates as they graze on the bacteria.

Onchocerciasis is a major cause of blindness in parts of Africa and South and Central America. This infestation by the parasite *Onchocerca volvulus* is called *river blindness* because its vector, the black simulian fly, breeds in swift-running mountain streams. Pairs of adult *Onchocerca* breed in characteristic nodules in the skin of infested individuals. The female worm releases myriad microfilariae that migrate to all parts of the body. Necrotic microfilariae incite focal inflammation. Microfilariae are often found in the corneal stroma where they produce keratitis with a characteristic nummular (coin-shaped) pattern. Secondary closed-angle glaucoma caused by anterior uveitis is a major cause of blindness in endemic areas. Chorioretinal degeneration, also an allergic reaction to the parasite, is another important cause of blindness. Slit lamp examination may disclose microfilariae in the anterior chamber in heavily infested patients. The tiny worms are photophobic, and they quickly swim behind the iris when the lamp is turned on. Patients are treated by the surgical removal of parasitic nodules and with the antihelminthic drug ivermectin.

PERIPHERAL CORNEAL ULCERS

Although bacterial and fungal ulcers usually involve the central cornea, a variety of ulcerations affect its periphery. Most important are the peripheral corneal ulcerations that may herald the presence of a systemic vasculitis such as Wegener granulomatosis, periarteritis nodosa, systemic lupus erythematosus, or rheumatoid arthritis.

A rapidly progressive, painful, ulcerative keratitis, **Mooren ulcer** begins peripherally and extends across the cornea.

The margin of the ulcer has a characteristic overhanging configuration (Fig. 6-10). Mooren ulcer usually is a unilateral disease of elderly patients in the United States. A severe, bilateral form of the disease affects young individuals in Africa. Autoimmunity is suspected in the pathogenesis of Mooren ulcer. Some cases have been linked to chronic hepatitis C infection.

Terrien ulcer is a slowly progressive bilateral trough-like thinning of the stroma that begins superiorly in men. The epithelium remains intact but Bowman membrane and the superficial stroma are lost. Vascularization and occasional lymphocytes and plasma cells are found in the ectatic stroma.

Toxins produced by staphylococci cause infiltrates and superficial ulcerations in the peripheral cornea.

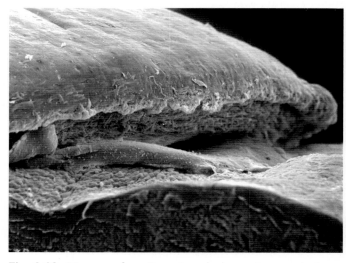

Fig. 6-10. Mooren ulcer. Scanning electron micrograph shows characteristic overhanging margin of ulcer. (SEM ×125)

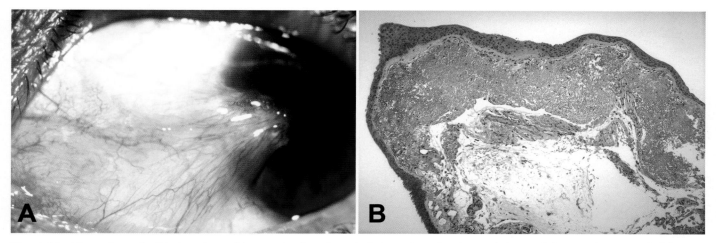

Fig. 6-11. Pterygium. A. Wedge-shaped ingrowth of conjunctival tissue invades the periphery of the nasal cornea. **B.** There is extensive actinic elastosis of the substantia propria in this example. (**A.** Clinical photo courtesy of Dr. Peter Laibson, Wills Eye Institute, **B.** H&E ×50)

PTERYGIUM

Pterygium (Fig. 6-11) is a degenerative disease of the cornea characterized by a wedge-shaped ingrowth of conjunctival tissue that slowly invades the peripheral cornea. The nasal limbus is usually affected, and both eyes are often involved. The name pterygium reflects the fanciful resemblance of the vascularized ingrowth to the membranous wing of an insect (pter is the Greek word for wing). Pterygium initially is a cosmetic blemish, but it can cause visual loss if it invades the pupillary axis. Pterygia arise from limbal conjunctiva exposed to light in the interpalpebral fissure. Prolonged exposure to UV-B is thought to play an important pathogenetic role by causing DNA mutations with resultant loss of cell cycle regulation. Increased expression and mutations in tumor-suppressing transcription factor p53 occur in pterygium cells but do not appear to be a prerequisite for pterygium formation. Focal limbal stem cell deficiency probably is an important factor in the transdifferentiation of cornea epithelium into conjunctival-like tissue. Pterygia are more common in southern latitudes and typically occur in individuals who work outdoors. Other environmental factors such as wind or dust could play a pathogenic role.

Histopathologically, pterygia resemble an ingrowth of conjunctiva onto the periphery of the cornea. Bowman membrane is absent, and the stroma shows increased vascularity. Actinic elastosis of collagen is often present but may be relatively inconspicuous or absent in some cases. The epithelium usually resembles conjunctival epithelium. Epithelial hyperplasia and even dysplasia occur rarely. Pterygia should be examined histopathologically to exclude the possibility of an unsuspected neoplasm. In addition to squamous malignancies, amelanotic melanomas occasionally are misdiagnosed clinically as pterygia.

OTHER CORNEAL DEGENERATIONS

Calcific band keratopathy is a superficial opacity that extends across the part of the cornea exposed in the interpalpebral fissure (Fig. 6-12). It is caused by calcification of Bowman membrane and the anterior stroma. A clear interval separates the band of superficial calcification from the limbus, and the opacity usually contains small circular holes. Calcific band keratopathy can complicate chronic uveitis or long-standing glaucoma, and also complicates systemic disorders of calcium metabolism including hypercalcemia, vitamin D intoxication, milk-alkali syndrome, hypophosphatemia and Fanconi syndrome. Histopathology discloses basophilic granules in Bowman membrane and the superficial stroma. The alizarin red and von Kossa stains for calcium are positive. The chelating agent EDTA is often used to treat calcific band keratopathy. A noncalcific form of band keratopathy related to chronic actinic keratopathy also occurs. The granules are larger and stain positively with the Verhoeff-van Gieson elastic stain (Fig. 6-12C).

Chronic actinic keratopathy (Fig. 6-13) and **climatic droplet keratopathy** are two of many names applied to a degenerative disorder that is marked by the deposition of multiple spherules of yellow hyaline material in the anterior cornea. The disorder is also called spheroidal degeneration and Labrador keratopathy. The degeneration is particularly prevalent in areas where intense glare is reflected from ice (Labrador) or sand (the Dahlac Islands in the Red Sea). Other synonyms such as oleoguttate dystrophy and degeneratio sphaerularis elaoides stress the resemblance of the corneal deposits to droplets of olive oil. In H&E-stained sections, the drop-like deposits of amorphous hyaline material usually are light gray or amphophilic. The material stains intensely with the Verhoeff-van Gieson elastic stain, and the positive reaction is not abolished by pretreatment with

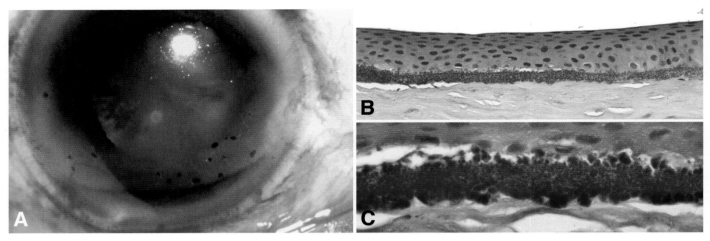

Fig. 6-12. Band keratopathy. A. Clinical photo shows band of superficial opacification involving the interpalpebral part of the cornea. **B.** Fine basophilic granules of calcium stipple Bowman layer. **C.** Elastic stain highlights larger granules of actinic elastosis in case with noncalcific component. (**B.** H&E ×100, **C.** Verhoeff-Van Gieson elastic stain ×250)

elastase such as the elastotic degeneration in pinguecula and pterygium. The hyaline deposits autofluoresce under ultraviolet light and are said to behave similarly when illuminated with the slit lamp's cobalt blue filter. In some cases, tiny globules of hyaline material are concentrated in Bowman membrane, mimicking calcific band keratopathy. Concurrent corneal scarring can severely decrease visual acuity in advanced cases.

Salzmann nodular degeneration was once called Salzmann nodular dystrophy. It is now recognized that this typically unilateral disorder is not heritable and is best classified as a secondary degenerative process of uncertain cause. Clinically, the corneal epithelium is focally elevated by white mounds of dense collagenous connective tissue. Salzmann nodular degeneration resembles a massive focal pannus histopathologically. Mounds of relatively acellular hyaline connective tissue elevate the corneal epithelium

anterior to the plane of Bowman membrane, which may be destroyed.

Lipid deposition occurs in the peripheral corneal stroma in **arcus senilis** (Fig. 6-29A) or gerontoxon, a relatively common aging change. Fat stains performed on frozen sections disclose a concurrent deposit in the perilimbal sclera which is inapparent clinically. Similar corneal deposition in a man younger than age forty may signify a hyperlipemic state that can predispose to cardiovascular disease. Lipid keratopathy is a secondary phenomenon caused by lipid deposition in a heavily vascularized stroma.

A **corneal keloid** (Fig. 6-14) is a hypertrophic scar that massively thickens the corneal stroma. Elevated and exposed, the corneal epithelium on the surface of the keloid typically undergoes epidermalization and transforms into opaque skin-like tissue. Large corneal keloids often develop in patients who have corneal staphylomas. In

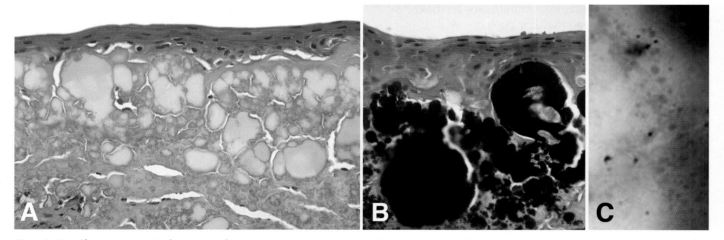

Fig. 6-13. Chronic actinic keratopathy. A. Anterior stroma contains amphophilic deposits of amorphous hyaline material. **B.** Material stains shows intensely with elastic stain. **C.** Material in scarred cornea resembles droplets of olive oil. (**A.** H&E ×100, **B.** Verhoeff-Van Gieson elastic stain ×125)

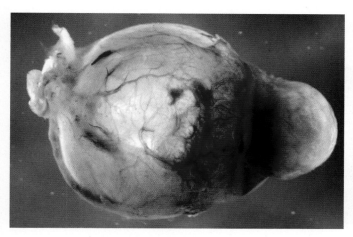

Fig. 6-14. Corneal staphyloma. The cornea is massively thickened by a hypertrophic scar (corneal keloid) that was lined internally by atrophic iris. The eye was enucleated from a child in Africa.

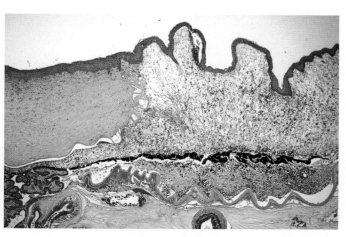

Fig. 6-15. Keratomalacia secondary to avitaminosis A. Incarcerated iris plugs sharply margined perforation in center of noninflamed cornea. Avitaminosis A was caused by dietary deficiency in chronic alcoholic. (H&E ×25)

such cases, the posterior surface of the cornea is lined by atrophic remnants of iris, mainly iris pigment. A **staphyloma** is an ectasia (area of thinning) lined by uveal tissue. Uveal is derived from the Latin word *uva* meaning grape. *Staphyle* means a "bunch of grapes" in Greek. The latter prefix signifies the involvement of uveal tissue. Corneal staphylomas and keloids are common sequelae of keratomalacia and measles keratitis in underdeveloped countries.

The tear film functions as the true anterior surface of the cornea, whose health depends on an adequate supply of properly constituted tears. Disorders of tear production and composition include deficiencies in the aqueous component, the mucinous wetting agent produced by the goblet cells, or abnormalities in the most superficial layer of lipid. Minor degrees of ocular drying are encountered often in clinical practice. If an eye is totally dry, the cornea becomes opaque.

Keratoconjunctivitis sicca is marked by corneal drying, superficial punctate keratopathy (punctate staining), and filamentary keratitis composed of strands of detached corneal epithelium and mucous. Keratoconjunctivitis sicca and xerostomia are characteristic features of the autoimmune disorder Sjögren syndrome. Drying of the mouth and eyes is caused by infiltration and destruction of the acini of the salivary and the main and accessory lacrimal glands by T lymphocytes. Myoepithelial islands persist in the lymphoid infiltrate (lymphoepithelial lesion of Godwin). About 10% of affected patients develop malignant lymphoma.

Corneal epithelial keratinization and epidermalization occur in severe **vitamin A deficiency**. Patients have xerophthalmia and night blindness caused by deficient rod photopigment. A process of bland corneal melting called keratomalacia frequently leads to corneal perforation (Fig. 6-15). Malnourished children in underdeveloped

countries and vitamin A–deficient alcoholics in the United States are at risk. Bitot spot, a clinical marker for xerophthalmia, is an elevated dry area of epithelium with a foamy appearance.

A corneal delle (pl. dellen) is a focal area of corneal thinning with superficial surface ulceration, which is located central to an elevated lesion at the limbus. Dellen probably are caused by focal dehydration of the corneal stroma related to deficient focal corneal wetting.

Neurotrophic or neuroparalytic keratopathy is a corneal epitheliopathy that may complicate V nerve lesions or corneal hypesthesia caused by herpetic eye disease or herpes zoster ophthalmicus. The keratopathy develops rapidly after surgical sectioning of the trigeminal nerve interrupts poorly understood trophic factors. Bland corneal ulceration may develop.

The term **pannus** is applied to a flat superficial scar of the anterior cornea (Fig. 6-16). Two types of pannus are recognized histopathologically. The paradigmatic inflammatory pannus occurs in trachoma and is marked by a subepithelial ingrowth of inflamed fibrovascular tissue from the limbus, which destroys Bowman membrane. Degenerative pannus occurs in chronically edematous corneas with bullous keratopathy. Microscopically, a layer of connective tissue is found interposed between the base of the epithelium and Bowman membrane, which remains intact (Fig. 6-16B). In contrast to an inflammatory pannus, the subepithelial scar of degenerative pannus does not necessarily grow in from the limbus. Cells, which probably are stromal fibroblasts, migrate into the space between Bowman membrane and the detached epithelium and synthesize collagen. This fibrous scar forms the pannus and may alleviate the painful bullous keratopathy at the expense of visual acuity. In rare instances, amyloid is deposited secondarily beneath the epithelium.

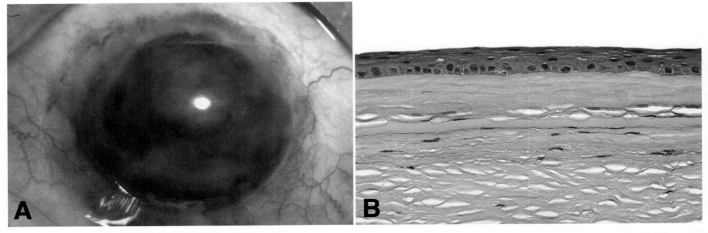

Fig. 6-16. Degenerative pannus, chronic corneal edema. A. Chronically edematous cornea is opacified by subepithelial fibrosis. **B.** A thick layer of relatively acellular connective tissue is interposed between the corneal epithelium and intact Bowman membrane. (**B.** H&E ×100)

KERATOCONUS

Keratoconus is an enigmatic bilateral degenerative disorder characterized by progressive thinning or ectasia of the central stroma that imparts a conical configuration to the cornea (Fig. 6-17). Keratoconus usually presents around puberty with visual loss caused by severe astigmatism. Most cases of keratoconus do not appear to be inherited, but the degeneration can complicate several systemic disorders including trisomy 21, Ehlers-Danlos syndrome, Leber congenital amaurosis, and atopic dermatitis. Keratoconus occurs in approximately 5% of patients with Down syndrome and frequently is associated with the acute onset of severe corneal edema called corneal hydrops. Keratoconus in patients with atopic dermatitis, Down syndrome, and Leber congenital amaurosis, a congenital photoreceptor degeneration, could be related to forceful eye rubbing or the oculodigital reflex. The latter is a behavioral pattern seen in visually and mentally handicapped children who repeatedly strike their eyes with their thumbs in order to mechanically induce flashes of light or phosphenes.

The consistency of the cornea in keratoconus is abnormal; the sectioned cornea almost invariably assumes an irregular wavy configuration on a microslide, which immediately suggests the diagnosis (Fig. 6-17B,C). Higher magnification discloses central or apical thinning of the stroma, which can be reduced to less than one-tenth normal thickness in exceptional cases. Characteristic dehiscences, which typically have a wavy configuration, occur in Bowman membrane. These probably are pathognomic for keratoconus and serve to confirm the diagnosis histopathologically (Fig. 6-17C,D). Some cases exhibit apical scarring with increased fibroblastic activity and new collagen production. The corneal epithelium usually is intact and irregular in caliber with areas of both thinning and compensatory hyperplasia. Descemet membrane usually is thin, and the endothelium is well preserved. A rupture in Descemet membrane is found if acute hydrops has occurred. If the hydrops had resolved prior to corneal transplantation, the gap in Descemet membrane is lined by a thin layer of new Descemet membrane synthesized by endothelial cells that have migrated into the defect. Special stains show iron deposition in the corneal epithelium encircling the cone. This deposit is evident clinically as a **Fleischer ring**, one of the several eponymic iron lines of the cornea (Fig. 6-17E–G). Other iron lines unassociated with keratoconus include the Hudson-Stähli line (across the low third of the cornea), the Stocker line (at the advancing head of a pterygium), and the Ferry line (next to a filtering bleb). The basic defect in keratoconus is uncertain but may be related to abnormal degradation of the corneal extracellular matrix. Abnormal levels of tissue metalloproteinase inhibitors and alcohol dehydrogenase have been identified in some cases.

Pellucid degeneration of the cornea resembles keratoconus histopathologically but is located in the periphery of the cornea.

CORNEAL DYSTROPHIES

Introduction

In classic ophthalmic usage, the term dystrophy usually denotes an inherited, relatively symmetric bilateral disease that is unassociated with vascularization or inflammation in its early stages. The pathology is or appears to be localized to an ocular tissue. Dystrophies usually are not evident at birth, but become clinically evident later in life. The etymological derivation of the word dystrophy is outdated

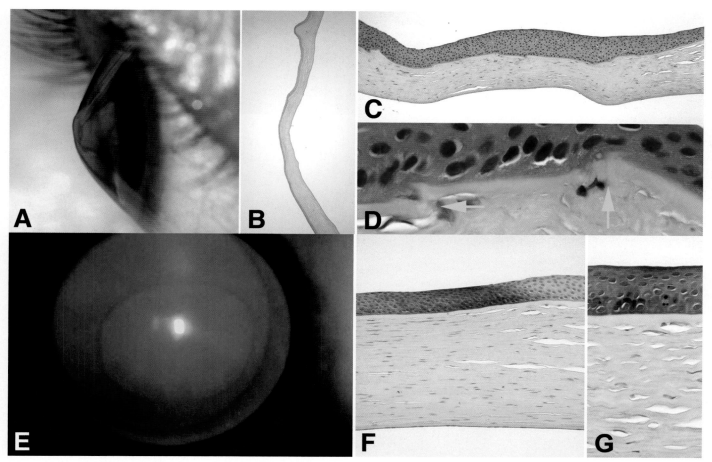

Fig. 6-17. Keratoconus. A. Clinical photo shows conical shape of cornea. **B.** Sectioned ectatic cornea has wavy configuration. **C.** Photomicrograph shows severe thinning of apical stroma, compensatory hyperplasia of the epithelium and multiple dehiscences in Bowman membrane. **D.** *Arrows* point to characteristic dehiscences in Bowman membrane. **E.** Cobalt blue illumination highlights Fleischer ring surrounding apex of cone. **F, G.** Iron stain of Fleischer ring shows focal deposition of iron in corneal epithelium surrounding cone. (**B.** H&E ×5, **C.** H&E ×25, **D.** H&E ×250, **F.** Iron stain ×100, **G.** Iron stain ×250)

because it refers to poor nutrition. The term usually is applied to hereditary diseases of the cornea and macula.

Advances in molecular biology have markedly increased our understanding of these rare, interesting disorders. Several corneal dystrophies currently are known to be caused by allelic mutations in the gene encoding a single corneal protein. Macular corneal dystrophy (MCD) appears to be the ocular manifestation of an otherwise innocuous systemic enzyme deficiency. Meesman epithelial dystrophy is caused by an abnormality in the genes for proteins that are only expressed in the corneal epithelium.

Corneal dystrophies are classified topographically as superficial, stromal, and endothelial based on the location of the clinical and pathologic findings. A new classification system called the IC3D Classification of Corneal Dystrophies was published in 2009. The new classification incorporates many aspects of the traditional definitions of corneal dystrophies with new genetic, clinical, and pathologic information. This new classification can be upgraded in the future as our understanding of molecular genetics increases.

Superficial Corneal Dystrophies

Meesman dystrophy (Fig. 6-18A) is a relatively benign autosomal dominantly inherited disorder of the corneal epithelium. The eponym Stocker-Holt dystrophy is applied to a somewhat similar disorder. Clinically, Meesman dystrophy is characterized by the presence of myriad small punctate vacuoles in the corneal epithelium, which are best seen in retroillumination. Fluorescein dye typically pools in the vacuoles that have migrated to the corneal surface. Although recurrent epithelial erosions are possible, good vision is the rule. Histopathologically, both the epithelium and its basement membrane are thickened, and the epithelium has a disorderly appearance. In addition to small intraepithelial cystoid spaces, the epithelium contains cells that have a hyalinized appearance. Electron microscopy has disclosed intracellular aggregates of fibrillogranular "peculiar substance" composed of mutated cytokeratin. Meesman corneal dystrophy is caused by mutations in either of the genes (KRT3 or KRT12) that encode cornea-specific cytokeratins. The mutations severely impair

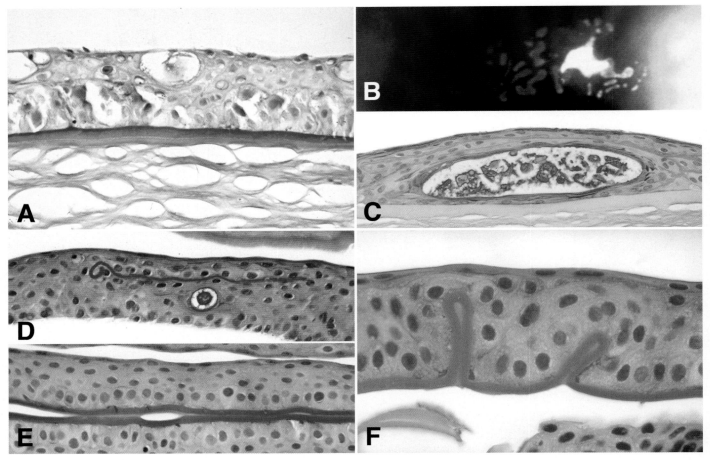

Fig. 6-18. Epithelial dystrophies. A. Meesman epithelial dystrophy. The epithelium is thickened and contains small cystoid spaces. The epithelial basement membrane is markedly thickened. **B.** Cogan microcystic dystrophy. Slit lamp discloses intraepithelial deposits of putty-like cellular debris. **C.** Photomicrograph of microcystic dystrophy shows devitalized cellular debris trapped by duplication of the epithelium. **D–F.** Map-dot-fingerprint dystrophy. Photomicrographs of corneal scrapings show small intraepithelial cyst and intraepithelial segment of basement membrane (**D**) and marked thickening of epithelial basement membrane (**E**). Folds of thickened basement membrane protrude into corneal epithelium. (**A.** PAS ×250, **C.** PAS ×100, **D.** PAS ×100, **E.** PAS ×100, **F.** PAS ×250)

cystoskeletal function and cause increased fragility of the corneal epithelium.

The terms **epithelial basement membrane dystrophy**, **anterior basement membrane dystrophy**, or **map-dot-fingerprint dystrophy** (Fig. 6-18B–F) have been applied to a corneal disorder marked by a spectrum of epithelial abnormalities including reduplication and intraepithelial segments of corneal epithelial basement membrane, intraepithelial cystoid spaces filled with devitalized cellular debris, and focal subepithelial scarring. Although rare familial cases with autosomal dominant inheritance have been reported, epithelial basement membrane dystrophy currently is not thought to be inherited. Most cases are sporadic and the disorder may be degenerative or secondary to trauma.

The clinical subtypes of the "dystrophy" often coexist. The microcystic form of the disorder (called Cogan microcystic dystrophy) shows multiple intraepithelial cysts filled with white putty-like cellular debris (Fig. 6-18B,C). The devitalized cells that fill the cystoid spaces are trapped

by duplication of the epithelium, which prevents their desquamation. Parallel relucent lines seen in the fingerprint subtype may represent basement membrane material separating sheets of duplicated epithelium (Fig. 6-18D–F). Irregular, geographically shaped areas of subepithelial scarring characterize map-like changes. The corneal epithelial basement membrane is often thickened.

Epithelial abnormalities that are similar to those found in map-dot-fingerprint dystrophy are found histopathologically in many chronically edematous corneas. Histopathologic evidence suggests that bullous detachment of the epithelium is the primary event that leads subsequently to secondary abnormalities such as reduplication and intraepithelial cyst formation. The rare, truly dystrophic cases of the disease might be caused by defective molecules involved in corneal epithelial adhesion. Several families with point mutations in the TGFBI gene have been reported.

Several corneal dystrophies including granular, lattice, Avellino, and Reis-Bücklers dystrophies are associated with distinct allelic mutations in the TGFBI (transforming growth factor induced gene) on the long arm of chromosome 5 (5q31). The TGFBI gene previously was called the Big-H3 gene. The TGFBI gene's protein product keratoepithelin is expressed in the corneal epithelium and keratocytes and numerous other tissues in the body. The different clinical manifestations of these dystrophies presumably reflect variations in the aggregation or precipitation of the several mutant forms of TGFBI protein in the cornea.

Reis-Bücklers dystrophy and **Thiel-Behnke honeycomb dystrophy** (Fig. 6-19) are two relatively similar disorders that primarily affect the epithelium, Bowman layer, and the anterior stroma of the cornea. Both dystrophies present with recurrent erosions in the first decade, and are characterized biomicroscopically by diffuse subepithelial scarring that markedly reduces visual acuity (Fig. 6-19A). Histopathologically, the epithelium in both dystrophies is irregular in caliber and has a saw-toothed appearance.

A thick multilaminar pannus composed of alternating layers of collagen and an abnormal material that has the same tinctorial characteristics as the deposits in granular corneal dystrophy elevates the epithelium anterior to the plane of Bowman layer (Fig. 6-19B,C, and E). Bowman layer usually is destroyed. The abnormal material is more eosinophilic than normal stromal collagen and stains intensely red with Masson trichrome (Fig. 6-9C,E). It initially collects beneath the epithelium and probably predisposes to recurrent erosions by interfering with epithelial adhesion. The multilaminated pannus probably results from repeated episodes of synthesis, epithelial detachment, and scarring. Inherited in an autosomal dominant fashion, Reis-Bucklers dystrophy is caused by a specific point mutation in the TGFBI gene (Arg124Leu), while Thiel-Behnke dystrophy is associated with a p. Arg555Gln TGFBI mutation.

Reis-Bücklers dystrophy and Thiel-Behnke dystrophy are distinguished histologically and electron microscopically

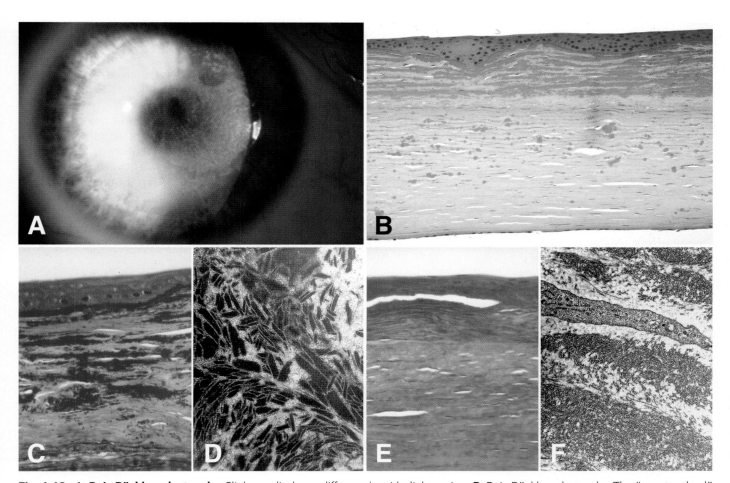

Fig. 6-19. A. Reis-Bücklers dystrophy. Slit lamp discloses diffuse subepithelial scarring. **B.** Reis-Bücklers dystrophy. The "saw-toothed" epithelium rests on a thick multilaminar pannus composed of alternating layers of collagen and more eosinophilic material. Bowman material has been destroyed. Smaller deposits of eosinophilic material are seen in the stroma. **C.** Reis-Bücklers dystrophy. Abnormal material comprising part of multilaminar pannus in Reis-Bücklers dystrophy stains red with Masson trichrome, similar to deposits in granular corneal dystrophy. **D.** Electron microscopy of Reis-Bücklers dystrophy shows osmiophilic crystalloids resembling deposits in granular corneal dystrophy. **E. Thiel-Behnke dystrophy.** Abnormal material in multilaminar pannus stains red with Masson trichrome. **F.** TEM shows that abnormal material in Thiel-Behnke dystrophy is composed of "curly filaments." (**A.** Clinical photo courtesy of Dr. Peter Laibson, Wills Eye Institute, **B.** H&E ×100, **C.** Masson trichrome ×250, **D.** TEM, **E.** Masson trichrome ×250, **F.** TEM)

by the morphology of the deposits of abnormal TGFBI protein. Reis-Bücklers dystrophy resembles a superficial variant of granular corneal dystrophy; the mutant keratoepithelin forms small, sharply angulated crystalloids that are intensely Masson trichrome-positive and osmophilic on transmission electron microscopy (Fig. 6-19C,D). The subepithelial deposits in Thiel-Behnke dystrophy are less pronounced, more amorphous, and less intensely acid-fuchsinophilic with Masson trichrome (Fig. 6-19E). The deposits are composed of proteinaceous "curly filaments" electron microscopically (Fig. 6-19F). Patients with the latter findings have been erroneously reported in the American literature as having Reis-Bücklers dystrophy. The European literature indicates that the patients who were reported by Reis and Bückler had a form of superficial granular dystrophy.

Primary gelatinous drop-like dystrophy or familial subepithelial corneal amyloidosis is a rare type of heritable corneal amyloidosis in which the amyloid accumulates as prominent milky-white gelatinous mulberry shaped nodules beneath the corneal epithelium (Fig. 6-20). The amyloid contains the antimicrobial protein lactoferrin but is not caused by mutations in the lactoferrin gene. The autosomal recessively inherited disorder is associated with mutations in the TACSTD2 gene that encodes tumor-associated calcium signal transducer 2. The gene was previously called M1S1. The TACSTD2 mutations affect corneal epithelial permeability, allowing amyloid to accumulate beneath the epithelium. Gelatinous drop-like dystrophy is severely debilitating and reoccurs rapidly after superficial keratectomy.

Stromal Dystrophies

Granular, macular, and lattice dystrophies are the three classic dystrophies of the corneal stroma (Figs. 6-21–6-23).

As noted above, lattice dystrophy type I (LCDI) granular dystrophy, a variant of granular dystrophy, called Avellino dystrophy, which combines features of both lattice and granular dystrophies, and Reis-Bücklers and Thiel-Behnke dystrophies are caused by disparate mutations in the TGFBI gene on the long arm of chromosome 5. All TGFBI dystrophies are inherited as autosomal dominant traits.

Granular corneal dystrophy (also known as Groenouw Type I) is the most benign of the corneal stromal dystrophies (Fig. 6-21). Visual loss develops relatively late in life. Slit lamp examination shows multiple white crumb, snowflake or ring-shaped opacities in the central cornea of both eyes (Fig. 6-21A). Most of the opacities are superficial. Visual acuity usually remains good because the opacities are separated by intervals of clear corneal stroma. Histologically, the deposits of mutant TGFBI protein resemble hyaline "rock candy." The material is more intensely eosinophilic and less PAS-positive than the surrounding normal stroma and exhibits intense acid fuchsinophilia (red staining) with Masson trichrome (Fig. 6-21B–D). The granular deposits also stain intensely with the myelin stain luxol fast blue, are negative for mucopolysaccharide, and are less birefringent on polarization microscopy than normal stromal collagen. Electron microscopy discloses electron-dense crystalloids, which may exhibit a regular periodicity. Granular corneal dystrophy can recur in the graft after corneal transplantation. When it does, the granular material typically accumulates in the anterior cornea beneath the epithelium. Classic granular corneal dystrophy (granular corneal dystrophy type I) is associated with a p. Arg555Trp mutation in TGFBI, while Avellino dystrophy (granular corneal dystrophy type II), which combines features of lattice and granular dystrophies, results from a p. Arg124His mutation. Lattice corneal dystrophy type I is also caused by a mutation at codon 124.

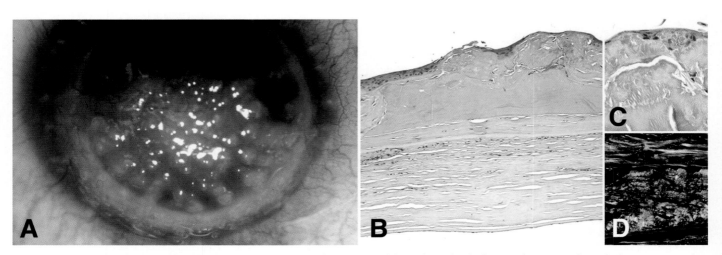

Fig. 6-20. Gelatinous drop-like dystrophy. A. Milky gelatinous nodules of amyloid elevate the corneal epithelium in case that recurred rapidly after penetrating keratoplasty. **B.** Massive subepithelial deposit of amorphous eosinophilic amyloid elevates irregular epithelium from Bowman material. Positive staining with Congo red (**C**) and characteristic apple-green birefringence with polarized light (**D**) confirms that material is amyloid. (**B.** H&E ×50, **C.** Congo red ×100, **D.** Congo red with crossed polarizers ×100)

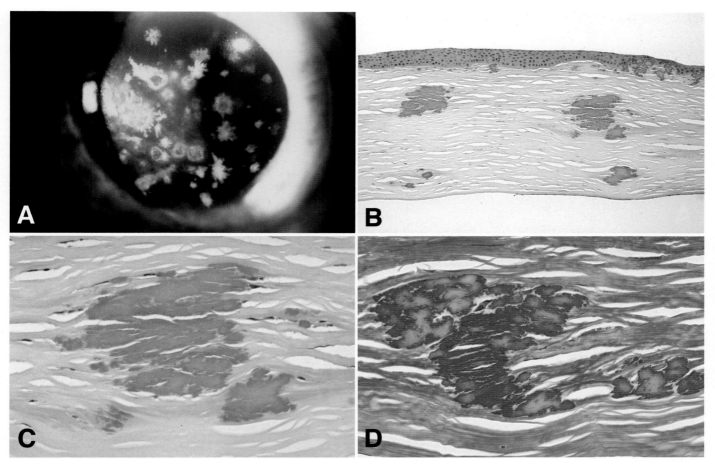

Fig. 6-21. Granular corneal dystrophy. A. Multiple white, crumb or ring-shaped opacities are present in the central cornea. The stroma is clear between the opacities. **B.** Granular corneal dystrophy. Irregular "rock candy" deposits of mutant TGFBI protein are more intensely eosinophilic than surrounding normal stroma. **C.** Irregular margins of granular deposits are distinct and angulated. **D.** Granular deposits show intense acid fuchsinophilia (*red staining*) with Masson trichrome. (**B.** H&E ×25, **C.** H&E ×100, **D.** Masson trichrome ×100)

Lattice corneal dystrophy, Type I (also known as Biber-Haab-Dimmer) is an autosomal dominantly inherited form of amyloidosis that is confined to the cornea (Fig. 6-22). The amyloid is composed of mutant TGFBI protein. Lattice corneal dystrophy typically begins in the first decade, and penetrating keratoplasty is indicated in the fourth or fifth decade. Surgery may be necessary earlier in cases with anterior amyloid deposition and scarring.

Clinically, the amyloid deposits form a characteristic latticework of branching relucent lines in the corneal stroma, which once were thought to be degenerating corneal nerves (Fig. 6-22A). Histopathology reveals smudgy round or oval deposits of eosinophilic amyloid material in the stroma, which stain positively with amyloid stains Congo red, crystal violet, and thioflavine T (Fig. 6-22B,C). The amyloid has a characteristic apple-green birefringence and dichroism when sections stained with Congo red are examined with polarization microscopy (Fig. 6-22D). The material is also PAS positive. Diffuse deposits of amyloid occur superficially and cause recurrent erosions in some cases, which may mimic Reis-Bücklers dystro-

phy. Lattice dystrophy recurs in the graft after penetrating keratoplasty. In the recurrent dystrophy, the amyloid first accumulates superficially beneath the epithelium and in suture tracts.

Lattice dystrophy type II (LCDII) is autosomal dominantly inherited form of systemic amyloidosis that includes fine lattice-like deposits in the cornea. It is unrelated to the more common form of lattice dystrophy (LCDI) caused by mutations in TGFBI. The linear deposits in LCDII are less numerous, more delicate, and more radially oriented than those in LCDI, and usually do not cause severe visual loss. In addition to the corneal manifestations, affected patients have a progressive bilateral cranial and peripheral neuropathy with dry, lax itchy skin and mask-like "hound dog" facies with pendulous ears and protruding lips. Amyloid deposits also occur in the heart, kidneys, skin, nerves, and other tissue. LCDII is caused by mutations in the GSN gene on chromosome 9q34, which encodes a protein called gelsolin that is involved in actin metabolism. LCDII is called the **Meretoja syndrome** or **familial amyloid polyneuropathy type IV**, Finnish or Meretoja type.

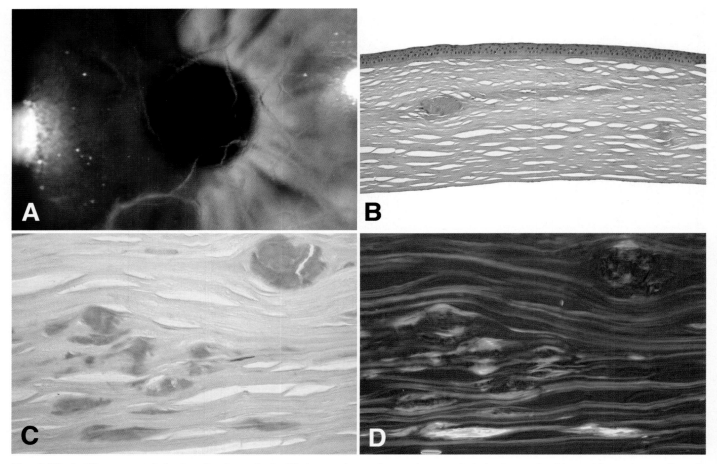

Fig. 6-22. Lattice corneal dystrophy, type I. A. Slit lamp photo shows characteristic latticework of branching relucent lines in corneal stroma. **B.** Corresponding stromal deposits of amyloid are eosinophilic but have more smudgy margins than deposits in granular dystrophy. **C.** Deposits stain positively with Congo red and show characteristic apple-green birefringence with polarized light (**D**). (**A.** Clinical photo courtesy of Dr. Irving Raber, Wills Eye Institute. **B.** H&E ×100. **C.** Congo red ×250, **D.** Congo red with crossed polarizers ×250)

Macular corneal dystrophy (MCD) is the most severe of the classic corneal stromal dystrophies (Fig. 6-23). Although rare in the United States, macular dystrophy is quite common in Saudi Arabia, India, and Iceland. Unlike the other classic stromal dystrophies, which are autosomal dominant, MCD is an autosomal recessive trait caused by a defective enzyme. Most patients develop severe visual loss by age 20 to 40 years and usually require corneal transplantation. The term macular refers to grayish opacities with indistinct borders that are found in the superficial stroma and begin axially (Fig. 6-23A). The macules are superimposed on a diffuse stromal haze that extends from limbus to limbus and involves the entire cornea.

Classified as a localized corneal mucopolysaccharidosis, MCD is caused by mutations in the CHST6 (*N*-acetylglucosamine-6-*O*-sulfotransferase) gene on chromosome 16q22. Mutations cause defective sulfonation of the proteoglycan keratan sulfate, a major constituent of the cornea's ground substance. The lack of sulfated keratan causes abnormal hydration of the stroma, which interferes

with collagen fibril spacing and destructive interference, degrading its optical properties. The hazy, poorly hydrated cornea in macular dystrophy is usually thinner than normal. This contrasts with the cloudy corneas in systemic mucopolysaccharidoses like Hurler disease, which usually are thickened. The abnormal nonsulfated keratan is insoluble and accumulates in the cytoplasm of keratocytes and corneal endothelial cells and as large extracellular deposits in the subepithelial stroma. The latter constitute the macules seen clinically. MCD appears to be the corneal manifestation of an otherwise innocuous systemic disease. Patients who have macular dystrophy type I are deficient in corneal keratan sulfate, and they also lack keratan sulfate in their serum and cartilage. Deficient keratan sulfate causes corneal opacification, but does not appear to have adverse consequences elsewhere.

Histopathologically, the cytoplasm of the keratocytes and endothelial cells has a frothy vacuolated appearance in routine H&E sections, and the extracellular deposits are comprised of vesicular granules that are mildly basophilic

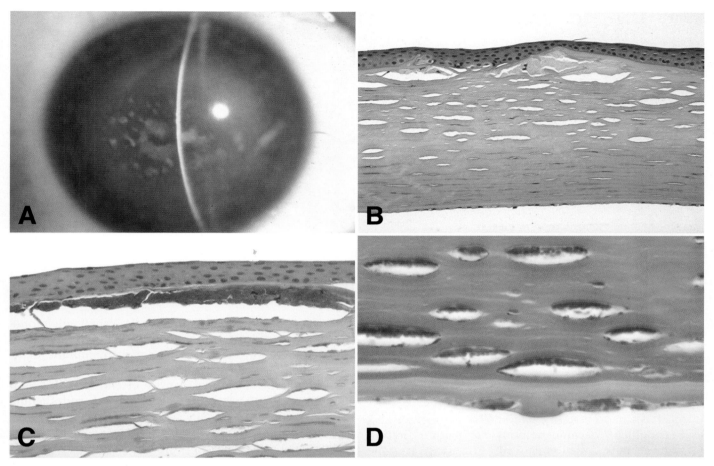

Fig. 6-23. Macular corneal dystrophy. A. The entire cornea is diffusely hazy. Grayish macules with indistinct borders are present axially. The cornea is not thickened. **B.** Large subepithelial extracellular deposits of abnormal nonsulfated keratan correspond to macules seen clinically. The stroma is thin. A few guttae stud Descemet membrane. **C.** Alcian blue stain for acid mucopolysaccharide stains large subepithelial extracellular deposit of nonsulfated keratan sulfate. Keratocytes also stain. **D.** Colloidal iron stain for acid mucopolysaccharide stains keratocytes and corneal endothelial cells. Note guttate excrescence on Descemet membrane. (**B.** H&E ×50, **C.** Alcian blue ×100, Colloidal iron ×250)

and PAS positive (Fig. 6-23B). The histochemical stains of choice for MCD are the colloidal iron and alcian blue stains for acid mucopolysaccharide (glycosaminoglycans) (Fig. 6-23C, D). Some cases of macular dystrophy have guttate excresences on Descemet membrane (Fig. 6-23D).

Schnyder crystalline dystrophy (SCD) is an autosomal dominantly inherited disorder caused by mutations in the UBIAD1 gene on the short arm of chromosome 1 (1p34.1-p36). The name crystalline dystrophy applied to the disorder refers to a deposition of polychromatic needle-shaped crystals of cholesterol in the anterior corneal stroma, which occur in approximately half of patients (Fig. 6-24A). Diffuse stromal haze and a prominent annulus lipoides senilis are other characteristic features. Central stromal opacification may necessitate penetrating keratoplasty in the fifth decade. Some patients have xanthelasmas and elevated serum lipids. A subtle pattern of stromal vacuolization is seen histopathologically in routine sections because the lipid is dissolved during processing (Fig. 6-24B). Stromal lipid deposition causes severe diffuse corneal clouding in

other rare heritable disorders of lipid metabolism including lecithin acyl transferase deficiency, fish eye disease, and Tangier disease. The histopathologic findings are relatively subtle.

François-Neetans fleck corneal dystrophy (FCD, dystrophie mouchetée) usually is an incidental finding clinically because visual acuity is unaffected. Patients have minute, asymptomatic fleck-like opacities in the deep stroma centrally, which have been likened to fly specks. Ultrastructurally, the keratocytes are swollen and contain GAGs and lipid. FCD is an autosomal dominantly inherited trait caused by mutations in the PIP5K gene (2q35).

Congenital hereditary stromal dystrophy is a stationary, autosomal dominantly inherited disorder marked by bilateral flaky or feathery clouding of the corneal stroma. The cornea is normal in thickness, but its disordered lamellae are composed of collagen fibers that are one-half normal diameter (15 nm), suggesting a defect in collagen fibrogenesis.

Deep filiform dystrophy and cornea farinata are now known to be manifestations of x-linked ichthyosis.

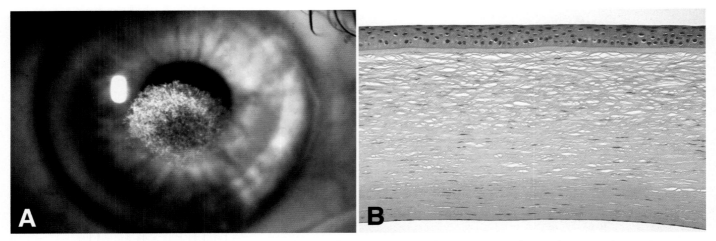

Fig. 6-24. Schnyder crystalline dystrophy. A. A deposit of cholesterol crystals is present in the axial stroma. A prominent arcus senilis is also present. **B.** Empty clefts and vacuoles that contained lipid *in vivo* are concentrated in the anterior stroma. No vessels or inflammation are present. (H&E ×50)

CORNEAL EDEMA, BULLOUS KERATOPATHY, AND THE ENDOTHELIAL DYSTROPHIES

Introduction

Corneal edema caused by endothelial damage or disease (endothelial decompensation) is a major indication for corneal transplantation (Fig. 6-25). In many cases, the endothelial damage is related to prior intraocular surgery (aphakic or pseudophakic bullous keratopathy) (Figs. 6-25 and 6-26). The edema also may be caused by primary endothelial disease. The endothelial dystrophies of the cornea include Fuchs dystrophy (FECD), which is relatively common, and congenital hereditary endothelial dystrophy (CHED) and posterior polymorphous dystrophy (PPMD), which are rare (Figs. 6-26 and 6-27).

The corneal endothelium is a relatively fragile monolayer of approximately 400,000 cells that synthesizes and rests upon a thick layer of basement membrane material called Descemet membrane (Figs. 1-8C,D and 6-26B). In the adult, the normal density of endothelial cells is 2,400 to 3,200 cells/mm². The corneal endothelium is derived embryologically from neural crest, as are the corneal stroma and most other anterior segment tissues. Mature endothelial cells do not divide, and the endothelium generally is incapable of regeneration or repair. Approximately 0.5% of the endothelial cells are lost yearly with increasing age.

The corneal endothelium plays an extremely important role in the maintenance of corneal transparency. The transparency and optical properties of the cornea depend on an exquisitely regular spacing of the collagen fibrils in the stroma that is necessary for destructive interference.

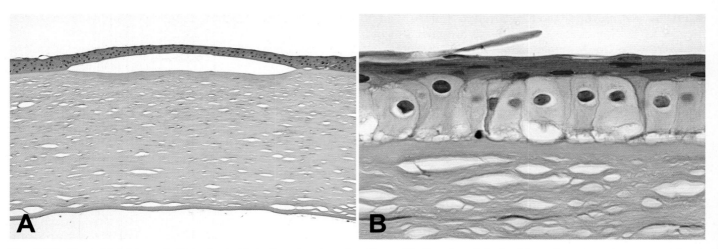

Fig. 6-25. Corneal edema. A. Pseudophakic bullous keratopathy. The epithelium has detached from the edematous cornea forming a bulla. Descemet membrane is regular in caliber. The endothelium is markedly atrophic. **B.** Basal edema, corneal epithelium. Cells comprising edematous basal cell layer of corneal epithelium have swollen lucent cytoplasm. (**A.** H&E ×25, **B.** H&E ×250)

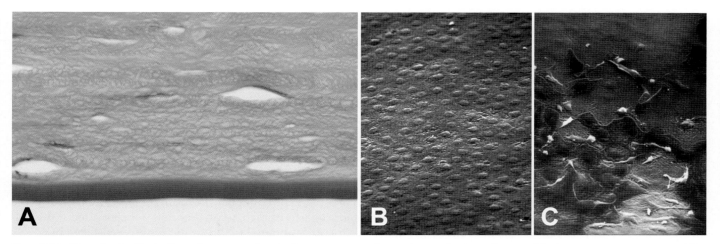

Fig. 6-26. **Pseudophakic bullous keratopathy** **A.** Descemet membrane is regular in caliber and lacks guttate excrescences. The endothelium is severely atrophic. Edematous stroma has cotton candy appearance and diminished clefts. **B.** Scanning electron micrograph of healthy endothelial mosaic in normal cornea. **C.** SEM of PBK shows focally denuded Descemet membrane. Residual cells comprising severely atrophic residual endothelium in PBK specimen are large and polymorphic. (**A.** PAS ×250, **B.** SEM ×320, **C.** SEM ×160)

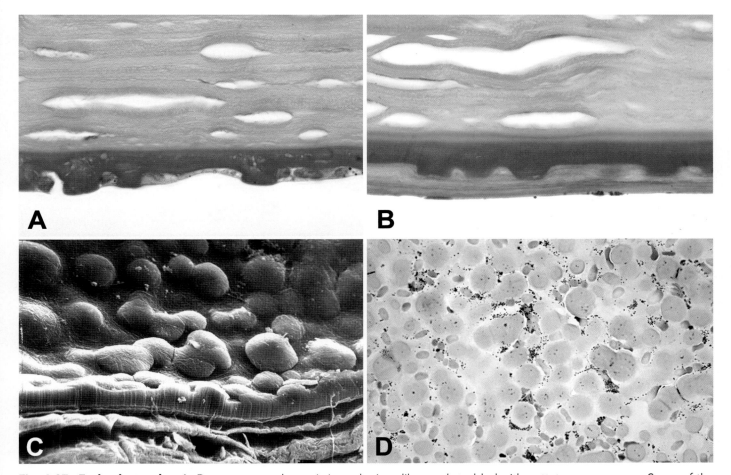

Fig. 6-27. **Fuchs dystrophy.** **A.** Descemet membrane is irregular in caliber and studded with guttate excrescences. Some of the residual endothelial cells contain melanin granules. **B.** Fuchs dystrophy, buried guttae. Guttae have been "buried" by a newly synthesized layer of extracellular matrix material. The endothelium is markedly atrophic. Buried guttae typically occur in the center of the cornea. **C.** Mushroom or anvil-shaped excrescences disclosed by scanning electron microscopy stud posterior surface of Descemet membrane. The specimen is oriented epithelial side down **D.** Flat preparation of Descemet membrane stripped from patient with FECD during DSEK procedure. Many endothelial cells between round pink guttae contain melanin granules. (**A.** PAS ×250, **B.** PAS ×250, SEM ×300, **D.** Whole mount flat preparation stained with H&E ×100)

This requires the stroma to be in a state of relative dehydration. The corneal endothelium maintains this state of relative stromal dehydration by acting as a barrier to aqueous humor and as an ion-fluid pump. If the endothelium is damaged or depleted, typically during surgery, aqueous humor enters the stroma, and the glycosaminoglycan-rich ground substance swells separating the collagen fibrils, causing edema, and degrading corneal transparency. The spacing of the neighboring collagen fibrils in the stroma must be < 200 nm for there to be transparency.

Histopathologically, an edematous cornea is thickened and may show partial obliteration of artifactitious interlamellar stromal clefts. The margins of the lamellae appear somewhat indistinct, and the edematous stroma is pale and may have a frothy appearance, which has been likened to cotton candy. As secondary epithelial edema develops, the basal cells often have a pale edematous appearance (Fig. 6-25B). Fluid accumulates in the spaces between cells and beneath the epithelium, forming focal bullous areas of epithelial detachment called bullous keratopathy (Fig. 6-25A). Bullous keratopathy is painful because the anterior cornea's rich supply of sensory nerve endings are exposed when the epithelial bullae rupture, which they often do. The cornea is also predisposed to infection because the normally protective epithelial layer has been compromised. A degenerative pannus (Fig. 6-16) develops in many corneas with chronic edema and bullous keratopathy. This opaque layer of connective tissue is interposed between the base of the epithelium and Bowman layer, which is intact. Secondary epithelial changes similar to those reported in epithelial basement membrane dystrophy are observed occasionally.

FUCHS DYSTROPHY

Fuchs dystrophy (FECD) presents in the fifth or sixth decade of life with corneal edema and bullous keratopathy, which are caused by a primary defect in the corneal endothelium (Fig. 6-27). By far, the most common corneal dystrophy in the United States, FECD affects 4% of individuals over age 40 and is more common and severe in women. This primary dystrophy of the corneal endothelium is readily diagnosed clinically and histopathologically by characteristic changes in Descemet membrane.

Descemet membrane in FECD typically is thickened and studded with anvil- or mushroom-shaped guttate excrescences of abnormal basement membrane material made by the dystrophic endothelial cells (Fig. 6-27A–D). The term cornea guttata ("drop-like cornea"; gutta = drop) is often applied to FECD and to cases of endothelial dystrophy prior to the onset of endothelial decompensation and bullous keratopathy. The guttae (*guttata* is an adjective!) are evident on slit lamp biomicroscopy as tiny drop-like relucencies on the posterior corneal surface. These appear as round or oval profiles in flat preparations of Descemet stripping endothelial keratoplasty (DSEK) specimens

(Fig. 6-27D). Histopathologically, guttae that have been buried by a newly elaborated posterior layer of Descemet membrane are often found, especially in the central cornea (Fig. 6-27B). Thickening and multilamination of Descemet membrane also is observed. In rare cases, Descemet membrane lacks guttate excrescences and is diffusely thickened instead. The endothelium typically is atrophic, but a significant number of corneal endothelial cells persists in many cases. The severe endothelial loss that characterizes pseudophakic bullous keratopathy (PBK) (Fig. 6-26) is quite unusual in FECD, and if present, suggests the superimposition of PBK on a pre-existent dystrophy. Granules of iris pigment epithelial melanin are typically found in the cytoplasm of the endothelial cells. Observation of this retrocorneal pigmentation in the fundus red reflex may suggest the diagnosis during ophthalmoscopy or retinoscopy. Unlike the vertically oriented Krukenberg spindle of pigmentary glaucoma, the endothelial pigmentation in FECD is irregular in shape, suggesting that the pattern of pigmentation is governed by an endothelial abnormality and not the circulation of aqueous humor.

FECD appears to be a complex inherited disorder caused by an interaction of genetic and environmental factors. Most cases lack a positive family history. In some instances, FECD appears to be an autosomal dominant disorder with incomplete penetrance. Mutations in the COL8A2 gene have been found in rare, early-onset cases.

PSEUDOPHAKIC BULLOUS KERATOPATHY

Pseudophakic bullous keratopathy (PBK) occurs in patients who have undergone cataract surgery with the implantation of a prosthetic intraocular lens (IOL) (pseudophacos) (Figs. 6-25 and 6-26). Aphakic bullous keratopathy (ABK) follows cataract surgery without IOL implantation. These iatrogenic forms of corneal edema result from direct or delayed damage to the corneal endothelium. In the past, PBK was one of the most common indications for corneal transplantation, but the incidence has decreased in recent years as IOL technology and surgical techniques have improved.

Descemet membrane in PBK is not thickened and is regular in caliber without guttate excrescences (Fig. 6-26). The endothelium usually is severely atrophic and may appear totally absent. Bullous keratopathy may be severe; some cases have total epithelial desquamation. Degenerative pannus formation is encountered less often than in FECD, probably because PBK has a more acute course.

An almost identical picture of corneal edema caused by severe endothelial decompensation occurs in most transplanted corneas that have failed necessitating repeat penetrating keratoplasty. An eosinophilic retrocorneal fibrous membrane is found on the posterior surface of Descemet membrane in many failed grafts. If a retrocorneal fibrous membrane is observed microscopically, the periphery of the edematous cornea should be examined carefully for surgical scars and suture tracts.

Massive corneal edema occurs in infants who have **congenital hereditary endothelial dystrophy (CHED)**. Autosomal dominant (CHED1) and recessive (CHED2) variants are recognized. CHED2 is caused by mutations in the SLC4A11 gene. Atrophic endothelium and massive thickening of Descemet membrane have been reported in some cases. However, recent reports have emphasized the association of massive corneal edema and normal-appearing endothelium. An inherited defect in endothelial function has been postulated in such cases.

POSTERIOR POLYMORPHOUS DYSTROPHY

Posterior polymorphous dystrophy (PPMD) is an autosomal dominantly inherited disorder characterized by the presence of irregular blebs or vacuoles at the level of Descemet membrane in the posterior cornea. These often are surrounded by a grayish area of mild opacification. The heterogenous spectrum of disease seen in some kindreds also includes congenital corneal clouding, trough- or gutter-shaped lesions of the posterior cornea, and peripheral anterior synechia formation that resembles that seen in the ICE syndrome, but is bilateral. The gutters can be confused with old Descemet membrane tears caused by obstetrical forceps injuries, but they lack relucent margins.

The corneal endothelial cells in PPMD have many properties of corneal epithelial cells (Fig. 6-28). They usually grow in a multilayered fashion, and electron microscopy discloses cytoplasmic tonofilaments and numerous surface microvilli. In addition, the endothelial cells express surface epithelial cytokeratins, particularly cytokeratin 7 and 19. Although some autosomal recessive cases have been reported, most cases of PPMD are inherited as an autosomal dominant trait. Mutations in the VSX1, COL8A2, and TCF8 genes have been implicated in PPMD, but evidence for transcription factor TCF8 is the most convincing.

Corneal edema occurs in some patients who have the iridocorneal endothelial or ICE syndrome, which is characterized by unilateral glaucoma and secondary iris abnormalities caused by a proliferation of abnormal corneal endothelial cells. This disease spectrum includes the Cogan-Reese and Chandler syndromes and essential iris atrophy. The ICE syndrome is discussed further in Chapter 8.

CORNEAL MANIFESTATIONS OF SYSTEMIC DISEASE

Copper deposition in the peripheral part of Descemet membrane is manifest clinically as a Kayser-Fleischer ring in patients with **Wilson hepatolenticular degeneration** (Fig. 6-29B). An analogous deposit of copper in the anterior lens capsule causes sunflower cataract (Fig. 4-12B). Corneal copper deposition has been reported in patients with primary biliary cirrhosis, familial cholestatic cirrhosis, monoclonal gammopathies associated with multiple myeloma, and pulmonary carcinoma.

Deposits of immunoglobulin in the cornea may herald the presence of protein dyscrasias such as multiple myeloma or Waldenstrom macroglobulinemia (Fig. 6-30). The corneal deposition is quite protean in its manifestations. Deep polymorphic infiltrates occur in some patients; others develop polychromatic crystals in the corneal epithelium.

Other causes of corneal crystals include SCD, cystinosis, gout, Bietti crystalline dystrophy, and injury by the sap of the tropical aroid plant Dieffenbachia that contains

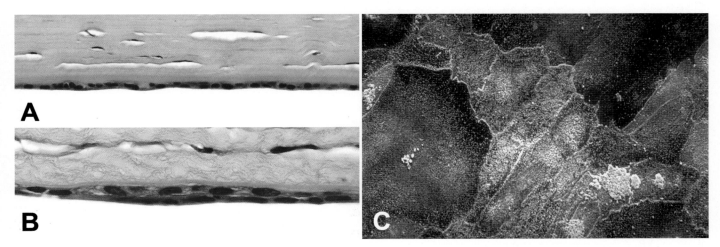

Fig. 6-28. Posterior polymorphous dystrophy. A. The corneal endothelium is hypercellular. **B.** Multilayered growth, a surface epithelial characteristic, is present. **C.** Endothelial cells disclosed by scanning electron microscopy vary markedly in size and shape. Numerous microvilli are present on the surface of the cells. (**A.** H&E ×100, **B.** H&E ×250, **C.** SEM ×1,000)

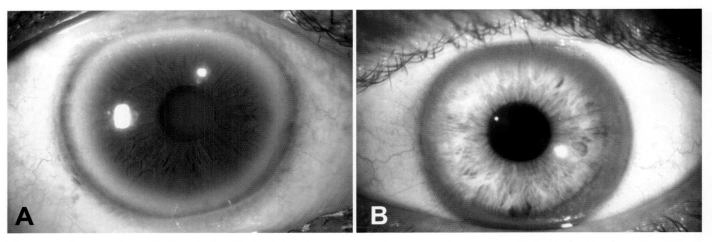

Fig. 6-29. Corneal rings. A. Annulus senilis. Peripheral cornea contains annular deposit of lipid. **B.** Kayser-Fleischer ring, Wilson disease. Brownish ring in peripheral cornea is caused by copper deposition in Descemet membrane.

crystalline raphides. Cystine crystals dissolve in water; preservation necessitates fixation of the cornea in absolute alcohol.

Cysts of the pars plana and pars plicata are quite common in multiple myeloma. The cysts in affected patients contain myeloma protein or Bence Jones protein, which is precipitated by fixation causing the cysts to become milky white (Fig. 9-23). Pars plana cysts found incidentally in elderly patients are filled with hyaluronic acid and are not opacified by fixation (Fig. 9-23).

CORNEAL TRANSPLANTATION

Corneal transplantation or penetrating keratoplasty involves the excision of a central disc or button of full-thickness cornea and its replacement with new

transparent tissue obtained postmortem from a donor. Corneal transplantation does not require systemic immunosuppression because the cornea is an avascular structure. Diseases with extensive corneal vascularization tend to do less well.

Corneal edema caused by endothelial damage or dystrophy is the most common indication for corneal transplantation in the United States. This category includes FECD and pseudophakic or aphakic bullous keratopathy. Most "failed grafts" also are edematous due to endothelial loss. Keratoconus is another very common indication for transplantation. Other diseases treated by penetrating keratoplasty include interstitial keratitis, visually disabling scars, corneal dystrophies, and infectious keratopathies including chronic HSV stromal keratitis and bacterial or fungal ulcers. Surgery is performed in acute keratitis when perforation has occurred or is imminent, or

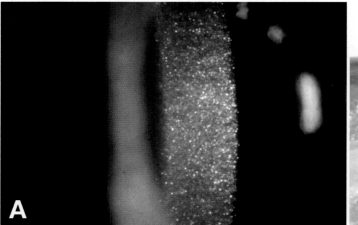

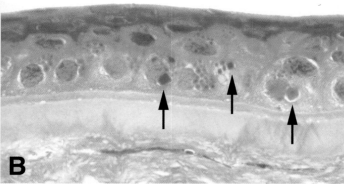

Fig. 6-30. Immunoglobulin deposits in protein dyscrasias. A. Corneal crystals, multiple myeloma. Myriad polychromatic crystals in the corneal epithelium were the presenting manifestation of multiple myeloma. (Photo courtesy of Dario Savino-Zari, Caracas, Venezuela.) **B.** *Arrows* denote square protein crystals in corneal epithelial cells. A verticillate epithelial deposit was the presenting manifestation of Waldenström macroglobulinemia. (**B.** Masson trichrome ×250)

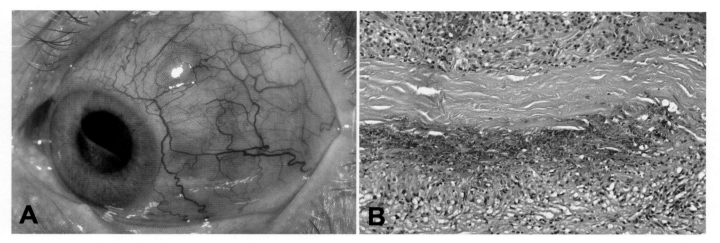

Fig. 6-31. Rheumatoid scleritis. A. Thinned areas of the sclera appear blue because there is increased visibility of the underlying uveal tract. **B.** A zonal pattern of granulomatous inflammation identical to that found in a rheumatoid nodule is seen. A palisading granuloma of epithelioid histiocytes surrounds a sequestrum of residual devitalized scleral collagen. Necrosis is evident as smudgy basophilic foci along the lower border of the sequestrum. (H&E ×50)

occasionally when the identity of the pathogenetic organism is uncertain.

Several forms of lamellar keratoplasty have become increasingly popular in recent years. These include Descemet stripping endothelial keratoplasty (DSEK) and deep lamellar anterior keratectomy (DALK).

DSEK is used to treat corneas with endothelial decompensation such as FECD or PBK. In this procedure, Descemet membrane and its dysfunctional endothelium are stripped from the posterior corneal surface. A graft of donor cornea tissue comprising healthy endothelium, Descemet membrane, and posterior corneal stroma is inserted in the anterior chamber. The graft adheres to posterior corneal surface without sutures. Patients recover vision faster and have significantly less astigmatism after DSEK compared to penetrating keratoplastiy. DSEK specimens can be sectioned routinely, or examined as flat mounts.

Deep anterior lamellar keratoplasty (DALK) is used to treat keratoconus and other anterior pathologies. A thick lamella of anterior corneal tissue including the epithelium, Bowman membane, and most of the stroma is excised and replaced with a new graft of donor tissue. Descemet membrane and endothelium, which typically are normal in keratoconus, are not affected. During the procedure, an injection of air is used to form a surgical plane. As a result, the stroma contains empty vacuoles called pneumatic artifact. The posterior surface of the anterior lamella is often irregular. Specimens from aborted DALK procedures include lamellas of anterior and posterior cornea.

The junction between the corneal flap and posterior stroma may be nearly invisible in corneal grafts after LASIK refractive surgery. Interface epithelialization complicates some cases.

THE SCLERA

Sclera specimens are relatively uncommon, and typically are inflammatory in nature. A superficial infiltrate of lymphocytes and plasma cells is seen in benign episcleritis. A necrotizing zonal pattern of granulomatous inflammation analogous to that seen in rheumatoid nodules characterizes the severe scleritis that complicates rheumatoid arthritis (Fig. 6-31). In nodular episcleritis, the granulomatous reaction is limited to the episcleral tissues. In severe cases of rheumatoid scleritis (scleromalacia perforans), areas of severe scleral thinning appear blue clinically because there is increased visibility of the underlying pigmented uvea. Patients who have rheumatoid scleritis are susceptible to the development of fatal cardiac and pulmonary manifestations of their rheumatoid disease. Posterior scleritis can mimic a primary uveal neoplasm. Scleritis and peripheral corneal ulceration can complicate systemic lupus erythematosus, polyarteritis nodosa, Wegener granulomatosis, and relapsing polychondritis. Focal plaques of scleral calcification called Cogan senile plaques occur anterior to the insertion of the rectus muscles in some elderly patients.

BIBLIOGRAPHY

General References

Rodrigues MM, Hidayat AA, Choe HS. Advances in corneal pathology. In: Grossniklaus HE, Margo CE, eds. *Advances in Ophthalmic Pathology. Ophthalmol Clin North Am* 1995;8:83–107.

Spencer WH. Cornea. In: Spencer WH, ed. *Ophthalmic Pathology: An Atlas and Textbook.* Philadelphia, PA: WB Saunders, 1985:229–388.

Starck T, Hersh PS, Kenyon KR. Corneal dysgeneses, dystrophies and degenerations. In: Albert DM, Jakobiec FA, eds. *Principles and Practice of Ophthalmology: Clinical Practice,* vol. 1, Philadelphia, PA: WB Saunders, 1994:13–77.

Developmental Lesions

Kanai A, Wood TC, Polack FM, et al. The fine structure of sclerocornea. *Invest Ophthalmol Vis Sci* 1971;10:687–694.

Kim T, Cohen EJ, Schnall BM, et al. Ultrasound biomicroscopy and histopathology of sclerocornea. *Cornea* 1998;17:443–445.

Mirzayans F, Pearce WG, MacDonald IM, et al. Mutation of the PAX6 gene in patients with autosomal dominant keratitis. *Am J Hum Genet* 1995;57:539–548.

Pearce WG, Mielke BW, Hassard DT, et al. Autosomal dominant keratitis: a possible aniridia variant. *Can J Ophthalmol* 1995;30:131–137.

Salmon JF, Wallis CE, Murray AD. Variable expressivity of autosomal dominant microcornea with cataract. *Arch Ophthalmol* 1988;106:505–510.

Simpson WA, Parsons MA. The ultrastructural pathological features of congenital microcoria. A case report. *Arch Ophthalmol* 1989;107:99–102.

Peters Anomaly

Alkemade P. *Dysgenesis Mesodermalis of the Iris and the Cornea.* Assen, Netherlands: Charles C Thomas, 1969.

Alward WL. Axenfeld-Rieger syndrome in the age of molecular genetics. *Am J Ophthalmol* 2000;130:107–115.

Espinoza HM, Cox CJ, Semina EV, et al. A molecular basis for differential developmental anomalies in Axenfeld-Rieger syndrome. *Hum Mol Genet* 2002;11:743–753.

Gomes J, Eagle RJ, Gomes A, et al. Recurrent keratopathy after penetrating keratoplasty for aniridia. *Cornea* 1996;15:457–462.

Green JS, Johnson GJ. Congenital cataract with microcornea and Peters' anomaly as expressions of one autosomal dominant gene. *Ophthalmic Paediatr Genet* 1986;7:187–194.

Hanson IM, Fletcher JM, Jordan T, et al. Mutations at the PAX6 locus are found in heterogeneous anterior segment malformations including Peters' anomaly. *Nat Genet* 1994;6:168–173.

Hanson IM, Fletcher JM, Jordan T, et al. Mutations at the PAX6 locus are found in heterogeneous anterior segment malformations including Peters' anomaly. *Nat Genet* 1994;6:168–173.

Henkind P, Siegel IM, Carr RE. Mesodermal dysgenesis of the anterior segment: Rieger's anomaly. *Arch Ophthalmol* 1965;73:810–817.

Hennekam RC, Van Schooneveld MJ, Ardinger HH, et al. The Peters'-Plus syndrome: description of 16 patients and review of the literature. *Clin Dysmorphol* 1993;2:283–300.

Heon E, Barsoum-Homsy M, Cevrette L, et al. Peters' anomaly. The spectrum of associated ocular and systemic malformations. *Ophthalmic Paediatr Genet* 1992;13:137–143.

Lines MA, Kozlowski K, Walter MA. Molecular genetics of Axenfeld-Rieger malformations. *Hum Mol Genet* 2002;11:1177–1184.

Maillette de Buy Wenniger-Prick LJ, Hennekam RC. The Peters' plus syndrome: a review. *Ann Genet* 2002;45:97–103.

Mirzayans F, Pearce WG, MacDonald IM, et al. Mutation of the PAX6 gene in patients with autosomal dominant keratitis. *Am J Hum Genet* 1995;57:539–548.

Myles WM, Flanders ME, Chitayat D, et al. Peters' anomaly: a clinicopathologic study. *J Pediatr Ophthalmol Strabismus* 1992;29:374–381.

Pearce WG, Mielke BW, Hassard DT, et al. Autosomal dominant keratitis: a possible aniridia variant. *Can J Ophthalmol* 1995;30:131–137.

Reese A, Ellsworth R. The anterior chamber cleavage syndrome. *Arch Ophthalmol* 1966;75:307–318.

Rieger H. Dysgenesis mesodermalis Corneae et Iridis. *Zeitschrift fur Augenheilk* 1935;86:333.

Shields M, Buckley E, Klintworth G, et al. Axenfeld-Rieger syndrome: a spectrum of developmental disorders. *Surv Ophthalmol* 1985;29:387–409.

Shields MB. Axenfeld-Rieger syndrome: a theory of mechanism and distinctions from the iridocorneal endothelial syndrome. *Trans Am Ophthalmol Soc* 1983;81:736–784.

Townsend WM, Font RL, Zimmerman LE. Congenital corneal leukomas. 2. Histopathologic findings in 19 eyes with central defect in Descemet's membrane. *Am J Ophthalmol* 1974;77:192–206.

Townsend WM. Congenital corneal leukomas. 1. Central defect in Descemet's membrane. *Am J Ophthalmol* 1974;77:80–86.

Traboulsi EI, Maumenee IH. Peters' anomaly and associated congenital malformations. *Arch Ophthalmol* 1992;110:1739–1742.

van Schooneveld MJ, Delleman JW, Beemer FA, et al. Peters'-plus: a new syndrome. *Ophthalmic Paediatr Genet* 1984;4:141–145.

Vieira V, David G, Roche O, et al. Identification of four new PITX2 gene mutations in patients with Axenfeld-Rieger syndrome. *Mol Vis* 2006;12:1448–1460.

Waring GO III, Rodrigues MM, Laibson PR. Anterior chamber cleavage syndrome. A stepladder classification. *Surv Ophthalmol* 1975;20:3–27.

Bacterial Keratitis

Bullington RH Jr, Lanier JD, Font RL. Nontuberculous mycobacterial keratitis. Report of two cases and review of the literature. *Arch Ophthalmol* 1992;110:519–524.

Dugel PU, Holland GN, Brown HH. Mycobacterium fortuitum keratitis. *Am J Ophthalmol* 1988;105:661–669.

Elder MJ, Stapleton F, Evans E, et al. Biofilm-related infections in ophthalmology. *Eye* 1995;9:102–109.

Elder MJ, Matheson M, Stapleton F, et al. Biofilm formation in infectious crystalline keratopathy due to *Candida albicans*. Cornea 1996;15:301–304.

Foroozan R, Eagle RC Jr, Cohen EJ. Fungal keratitis in a soft contact lens wearer. *Clao J* 2000;26:166–168.

Hunts JH, Matoba AY, Osato MS, et al. Infectious crystalline keratopathy. The role of bacterial exopolysaccharide. *Arch Ophthalmol* 1993;111:528–530.

Meisler DM, Langston RH, Naab TJ, et al. Infectious crystalline keratopathy. *Am J Ophthalmol* 1984;97:337–343.

Rhem MN, Wilhelmus KR, Font RL. Infectious crystalline keratopathy caused by *Candida parapsilosis*. *Cornea* 1996;15:543–545.

Herpetic Keratitis

Cook SD, Hill JH. Herpes simplex virus: molecular biology and the possibility of corneal latency. *Surv Ophthalmol* 1991;36:140–148.

Dawson CR, Togni B, Moore TE Jr. Structural changes in chronic herpetic keratitis studied by light and electron microscopy. *Arch Ophthalmol* 1968;79:740–747.

Font RL. Chronic ulcerative keratitis caused by herpes simplex virus. *Arch Ophthalmol* 1973;90:382–385.

Hendricks RL. An immunologist's view of herpes simplex keratitis: Thygeson Lecture 1996. *Cornea* 1997;16:503–506.

Lee SY. Herpes simplex virus ocular infections. *Drugs Today (Barc)* 1998;34:241–249.

Liesgang TJ. Biology and molecular aspects of herpes simplex and varicella-zoster virus infections. *Ophthalmology* 1992;99:781–799.

Pepose JS. Herpes simplex keratitis: role of viral infection versus immune response. *Surv Ophthalmol* 1991;35:345–352.

Piebenga LW, Laibson PR. Dendritic lesions in herpes zoster ophthalmicus. *Arch Ophthalmol* 1973;90:268–270.

Zhao Z-S, Granucci F, Yeh L, et al. Molecular mimicry by herpes simplex virus-type I: autoimmune disease after viral infection. *Science* 1998;279:1344–1347.

Epidemic Keratoconjunctivitis

Dawson CR, Hanna L, Wood TR, et al. Adenovirus type 8 keratoconjunctivitis in the United States. III. Epidemiological, clinical and microbiologic features. *Am J Ophthalmol* 1970;69:473–480.

Laibson PR, Dhiri S, Oconer J, et al. Corneal infiltrates in epidemic keratoconjunctivitis: response to double-blind corticosteroid therapy. *Arch Ophthalmol* 1970;84:36–40.

Wilhelmus KR, Font RL, Lehmann RP, et al. Cytomegalovirus keratitis in acquired immunodeficiency syndrome. *Arch Ophthalmol* 1996;114:869–872.

Interstitial Keratitis

Char DH, Cogan DG, Sullivan WR. Immunologic study of non-syphilitic interstitial keratitis with vestibulo-auditory symptoms. *Am J Ophthalmol* 1975;80:491–494.

Chynn EW, Jakobiec FA. Cogan's syndrome: ophthalmic, audiovestibular, and systemic manifestations and therapy. *Int Ophthalmol Clin* 1996;36:61–72.

Waring GO, Font RL, Rodrigues MM, et al. Alterations of Descemet's membrane in interstitial keratitis. *Am J Ophthalmol* 1976;81:773–785.

Acanthamoeba Keratitis

Auran JD, Starr MB, Jakobiec FA. Acanthamoeba keratitis: a review of the literature. *Cornea* 1987;62:2–26.

Chan CC, Ottesen EA, Awadzi K, et al. Immunopathology of ocular onchocerciasis. I. Inflammatory cells infiltrating the anterior segment. *Clin Exp Immunol* 1989;77:367–372.

Clarke DW, Niederkorn JY. The pathophysiology of Acanthamoeba keratitis. *Trends Parasitol* 2006;22:175–180.

Font RL, Su GW, Matoba AY. Microsporidial stromal keratitis. *Arch Ophthalmol* 2003;121:1045–1047.

Garner A. Pathogenesis of acanthamoebic keratitis: hypothesis based on a histological analysis of 30 cases. *Br J Ophthalmol* 1993;77:366–370.

Hall LR, Pearlman E. Pathogenesis of onchocercal keratitis (River blindness). *Clin Microbiol Rev* 1999;12:445–453.

Kremer I, Cohen EJ, Eagle RC Jr, et al. Histopathologic evaluation of stromal inflammation in Acanthamoeba keratitis. *Clao J* 1994;20:45–48.

Marines HC, Osato MS, Font RL. The value of calcofluor white in the diagnosis of mycotic and *Acanthamoeba* infections of the eye and ocular adnexa. *Ophthalmology* 1987;94:23–26.

Mathers W, Stevens G Jr, Rodrigues M, et al. Immunopathology and electron microscopy of Acanthamoeba keratitis. *Am J Ophthalmol* 1987;103:626–635.

Mietz H, Font RL. Acanthamoeba keratitis with granulomatous reaction involving the stroma and anterior chamber. *Arch Ophthalmol* 1997;115:259–263.

Paul EV, Zimmerman LE. Some observations on the ocular pathology of onchocerciasis. *Hum Pathol* 1970;1:581–594.

Pearlman E, Gillette-Ferguson I. Onchocerca volvulus, Wolbachia and river blindness. *Chem Immunol Allergy* 2007;92:254–265.

Pearlman E, Hall LR, Higgins AW, et al. The role of eosinophils and neutrophils in helminth-induced keratitis. *Invest Ophthalmol Vis Sci* 1998;39:1176–1182.

Thebpatiphat N, Hammersmith KM, Rocha FN, et al. Acanthamoeba keratitis: a parasite on the rise. *Cornea* 2007;26:701–706.

Vemuganti GK, Pasricha G, Sharma S, et al. Granulomatous inflammation in Acanthamoeba keratitis: an immunohistochemical study of five cases and review of literature. *Indian J Med Microbiol* 2005;23:231–238.

Peripheral Corneal Ulcerations

Ahmed M, Niffenegger JH, Jakobiec FA, et al. Diagnosis of limited ophthalmic Wegener granulomatosis: distinctive pathologic features with ANCA test confirmation. *Int Ophthalmol* 2008;28:35–46.

Austin P, Green WR, Sallyer DC, et al. Peripheral corneal degeneration and occlusive vasculitis in Wegener's granulomatosis. *Am J Ophthalmol* 1978;85:311–317.

Brown SI, Mondino BJ, Rabin BS. Autoimmune phenomenon in Mooren's ulcer. *Am J Ophthalmol* 1976;82:835–840.

Brown SI. Mooren's ulcer. Histopathology and proteolytic enzymes of adjacent conjunctiva. *Br J Ophthalmol* 1975;59:670–674.

Frayer WC. The histopathology of perilimbal ulceration in Wegener's granulomatosis. *Arch Ophthalmol* 1960;64:88–94.

Guyer DR, Barraquer J, McDonnell PJ, et al. Terrien's marginal degeneration: clinicopathologic case reports. *Graefes Arch Clin Exp Ophthalmol* 1987;225:19–27.

Moazami G, Auran JD, Florakis GJ, et al. Interferon treatment of Mooren's ulcers associated with hepatitis C. *Am J Ophthalmol* 1995;119:365–366.

Corneal Degenerations

Austin P, Jakobiec FA, Iwamoto T. Elastodysplasia and elastodystrophy as the pathologic bases of ocular pterygia and pinguecula. *Ophthalmology* 1983;90:96–109.

Barchiesi BJ, Eckel RH, Ellis PP. The cornea and disorders of lipid metabolism. *Surv Ophthalmol* 1991;36:1–22.

Cogan DG, Albright F, Bartter FC. Hypercalcemia and band keratopathy. Report of nineteen cases. *Arch Ophthalmol* 1940;40:624–638.

Cursino JW, Fine BS. A histologic study of calcific and noncalcific band keratopathy. *Am J Ophthalmol* 1976;82:395–404.

Detorakis ET, Spandidos DA. Pathogenetic mechanisms and treatment options for ophthalmic pterygium: trends and perspectives (Review). *Int J Mol Med* 2009;23(4):439–447.

Dua HS, Miri A, Said DG. Contemporary limbal stem cell transplantation—a review. *Clin Experiment Ophthalmol* 2010;38:104–117.

Dua HS, Saini JS, Azuara-Blanco A, et al. Limbal stem cell deficiency: concept, aetiology, clinical presentation, diagnosis and management. *Indian J Ophthalmol* 2000;48:83–89.

Dua HS, Shanmuganathan VA, Powell-Richards AO, et al. Limbal epithelial crypts: a novel anatomical structure and a putative limbal stem cell niche. *Br J Ophthalmol* 2005;89:529–532.

Dushku N, Hatcher SL, Albert DM, et al. p53 expression and relation to human papillomavirus infection in pinguceulae, pterygia, and limbal tumors. *Arch Ophthalmol* 1999;117:1593–1599.

Eagle RC Jr, Dillon EC, Laibson PR. Compensatory epithelial hyperplasia in human corneal disease. *Trans Am Ophthalmol Soc* 1992;90:265–273, discussion 74–76.

Freedman A. Climatic droplet keratopathy. I. Clinical aspects. *Arch Ophthalmol* 1973;89:193–197.

Freedman A. Labrador keratopathy and related diseases. *Can J Ophthalmol* 1973;8:286–290.

Gray RH, Johnson GJ, Freedman A. Climatic droplet keratopathy. *Surv Ophthalmol* 1992;36:241–253.

Hida T, Kigasawa K, Tanaka E, et al. Primary band-shaped spheroidal degeneration of the cornea: three cases from two consanguineous families. *Br J Ophthalmol* 1986;70:347–353.

Hogan MJ, Alvarado J. Pterygium and pinguecula: electron microscopic study. *Arch Ophthalmol* 1967;78:174–186.

Klintworth GK. Chronic actinic keratopathy—a condition associated with conjunctival elastosis (pinguceulae) and typified by characteristic extracellular concretions. *Am J Pathol* 1972;67:327–342.

Nevyas AS, Raber IM, Eagle RC Jr, et al. Acute band keratopathy following intracameral Viscoat. *Arch Ophthalmol* 1987;105:958–964.

Ormerod LD, Dahan E, Hagele JE, et al. Serious occurrences in the natural history of advanced climatic keratopathy. *Ophthalmology* 1994;101:448–453.

Rodrigues MM, Laibson PR, Weinreb S. Corneal elastosis. Appearance of band-like keratopathy and spheroidal degeneration. *Arch Ophthalmol* 1975;93:111–114.

Secker GA, Daniels JT. Corneal epithelial stem cells: deficiency and regulation. *Stem Cell Rev* 2008;4:159–168.

Tsai YY, Chang KC, Lin CL, et al. p53 Expression in pterygium by immunohistochemical analysis: a series report of 127 cases and review of the literature. *Cornea* 2005;24(5):583–586.

Vannas A, Hogan MJ, Wood I. Salzmann's nodular degeneration of the cornea. *Am J Ophthalmol* 1975;79:211–219.

Vitamin A Deficiency

Sjögren H, Bloch K. Keratoconjunctivitis sicca and the Sjögren syndrome. *Surv Ophthalmol* 1971;16:145–159.

Smith RS, Farrell T, Bailey T. Keratomalacia. *Surv Ophthalmol* 1975;20:213–219.

Suan EP, Bedrossian EH Jr, Eagle RC Jr, et al. Corneal perforation in patients with vitamin A deficiency in the United States. *Arch Ophthalmol* 1990;108:350–353.

Venkataswamy G. Ocular manifestations of vitamin A deficiency. *Br J Ophthalmol* 1967;51:854–859.

Keratoconus

Barraquer-Somers E, Chan CC, Green WR. Corneal epithelial iron deposition. *Ophthalmology* 1983;90:729–734.

Cremona FA, Ghosheh FR, Rapuano CJ, et al. Keratoconus associated with other corneal dystrophies. *Cornea* 2009;28:127–135.

Heher KL, Traboulsi EI, Maumenee IH. The natural history of Leber's congenital amaurosis. Age-related findings in 35 patients. *Ophthalmology* 1992;99:241–245.

Kenney MC, Chwa M, Opbroek AJ, et al. Increased gelatinolytic activity in keratoconus keratocyte cultures. A correlation to an altered matrix metalloproteinase-2/tissue inhibitor of metalloproteinase ratio. *Cornea* 1994;13:114–124.

Kenney MC, Nesburn AB, Burgeson RE, et al. Abnormalities of the extracellular matrix in keratoconus corneas. *Cornea* 1997;16: 345–351.

Klintworth GK, Damms T. Corneal dystrophies and keratoconus. *Curr Opin Ophthalmol* 1995;6:44–56.

Krachmer JH, Feder RS, Belin MW. Keratoconus and related noninflammatory corneal thinning disorders. *Surv Ophthalmol* 1984;28:293–322.

Kremer I, Eagle RC, Rapuano CJ, et al. Histologic evidence of recurrent keratoconus seven years after keratoplasty. *Am J Ophthalmol* 1995;119:511–512.

Whitelock RB, Fukuchi T, Zhou L, et al. Cathepsin G, acid phosphatase, and alpha 1-proteinase inhibitor messenger RNA levels in keratoconus corneas. *Invest Ophthalmol Vis Sci* 1997;38:529–534.

Whitelock RB, Li Y, Zhou LL, et al. Expression of transcription factors in keratoconus, a cornea-thinning disease. *Biochem Biophys Res Commun* 1997;235:253–258.

Corneal Dystrophies

Kannabiran C, Klintworth GK. TGFBI gene mutations in corneal dystrophies. *Hum Mutat* 2006;27:615–625.

Klintworth GK. Advances in the molecular genetics of corneal dystrophies. *Am J Ophthalmol* 1999;128:747–754.

Klintworth GK. The molecular genetics of the corneal dystrophies—current status. *Front Biosci* 2003;8:d687–d713.

Klintworth GK. Corneal dystrophies. *Orphanet J Rare Dis* 2009;4:7.

Weiss JS, Moller HU, Lisch W, et al. The IC3D classification of the corneal dystrophies. *Cornea* 2008;27(Suppl 2):S1–S83.

Epithelial and Bowman's Membrane Dystrophies

Burns RP. Meesman's corneal dystrophy. *Trans Am Ophthalmol Soc* 1968;66:530–635.

Corden L. Molecular genetics of Meesmann's corneal dystrophy: ancestral and novel mutations in keratin 12 (K12) and complete sequence of the human KRT12 gene. *Exp Eye Res* 2000;70: 41–49.

Dota A, Nishida K, Honma Y, et al. Gelatinous drop-like corneal dystrophy is not one of the beta ig-h3- mutated corneal amyloidoses. *Am J Ophthalmol* 1998;126:832–833.

Irvine AD, Corden LD, Swensson O, et al. Mutations in cornea-specific keratin K3 or K12 genes cause Meesmann's corneal dystrophy. *Nat Genet* 1997;16:184–187.

Klintworth GK, Sommer JR, Obrian G, et al. Familial subepithelial corneal amyloidosis (gelatinous drop-like corneal dystrophy): exclusion of linkage to lactoferrin gene. *Mol Vis* 1998;4:31.

Klintworth GK, Valnickova Z, Kielar RA, et al. Familial subepithelial corneal amyloidosis—a lactoferrin-related amyloidosis. *Invest Ophthalmol Vis Sci* 1997;38:2756–2763.

Kuchle M, Green WR, Volcker HE, et al. Reevaluation of corneal dystrophies of Bowman's layer and the anterior stroma (Reis-Bucklers and Thiel-Behnke types): a light and electron microscopic study of eight corneas and a review of the literature. *Cornea* 1995;14:333–354.

Kuwabara T, Ciccarelli EC. Meesmann's corneal dystrophy. A pathological study. *Arch Ophthalmol* 1964;71:676–682.

Li S, Edward DP, Ratnakar KS, et al. Clinicohistopathological findings of gelatinous droplike corneal dystrophy among Asians. *Cornea* 1996;15:355–362.

Nishida K, Honma Y, Dota A, et al. Isolation and chromosomal localization of a cornea-specific human keratin 12 gene and detection of four mutations in Meesmann corneal epithelial dystrophy. *Am J Hum Genet* 1997;61:1268–1275.

Perry HD, Fine BS, Caldwell DR. Reis-Bücklers dystrophy: a study of eight cases. *Arch Ophthalmol* 1979;97:664–670.

Quantock AJ, Nishida K, Kinoshita S. Histopathology of recurrent gelatinous drop-like corneal dystrophy. *Cornea* 1998;17:215–221.

Rodrigues MM, Fine BS, Laibson PR, et al. Disorders of the corneal epithelium—a clinicopathologic study of dot, geographic and fingerprint patterns. *Arch Ophthalmol* 1974;92:475–482.

Small KW, Mullen L, Barletta J, et al. Mapping of Reis-Bucklers' corneal dystrophy to chromosome 5q. *Am J Ophthalmol* 1996;121:384–390.

Sullivan LS, Baylin EB, Font R, et al. A novel mutation of the Keratin 12 gene responsible for a severe phenotype of Meesmann's corneal dystrophy. *Mol Vis* 2007;13:975–980.

Tsujikawa M, Kurahashi H, Tanaka T, et al. Homozygosity mapping of a gene responsible for gelatinous drop-like corneal dystrophy to chromosome 1p. *Am J Hum Genet* 1998;63:1073–1077.

Waring GO, Rodrigues MM, Laibson PR. Corneal dystrophies. I. Dystrophies of the epithelium, Bowman's layer and stroma. *Surv Ophthalmol* 1978;23:71–122.

Weber FL, Babel J. Gelatinous drop-like dystrophy. A form of primary corneal amyloidosis. *Arch Ophthalmol* 1980;98:144–148.

Yee RW, Sullivan LS, Lai HT, et al. Linkage mapping of Thiel-Behnke corneal dystrophy (CDB2) to chromosome 10q23-q24. *Genomics* 1997;46:152–154.

Stromal Dystrophies

Belliveau MJ, Brownstein S, Agapitos P, et al. Ultrastructural features of posterior crocodile shagreen of the cornea. *Surv Ophthalmol* 2009;54:569–575.

Edward DP, Thonar EJ, Srinivasan M, et al. Macular dystrophy of the cornea: a systemic disorder of keratan sulfate metabolism. *Ophthalmology* 1990;97:1194–1200.

Garner A, Tripathi RC. Hereditary crystalline stromal dystrophy of Schnyder. II. Histopathology and ultrastructure. *Br J Ophthalmol.* 1972;56:400–408.

Gaynor PM, Zhang WY, Weiss JS, et al. Accumulation of HDL apolipoproteins accompanies abnormal cholesterol accumulation in Schnyder's corneal dystrophy. *Arterioscler Thromb Vasc Biol* 1996;16:992–999.

Haltia M, Levy E, Meretoja J, et al. Gelsolin gene mutation—at codon 187—in familial amyloidosis, Finnish: DNA-diagnostic assay. *Am J Med Genet* 1992;42:357–359.

Hassell JR, Klintworth GK. Serum sulfotransferase levels in patients with macular corneal dystrophy type I. *Arch Ophthalmol* 1997;115:1419–1421.

Hirano K, Klintworth GK, Zhan Q, et al. Beta ig-h3 is synthesized by corneal epithelium and perhaps endothelium in Fuchs dystrophic corneas. *Curr Eye Res* 1996;15:965–972.

Hogan MJ, Albarado J. Ultrastructure of lattice dystrophy of the cornea. A case report. *Am J Ophthalmol* 1967;64:656–660.

Jonasson F, Oshima E, Thonar EJ, et al. Macular corneal dystrophy in Iceland. A clinical, genealogic, and immunohistochemical study of 28 patients. *Ophthalmology* 1996;103:1111–1117.

Jones ST, Zimmerman LE. Histopathologic differentiation of granular, macular, and lattice dystrophies of the cornea. *Am J Ophthalmol* 1961;51:394–410.

Karp CL, Scott IU, Green WR, et al. Central cloudy corneal dystrophy of Francois. A clinicopathologic study. *Arch Ophthalmol* 1997;115:1058–1062.

Kivela T, Tarkkanen A, Frangione B, et al. Ocular amyloid deposition in familial amyloidosis, Finnish: an analysis of native and variant gelsolin in Meretoja's syndrome. *Invest Ophthalmol Vis Sci* 1994;35:3759–3769.

Kivela T, Tarkkanen A, McLean I, et al. Immunohistochemical analysis of lattice corneal dystrophies types I and II. *Br J Ophthalmol* 1993;77:799–804.

Klintworth Chang TS, Culbertson WW. Central cloudy corneal dystrophy of Francois. A clinicopathologic study. *Arch Ophthalmol* 1997;115:1058–1062.

Klintworth GK. Lattice corneal dystrophy. An inherited variety of amyloidosis restricted to the cornea. *Am J Pathol* 1967;50:371–399.

Klintworth GK, Oshima E, al-Rajhi A, et al. Macular corneal dystrophy in Saudi Arabia: a study of 56 cases and recognition of a new immunophenotype. *Am J Ophthalmol* 1997;124:9–18.

Liu NP, Baldwin J, Lennon F, et al. Coexistence of macular corneal dystrophy types I and II in a single sibship. *Br J Ophthalmol* 1998;82:241–244.

Loeffler KU, Edward DP, Tso MO. An immunohistochemical study of gelsolin immunoreactivity in corneal amyloidosis. *Am J Ophthalmol* 1992;113:546–554.

Mannis MJ, Krachmer JH, Rodrigues MM, et al. Polymorphic amyloid degeneration of the cornea. A clinical and histopathologic study. Arch Ophthalmol 1981;99:1217–1223.

McCarthy M, Innis S, Dubord P, et al. Panstromal Schnyder corneal dystrophy: a clinical pathologic report with quantitative analysis of corneal lipid composition. *Ophthalmology* 1994;101:895–901.

Meretoja J. Familial systemic paramyloidosis with lattice dystrophy of the cornea, progressive cranial neuropathy, skin changes and various internal symptoms. A previously unrecognized heritable syndrome. *Ann Clin Res* 1969;1:314–324.

Meyer JC, Quantock AJ, Thonar EJ, et al. Characterization of a central corneal cloudiness sharing features of posterior crocodile shagreen and central cloud dystrophy of Francois. *Cornea* 1996;15:347–354.

Munier FL, Korvatska E, Djemai A, et al. Kerato-epithelin mutations in four 5q31-linked corneal dystrophies. *Nat Genet* 1997;15:247–251.

Nicholson DH, Green WR, Cross HE, et al. A clinical and histopathological study of François-Neetens speckled corneal dystrophy. *Am J Ophthalmol* 1977;83:554–560.

Purcell JJ Jr, Rodrigues M, Chishti MI, et al. Lattice corneal dystrophy associated with familial systemic amyloidosis (Meretoja's syndrome). *Ophthalmology* 1983;90:1512–1517.

Shearman AM, Hudson TJ, Andresen JM, et al. The gene for schnyder's crystalline corneal dystrophy maps to human chromosome 1p34.1-p36. *Hum Mol Genet* 1996;5:1667–1672.

Starck T, Kenyon KR, Hanninen LA, et al. Clinical and histopathologic studies of two families with lattice corneal dystrophy and familial systemic amyloidosis (Meretoja syndrome). *Ophthalmology* 1991;98:1197–1206.

Stone EM, Mathers WD, Rossenwasser GOD, et al. Three autosomal dominant corneal dystrophies map to chromosome 5q. *Nature Genetics* 1994;6:47–51.

Streeten BW, Qi Y, Klintworth GK, et al. Immunolocalization of beta ig-h3 protein in 5q31-linked corneal dystrophies and normal corneas. *Arch Ophthalmol* 1999;117:67–75.

Vance JM, Jonasson F, Lennon F, et al. Linkage of a gene for macular corneal dystrophy to chromosome 16. *Am J Hum Genet* 1996;58:757–762.

Varssano D, Cohen EJ, Nelson LB, et al. Corneal transplantation in Maroteaux-Lamy syndrome. *Arch Ophthalmol* 1997;115:428–429.

Weiss JS. Schnyder crystalline dystrophy sine crystals. Recommendation for a revision of nomenclature. *Ophthalmology* 1996;103:465–473.

Weller RO, Rodger FC. Crystalline stromal dystrophy: histochemistry and ultrastructure of the cornea. *Br J Ophthalmol* 1980;64:46–52.

Wilson DJ, Weleber RG, Klein ML, et al. Bietti's crystalline dystrophy. A clinicopathologic correlative study. *Arch Ophthalmol* 1989;107:213–221.

Endothelial Dystrophies

Adamis AP, Filatov V, Tripathi Bj, et al. Fuchs endothelial dystrophy of the cornea. *Surv Ophthalmol* 1993;38:149–168.

Chan C, Green WR, Barraquer J. Similarities between posterior polymorphous and congenital hereditary endothelial dystrophies: a study of 14 buttons in 11 cases. *Cornea* 1982;1:155–172.

Cibis G, Krachmer J, Phelps C, et al. Iridocorneal adhesions in posterior polymorphous dystrophy. *Trans Am Acad Ophthalmol Otolaryngol* 1976;81:770–777.

Cibis G, Krachmer J, Phelps C, et al. The clinical spectrum of posterior polymorphous dystrophy. *Arch Ophthalmol* 1977;95:1529–1527.

Ehlers N, Modis L, Moller-Pedersen T. A morphological and functional study of congenital hereditary endothelial dystrophy. *Acta Ophthalmol Scand* 1998;76:314–318.

Hanna C, Fraunfelder FT, McNair JR. An ultrastructure study of posterior polymorphous dystrophy of the cornea. *Ann Ophthalmol* 1977;9:1371–1378.

Heon E, Mathers WD, Alward WL, et al. Linkage of posterior polymorphous corneal dystrophy to 20q11. *Hum Mol Genet* 1995;4:485–488.

Hirst LW, Bancroft J, Yamauchi K, et al. Immunohistochemical pathology of the corneal endothelium in iridocorneal endothelial syndrome. *Invest Ophthalmol Vis Sci* 1995;36:820–827.

Jirsova K, Merjava S, Martincova R, et al. Immunohistochemical characterization of cytokeratins in the abnormal corneal endothelium of posterior polymorphous corneal dystrophy patients. *Exp Eye Res* 2007;84:680–686.

Levy SG, Moss J, Noble BA, et al. Early-onset posterior polymorphous dystrophy. *Arch Ophthalmol* 1996;114:1265–1268.

Levy SG, Moss J, Sawada H, et al. The composition of wide-spaced collagen in normal and diseased Descemet membrane. *Curr Eye Res* 1996;15:45–52.

Lisch W, Buob M, Steuhl KP. Cornea guttata and Fuchs' endothelial-epithelial dystrophy. Clinico-histologic study of 73 patients. *Klin Monatsbl Augenheilkd* 1991;198:83–86.

McCartney AC, Kirkness CM. Comparison between posterior polymorphous dystrophy and congenital hereditary endothelial dystrophy of the cornea. *Eye* 1988;2:63–70.

Molia LM, Lanier JD, Font RL. Posterior polymorphous dystrophy associated with posterior amyloid degeneration of the cornea. *Am J Ophthalmol* 1999;127:86–88.

Ross JR, Foulks GN, Sanfilippo FP, et al. Immunohistochemical analysis of the pathogenesis of posterior polymorphous dystrophy. *Arch Ophthalmol* 1995;113:340–345.

Sekundo W, Lee WR, Kirkness CM, et al. An ultrastructural investigation of an early manifestation of the posterior polymorphous dystrophy of the cornea. *Ophthalmology* 1994;101:1422–1431.

Toma NM, Ebenezer ND, Inglehearn CF, et al. Linkage of congenital hereditary endothelial dystrophy to chromosome 20. *Hum Mol Genet* 1995;4:2395–2398.

The Cornea in Systemic Disease

Auran JD, Donn A, Hyman GA. Multiple myeloma presenting as vortex crystalline keratopathy and complicated by endocapsular hematoma. *Cornea* 1992;11:584–585.

Ayres BD, Rapuano CJ. Excimer laser phototherapeutic keratectomy. *Ocul Surf* 2006;4:196–206.

Barr CC, Gelender H, Font RL. Corneal crystalline deposits associated with dysproteinemia. Report of two cases and review of the literature. *Arch Ophthalmol* 1980;98:884–889.

Font RL, Matoba AY, Prabhakaran VC. IgG-kappa immunoglobulin deposits involving the predescemetic region in a patient with multiple myeloma. *Cornea* 2006;25:1237–1239.

Ghosheh FR, Cremona F, Ayres BD, et al. Indications for penetrating keratoplasty and associated procedures, 2001–2005. *Eye Contact Lens* 2008;34:211–214.

Graichen DF, Perez E, Jones DB, et al. kappa-Immunoglobulin corneal deposits associated with monoclonal gammopathy. Immunohistochemical and electron microscopic findings. *Ger J Ophthalmol* 1994;3:54–57.

Gu X, Barrios R, Cartwright J, et al. Light chain crystal deposition as a manifestation of plasma cell dyscrasias: the role of immunoelectron microscopy. *Hum Pathol* 2003;34:270–277.

Liu M, Cohen EJ, Brewer GJ, et al. Kayser-Fleischer ring as the presenting sign of Wilson disease. *Am J Ophthalmol* 2002;133:832–834.

Lois N, Kowal VO, Cohen EJ, et al. Indications for penetrating keratoplasty and associated procedures, 1989–1995. *Cornea* 1997;16:623–629.

Marcon AS, Cohen EJ, Rapuano CJ, et al. Recurrence of corneal stromal dystrophies after penetrating keratoplasty. *Cornea* 2003;22:19–21.

Perry HD, Donnenfeld ED, Font RL. Intraepithelial corneal immunoglobulin crystals in IgG-kappa multiple myeloma. *Cornea* 1993;12:448–450.

Ramsay AS, Lee WR, Mohammed A. Changing indications for penetrating keratoplasty in the west of Scotland from 1970 to 1995. *Eye* 1997;11:357–360.

Ramsay AS, Lee WR, Mohammed A. Changing indications for penetrating keratoplasty in the west of Scotland from 1970 to 1995. *Eye* 1997;11(Pt 3):357–360.

Stirling JW, Henderson DW, Rozenbilds MA, et al. Crystalloidal paraprotein deposits in the cornea: an ultrastructural study of two new cases with tubular crystalloids that contain IgG kappa light chains and IgG gamma heavy chains. *Ultrastruct Pathol* 1997;21:337–344.

Tso MO, Fine BS, Thorpe HE. Kayser-Fleischer ring and associated cataract in Wilson's disease. *Am J Ophthalmol* 1975;79:479–488.

Tzelikis PF, Laibson PR, Ribeiro MP, et al. Ocular copper deposition associated with monoclonal gammopathy of undetermined significance: case report. *Arq Bras Oftalmol* 2005;68:539–541.

Sclera

Arevalo JF, Shields CL, Shields JA. Giant nodular posterior scleritis simulating choroidal melanoma and birdshot retinochoroidopathy. *Ophthalmic Surg Lasers Imaging* 2003;34:403–405.

Benson WE, Shields JS, Tasman W, et al. Posterior scleritis, a cause of diagnostic confusion. *Arch Ophthalmol* 1979;97:1482–1486.

Ferry AP. The histopathology of rheumatoid episcleral nodules: an extra-articular manifestation of rheumatoid arthritis. *Arch Ophthalmol* 1969;82: 77–88.

Foster CS, Forstot SL, Wilson LA. Mortality rate in rheumatoid arthritis patients developing necrotizing scleritis peripheral ulcerative keratitis: effects of systemic immunosuppression. *Ophthalmology* 1984;91:1253–1263.

Norn MS. Scleral plaques. I. Incidence and morphology. *Acta Ophthalmol (Copenh)* 1974;52:96–106.

Palamar M, Thangappan A, Shields CL, et al. Necrotic choroidal melanoma with scleritis and choroidal effusion. *Cornea* 2009;28:354–356.

Rao NA, Marak GE, Hidayat AA. Necrotizing scleritis. A clinicopathologic study of 41 cases. *Ophthalmology* 1985;92:1542–1549.

Riono WP, Hidayat AA, Rao NA. Scleritis: a clinicopathologic study of 55 cases. *Ophthalmology* 1999;106:1328–3133.

Shields JA, Shields CL. CME review: sclerochoroidal calcification: the 2001 Harold Gifford Lecture. *Retina* 2002;22:251–261.

Watson PG, Hayreh SS. Scleritis and episcleritis. *Br J Ophthalmol* 1976;60:163–191.

Wilhelmus KR, Yen MT, Rice L, et al. Necrobiotic xanthogranuloma with posterior scleritis. *Arch Ophthalmol* 2006;124:748.

7 The Lens

The structure and embryology of the lens are discussed in Chapter 1.

CONGENITAL ANOMALIES OF THE LENS

The posterior surface of the lens in an infant's eye often has a dimpled configuration called **posterior umbilication** (Fig. 7-1A). Posterior umbilication is an artifact caused by fixation and is not present *in vivo*.

The surface of the lens has a conical configuration in lenticonus. Lenticonus can be anterior or posterior, and probably is caused by focal thinning of the lens capsule. Anterior lenticonus usually is bilateral, and may be associated with Alport syndrome of hereditary hemorrhagic nephritis and deafness, which is caused by mutations in several genes for Type IV or basement membrane collagen. The lens capsule in Alport syndrome is thin and has linear dehiscences. The renal disease presumably is caused by analogous abnormalities in the glomerular basement membrane. Many cases of Alport syndrome are caused by mutations in the COL4A5 gene on the X chromosome and show X-linked inheritance.

Posterior lenticonus usually is a unilateral sporadic condition that is not associated with other ocular or systemic disease. When the lens is retro-illuminated, the lenticonus often appears as an "oil droplet" (Fig. 7-1B).

Lens coloboma (lens notching) is a secondary phenomenon caused by a focal absence of zonular fibers in a contiguous coloboma of the ciliary body. Rarely, lens coloboma can herald the presence of a pediatric ciliary body neoplasm, usually a medulloepithelioma.

Congenital or developmental cataracts (Fig. 7-2) occur in isolation or in association with systemic or ocular anomalies. Approximately one third of congenital cataracts are inherited, one third are idiopathic, and the remaining third have systemic associations. Most hereditary cataracts are inherited in an autosomal dominant fashion with high penetrance. At least 39 loci for isolated or primary congenital cataracts have been identified. These include genes for a variety of lens crystallins, gap junction and membrane proteins, and growth and transcription factors.

Developmental cataracts can affect different parts of the lens. **Anterior pyramidal cataract** (Fig. 7-2B) is a congenital form of anterior subcapsular cataract. The opacity beneath the anterior lens capsule is a white plaque of dense collagen.

A spectrum of opacities that involve the posterior pole of the lens is related to faulty resorption of the embryonic hyaloid vascular system that nourishes the developing lens *in utero*. An innocuous spot called a Mittendorf dot marks the site where the hyaloid artery was attached to the posterior lens capsule. Mittendorf is found in about 25% of normal individuals and is best seen on retroillumination. A patent hyaloid artery may persist in some adults. Posterior remnants of the hyaloid artery and Bergmeister papilla may be evident as vascular loops and glial veils on the optic disc.

The most severe condition related to incomplete resorption of the embryonic vasculature is **persistent hyperplastic**

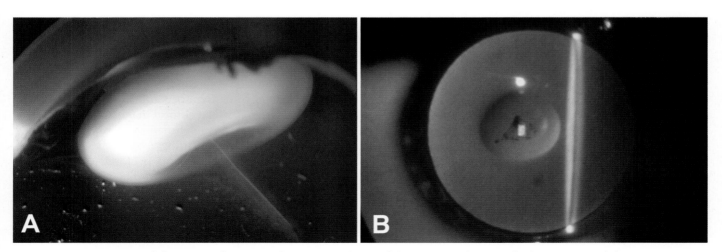

Fig. 7-1. A. Posterior umbilication, infant eye. The concave shape of the posterior lens is called posterior umbilication. Posterior umbilication is a fixation artifact that affects the lens in infants. The hyaloid artery persists in this specimen. **B. Posterior lenticonus.** Posterior lenticonus appears as "oil droplet" in retroillumination. Anomaly occurred unilaterally in healthy patient.

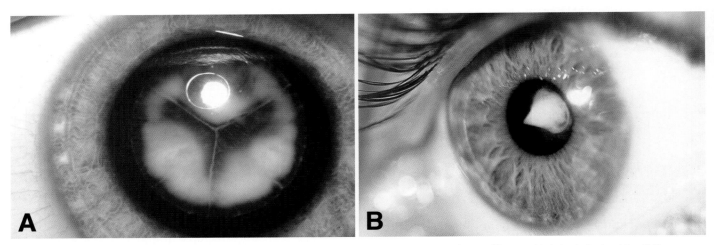

Fig. 7-2. Developmental cataracts. A. Congenital opacity involves embryonic nucleus of lens, which is delimited by "Y" sutures. **B.** Anterior pyramidal cataract. Cone of collagenous connective tissue projects from anterior surface of lens. Anterior pyramidal cataract is a development variant of anterior subcapsular cataract.

primary vitreous (PHPV) or **persistent fetal vasculature (PFV)**, a congenital anomaly that often is found in microophthalmic eyes (Fig. 12-17). PHPV/PFV is characterized by a retrolental plaque of vascularized connective tissue that is thought to represent a residuum of the embryonic primary vitreous. The tips of the ciliary processes are attached to the margins of this retrolental plaque. As the eye enlarges, the ciliary processes are drawn centrally and stretched, and may be seen clinically when the pupil is dilated. PHPV/PFV produces leukocoria (a white pupil), and is an important lesion in the differential diagnosis of the childhood retinal malignancy retinoblastoma. Goldberg applied the term PFV to this syndrome to emphasize the involvement of other fetal ocular vessels such as iris shunts.

Zonular cataracts are marked by the opacification of a single zone of lens fibers. Lamellar cataract is a form of zonular cataract that results when a group of lens fibers are opacified at one point during development and subsequently are buried by the formation of new, healthy clear cortex. Damage to developing lens fibers during an attack of neonatal tetany is a classic cause of lamellar cataract. Analogous to tree rings in chronodendrology, the opacified fibers serve as a clinical marker that allows one to roughly estimate when an insult occurred during lens development.

Cataracts occur in patients who have a bewildering number of genetic syndromes, genetic diseases, and developmental disorders. A search for cataract on the Online Mendelian Inheritance in Man (OMIM) Web site in 2010 retrieved 364 separate items. Rare syndromic associations include chondrodysplasia punctata and the Hallermann-Streiff, Nance-Horan, Rothmund-Thomson, Marinesco-Sjogren, and hyperferritinemia-cataract syndromes.

Congenital cataract and glaucoma occur together in patients who have **Lowe syndrome**, an X-linked oculo-cerebrorenal syndrome characterized by renal rickets and amino aciduria. The lens in Lowe syndrome is small and discoid in shape, and may have lens capsular incresences.

Obligate female carriers of Lowe syndrome may have punctate opacities and plaque-like posterior subcapsular cataracts. Thirteen percent of patients with Down syndrome (trisomy 21) have cataracts.

The clinical triad that comprises Gregg syndrome of **rubella embryopathy** includes cataract, deafness, and cardiac anomalies such as patent ductus arteriosus. Rubella cataracts are typically dense, pearly-white and nuclear. Lens epithelial nuclei may persist for decades in the embryonic nucleus of a rubella cataract. Virus has been cultured from rubella cataracts several years after birth.

CATARACT

Cataract is opacification or optical dysfunction of the crystalline lens. Cataract is an extremely common and economically important cause of visual loss. Derived from the Greek word for waterfall, the term cataract probably refers to the white appearance of some senile cataracts that was likened to rapidly flowing "white water."

Cataract is the end stage or final common pathway of lens pathology. Although lens opacification often occurs as the result of aging, a host of other factors can cause cataracts, including trauma, drugs, toxins, radiation, inborn errors of metabolism, and concurrent ocular or systemic disease.

Cataract is essentially a clinical diagnosis denoting loss of optical function. Visual function is best determined by the ophthalmologist during a clinical examination. In most institutions, cataracts are no longer submitted to pathology. It actually is difficult to diagnose cataract histopathologically in many cases, especially when modern surgical techniques of extracapsular lens extraction such as phacoemulsification have been used. After the contents of the optically dysfunctional lens have been removed, a prosthetic intraocular lens (IOL) is inserted in the lens capsular bag. The "IOL" obviates the need for aphakic spectacles postoperatively (Fig. 7-3).

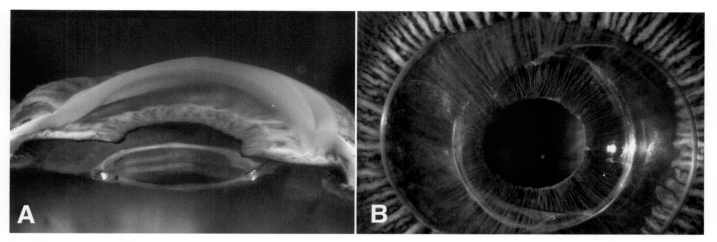

Fig. 7-3. Pseudophakia. A. Optic of posterior chamber IOL is seen within lens capsular bag in posterior chamber. Some residual lens cortical material is present. Eye was enucleated for uveal melanoma. **B.** Blue haptics of older three-piece posterior chamber IOL are confined to lens capsular bag. Iris pigment epithelium and ring of ciliary processes are evident.

Although a bewildering variety of lens opacities have been described clinically, the pathologist is able to recognize only four basic types of cataract histopathologically: cortical, nuclear, anterior subcapsular and posterior subcapsular cataracts. Each differs in its pathogenesis and histology.

Some degree of **nuclear sclerosis** (Fig. 7-4) develops in all individuals as they age. The inevitability of nuclear sclerotic cataract is inherent in the lens' normal pattern of growth and development. The lens is derived from surface ectoderm, and, like the skin, it grows continuously, albeit slowly, throughout life. Growth of the lens results from the continuous accretion of new secondary lens fibers around its circumference. The formation of the new lens fibers buries the older fibers, which are sequestered centrally in the lens nucleus. (Mature skin cells are desquamated.) With the passage of years, the older cells gradually degenerate. This is not surprising because mature lens cells are anucleate and lack the metabolic machinery for protein synthesis and repair. Eventually, the highly specialized lens proteins called crystallins become denatured, and the cytoplasm of the lens fibers becomes increasingly dehydrated. The degenerative process is also marked by the accumulation of a yellow-brown pigment called urochrome that is probably related to photo-oxidation (Fig. 7-4B).

Histopathologically, nuclear sclerosis is marked by increased eosinophilia and homogeneity of the lens nucleus, and an absence of the artifactitious cracks that normally occur between lens fibers during microtomy (Fig. 7-4C). As the nucleus becomes denser, its index of refraction, and hence refractive power, increase, causing lenticular myopia (*grandma's second sight*). Presbyopic patients often find that they are able to read without their reading glasses, as they develop nuclear sclerosis and become progressively

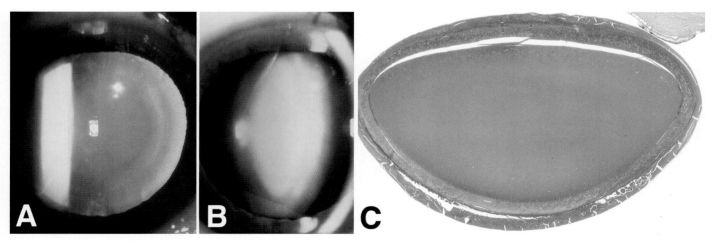

Fig. 7-4. Nuclear sclerosis. A. Sclerotic nucleus is evident as oil droplet in *red* reflex. Patient developed cataract after filtering surgery. **B.** Slit beam discloses *yellow* urochrome pigment in nucleus. **C.** Artifactitious clefts delimit boundary between the sclerotic lens nucleus and the cortex. The nucleus is more eosinophilic than the cortex and lacks the artifactitious clefts that normally form when the lens is sectioned. (H&E ×10)

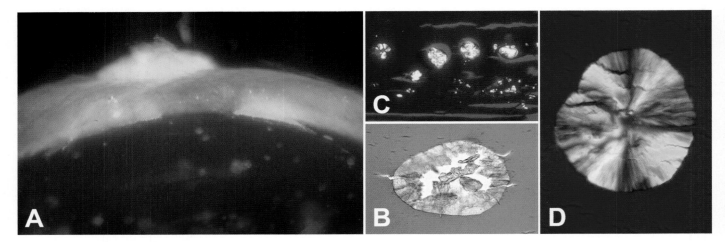

Fig. 7-5. Oxalate crystals, nuclear sclerosis. A. Oxalate crystals are evident as orange sperules in severely scerotic, brunescent nucleus. Peripheral degenerated cortex contains foci of calcification. **B–D.** Polarization microscopy highlights oval birefringent crystals of calcium oxalate in nuclear sclerotic cataract. The crystal in **part D** exhibits vivid rainbow-like pattern of birefringence. (**A.** H&E with crossed polarizers ×25, **B.** H&E ×100, **C.** H&E with crossed polarizers ×250)

myopic. Nuclear sclerosis also distorts color vision because of the yellow-brown urochrome pigment, which accumulates in the lens and filters out blue wavelengths of light. After nuclear sclerotic cataracts are removed, patients may complain about *blue vision*. In advanced nuclear sclerosis, cataracts may be amber-colored (brunescent) or even black (*cataracta nigra*). Calcium oxalate crystals occasionally are found in lenses with nuclear sclerosis. These oval crystals exhibit vivid rainbow-like birefringence during polarization microscopy (Fig. 7-5).

Cortical cataract (or soft cataract) is marked by degeneration of the fiber cells comprising the lens cortex. The incipient stage of cortical cataract is marked clinically by the development of vacuoles or clefts containing clear watery fluid (water clefts). As the disease progresses, the foci of degenerated cortical material appear white in direct illumination and are seen as black shadows in retroillumination.

The cortical opacities often begin near the equator, and may involve a wedge-shaped sector of cortex. Sparkling crystals of cholesterol and insoluble amino acids develop in some cases. The term *Christmas tree cataract* is applied to cataracts that contain many crystals.

Histopathologically, cortical degeneration is marked by clefts and spaces in the cortex filled with liquefied cortical material, which oozes from fractured lens fibers. Spherules of degenerated lens cytoplasm called morgagnian globules typically are seen (Fig. 7-6). Total cortical liquefaction occurs in morgagnian cataracts (Fig. 7-7). **Morgagnian cataracts** are typically swollen and intumescent because the osmotic effect of the degenerated cortical material causes the lens to imbibe aqueous humor. In some patients, the swollen lens may precipitate closed angle glaucoma (phacomorphic glaucoma). The sclerotic nucleus typically resists liquefaction and sinks inferiorly in the capsular bag

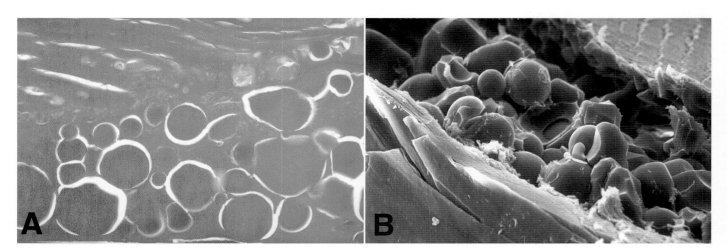

Fig. 7-6. Cortical cataract, morgagnian globules. A. Liquefied cortex and morgagnian globules fill cleft in cortical cataract. Morgagnian globules are spherules of degenerated lens protein that have leaked from fragmented lens fibers. **B.** Scanning electron micrograph of cortical cataract showing morgagian globules in cleft. (**A.** H&E ×100, **B.** SEM ×320)

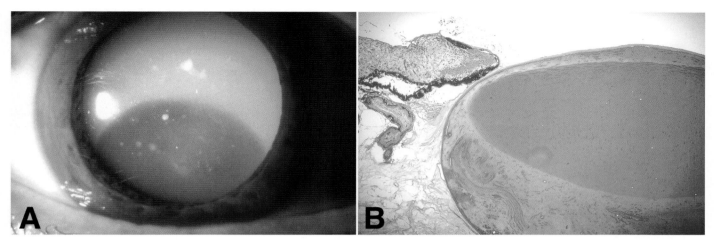

Fig. 7-7. Morgagnian cataract. A. Morgagnian cataract results when the lens cortex undergoes total liquefaction. The densely sclerotic nucleus is resistant to liquefaction and sinks to the bottom of the bag of liquefied cortex. Calcium oxalate crystals are evident as lighter spherules in the amber nucleus. (Photo courtesy of Prof. Dr. med. Wolfgang Lieb, University of Würzburg.) **B.** Degenerated lens cortex surrounds the intensely eosinophilic sclerotic nucleus. Although most of the cortex has liquefied, a few curved disrupted lens fibers are seen posteriorly. (H&E ×10)

of liquefied cortex (Fig. 7-7A). The milky, fluid cortex often contains crystals of cholesterol. The denatured lens protein can leak through the intact lens capsule in advanced cases and stimulate a bland macrophagic response. This may lead to a variety of secondary open angle glaucoma called phacolytic glaucoma, which is caused by obstruction of the trabecular meshwork by macrophages that have ingested lens material and free high molecular weight lens protein, as well (Figs. 3-6B and 8-15A,B). Dystrophic calcification is often found in the degenerated cortex of long-standing cataracts. Blind painful eyes occasionally contain totally calcified lenses that are rock-hard and cannot be sectioned without prior decalcification.

The two other histologic subtypes of cataract, anterior subcapsular cataract and posterior subcapsular cataract are caused by abnormalities in the anterior lens epithelium. **Anterior subcapsular cataract** is marked histopathologically by a white plaque of dense collagenous connective tissue that forms beneath the anterior lens capsule (Fig. 7-8). Contraction of the fibrous tissue causes characteristic sinuous folds in the anterior capsule (Fig. 7-8B). The subcapsular collagen is synthesized by lens epithelial cells. The cells are found within the plaque surrounded by capsules of basement membrane material that evidence their lens epithelial lineage (Fig. 7-8C). In some instances, a second, delicate, new layer of lens capsule is found beneath

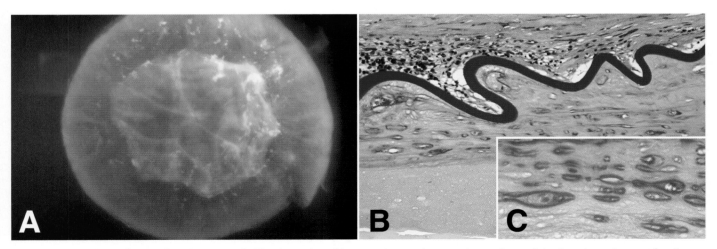

Fig. 7-8. Anterior subcapsular cataract. A. The irregular white opacity on the anterior surface of the lens is a plaque of collagen that has been synthesized by lens epithelial cells. The anterior lens capsule is folded and the lens nucleus is sclerotic. **B.** Sinuously folded anterior lens capsule covers anterior surface of fibrous plaque made by lens epithelial cells irritated by inflammatory membrane in posterior chamber. **C.** Lens epithelial cells within the plaque surrounded by capsules of PAS-positive basement membrane. (**B.** PAS ×100, **C.** PAS ×250)

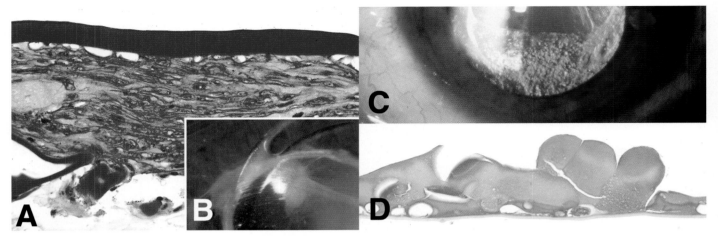

Fig. 7-9. A. Capsular fibrosis, post-extracapsular cataract extraction (post-ECCE). Lens capsular bag contains mass of collagenous connective tissue made by residual lens epithelial cells that reside in basement membrane capsules. Anterior capsule is above, posterior capsule below. **B.** Macrophoto in inset shows capsular folds and opacification near edge of IOL. **C.** Elschnig pearls, post-ECCE. Relucent spherules derived from residual lens epithelial cells are seen within lens capsule after extracapsular cataract extraction. **D.** Elschnig pearls are analogous to bladder cells found in posterior subcapsular cataract (PSC). Nuclei of Elschnig pearls on posterior capsule (below) are not evident in this plane of section. (**A.** PAS ×100, **D.** H&E ×100)

the anterior subcapsular fibrous plaque. This is made by lens epithelial cells that have migrated beneath the plaque. Adhesions between the iris and lens (posterior synechiae) and/or anterior segment inflammation often stimulates the proliferation and fibrous transformation of the lens epithelium. Although anterior subcapsular cataracts frequently are found in blind painful eyes in the ophthalmic pathology laboratory, they are not observed clinically very often because they typically are obscured by posterior synechiae and pupillary membranes. **Capsular fibrosis**, which causes posterior capsular opacification and wrinkling after planned extracapsular cataract surgery, reflects an identical process of lens epithelial proliferation and fibrous transformation (Fig. 7-9A,B).

In **posterior subcapsular cataract**, lens epithelial cells migrate posteriorly beneath the lens capsule behind the lens equator where the monolayer of anterior lens epithelium normally terminates. Noxae such as inflammation or ciliary body tumors stimulate the abnormal epithelial migration. Situated aberrantly at the posterior pole of the lens, the lens epithelial cells attempt to form new secondary lens fibers, but abortive lens fibers called Wedl or bladder cells result (Fig. 7-10). Filled with lens protein, the Wedl cells are large and round or oval and have a single nucleus. Posterior subcapsular cataracts tend to interfere with near vision early because the opacity is located near the nodal point of the eye's visual system. Patients with posterior subcapsular cataract also are prone to develop severe glare

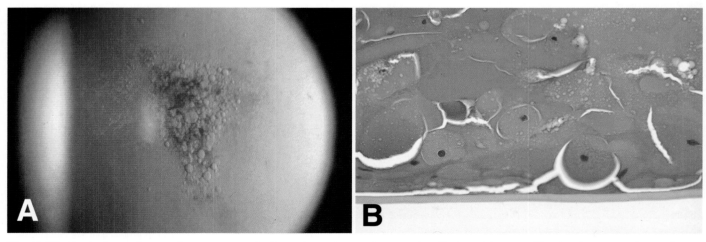

Fig. 7-10. Posterior subcapsular cataract. A. Posterior subcapsular opacity disclosed by retroillumination comprises relucent spherules consistent with bladder cells. **B.** Wedl or bladder cells represent abortive attempts by lens epithelial cells to form new lens fibers. They develop from aberrantly situated lens epithelial cells that have migrated posteriorly. Several of the bladder cells contain nuclei. The nuclei in some of the other large cells are not present in this plane of section. (**B.** H&E ×100)

symptoms, especially during night driving. The nuclei of bladder or Wedl cells serve to distinguish them from morgagnian globules, which are round anucleate spherules of degenerated lens protein.

Cells analogous to Wedl cells can form on, or within, the lens capsular bag after planned extracapsular surgery. Large spherical aggregates of these proliferating cells are called Elschnig pearls. Clinically, the pearls may resemble a mass of fish eggs (Fig. 7-9C,D).

COMPLICATED CATARACTS

Complicated cataracts (cataracta complicata) are caused by concurrent ocular disease. Cataract formation can complicate chronic uveitis in patients who have sarcoidosis or the pauciarticular, RF-seronegative, ANA-positive type of juvenile rheumatoid arthritis. Unilateral cataract, mild asymptomatic uveitis, and depigmentation of the iris stroma are the classic clinical manifestations of Fuchs heterochromic cyclitis (Fig. 7-11). There is some evidence linking Fuchs heterochromic cyclitis with rubella infection.

Posterior subcapsular cataracts form in nearly 50% of patients who have retinitis pigmentosa. It is unclear how cataract formation is related to heritable defects in photopigments such as rhodopsin.

Intraocular tumors, particularly ciliary body malignant melanomas, should be excluded in patients with unilateral or asymmetrical cataracts. Ciliary body tumors can directly impinge upon and deform the periphery of the lens and stimulate posterior migration of lens epithelium as well.

Cataract also can complicate long-standing glaucoma. Some cases probably are related to chronic miotic therapy. In the past, anterior subcapsular vacuoles were reported in patients receiving strong topical anticholinesterase agents. Filtering surgery for glaucoma accelerates cataract formation. Scattered focal subcapsular lens opacities called glaukomflecken are observed in some patients who have had a prior attack of acute closed angle glaucoma. These small grayish opacities are thought to represent focal areas of lens epithelial necrosis and cortical degeneration and may be caused by hypothetical toxins in the stagnant aqueous humor.

SUGAR CATARACTS—DIABETES MELLITUS AND GALACTOSEMIA

The accumulation of sugar alcohol in lens cells is hypothesized to produce osmotic cataracts in patients who have disorders of sugar metabolism such as diabetes mellitus. Rarely, patients with previously undiagnosed diabetes mellitus may present with a characteristic type of diabetic cataract caused by markedly elevated levels of serum glucose. Such cataracts may resorb partially when diabetic therapy is instituted. Diabetics are also prone to develop typical senile nuclear and cortical cataracts at a much earlier age than the normal population.

The sugar alcohols that cause osmotic cataracts in patients with diabetes and galactosemia are formed by the enzyme aldose reductase in the alternative hexose monophosphate shunt when the normal glycolytic pathway is overwhelmed by high levels of serum glucose or galactose. Sorbitol, the sugar alcohol of glucose, accumulates in the lens cells of diabetics because it is unable to pass through cellular membranes. Similarly, the sugar alcohol of galactose called galactolol or dulcitol accumulates in the lens cells of galactosemic infants who are deficient in the enzyme galactose-1-phosphate uridylyltransferase. Galactosemic cataracts often have a central oil droplet configuration, may be the first clinical manifestation of galactosemia, and are partially reversible if dietary therapy is promptly instituted. Presenile cataracts also occur in patients who are deficient in galactokinase.

CATARACT AND SYSTEMIC DISEASE

Patients with **myotonic dystrophy** develop presenile cataract as well as myotonia, muscular dystrophy, frontal baldness, and testicular atrophy. Myotonic cataracts classically have an "iridescent dust" of multiple polychromatic crystals in the anterior and posterior subcapsular cortex and a stellate grouping of opacities along suture lines in the posterior cortex, which develops later.

The sunflower cataract of **Wilson disease** (hepatolenticular degeneration) is caused by the deposition of copper

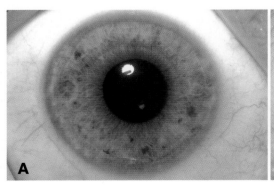
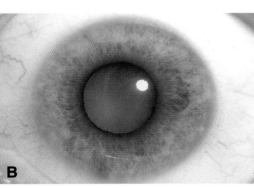

Fig. 7-11. A, B. Fuchs heterochromic cyclitis. Affected eye (**B**) has developed cataract and hypochromic heterochromia iridum.

in the lens capsule. The familiar Kayser-Fleischer ring in the periphery of the cornea results from an analogous deposition of copper in Descemet membrane. The central disc of the "sunflower" corresponds to the diameter of the undilated pupil, while the large radial ridges on the back of the iris probably govern the formation of the "petals." An identical cataract may occur in patients who have retained intraocular copper foreign bodies (chalcosis lentis) (Fig. 4-12B). In fact, the similarity between traumatic chalcosis and Wilson disease led German ophthalmologists to suggest that copper metabolism was abnormal in Wilson disease.

Posterior spoke-like lens opacities occur in **Fabry disease**, an X-linked deficiency of the enzyme α-galactosidase A, which causes the storage of ceramide trihexoside in tissues. A vortex pattern of pigment deposition called cornea verticillata occurs in affected men.

It is not surprising that cataracts occur in patients who have certain skin diseases, because both the lens and skin are derived from surface ectoderm. Most important is the syndermatotic cataract that occurs in atopic dermatitis, an association called Andogsky syndrome. Patients with atopic cataract may do poorly after cataract surgery.

TRAUMATIC CATARACTS

Total opacification of the lens can develop several days after rupture or laceration of the lens capsule. The entire cortex can undergo liquefaction in young individuals, in whom total spontaneous resorption of the lens cortical material occasionally occurs. The iris can seal small lacerations. If the capsule reforms, only a small focal opacity may result. Severe contusion injuries can rupture the lens. Less severe contusions often produce a superficial type of cataract with a distinctly floral appearance called a petalliform cataract or **contusion rosette** (Fig. 4-7A). Such cataracts may cause minimal visual loss, but are an important clinical marker for prior ocular contusion injury. If a contusion rosette is found during biomicroscopy, gonioscopy should be performed to rule out postcontusion angle deformity, which predisposes to glaucoma.

Vossius ring is an annulus of pigment on the anterior lens capsule caused by a forceful imprint of the iris pigment epithelium during a contusion injury. Chronically retained intraocular iron foreign bodies can cause **siderosis lentis**. Siderotic cataract is marked by scattered foci of rust-colored material on the anterior surface of the lens and often is associated with iris heterochromia caused by the deposition of iron pigment in the iris stroma. Histopathology shows subepithelial plaques of lens epithelial cells that contain large quantities of iron pigment. The siderosis or hemosiderosis lentis (iron from intraocular hemorrhage) is evident as a yellowish or yellowish-brown discoloration of the anterior lens epithelium in routine sections stained with hematoxlin and eosin. Special iron stains that employ the Prussian blue reaction are used to confirm the presence of iron (Fig. 4-7B,C). Chalcosis lentis is discussed above.

The crystalline lens is very sensitive to relatively low doses of ionizing radiation. Doses of ionizing radiation as low as 250 cGy can cause cataract. Hence, the lens should be carefully shielded during radiotherapy.

Soemmerring ring cataract is a donut of residual cortical material that remains in the equatorial part of the lens capsular bag after expulsion of the lens nucleus during a perforating corneal or scleral injury. Most eyes that are examined pathologically after planned extracapsular cataract surgery have a Soemmerring ring of residual lens cortex (Fig. 7-12).

Electrical cataracts are caused by lightning strikes or severe electrical injuries. A thin lamella of anterior or posterior subcapsular cortex usually is opacified in this rare type of cataract. Lightning often opacifies the posterior subcapsular cortex because the electrical current passes down the neuraxis. Industrial injuries usually cause anterior opacification because the extremities are the path of the current. The onset of electrical cataract after injury may be delayed.

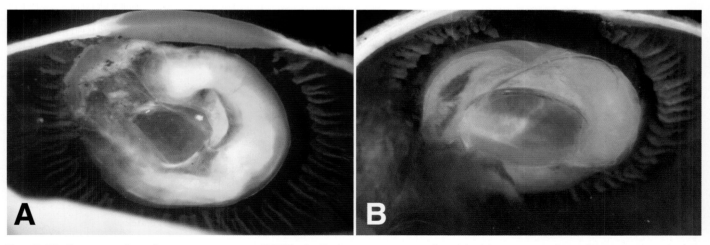

Fig. 7-12. Soemmerring ring cataract, post-ECCE. A, B. Large amounts of residual lens cortex form Soemmerring ring in equatorial part of lens capsular bag. The lens in (**B**) was found in an eye with a uveal melanoma.

The blue wavelengths of the argon blue-green laser are absorbed by the yellow urochrome pigment in nuclear cataract. In the past, lenticular burns occurred during retinal photocoagulation of patients with advanced nuclear sclerosis. This complication can be avoided by the use of red laser light, that is, krypton red. Absorption of laser energy by the iris pigment epithelium can cause focal thermal opacities in the underlying lens during transpupillary thermotherapy of posterior segment tumors.

TOXIC CATARACT

A variety of drugs and toxins can cause cataract. The most important drug-induced cataract is the posterior subcapsular cataract that develops in patients receiving chronic therapy with high doses of systemic corticosteroids. The dose of steroids necessary to produce cataract is uncertain. One study found that cataracts develop in approximately one third of patients who receive a chronic daily dose of 10 mg of prednisilone. Fifteen milligram of oral prednisone daily for more than 1 year leads to cataract formation in 75% of patients. All patients with fluocinolone acetate intravitreal implants are expected to require cataract surgery within 3-year lifetime of the implant.

Other toxins and drugs that produce cataract include naphthalene, dinitrophenol, mercury, phenothiazine, anticholinesterase agents, triparanol, and cigarette smoke.

LENS CAPSULAR ABNORMALITIES

True exfoliation of the lens capsule or capsular delamination is marked by a split in the lens capsule that leads to the formation of relucent scrolls on the anterior surface of the lens. True exfoliation is quite rare. Although it classically is associated with occupational exposure to infrared radiation (e.g., in glass blowers or steel puddlers), most cases are associated with aging. True exfoliation does not predispose to glaucoma.

Pseudoexfoliation (PXE) of the lens capsule, or exfoliation syndrome, is a relatively common disease that causes a variety of secondary open angle glaucoma called capsular glaucoma in about half of affected patients. Dvorak-Theobald first used the term pseudoexfoliation to differentiate this disorder from true exfoliation, which does not cause glaucoma. PXE is an extremely important cause of glaucoma in some populations.

Clinically, PXE is marked by the deposition of a complex mucoprotein on the anterior lens capsule, as well as on all of the aqueous-bathed surfaces of the anterior segment, including the ciliary processes, zonule, vitreous face, and the posterior iris. On the anterior lens capsule, the PXE material forms a central disc of granular white material whose diameter corresponds to that of the undilated pupil (Fig. 7-13A). Surrounding the central disc is a clear zone wiped clean of PXE by the motion of the pupil. A granular zone marked by areas of rarefaction that correspond to radial macroridges on the posterior iridic surface is found peripherally. PXE may be relatively inconspicuous in an undilated patient. Observation of a few, white, dandruff-like flakes at the pupillary margin should always prompt a dilated exam.

The PXE material on the anterior surface of the lens is synthesized by the lens epithelium and extruded through the lens capsule, forming clumps of eosinophilic material called Busacca deposits. The light microscopic appearance of these deposits has been likened to magnetized iron filings (Fig. 7-13B,C). Coarser, more irregular clumps of PXE are found on the zonular fibers, ciliary processes,

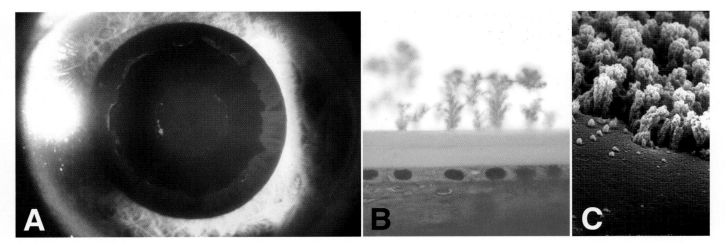

Fig. 7-13. PXE of the lens capsule. A. Grayish-white pseudoexfoliative material forms a "target" on the anterior lens capsule. A PXE-free zone wiped clean by the iris surrounds the central bull's eye whose diameter corresponds to the miotic pupil. The peripheral granular zone contains radial erosions caused by large radial folds on the posterior iris. Focal outward peeling of the margin of the peripheral zone is present. **B.** Eosinophilic bush-like Busacca deposits of PXE material are seen on the anterior lens capsule. The appearance of the material has been likened to iron filings on a magnet. **C.** Scanning electron microscopy of PXE on anterior lens capsule. (**B.** H&E ×250, **C.** SEM ×320)

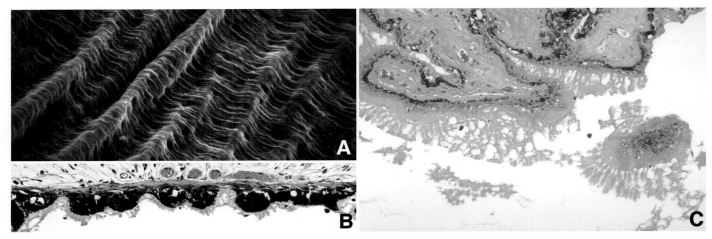

Fig. 7-14. PXE syndrome, iris pigment epithelium. Scanning electron microscopy (**A**) and light microscopy (**B**) shows coarse "saw-toothed" appearance of the iris pigment epithelium caused by coalescence of circumferential ridges. PXE material festoons the ridges. **C.** Extensive deposits of PXE are found on the ciliary processes and zonular fibers. (**A.** SEM ×80, **B.** H&E ×100, **C.** H&E ×100)

and iris pigment epithelium (Fig. 7-14A–C). Material is also found in the iris stroma, the anterior chamber, and the trabecular meshwork. Secondary open angle glaucoma is caused by obstruction of the trabecular meshwork. Recent electron microscopic studies suggest that some of the PXE actually may be synthesized within the meshwork. PXE has been found in the conjunctiva, orbit, skin, lung, liver, and heart with electron microscopy. The extraocular material is always associated with elastic fibers, and it shows immunoreactivity with antibodies against elastic microfibrils. Such observations suggest that PXE of the lens capsule may be the ocular manifestation of a presumably innocuous systemic disorder of elastic tissue.

Involvement of the zonule by PXE predisposes to dislocation of the lens or lens capsular bag after extracapsular cataract surgery. Cataract surgery may also be complicated by poor pupillary dilation and an abnormal leathery consistency of the iris. Histopathologically, one finds "sawtoothing" of the iris pigment epithelium caused by coarsening and coalescence of its circumferential ridges, which are festooned with pseudoexfoliative material (Fig. 7-14A,B). The iris pigment epithelial changes often suggest the diagnosis under low magnification microscopy. Many patients have extensive pigment dispersion, not unlike that found in pigmentary glaucoma.

ZONULAR FIBERS AND ECTOPIA LENTIS

The lens is suspended in the posterior chamber by zonular fibers, which are composed largely of elastic microfibrils (Fig. 1-7). The zonular fibers arise from the peripheral pars plana and the inner surface of the peripheral retina, and extend as a sheet anteriorly across the pars plana (Fig. 1-7A). At the posterior aspect of the pars plicata, the sheet divides into bundles that pass through the valleys between the ciliary processes (Fig. 1-7B). The zonular fibers are attached to the inner surface of the pars plicata, which acts as a fulcrum. Two groups of zonular fibers extend from the ciliary body and insert onto the anterior and posterior surface of the lens capsule. They enclose a triangular space called the canal of Hannover (Fig. 1-7D).

Trauma, for example, contusion injury, is the most common cause of lens dislocation. Spontaneous dislocation also occurs in patients with tertiary syphilis. **Ectopia lentis** also occurs in a variety of heritable diseases of connective tissue including **Marfan syndrome**, **homocystinuria**, and the **Weill-Marchesani syndrome**. In most cases the ectopia lentis has been linked to mutations in the FBN1 gene for the microfibrillar glycoprotein fibrillin-1, which is located on the long arm of chromosome 15 (15q21.1), or by other metabolic disorders that affect the structure of fibrillin secondarily. Fibrillin-1 is a major component of the zonular fibers and also is involved in the formation of elastic tissue throughout the body.

Seventy percent of cases of heritable ectopia lentis occur in patients with **Marfan syndrome**, which has been linked to more than 50 mutations in the fibrillin-1 gene. The major manifestations of Marfan syndrome are ocular, skeletal, and cardiovascular. Bilateral lens dislocation occurs in 50% to 80% of patients and classically is superotemporal in direction (Fig. 7-15A). Patients are tall and have arachnodactyly (long spidery fingers and toes), dolichostenomelia, scoliosis, and pectus excavatum or carinatum. Cardiovascular disease is caused by defective elastic tissue and includes fatal dissecting aortic aneurysms and aortic valve defects. Other ocular defects include high myopia, large flat corneas, and a tendency to develop retinal detachment. Fibrillin-1 defects, which presumably are relatively innocuous, also have been identified in families that inherit isolated or simple ectopia lentis as autosomal dominant trait. The autosomal dominant form of

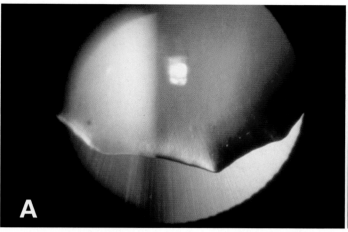 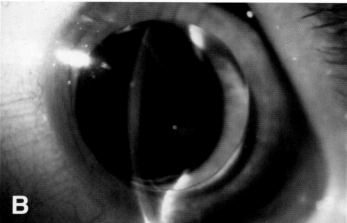

Fig. 7-15. Ectopia lentis. A. Marfan syndrome. Lens is dislocated superiorly. Stretched zonular fibers are seen in red reflex. **B.** Weill-Marchesani syndrome. Microspherophakic lens has dislocated into anterior chamber, causing pupillary block glaucoma. (Photo courtesy of Dr. Dario Savino-Zari, Caracas, Venezuela.)

Weill-Marchesani syndrome also has been linked to the FBN1 gene.

The classic manifestations of the **Weill-Marchesani syndrome** are microspherophakia and brachydactyly. Patients are short and muscular and have short fingers, broad hands, limited joint mobility, and hearing defects. The most debilitating aspects of this syndrome are ocular. Patients typically present with 15 to 20 diopters of lenticular myopia, and often develop axial lens dislocation in their teens (Fig. 7-15B). Lens dislocation often causes secondary closed angle glaucoma due to papillary block. The volume of the small, microspherophakic lens is 20% to 40% less than normal.

The heritable disorders that cause secondary abnormalities in fibrillin-1 are caused by defects in the metabolism of sulfur-containing amino acids. These disorders interfere with the formation of important disulfide bonds that serve to determine the conformation and aggregation of fibrillin-1. They include homocystinuria, sulfite oxidase deficiency, and molybdenum cofactor deficiency.

Many cases of **homocystinuria** are caused by a recessively inherited deficiency in cystathionine beta-synthase (21q22.3), an enzyme that catalyses the condensation of homocysteine with serine to form cystathionine, an important precursor of cysteine and cystine. Homocystinuric patients tend to be fair skinned and blonde and have a tall marfanoid habitus. About half develop progressive mental retardation, and nearly 75% die by age 30 from venous and arterial thromboses. The latter may be related to the endothelial protein thrombomodulin, which also contains structurally important disulfide bonds. Patients are at increased risk for thromboembolic complications during general anesthesia. Lens dislocation occurs in about 90% of patients. The lens usually dislocates inferiorly, or into the anterior chamber. It never dislocates superiorly as in Marfan syndrome, a clinical feature that differentiates homocystinuric patients who are marfanoid. Patients may

present with acute pupillary block glaucoma. High myopia, retinal detachment, and peripheral retinal pigment epithelium (RPE) degeneration are other ocular manifestations. A thick layer of periodic acid-Schiff (PAS)-positive zonular material has been found histopathologically on the surface of the ciliary body.

Sulfite oxidase deficiency usually presents with seizures shortly after birth in infants who have severe neurological findings. Lens dislocation occurs in about half, and typically is found in older infants. Affected patients are unable to convert sulfite to sulfate. This leads to an accumulation of sulfite which destroys sulfhydryl groups and disulfide bonds. Most patients with sulfite oxidase deficiency actually have a deficiency in a molybdenum cofactor that is also shared by xanthine dehydrogenase and aldehyde oxidase. The manifestations of the latter two enzyme deficiencies are relatively innocuous.

Ectopia lentis occurs rarely in other hereditary disorders including hyperlysinemia and Ehlers-Danlos syndrome.

BIBLIOGRAPHY

The Lens

Eagle RC, Spencer WH. The Lens. In: Spencer W, ed. *Ophthalmic Pathology: An Atlas and Textbook*, 4th ed., vol. 1. Philadelphia, PA: WB Saunders, 1996:372–437.

Hockwin O, Kojima M, Muller-Breitenkamp U, et al. Lens and cataract research of the 20th century: a review of results, errors and misunderstandings. *Dev Ophthalmol* 2002;35:1–11.

Developmental Anomalies

Bellows JG. Phakochronology. The study of dating structural changes in the lens. *Br J Ophthalmol* 1968;52:540–545.

Brownell RD, Wolter JR. Anterior lenticonus in familial hemorrhagic nephritis. *Arch Ophthalmol* 1964;71:481–483.

de Gottrau P, Schlotzer-Schrehardt U, Dorfler S, et al. Congenital zonular cataract. Clinicopathologic correlation with electron microscopy and review of the literature. *Arch Ophthalmol* 1993;111:235–239.

Goldberg MF. Persistent fetal vasculature (PFV): an integrated interpretation of signs and symptoms associated with persistent hyperplastic primary vitreous (PHPV). LIV Edward Jackson Memorial Lecture. *Am J Ophthalmol* 1997;124:587–626.

Jampol LM, Kass M, Dueker D, et al. Anterior polar cataracts. *Am J Ophthalmol* 1974;78:95–97.

Khalil M, Saheb N. Posterior lenticonus. *Ophthalmology* 1984;91: 1429–1430.

Lambert SR, Drack AV. Infantile cataracts. *Surv Ophthalmol* 1996; 40:427–458.

Leonard A, Bernard P, Hiel AL, et al. Prenatal diagnosis of fetal cataract: case report and review of the literature. *Fetal Diagn Ther* 2009;26:61–67.

Meisels H, Goldberg M. Vascular anastomoses between the iris and persistent primary vitreous. *Am J Ophthalmol* 1979;88:179–185.

Roche O, Beby F, Orssaud C, et al. Congenital cataract: general review. *J Fr Ophtalmol* 2006;29:443–455.

Sabates R, Krachmer JH, Weingeist TA. Ocular findings in Alport syndrome. *Ophthalmologia* 1983;186:204–210.

Streeten BW, Robinson MR, Wallace RN, et al. Lens capsule abnormalities in Alport syndrome. *Arch Ophthalmol* 1987;105:1693–1697.

Yanoff M, Fine BS, Schaffer DB. Histopathology of transient neonatal lens vacuoles. *Am J Ophthalmol* 1973;76:363–370.

Rubella Cataract

Boniuk M, Zimmerman LE. Ocular pathology in the rubella syndrome. *Arch Ophthalmol* 1967;17:455–473.

Roy FH, Fuste F, Hiatt RL, et al. The congenital rubella syndrome with virus recovery. Ocular pathology and literature review. *Am J Ophthalmol* 1966;62:222–232.

Yanoff M, Schaffer DB, Scheie HG. Rubella ocular syndrome. Clinical significance of viral and pathologic studies. *Trans Am Acad Ophthalmol Otolaryngol* 1968;72:896–902.

Zimmerman LE. Histopathologic basis for ocular manifestations of congenital rubella syndrome. The Eighth William Hamlin Wilder Memorial Lecture. *Am J Ophthalmol* 1968;65:837–862.

Cataract in Genetic Syndromes

Cogan DG, Kuwabara T. Pathology of cataracts in mongoloid idiocy: a new pathogenesis of cataracts of the coronary-cerulean type. *Doc Ophthalmol* 1962;16:73–80.

Curtin VT, Joyce EE, Ballin N. Ocular pathology in the oculo-cerebro-renal syndrome of Lowe. *Am J Ophthalmol* 1967;64 (Pt II):533–543.

Robb RM, Marchevsky A. Pathology of the lens in Down's syndrome. *Arch Ophthalmol* 1978;96:1039–1042.

Wadelius C, Fagerholm P, Pettersson U, et al. Lowe oculocerebrorenal syndrome: DNA-based linkage of the gene to Xq24-q26, using tightly linked flanking markers and the correlation to lens examination in carrier diagnosis. *Am J Hum Genet* 1989;44:241–247.

Wolter JR, Jones DH. Spontaneous cataract absorption in Hallermann-Streiff syndrome. *Ophthalmologica* 1965;150:401–408.

Senile Cataract

Benedek GB. Cataract as a protein condensation disease. *Invest Ophthalmol Vis Sci* 1997;38:1911–1921.

Boyle DL, Takemoto LJ. Confocal microscopy of human lens membranes in aged normal and nuclear cataracts. *Invest Ophthalmol Vis Sci* 1997;38:2826–2832.

Fledelius H. Cataracta ossea and other intraocular ossifications. A case report and a thirty-year Danish material. *Acta Ophthalmol (Copenh)* 1975;53:790–797.

Flocks M, Littwin CS, Zimmerman LE. Phacolytic glaucoma: a clinicopathologic study of 138 cases of glaucoma associated with hypermature cataract. *Arch Ophthalmol* 1955;54:37–45.

Font RL, Brownstein S. A light and electron microscopic study of anterior subcapsular cataracts. *Am J Ophthalmol* 1974;78:972–984.

Henkind P, Prose P. Anterior polar cataract. Electron-microscopic evidence of collagen. *Am J Ophthalmol* 1967;63:768–771.

Jensen OA, Laursen AB. Human senile cataract. Light- and electron-microscopic studies of the morphology of the anterior lens structures, with special reference of anterior capsular/subcapsular opacity. *Acta Ophthalmol (Copenh)* 1980;58:481–495.

Klintworth GK, Garner A. The causes, types, and morphology of cataracts. In: Garner A, Klintworth GK, eds. *Pathobiology of Ocular Disease: A Dynamic Approach*, 2nd ed., Part A. New York, NY: Marcel Dekker, 1994:481–532.

Kluxen G, Wolf E, Kalisch M, et al. Color vision disorders caused by yellow coloration of lenses. *Fortschr Ophthalmol* 1984;81: 180–182.

Zimmerman LE, Johnson FB. Calcium oxalate crystals within ocular tissues. *Arch Ophthalmol* 1958;60:372–383.

Posterior Capsular Opacification

Apple DJ, Solomon KD, Tetz MR, et al. Posterior capsule opacification. *Surv Ophthalmol* 1992;37:73–116.

Green WR, McDonnell PJ. Opacification of the posterior capsule. *Trans Ophthalmol Soc U K* 1985;104:727–739.

McDonnell PJ, Zarbin MA, Green WR. Posterior capsular opacification in pseudophakic eyes. *Ophthalmology* 1984;90:1548–1553.

Posterior Subcapsular Cataract

Greiner JV, Chylack LT Jr. Posterior subcapsular cataracts: histopathologic study of steroid-associated cataracts. *Arch Ophthalmol* 1979;97:135–144.

Streeten BW, Eshaghian J. Human posterior subcapsular cataract: a gross and flat preparation study. *Arch Ophthalmol* 1978;96:1653–1658.

Cataracts Caused by Ocular Disease (Complicated Cataracts)

Axelsson U. Glaucoma, miotic therapy and cataract. I. The frequency of anterior subcapsular vacuoles in glaucoma eyes treated with echothiophate (Phospholine Iodide), pilocarpine or pilocarpine-eserine, and in nonglaucomatous untreated eyes with common senile cataract. *Acta Ophthalmol (Copenh)* 1968;46:83–98.

Fagerholm PP, Philipson BT. Cataract in retinitis pigmentosa. An analysis of cataract surgery results and pathological lens changes. *Acta Ophthalmol (Copenh)* 1985;63:50–58.

Fisher RF. The lens in uveitis. *Trans Ophthalmol Soc U K* 1981;101:317–320.

Loewenfeld IE, Thompson HS. Fuchs's heterochromic cyclitis: a critical review of the literature. I. Clinical characteristics of the syndrome. *Surv Ophthalmol* 1973;17:394–457.

Sugar Cataracts

Beigi B, O'Keefe M, Bowell R, et al. Ophthalmic findings in classical galactosaemia—prospective study. *Br J Ophthalmol* 1993;77: 162–164.

Bron AJ, Sparrow J, Brown NAP, et al. The lens in diabetes. *Eye* 1993;7:260–275.

Kinoshita JH. Cataracts in galactosemia. *Invest Ophthalmol* 1965;4:786–799.

Stambolian D, Scarpino-Myers V, Eagle RC Jr, et al. Cataracts in patients heterozygous for galactokinase deficiency. *Invest Ophthalmol Vision Sci* 1986;27:429–433.

Cataracts Associated with Systemic Disease

Bullock JD, Howard RO. Werner syndrome. *Arch Ophthalmol* 1973;90:53–56.

Burns CA. Ocular histopathology of myotonic dystrophy. A clinicopathologic case report. *Am J Ophthalmol* 1969;68:416–422.

Chen CC, Huang JL, Yang KD, et al. Atopic cataracts in a child with atopic dermatitis: a case report and review of the literature. *Asian Pac J Allergy Immunol* 2000;18:69–71.

Dark AJ, Streeten BW. Ultrastructural study of cataract in myotonia dystrophica. *Am J Ophthalmol* 1977;84:666–674.

Eshaghian J, March WF, Goossens W, et al. Ultrastructure of cataract in myotonic dystrophy. *Invest Ophthalmol Vis Sci* 1978;17: 289–293.

Fagerholm P, Palmquist BM, Philipson B. Atopic cataract: changes in the lens epithelium and subcapsular cortex. *Graefes Arch Clin Exp Ophthalmol* 1984;221:149–152.

Racz P, Kovacs B, Varga L, et al. Bilateral cataract in acrodermatitis enteropathica. *J Pediatr Ophthalmol Strabismus* 1979;16:180–182.

Seland JH. The nature of capsular inclusions in lenticular chalcosis. Report of a case. *Acta Ophthalmol (Copenh)* 1976;54:99–108.

Spaeth GL, Frost P. Fabry's disease. Its ocular manifestations. *Arch Ophthalmol* 1965;74:760–769.

Tso MO, Fine BS, Thorpe HE. Kayser-Fleischer ring and associated cataract in Wilson's disease. *Am J Ophthalmol* 1975;79:479–488.

Traumatic Cataract

Fraunfelder FT, Hanna C. Electric cataracts. I. Sequential changes, unusual and prognostic findings. *Arch Ophthalmol* 1972;87: 179–183.

Hanna C, Fraunfelder FT. Electric cataracts. II. Ultrastructural lens changes. *Arch Ophthalmol* 1972;87:184–191.

Hanna C, Fraunfelder FT. Lens capsule change after intraocular copper. *Ann Ophthalmol* 1973;5:9–12.

Jongebloed WL, Dijk F, Kruis J, et al. Soemmering's ring, an aspect of secondary cataract: a morphological description by SEM. *Doc Ophthalmol* 1988;70:165–174.

Masciulli L, Andersen DR, Charles S. Experimental ocular siderosis in the squirrel monkey. *Am J Ophthalmol* 1972;74:638–661.

McCanna P, Chandra SR, Stevens TS, et al. Argon laser induced cataract as a complication of retinal photocoagulation. *Arch Ophthalmol* 1982;100:1071–1073.

Rafferty NS, Goossens W, March WF. Ultrastructure of human traumatic cataract. *Am J Ophthalmol* 1974;78:985–995.

Reddy SC. Electric cataract: a case report and review of the literature. *Eur J Ophthalmol* 1999;9:134–138.

Talamo JH, Topping TM, Maumenee AE, et al. Ultrastructural studies of cornea, iris and lens in a case of siderosis bulbi. *Ophthalmology* 1985;92:1675–1680.

Toxic Cataract

Hamming NA, Apple DJ, Goldberg MF. Histopathology and ultrastructure of busulfan-induced cataract. *Albrecht Von Graefes Arch Klin Exp Ophthalmol* 1976;200:139–147.

Hiller R, Sperduto RD, Podgor MJ, et al. Cigarette smoking and the risk of development of lens opacities. The Framingham studies. *Arch Ophthalmol* 1997;115:1113–1118.

Kirby TJ. Cataracts produced by triparanol. (MER-29). *Trans Am Ophthalmol Soc* 1967;65:494–543.

West S, Munoz B, Schein OD, et al. Cigarette smoking and risk for progression of nuclear opacities. *Arch Ophthalmol* 1995;113:1377–1380.

True Exfoliation of the Lens Capsule

Anderson IL, van Bockxmeer FM. True exfoliation of the lens capsule. A clinicopathological report. *Aust N Z J Ophthalmol* 1985;13:343–347.

Brodrick JD, Tate GW Jr. Capsular delamination (true exfoliation) of the lens. Report of a case. *Arch Ophthalmol* 1979;97: 1693–1698.

Burde RM, Bresnick G, Uhrhammer J. True exfoliation of the lens cpsule. An electron microscopic study. *Arch Ophthalmol* 1969;82:651–653.

Cashwell LF Jr, Holleman IL, Weaver RG, et al. Idiopathic true exfoliation of the lens capsule. *Ophthalmology* 1989;96:348–351.

Pseudoexfoliation of the Lens Capsule

Schlotzer-Schrehardt U, Koca M, Naumann G, et al. Pseudoexfoliation syndrome. Ocular manifestation of a systemic disorder? *Arch Ophthalmol* 1992;110:1752–1756.

Schlotzer-Schrehardt UM, Dorfler S, Naumann GO. Corneal endothelial involvement in pseudoexfoliation syndrome. *Arch Ophthalmol* 1993;111:666–674.

Schlotzer-Schrehardt U, Naumann GO. A histopathologic study of zonular instability in pseudoexfoliation syndrome. *Am J Ophthalmol* 1994;118:730–743.

Schlotzer-Schrehardt U. Molecular pathology of pseudoexfoliation syndrome/glaucoma—new insights from LOXL1 gene associations. *Exp Eye Res* 2009;88:776–785.

Schlotzer-Schrehardt U, Naumann GO. Ocular and systemic pseudoexfoliation syndrome. *Am J Ophthalmol* 2006;141:921–937.

Schlotzer-Schrehardt U, Pasutto F, Sommer P, et al. Genotype-correlated expression of lysyl oxidase-like 1 in ocular tissues of patients with pseudoexfoliation syndrome/glaucoma and normal patients. *Am J Pathol* 2008;173:1724–1735.

Schlotzer-Schrehardt U, von der Mark K, Sakai LY, et al. Increased extracellular deposition of fibrillin-containing fibrils in pseudoexfoliation syndrome. *Invest Ophthalmol Vis Sci* 1997;38:970–984.

Streeten BW, Dark AJ. Pseudoexfoliation syndrome. In: Garner A, Klintworth GK, eds. *Pathobiology of Ocular Disease: A Dynamic approach*, 2nd ed., Part A. New York, NY: Marcel Dekker, 1994:591–629.

Streeten BW, Li Zy, Wallace RN, et al. Pseudoexfoliative fibrillopathy in visceral organs of a patient with pseudoexfoliation syndrome. *Arch Ophthalmol* 1992;110:1757–1762.

Heritable Lens Dislocation (Ectopia Lentis)

Edwards MJ, Challinor CJ, Colley PW, et al. Clinical and linkage study of a large family with simple ectopia lentis linked to FBN1. *Am J Med Genet* 1994;53:65–71.

Fujiwara H, Takigawa Y, Ueno S, et al. Histology of the lens in the Weill-Marchesani syndrome. *Br J Ophthalmol* 1990;74:631–634.

Hayward C, Brock DJ. Fibrillin-1 mutations in Marfan syndrome and other type-1 fibrillinopathies. *Hum Mutat* 1997;10:415–423.

Henkind P, Ashton N. Ocular pathology in homocystinuria. *Trans Ophthalmol Soc U K* 1965;85:21–38.

Hollister DW, Godfrey M, Sakai LY, et al. Immunohistologic abnormalities of the microfibrillar-fiber system in the Marfan syndrome. *N Engl J Med* 1990;323:152–159.

Lueder GT, Steiner RD. Ophthalmic abnormalities in molydenum cofactor deficiency and isolated sulfite oxidase deficiency. *J Pediatr Ophthalmol Strabismus* 1995;32:334–337.

Maumenee IH. The eye in the Marfan syndrome. *Trans Am Ophthalmol Soc* 1981;79:684–733.

Maumenee IH. The Marfan syndrome is caused by a point mutation in the fibrillin gene. *Arch Ophthalmol* 1992;110:472–473.

Maumenee IH. The Weill-Marchesani syndrome. In: Beighton P, ed. *McCusick's Heritable Disorders of Connective Tissue*. St. Louis, MO: Mosby, 1993:179–187.

Pyeritz, RE. Homocystinuria. In: Beighton P, ed. *McCusick's Heritable Disorders of Connective Tissue*. St. Louis, MO: Mosby, 1993:137–178.

Schienle HW, Seitz R, Nawroth P, et al. Thrombomodulin and ristocetincofactor in homocystinuria: a study in two siblings. *Thromb Res* 1995;77:79–86.

Shih VE, Abroms IF, Johnson JL, et al. Sulfite oxidase deficiency. Biochemical and clinical investigations of a hereditary metabolic disorder in sulfur metabolism. *N Engl J Med* 1977;297:1022–1028.

Smith TH, Holland MG, Woody NC. Ocular manifestations of familial hyperlysinemia. *Trans Am Acad Ophthalmol Otolaryngol* 1971;75:355–360.

Thomas C, Cordier J, Algan B. Les altérations oculaires de la maladie d'Ehlers-Danlos. *Arch Ophthalmol (Paris)* 1954;14:691–697.

Wirtz MK, Samples JR, Kramer PL, et al. Weill-Marchesani syndrome—possible linkage of the autosomal dominant form to 15q21.1. *Am J Med Genet* 1996;65:68–75.

8

Glaucoma

INTRODUCTION

Visual loss in glaucoma is caused by the death of the retinal ganglion cells and their axons that constitute the nerve fiber layer of the retina and the optic nerve (Fig. 8-1A). The optic nerve head has a characteristic cupped or excavated configuration in glaucoma (Figs. 8-1B, 8-2, and 8-3B). Cupping distinguishes glaucomatous optic atrophy from primary optic atrophy, in which loss of retinal ganglion cells and nerve fibers also occurs. Cupping of the optic disc suggests that elevated intraocular pressure is a major risk factor in the pathogenesis of glaucomatous optic atrophy.

How elevated intraocular pressure kills retinal ganglion cells is not clear. Experimental evidence suggests that it may be related to ischemia and/or blockage of axoplasmic flow caused by mechanical compression of axons in the pores of the lamina cribrosa, which are distorted by high levels of intraocular pressure. The blockage of axoplasmic flow may deprive cells of brain-derived neurotrophic factor whose absence triggers programmed cell death. Glial cell activation, TNF-α, and neuroinflammatory processes are thought to be important mediators of retinal ganglion cell damage.

Glaucoma has been defined as *a syndrome characterized by an elevation of intraocular pressure of sufficient degree or chronicity to produce ocular tissue damage* (Yanoff) or as *an optic neuropathy associated with a characteristic excavation of the optic disc and a progressive loss of visual field sensitivity* (Quigley). The first definition emphasizes that tissue damage, usually nerve fiber atrophy or optic nerve cupping is a requisite for the diagnosis. The term syndrome indicates that there are many mechanisms that can raise intraocular pressure. The first definition also implies that a single elevated pressure reading is not glaucoma. The second newer definition does not mention intraocular pressure because authorities recently have stressed that elevation of intraocular pressure is only one of the risk factors that are responsible for neuronal loss in glaucoma. The latter definition includes so-called low-tension glaucoma that develops in patients whose optic nerves seem to be especially vulnerable to damage. Most glaucomatous eyes examined in the ophthalmic pathology laboratory have had elevated intraocular pressure. In nearly all cases of glaucoma, the elevated intraocular pressure is caused by obstruction of aqueous outflow.

As noted earlier (see Chapter 1), intraocular pressure is governed by a delicate balance between the production of aqueous humor by the nonpigmented ciliary epithelial cells and its egress or outflow from the eye via the trabecular meshwork and the canal of Schlemm, which are located in the anterior chamber angle formed by the cornea and peripheral iris (Figs. 1-9 and 8-4). Lesser amounts of aqueous exit through nontraditional pathways that include iris vessels and posterior uveoscleral outflow via the ciliary body and the vortex veins.

The trabecular meshwork is a sieve-like structure that is nestled in the anterior crotch of the scleral spur (Fig. 1-9C,D). It is composed of an interconnected network of small collagenous beams or trabeculae enveloped by trabecular endothelial cells. A thin layer of extracellular matrix material called the juxtacanalicular connective tissue (JXT) is interposed between the interstices of the meshwork

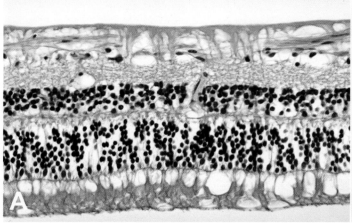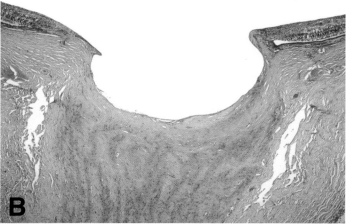

Fig. 8-1. A. Glaucomatous retinal atrophy. The ganglion cell and nerve fiber layers of the retina are atrophic. The inner plexiform and inner nuclear layers are well preserved excluding inner ischemic retinal atrophy. **B. Glaucomatous optic atrophy.** The nerve head is massively cupped, and the lamina cribrosa is bowed posteriorly. The nerve fiber layer of the retina is markedly atrophic. (**A.** H&E ×10, **B.** H&E ×100)

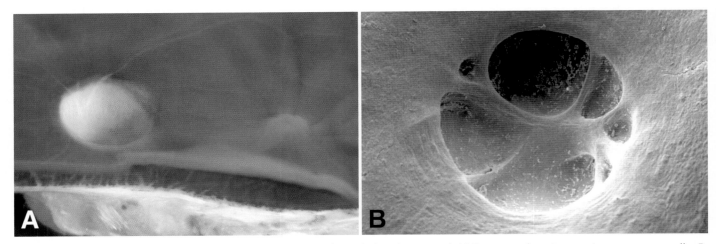

Fig. 8-2. A. Glaucomatous optic atrophy. The disc is pale and deeply cupped. *Yellow macular pigment* is seen temporally. **B.** Scanning electron microscopy of deeply cupped optic nerve.

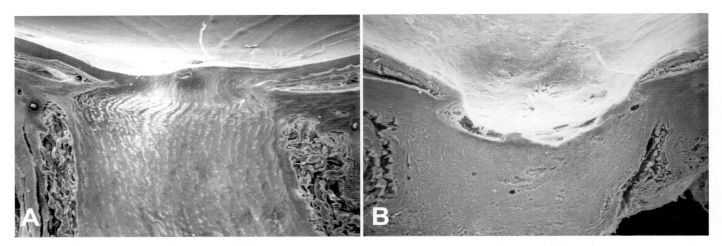

Fig. 8-3. Glaucomatous optic atrophy, SEM. A. Longitudinally sectioned normal nerve shows mild physiologic cupping. Lamina cribrosa is visible. **B.** Longitudinal section of nerve with severe glaucomatous cupping. Retina at margin of cup is severely atrophic.

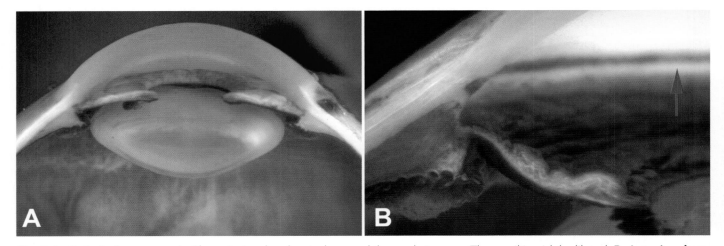

Fig. 8-4. A. Anterior segment. The anterior chamber is deep and the angle is open. The pupil is widely dilated. **B. Anterior chamber angle.** Trabecular meshwork is pigmented band directly in front of lighter scleral spur, which is marked by *arrow*. The meshwork is heavily pigmented in this eye.

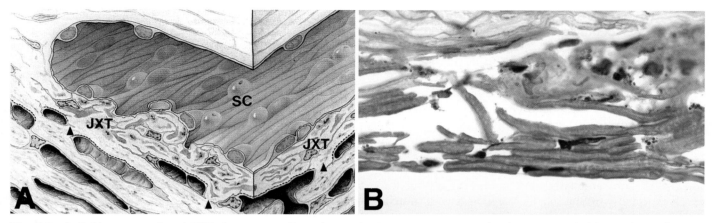

Fig. 8-5. A. Schlemm canal and JXT. Aqueous outflow obstruction in primary open angle glaucoma probably resides in the JXT, which borders the inner wall of Schlemm canal. Alvarado has shown that the area of the trabecular culs-de-sac is markedly reduced in primary open-angle glaucoma. These trabecular culs-de-sac, which abut the JXT, are responsible for a major proportion of normal outflow resistance. (From Alvarado JA, Murphy CG. Outflow obstruction in pigmentary and primary open angle glaucoma. *Arch Ophthalmol* 1992;110:1769–1778. Copyright 1992, American Medical Association.) **B. Trabecular meshwork, primary open-angle glaucoma.** Trabeculectomy specimen from patient with primary open-angle glaucoma shows decreased cellularity of trabecular endothelium and fusion of beams in inner meshwork. These changes may be artifactitious. (PAS ×250)

and the lumen of Schlemm canal, which is lined by a continuous layer of endothelial cells (Fig. 8-5A). A modified vein, Schlemm canal runs circumferentially around the chamber angle, giving off branches or collector channels that traverse the sclera and discharge their contents into the epibulbar veins via the aqueous veins of Ascher.

CLASSIFICATION OF THE GLAUCOMAS

The glaucomas are classified into developmental, primary or idiopathic, and secondary types. Primary and secondary glaucomas are subclassified into open-angle and closed-angle variants depending on whether the angle is open or closed. Angle-closure glaucoma is marked by the apposition or adherence of the peripheral iris to the trabecular meshwork (Fig. 8-6). Developmental glaucomas present in infancy or childhood and may be inherited or are associated with other ocular anomalies or systemic disorders.

Developmental Glaucoma

Developmental glaucomas are caused by developmental abnormalities or dysembryogenesis of the aqueous outflow pathways. **Primary congenital glaucoma** is a bilateral disorder that is often inherited as an autosomal recessive

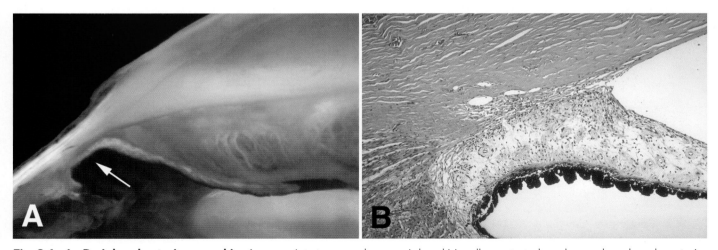

Fig. 8-6. A. Peripheral anterior synechia. *Arrow* points to area where peripheral iris adheres to trabecular meshwork and posterior cornea. The anterior iridic surface is flattened by a subtle neovascular membrane. **B.** Peripheral anterior synechia. The peripheral iris adheres to the inner surface of the trabecular meshwork, blocking the outflow of aqueous humor. A neovascular membrane flattens the anterior iridic surface. (H&E ×25)

trait. Autosomal recessively inherited congenital glaucoma is caused by mutations in the cytochrome P4501B1 gene (CYP1B1) on chromosome 2 (2p22-p21). Forty percent of cases are present at birth and eighty-six percent become evident during the first year of life. Affected infants often have light sensitivity (photophobia), blepharospasm, and tearing and may be misdiagnosed as having nasolacrimal duct obstruction. Ocular enlargement (buphthalmos or "ox eye") is the clinical hallmark of congenital glaucoma. Elevation of intraocular pressure only causes ocular enlargement during childhood when the sclera is relatively thin and elastic. Corneal enlargement and ectasia of limbal tissues is especially striking (Fig. 8-7A). As the cornea stretches, Descemet membrane may rupture spontaneously, causing corneal edema and opacification. Old healed ruptures in Descemet membrane in patients with congenital glaucoma are called Haab striae (Fig. 8-7). Haab striae usually are oriented horizontally or concentric to the limbus in the peripheral cornea. This distinguishes them from traumatic ruptures caused by obstetrical forceps, which usually are oriented obliquely.

Hypothetical mechanisms involved in the pathogenesis of congenital glaucoma include an imperforate mesodermal sheet covering the trabecular meshwork called Barkan membrane, congenital absence of Schlemm canal, and persistence of a fetal angle configuration. Histopathologically, the fetal angle is characterized by anterior insertion of the iris root and ciliary processes, the presence of mesenchymal tissue in the angle, and continuity of ciliary muscle fibers with trabecular beams. The anterior chamber usually is quite deep in eyes with congenital glaucoma. The angle is open gonioscopically, and there is a high insertion of the iris root.

Developmental glaucoma occasionally occurs in association with other ocular abnormalities or congenital syndromes including aniridia, the Axenfeld-Rieger syndrome, and Peters anomaly. Glaucoma also complicates von Recklinghausen neurofibromatosis (NF I) and Sturge-Weber syndrome, particularly if the upper eyelid is involved by the hamartomatous process: a plexiform or diffuse neurofibroma in NF-1 or a nevus flammeus in Sturge-Weber syndrome (Fig. 2-8). Hamartomatous infiltration of the angle may produce a distinctive gonioscopic appearance in neurofibromatosis. The angle is blanketed by a uniform layer of tan tissue which obscures normal trabecular landmarks. Glaucoma and cataract occur concurrently in Lowe syndrome. Other syndromes that may have congenital glaucoma include Gregg congenital rubella syndrome, Stickler syndrome, Hallermann-Streiff syndrome, Hurler syndrome, Turner syndrome, and trisomies 21 and 13.

Primary Open-Angle Glaucoma

Primary or idiopathic open-angle glaucoma (POAG) is the most common type of glaucoma and affects an estimated 1% to 3% of the population. POAG is an insidious disease that causes asymptomatic painless visual loss. By definition, the angle is open on gonioscopic examination. POAG usually is a bilateral disease, and affected patients frequently have a positive family history. The genetics of POAG are complex; the disorder has been linked to 14 genes, most notably the myocilin (MYOC) gene on chromosome 1. Mutations in myocilin are found in 3% to 5% of patients with adult-onset POAG.

The cause of aqueous outflow obstruction in POAG remains uncertain, but the area of obstruction may be located in the JXT in the deepest part of the trabecular meshwork bordering Schlemm canal. Several pathogenetic theories involve obstruction of the meshwork or JXT by

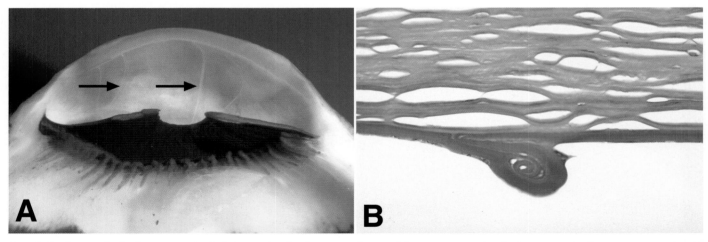

Fig. 8-7. Congenital glaucoma. A. Ridges on back of cornea denoted by *arrows* are healed ruptures in Descemet membrane (Haab striae). The cornea is large, the anterior chamber is deep, and the limbal tissues are somewhat ectatic. Depigmentation of ciliary body was caused by a prior cyclodestructive procedure. **B.** Haab stria, congenital glaucoma. A thickened ridge of hypertrophic coiled Descemet membrane has formed at the site of a rupture caused by corneal enlargement. Intrinsically elastic, Descemet membrane often coils up when lacerated or ruptured. (PAS ×100)

glycosaminoglycans or other abnormal extracellular matrix material. Loss of trabecular endothelial cells could lead to fusion of trabecular beams and decreased porosity of the meshwork (Fig. 8-5B). Electron microscopy has shown that the density of trabecular endothelial cells is decreased in patients with POAG. Trabecular endothelial cell death in patients with mutations in the MYOC gene may be related to the intracellular accumulation of abnormal myocilin. Another study showed that the area of the trabecular culs-de-sac, which provide a major proportion of normal outflow resistance, is markedly reduced in POAG (Fig 8-5A). Other hypothetical pathogenetic mechanisms include abnormalities in the formation of giant vacuoles in the endothelial lining of Schlemm canal, or age-related sclerosis in the scleral spur that impedes posterior uveoscleral outflow.

Primary Closed-Angle Glaucoma

Primary closed-angle glaucoma (acute angle-closure glaucoma or acute congestive glaucoma) is caused by functional apposition or blockage of the trabecular meshwork by the peripheral iris. The resultant acute rise in intraocular pressure produces major symptoms including severe ocular pain, headache, and gastrointestinal symptoms (nausea and vomiting) caused by a vagal oculogastric reflex. The involved eye is injected and classically has a fixed, dilated pupil during an acute attack of closed-angle glaucoma. The vision usually is diminished by corneal epithelial edema evident clinically as "bedewing," or possibly by posterior segment ischemia. Primary closed-angle glaucoma usually is unilateral and classically occurs in hyperopic ("far-sighted") patients whose small eyes have shallow, crowded anterior chambers. Primary closed-angle glaucoma is extremely rare in myopes (near-sighted individuals) and younger patients less than age 40. Progressive growth of the lens or development of an intumescent cataract can precipitate an acute attack of closed-angle glaucoma in elderly patients (phacomorphic glaucoma). Acute angle-closure glaucoma is more prevalent in certain racial groups (e.g., Asians and Inuits) and often occurs in nanophthalmic eyes that are markedly hyperopic and prone to develop exudative ciliochoroidal detachment. Most patients with angle closure have an asymptomatic course and do not suffer acute attacks. Quigley has hypothesized that disturbed physiological mechanisms contribute to angle closure and angle-closure glaucoma in many cases. Such factors include diminished loss of iris volume during pupillary dilation and expansion of choroidal volume.

Functional pupillary block is involved in the pathogenesis of primary closed-angle glaucoma. When the pupil is mid-dilated, the iris pigment epithelium near the pupil is pressed firmly against the anterior surface of the lens, impeding the flow of aqueous humor into the anterior chamber. The pupillary block is functional because actual adhesions between the iris and lens called posterior synechiae have not formed. Continual production of aqueous humor behind the iris produces a pressure gradient that bows the peripheral part of the iris forward, obstructing the trabecular meshwork. If this functional papillary block is not relieved expeditiously, permanent adhesions between peripheral iris and trabecular meshwork called peripheral anterior synechiae eventually develop. Acute closed-angle glaucoma is cured by making a full-thickness hole in the iris. This equalizes the pressure in the anterior and posterior chambers and allows the iris to fall back into its normal position. The iridotomy usually is performed with a surgical laser.

High levels of intraocular pressure can cause permanent damage to anterior segment structures during an attack of acute closed-angle glaucoma. Ischemic in nature, these changes persist as stigmata of a prior "acute attack" and include permanent dilation and unreactivity of the pupil caused by necrosis of the sphincter muscle, patchy atrophy of the iris stroma, and small grayish anterior subcapsular lens opacities called glaukomflecken. Glaukomflecken probably represent focal areas of lens epithelial necrosis and cortical degeneration.

Secondary Closed-Angle Glaucoma

Secondary glaucomas are caused by concurrent ocular or systemic disease. Both closed-angle and open-angle varieties of secondary glaucoma occur. Many blind glaucomatous eyes examined in the ophthalmic pathology laboratory have secondary closed-angle glaucoma. Secondary closed-angle glaucoma is characterized by the formation of permanent adhesions between iris and trabecular meshwork called **peripheral anterior synechiae** (Figs. 8-6–8-9). There are many causes of secondary

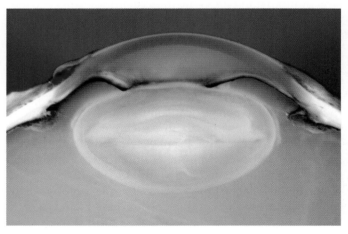

Fig. 8-8. Iris bombé. Pupil is secluded by 360-degree posterior synechiae. Peripheral iris is bowed anteriorly forming broad secondary peripheral anterior synechiae.

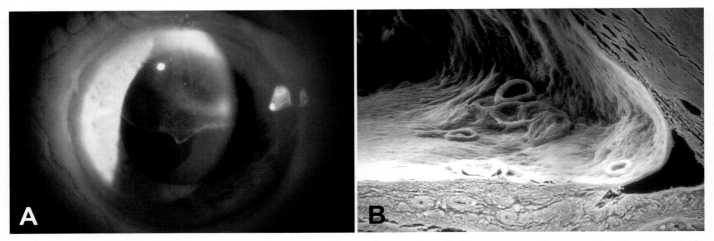

Fig. 8-9. Epithelial downgrowth. A. Slit lamp discloses sheet of corneal epithelium on posterior corneal surface superiorly. **B.** SEM shows sheet of surface epithelium introduced by trauma lining the posterior cornea, trabecular meshwork, and anterior surface of the iris. The epithelial membrane flattens the anterior surface of the iris. (SEM ×80)

closed-angle glaucoma. Permanent peripheral anterior synechiae can form in untreated primary closed-angle glaucoma and often develop in the late stages of retinopathy of prematurity or persistent hyperplastic primary vitreous (PHPV). Posterior segment tumors usually cause secondary closed-angle glaucoma by stimulating iris neovascularization or by a pupillary block mechanism.

The role of functional pupillary block in primary closed-angle glaucoma has been discussed earlier. Pupillary block also is important in several types of secondary closed-angle glaucoma. Inflammatory adhesions between the pupillary part of the iris and the anterior lens capsule called posterior synechiae readily form in the sticky, fibrin-rich milieu of iritis or iridocyclitis. The entire circumference of the pupil may become firmly bound to the lens (seclusio pupillae), totally blocking the flow of aqueous humor into the anterior chamber. The elevated pressure in the posterior chamber bows the peripheral part of the iris forward (**iris bombé**) and blocks the trabecular meshwork secondarily (Fig. 8-8). Cycloplegic medications such as atropine or scopolamine relieve the pain of pupillary and ciliary spasm in uveitis and help to prevent posterior synechiae by dilating the pupil. The lens or vitreous can also block the pupil. Anterior displacement of the microspherophakic lens in Weill-Marchesani Syndrome readily occludes the pupil, causing pupillary block glaucoma (Fig. 7-15B). Pupillary block glaucoma also occurs in patients with traumatic or heritable lens dislocation. Prophylactic peripheral iridectomies were performed routinely during intracapsular cataract surgery to prevent postoperative blockage of the pupil by the anterior face of the vitreous. Pupillary block caused by anterior movement of the lens-iris diaphragm is a common cause of secondary closed-angle glaucoma in eyes that have large posterior segment tumors or extensive bullous retinal detachments.

Several clinically important types of secondary closed-angle glaucoma are caused by the proliferation of cells on anterior chamber structures. These secondary proliferative glaucomas include epithelial downgrowth or ingrowth caused by proliferation of ocular surface epithelium after surgical or nonsurgical trauma, the iridocorneal endothelial (ICE) syndrome caused by proliferation of abnormal corneal endothelial cells, and neovascular glaucoma (NVG) caused by iris neovascularization. **Epithelial downgrowth is discussed in Chapter 3** (Figs. 4-15A and 8-9).

Neovascular Glaucoma

Many blind painful eyes accessioned by ophthalmic pathology laboratories have NVG (Figs. 8-10–8-12). Peripheral anterior synechia formation in NVG is caused by the proliferation of fibrovascular tissue on the anterior surface of the iris and angle. Angiogenic factors such as vascular endothelial growth factor (VEGF) produced by ischemic parts of the retina or intraocular tumor cells stimulate the iris neovascularization. VEGF levels in the aqueous humor are significantly increased in NVG. Clinically, conditions most commonly associated with NVG include retinal vein and artery occlusions, proliferative diabetic retinopathy, and intraocular tumors, particularly retinoblastoma.

Severe iris neovascularization (NVI, rubeosis iridis) flattens the anterior surface of the iris, effacing normal architectural details such as contraction furrows (Fig. 8-10). The anterior border layer of the iris normally is a totally avascular site. Any vessels found here during histopathologic examination are abnormal. The new vessels have thin walls and lack the thick mantle of collagen fibers that normally envelops iris stromal vessels. The new vessels are located deep to a flat, delicate sheet of contractile myofibroblasts, which is transparent clinically (Fig. 8-11). The surface layer of myofibroblasts may provide the motive force for synechial closure of the angle and formation of pigment epithelial ectropion (ectropion iridis) (Fig. 8-12). In ectropion iridis, the iris pigment epithelium is dragged around the

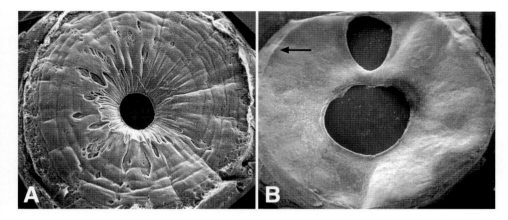

Fig. 8-10. Neovascular glaucoma. A. Scanning electron microscopy of normal iris shows collarette, crypts, and contraction furrows. **B.** Neovascular glaucoma. Neovascular membrane flattens and effaces normal architecture of anterior iridic surface. A peripheral iridectomy is present. Peripheral ridge (*arrow*) marks site of ruptured anterior synechia. (**A.** SEM ×10, **B.** SEM ×10)

pupillary margin onto the anterior surface of the iris by the contracting sheet of neovascular tissue. An associated ectropion of the pupillary sphincter muscle is often present.

Fewer eyes with NVG are being enucleated and submitted to ophthalmic pathology laboratories in recent years. This reflects the availability of effective new therapies such as pan-retinal photocoagulation (PRP) that prevent the development of proliferative retinopathy and iris neovascularization in patients who have diabetes and other ischemic retinopathies. PRP uses hundred of laser burns to kill outer retinal cells. Hypothetically, this diminishes the production of angiogenic factors by decreasing the demand for oxygen and nutrients or increases the supply of metabolites by disrupting the outer part of the blood–retinal barrier. PRP does not reverse synechiae after they have formed. Specialized filtering operations using plastic setons or tube shunts, or transscleral cycloablation procedures that use intense cold or laser energy to reduce aqueous production can be used to treat established cases of NVG. VEGF-inhibitors

Ranibizumab and Bevacizumab currently are being evaluated as an adjunctive therapy for NVI.

The Iridocorneal Endothelial Syndrome

Proliferation of abnormal corneal endothelial cells, possibly transformed by viral infection, causes unilateral closed-angle glaucoma and a characteristic spectrum of iris abnormalities in patients who have the ICE syndrome (Figs. 8-13 and 8-14). The iris abnormalities include distortion of the pupil, which typically is drawn toward a synechia that develops in the otherwise open angle, marked degrees of iris pigment epithelial ectropion, flattening and effacement of the anterior iridic surface with multiple pigmented iris nodules, and the formation of full-thickness tractional iris holes (Fig. 8-13). The name iridocorneal endothelial or ICE syndrome stresses the role of endothelial proliferation in the pathogenesis of the iris abnormalities. Several conditions that form the ICE syndrome are distinguished by the

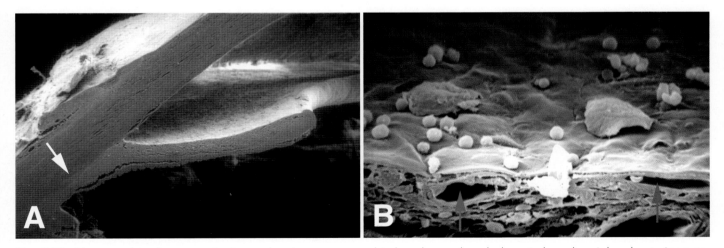

Fig. 8-11. Neovascular glaucoma. A. *Arrow* denotes compressed trabecular meshwork deep to broad peripheral anterior synechia in eye with NVG secondary to central retinal vein occlusion. The anterior surface of the iris is flattened. **B.** Iris neovascularization. *Arrows* point to new vessels on iris beneath surface sheet of myofibroblasts. (From John T, Sassani JW, Eagle RC. The myofibroblastic component of rubeosis iridis. *Ophthalmology* 1983;90:721–728. Courtesy of *Ophthalmology*.) (**A.** SEM ×20, SEM ×640)

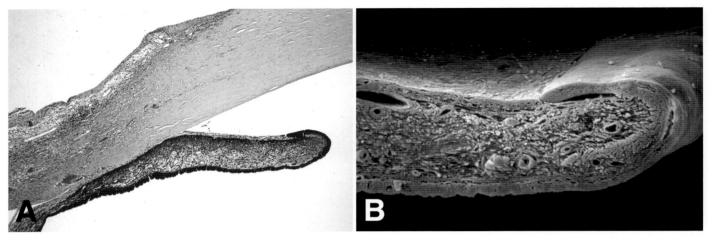

Fig. 8-12. Neovascular glaucoma. A. A broad peripheral anterior synechia is present. The free surface of the iris is flattened by a florid neovascular membrane that is causing ectropion of the iris pigment epithelium and sphincter muscle. **B.** Ectropion iridis, NVG. SEM discloses a florid fibrovascular membrane that flattens the anterior surface of the iris, which normally is an avascular site. Traction has pulled the iris pigment epithelium and sphincter muscle onto the front of the iris. (**A.** H&E ×10, **B.** SEM ×80)

nature of their iris abnormalities. Full-thickness iris holes are a characteristic feature of essential iris atrophy but typically do not develop in the Cogan-Reese or iris nevus syndrome, in which the iris is covered by endothelium and flattened by ectopic Descemet membrane studded with pigmented nodules (Fig. 8-13A). Corneal edema overshadows iris abnormalities in the variant of essential iris atrophy described by Chandler (Chandler syndrome).

Normal corneal endothelium does not proliferate during adult life, but the abnormal endothelial cells in the ICE syndrome are able to multiply and extend across the trabecular meshwork onto the iris where they elaborate large quantities of extracellular matrix material including new Descemet membrane (Fig. 8-14). The matrix material thickens trabecular beams and welds the flattened iris to the posterior cornea. The iris nodules that characterize Cogan-Reese syndrome and some cases of essential iris atrophy are formed when the sheets of migrating endothelial cells encircle and "pinch-off" knuckles of iris stroma (Fig. 8-13B). Endothelialization and descemetization of fistulas and filtering blebs leads to failure of glaucoma surgery.

Corneal endothelial abnormalities often are evident on clinical specular microscopy as "dark-light" reversal and the presence of two sharply demarcated populations of

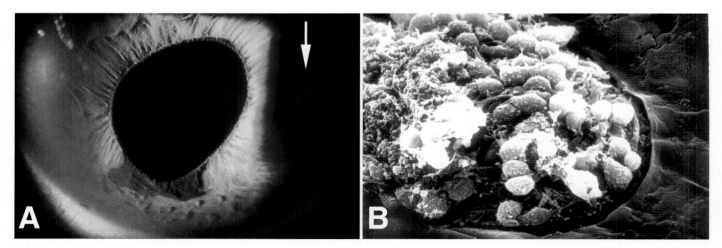

Fig. 8-13. A. Essential iris atrophy. Distorted pupil is drawn toward synechia in inferior angle. *Arrow* points to full-thickness iris hole. Multiple iris nodules are seen in flattened endothelialized zone of iris bordering synechia and ectropion iridis. **B. Iris nodule, ICE syndrome.** Sheet of endothelial cells encircles knuckle of iris stromal melanocytes forming iris nodule. (**A.** From Eagle RC Jr. Congenital, developmental and degenerative disorders of the iris and ciliary body. In: Albert DM, Jakobiec FA, eds. *Principles and Practice of Ophthalmology. Clinical Practice,* vol. 1. Philadelphia, PA: Saunders, 1993:368–389; **B.** SEM ×640 [From Eagle RC, Font RL, Yanoff M, et al. The iris nevus (Cogan-Reese) syndrome: light and electron microscopic observations. *Br J Ophthalmol* 1980;64:446–452.])

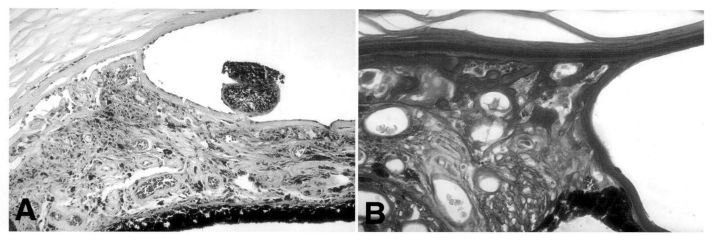

Fig. 8-14. A. ICE syndrome, Cogan-Reese variant. Pigmented iris nodule and thick layer of ectopic Descemet membrane are seen on anterior surface of iris in section from initial case reported by Cogan and Reese. Basement membrane material also is interposed between iris and cornea in area of synechial closure. **B. ICE syndrome, essential iris atrophy variant.** Rodlets and tubules of new Descemet membrane material are seen within area of synechia closure excluding secondary reactive endothelialization. Thick layer of ectopic Descemet membrane lines anterior surface of severely stretched iris at right. (**A.** H&E ×50, PAS ×100)

endothelial cells that vary in size and shape. What causes the corneal endothelium to transform into a new species of cells capable of proliferation is unclear. Theories include viral transformation of cells, an endothelial neoplasm, or abnormalities in terminal differentiation of neural crest cells.

Secondary Open-Angle Glaucoma

The angle appears open on gonioscopic examination in patients who have secondary open-angle glaucoma. Causes of secondary open-angle glaucoma include obstruction of the trabecular meshwork by cells, pigment, debris or other material, damage or scarring of outflow pathways, or systemic or local conditions that elevate episcleral venous pressure.

Substances that can obstruct the trabecular meshwork include blood, inflammatory cells, particles of lens material, melanin pigment, and an abnormal form of matrix material called pseudoexfoliation that is found in some elderly patients (see lens chapter). Glaucoma complicates large anterior chamber hemorrhages caused by contusion injuries ("eight-ball" or "black ball" hyphemas). Patients with sickle hemoglobinopathies who develop hyphemas are at particular risk for glaucoma because their erythrocytes sickle in the low-oxygen environment and the sickled cells, which are less pliable, become trapped in the trabecular meshwork.

Infiltration of the trabecular meshwork by inflammatory cells ("trabeculitis") occasionally causes elevated intraocular pressure in eyes with iridocyclitis. Frequently, however, disruption of the blood-aqueous barrier by the inflammation leads to "shut-down" of aqueous production by the ciliary body.

Several rare types of secondary glaucoma are caused by physical obstruction of the trabecular meshwork by macrophages. **Phacolytic glaucoma** (Fig. 8-15A,B) is caused by macrophages that have ingested degenerated lens material that has leaked through the capsule of a mature cortical cataract. Free high molecular weight lens protein also contributes to trabecular meshwork blockage. Patients who have phacolytic glaucoma often have undergone successful cataract surgery in their fellow eye and have forgone additional surgery because they are satisfied with uniocular vision. Many eyes with phacolytic glaucoma were enucleated in the past before the condition was widely recognized. Now most cases respond to lens extraction and anterior chamber lavage.

The trabecular meshwork in **hemolytic glaucoma** is obstructed by macrophages laden with blood breakdown products including globules of the golden-brown pigment hemosiderin and erythrocyte ghost cells (Fig. 8-15C). Hemolytic glaucoma usually occurs in patients who have chronic vitreous hemorrhage. Microscopic examination of the khaki or yellow ochre-colored vitreous blood discloses small eosinophilic hemoglobin spherules, macrophages laden with hemosiderin and other blood breakdown products and erythrocyte ghost cells. Ghost cells or erythroclasts are red blood cells that have lost their hemoglobin. The inner surface of the empty cell membranes is studded with dots called Heinz bodies. All of these blood breakdown products occasionally are able to enter the anterior segment through defects in the vitreous face or zonule. A relatively pure population of ghost cells blocks the meshwork in the variant of hemolytic glaucoma called ghost cell glaucoma. The clinical findings in ghost cell glaucoma may be quite subtle; the ghost cells usually form a faint, inconspicuous khaki-colored layer in the inferior chamber angle.

Macrophages that have ingested melanin pigment released from necrotic pigmented tumors cause **melanomalytic glaucoma** and **melanocytomalytic glaucoma**

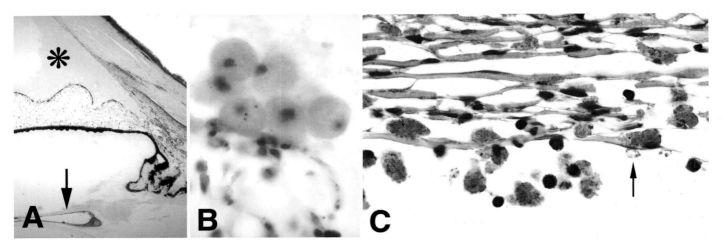

Fig. 8-15. Secondary open-angle glaucoma. A. Phacolytic glaucoma. *Asterisk* labels lens protein-rich fluid in open angle. *Arrow* points to empty lens capsule. Postcontusion angle recession is present. **B.** Aggregate of macrophages laden with lens material is seen on anterior iridic surface. **C. Hemolytic glaucoma.** Macrophages that have ingested hemosiderin and erythrocyte ghost cells (*arrow*) infiltrate trabecular meshwork. (**A.** H&E ×10, **B.** H&E ×250, **C.** H&E ×100)

(Fig. 8-16). Magnocellular nevi called melanocytomas are particularly prone to undergo spontaneous necrosis. Several cases of melanocytomalytic glaucoma caused by necrosis of iris melanocytomas have been reported. Gonioscopy discloses heavy pigmentation of the trabecular meshwork.

Particles of degenerated lens material dispersed by lens injuries or surgery can cause secondary open-angle glaucoma (lens particle glaucoma). Rare cases of alpha-chymotrypsin glaucoma were reported in the era of intracapsular cataract surgery. The enzymatic zonulysis released zonular fragments and debris, causing temporary obstruction of the trabecular meshwork. Secondary trabecular obstruction by photoreceptor outer segments in eyes with chronic rhegmatogenous retinal detachments is called the Schwartz-Matsuo syndrome.

A relatively common type of secondary open-angle glaucoma called *capsular glaucoma* occurs in elderly patients who have **pseudoexfoliation (PXE) of the lens capsule** (see lens chapter). PXE dispersed by the aqueous physically blocks the trabecular meshwork, and additional material actually may be synthesized within the meshwork by the trabecular endothelial cells. Iris pigment epithelial abnormalities also lead to dispersal of iris pigment epithelial melanin throughout the anterior segment.

Granules of melanin pigment released from the iris pigment epithelium accumulate in the trabecular meshwork and interfere with aqueous outflow in **pigmentary glaucoma** (Fig. 8-17). Pigmentary glaucoma is particularly common in young to middle-aged men who are myopic and have a deep anterior chamber and a tremulous iris (iridodonesis).

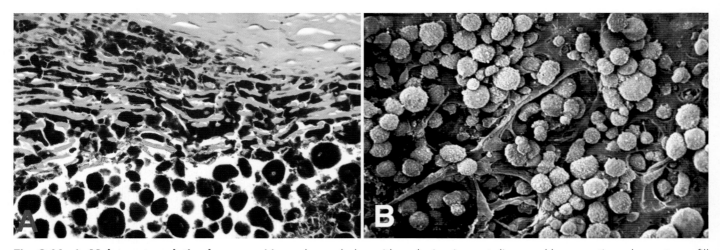

Fig. 8-16. A. Melanocytomalytic glaucoma. Macrophages laden with melanin pigment dispersed by necrotic melanocytoma fill peripheral anterior chamber and infiltrate trabecular meshwork. **B.** Scanning electron micrograph graphically depicts melanophages obstructing trabecular meshwork. (**A.** H&E ×100, **B.** SEM ×160 [From Fineman MS, Eagle RC Jr, Shields JA, et al. Melanocytomalytic glaucoma in eyes with necrotic iris melanocytoma. *Ophthalmology* 1998;105:492–496. Courtesy of *Ophthalmology*.])

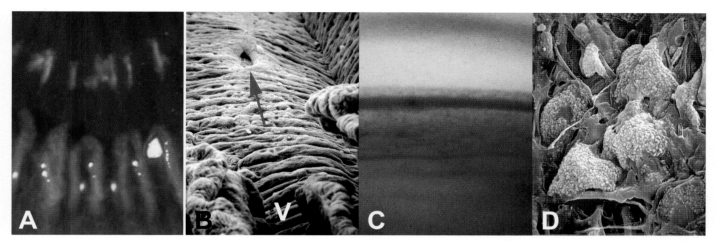

Fig. 8-17. Pigmentary glaucoma. A. Depigmented foci on posterior surface of iris correspond to erosions in iris pigment epithelium (*arrow*) thought to be caused by zonular bundles, which pass through valleys between ciliary processes. **B.** *Arrow* points to defect in iris pigment epithelium that lines up with valley (*V*). **C.** Trabecular meshwork of open angle is heavily pigmented. **D.** Cytoplasm of trabecular endothelial cells is replete with large round oval granules of iris pigment epithelial melanin. (**A.** Macrophoto courtesy of Dr. Myron Yanoff, **B.** SEM ×40, **C.** SEM ×1,250)

Campbell proposed that abrasion by bundles of zonular fibers causes release of melanin from the iris pigment epithelium. An inverse pupillary block mechanism appears to bow the peripheral iris against the zonules in some patients. The zonular abrasions cause defects in the pigment epithelium that are evident during transillumination as characteristic radially oriented areas of increased light transmission. Biomicroscopy discloses pigment-laden macrophages (clump cells of Koganei type I) in the superficial iris stroma overlying the defects. Iris pigment phagocytized by the corneal endothelium is seen clinically as a vertically oriented Krukenberg spindle. The orientation of the spindle is governed by convection currents in the aqueous humor. The trabecular meshwork is heavily pigmented. Large round melanin granules consistent with iris pigment epithelial origin are found within the cytoplasm of the trabecular endothelial cells. Chronic pigmentation is thought to induce trabecular scarring. Only about half of patients with pigment dispersion actually develop glaucoma.

Malignant tumors, particularly malignant melanomas of the ciliary body and/or iris can cause secondary open-angle glaucoma by diffusely seeding the trabecular meshwork with tumor cells, or by proliferating circumferentially around the angle as a "ring melanoma" (Fig. 8-18). Anterior segment tumors generally cause secondary open-angle glaucoma. Posterior tumors, especially large choroidal melanomas or exophytic retinoblastomas with extensive bullous retinal detachments cause secondary closed angle glaucoma (Fig. 8-19). Angiogenesis factors such as VEGF produced by tumors can also cause NVG.

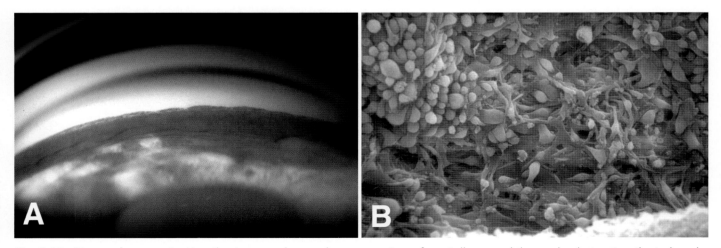

Fig. 8-18. Ring melanoma. A. Heavily pigmented tumor has grown circumferentially around the angle obstructing the trabecular meshwork. **B.** Melanoma cells infiltrating trabecular meshwork. Patient had unilateral glaucoma. Round or oval cells are epithelioid melanoma cells. Bipolar spindle cells also are present. (**B.** SEM ×160)

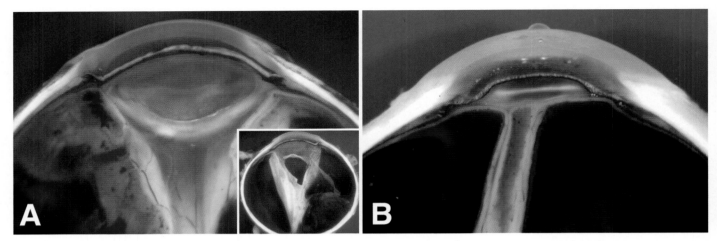

Fig. 8-19. Secondary closed-angle glaucoma in eyes with choroidal melanomas and total retinal detachments. A. Anterior displacement of lens-iris diaphragm has caused secondary closed-angle glaucoma. **Inset** shows large posterior choroidal melanoma and total retinal detachment. **B.** Another eye with posterior melanoma, total high bullous retinal detachment, and secondary closed-angle glaucoma caused by anterior displacement of lens iris diaphragm. A tumor must be excluded in any eye with glaucoma and a total retinal detachment.

Glaucoma often occurs in eyes that have diffuse iris melanomas that typically are composed of poorly cohesive epithelioid cells. Aqueous dispersion of tumor cells throughout the anterior chamber may cause a progressive darkening of the involved iris (hyperchromic heterochromia iridum). Unilateral glaucoma and a subtle change in the color of the iris may be the only indications that a patient harbors a diffuse iris melanoma (Fig. 8-20).

Ocular trauma is another cause of secondary open-angle glaucoma. Chronic inflammation or repeated anterior chamber hemorrhage can cause scarring of the trabecular meshwork. Iron released from retained iron intraocular foreign bodies (siderosis) or recurrent intraocular hemorrhages (hemosiderosis) can have toxic effects on the trabecular endothelial cells as well as on the retinal photoreceptors.

Post contusion angle recession, a well-recognized cause of unilateral glaucoma, is discussed in Chapter 3.

An important factor that determines the outflow of aqueous humor from the eye is the difference between the intraocular pressure and the pressure in the episcleral veins (episcleral venous pressure). Diseases that cause venous obstruction such as cavernous sinus thromboses or mediastinal syndromes can cause glaucoma by elevating episcleral venous pressure. Arterialization of episcleral veins markedly elevates episcleral venous pressure in some patients with carotid cavernous fistulas. The resultant glaucoma is difficult to manage.

Orbital pathology, for example, orbital tumors or the enlarged extraocular muscles of thyroid ophthalmopathy, can raise intraocular pressure by directly compressing the globe.

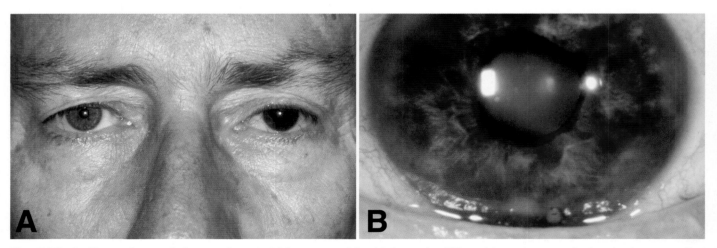

Fig. 8-20. A. Hyperchromatic heterochromia iridum caused by high-grade diffuse iris melanoma. Patient had uncontrolled unilateral glaucoma. **B.** Tumor dispersed by aqueous humor blankets anterior surface of left iris. Eye previously was blue prior to development of unilateral glaucoma.

OCULAR TISSUE CHANGES IN GLAUCOMATOUS EYES

The histopathologic diagnosis of glaucoma requires the demonstration of ocular tissue damage, typically glaucomatous retinal and optic atrophy. **Glaucomatous retinal atrophy** is characterized by atrophy of the retinal ganglion and nerve fiber layer, which is composed of the axons of the ganglion cells (Fig. 8-1A). The atrophic nerve fiber layer is often gliotic. Involvement of the inner plexiform layer and the inner part of the inner nuclear layer distinguish inner ischemic retinal atrophy that follows retinal artery occlusion from glaucomatous retinal atrophy. Gliosis typically is absent in ischemic atrophy, and the inner retinal layers may have a hyalinized appearance.

Cupping of the optic disc is the characteristic feature of **glaucomatous optic atrophy** (Figs. 8-1B, 8-2, and 8-3B). There is posterior bowing and distortion of the collagenous lamina cribrosa, and loss of nerve tissue anterior to the lamina. The pia and pial septa and subarachnoid space are widened. Schnabel cavernous optic atrophy occasionally occurs in eyes with severe glaucoma. Clear cavernous spaces filled with hyaluronic acid are found in the retrolaminar part of the nerve (Fig. 15-5).

Focal areas of scleral thinning may develop in eyes with chronically elevated intraocular pressure. These scleral ectasias are called staphylomas if they are lined by uveal tissue (*staphylo* and *uva* mean grape in Greek and Latin, respectively). Corneal changes found in eyes with chronic glaucoma include calcific band keratopathy, vascularization, corneal edema, bullous keratopathy, and degenerative pannus formation. Chronically edematous corneas are at risk for infection. Perforation of corneal ulcers in hypertensive eyes can cause spontaneous expulsive choroidal hemorrhage.

BIBLIOGRAPHY

General Reference

Spencer WH. Glaucoma. In: Spencer W, ed. *Ophthalmic Pathology: An Atlas and Textbook*, 4th ed., vol. 1. Philadelphia, PA: WB Saunder, 1996:438–512.

Optic Nerve Damage

Anderson DR. Glaucoma: the damage caused by pressure. XLVI Edward Jackson memorial lecture. *Am J Ophthalmol* 1989;108:485–495.

Kerrigan LA, Zack DJ, Quigley HA, et al. TUNEL-positive ganglion cells in human primary open-angle glaucoma. *Arch Ophthalmol* 1997;115:1031–1035.

Quigley HA, Addicks EM, Green WR, et al. Optic nerve damage in human glaucoma. II. The site of injury and susceptibility to damage. *Arch Ophthalmol* 1981;99:635–649.

Quigley HA, Addicks EM, Green WR. Optic nerve damage in human glaucoma. III. Quantitative correlation of nerve fiber loss and visual field defect in glaucoma, ischemic neuropathy, papilledema, and toxic neuropathy. *Arch Ophthalmol* 1982;100:135–146.

Quigley HA, Green WR. The histology of human glaucoma and nerve damage: clinicopathologic correlation in 21 eyes. *Ophthalmology* 1979;86:1803–1827.

Tripathi RC, Tripathi BJ. Functional anatomy of the anterior chamber angle. In: Jakobiec FA, ed. *Ocular Anatomy, Embryology and Teratology*. Philadelphia, PA: Harper & Row, 1982:197–284.

Developmental Glaucoma

Anderson DR. The development of the trabecular meshwork and its abnormality in primary infantile glaucoma. *Trans Am Ophthalmol Soc* 1981;79:458–485.

Boniuk M. Glaucoma in the congenital rubella syndrome. *Int Ophthalmol Clin* 1972;12:121–136.

Broughton WL, Fine B, Zimmerman LE. A histologic study of congenital glaucoma associated with a chromosome defect. *Arch Ophthalmol* 1981;99:481–486.

Curtin VT, Joyce EE, Ballin N. Ocular pathology in the oculo-cerebro-renal syndrome of Lowe. *Am J Ophthalmol* 1967;64 (Pt II):533–543.

François J, Hanssens M. Syndrome oculo-cerebro-renal de Lowe: Examen histopathogique oculaire. *Bull Soc Belge Ophtalmol* 1963;135:412–431.

Furuyoshi N, Furuyoshi M, Futa R, et al. Ultrastructural changes in the trabecular meshwork of juvenile glaucoma. *Ophthalmologica* 1997;211:140–146.

Grant WM, Walton DS. Distinctive gonioscopic findings in glaucoma due to neurofibromatosis. *Arch Ophthalmol* 1968;79:127–134.

Grant WM, Walton DS. Progressive changes in the angle in congenital aniridia, with development of glaucoma. *Trans Am Ophthalmol Soc* 1974;72:207–228.

Honig MA, Barraquer J, Perry HD, et al. Forceps and vacuum injuries to the cornea: histopathologic features of twelve cases and review of the literature. *Cornea* 1996;15:463–472.

Lichter PR. Genetic clues to glaucoma's secrets: the L. Edward Jackson Memorial Lecture. Part 2. *Am J Ophthalmol* 1994;117: 706–727.

Maul E, Strozzi L, Munro C, et al. The outflow pathway in congenital glaucoma. *Am J Ophthalmol* 1980;89:667–675.

Maumenee AE. The pathogenesis of congenital glaucoma: a new theory. *Trans Am Ophthalmol Soc* 1958;56:507–570.

Phelps CD. The pathogenesis of glaucoma in Sturge-Weber syndrome. *Trans Am Acad Ophthalmol Otolaryngol* 1978;85:276–286.

Sarfarazi M. Recent advances in molecular genetics of glaucomas. *Hum Mol Genet* 1997;6:1667–1677.

Shaffer RN. Pathogenesis of congenital glaucoma: Gonioscopic and microscopic anatomy. *Trans Am Acad Ophthalmol Otolaryngol* 1955;59:297–300.

Shields B. Axenfeld-Rieger syndrome: a theory of mechanism and distinctions from the iridocorneal endothelial syndrome. *Trans Am Ophthalmol Soc* 1983;81:736–784.

Stoilova D, Child A, Brice G, et al. Identification of a new 'TIGR' mutation in a family with juvenile-onset primary open angle glaucoma. *Ophthalmic Genet* 1997;18:109–118.

Traboulsi E, Maumenee IH. Peters' anomaly and associated congenital malformations. *Arch Ophthalmol* 1992;110:1739–1742.

Wiggs JL, Del Bono EA, Schuman JS, et al. Clinical features of five pedigrees genetically linked to the juvenile glaucoma locus on chromosome 1q21-q31. *Ophthalmology* 1995;102:1782–1789.

Primary Open Angle Glaucoma

Alvarado J, Murphy C, Polansky J, et al. Age-related changes in trabecular meshwork cellularity. *Invest Ophthalmol Vis Sci* 1981;21:714–727.

Alvarado JA, Murphy CG. Outflow obstruction in pigmentary and primary open angle glaucoma. *Arch Ophthalmol* 1992;110:1769–1778.

Alvarado JA, Murphy CG, Juster R. Trabecular meshwork cellularity in primary open-angle glaucoma and nonglaucomatous normals. *Ophthalmology* 1984;91:564–579.

Alvarado JA, Yun AJ, Murphy CG. Juxtacanalicular tissue in primary open angle glaucoma and in nonglaucomatous normals. *Arch Ophthalmol* 1986;104:1517–1528.

Murphy CG, Johnson M, Alvarado JA. Juxtacanalicular tissue in pigmentary and open angle glaucoma: the hydrodynamic role of pigment and other constituents. *Arch Ophthalmol* 1992;110: 1779–1785.

Pesin SR, Katz LJ, Augsburger JJ, et al. Acute angle-closure glaucoma from acute spontaneous massive hemorrhagic retinal or choroidal detachment. An updated diagnostic and therapeutic approach. *Ophthalmology* 1990;97:76–84.

Quigley HA. Angle-closure glaucoma-simpler answers to complex mechanisms: LXVI Edward Jackson Memorial Lecture. *Am J Ophthalmol* 2009;148(5):657–669.

Neovascular Glaucoma

Aiello LP, Avery RL, Arrigg PG, et al. Vascular endothelial growth factor in ocular fluid of patients with diabetic retinopathy and other retinal disorders. *N Engl J Med* 1994;331:1519–1520.

Colosi NJ, Yanoff M. Reactive corneal endothelialization. *Am J Ophthalmol* 1977;83:219–224.

John TJ, Sassani JW, Eagle RC Jr. The myofibroblastic component of rubeosis iridis. *Ophthalmology* 1983;90:721–728.

Madsen PH. Rubeosis of the iris and hemorrhagic glaucoma in patients with proliferative diabetic retinopathy. *Br J Ophthalmol* 1971;55: 368–371.

The Iridocorneal Endothelial (ICE) Syndrome

Alvarado JA, Murphy CG, Juster RP, et al. Pathogenesis of Chandler's syndrome, essential iris atrophy and the Cogan-Reese syndrome. II. Estimated age at disease onset. *Invest Ophthalmol Vis Sci* 1986;27:873–882.

Alvarado JA, Underwood JL, Green WR, et al. Detection of herpes simplex viral DNA in the iridocorneal endothelial syndrome. *Arch Ophthalmol* 1994;112:1601–1609.

Bourne W, Brubaker R. Decreased endothelial permeability in the iridocorneal endothelial syndrome. *Ophthalmology* 1982;89:591–595.

Bourne WM, Brubaker RF. Progression and regression of partial corneal involvement in the iridocorneal endothelial syndrome. *Am J Ophthalmol* 1992;114:171–181.

Campbell DG, Shields BM, Smith TR. The corneal endothelium and the spectrum of essential iris atrophy. *Am J Ophthalmol* 1978;86:317–324.

Chandler P. Atrophy of the stroma of the iris, endothelial dystrophy, corneal edema and glaucoma. *Am J Ophthalmol* 1956;41:607–615.

Cogan D, Reese A. A syndrome of iris nodules, ectopic Descemet's membrane and unilateral glaucoma. *Doc Ophthalmol* 1969;26:424–433.

Eagle RJ, Font R, Yanoff M, et al. The iris naevus (Cogan-Reese) syndrome: light and electron microscopic observations. *Br J Ophthalmol* 1980;64:446–452.

Eagle RC Jr, Font RL, Yanoff M, et al. Proliferative endotheliopathy with iris abnormalities. The iridocorneal endothelial syndrome. *Arch Ophthalmol* 1979;97:2104–2111.

Eagle RJ, Shields J. Iridocorneal endothelial syndrome with contralateral guttate endothelial dystrophy. *Ophthalmology* 1987;94:862–870.

Hirst L, Quigley H, Stark W, et al. Specular microscopy of iridocorneal endothelial syndrome. *Am J Ophthalmol* 1980;89:11–21.

Hirst LW, Bancroft J, Yamauchi K, et al. Immunohistochemical pathology of the corneal endothelium in iridocorneal endothelial syndrome. *Invest Ophthalmol Vis Sci* 1995;36:820–827.

Kramer TR, Grossniklaus HE, Vigneswaran N, et al. Cytokeratin expression in corneal endothelium in the iridocorneal endothelial syndrome. *Invest Ophthalmol Vis Sci* 1992;33:3581–3585.

Lee WR, Marshall GE, Kirkness CM. Corneal endothelial cell abnormalities in an early stage of the iridocorneal endothelial syndrome. *Br J Ophthalmol* 1994;78:624–631.

Levy SG, McCartney AC, Baghai MH, et al. Pathology of the iridocorneal-endothelial syndrome. The ICE-cell. *Invest Ophthalmol Vis Sci* 1995;36:2592–2601.

Neubauer L, Lund O, Leibowitz H. Specular microscopic appearance of the corneal endothelium in the iridocornal endothelial syndrome. *Arch Ophthalmol* 1983;101:916–918.

Scheie H, Yanoff M. Iris nevus (Cogan-Reese) syndrome. A cause of unilateral glaucoma. *Arch Ophthalmol* 1975;93:963–970.

Shields M. Progressive essential iris atrophy, Chandler's syndrome, and the iris nevus (Cogan-Reese) syndrome. A spectrum of disease. *Surv Ophthalmol* 1979;24:3–20.

Shields M, Campbell D, Simmons R. The essential iris atrophies. *Am J Ophthalmol* 1978;85:749–759.

Yanoff M. Iridocorneal endothelial syndrome. Unification of a disease spectrum. *Surv Ophthalmol* 1979;24:1–2.

Phacolytic Glaucoma

Flocks M, Littwin CS, Zimmerman LE. Phacolytic glaucoma: a clinicopathologic study of 138 cases of glaucoma associated with hypermature cataract. *Am J Ophthalmol* 1955;54:37–45.

Rosenbaum JT, Samples JR, Seymour B, et al. Chemotactic activity of lens proteins and the pathogenesis of phacolytic glaucoma. *Arch Ophthalmol* 1987;105:1582–1584.

Smith ME, Zimmerman LE. Contusive angle recession in phacolytic glaucoma. *Arch Ophthalmol* 1965;74:799–804.

Volcker HE, Naumann G. Clinical findings in phakolytic glaucoma. *Klin Monatsbl Augenheilkd* 1975;166:613–618.

Yanoff M, Scheie HG. Cytology of human lens aspirate. Its relationship to phacolytic glaucoma and phacoanaphylactic endophthalmitis. *Arch Ophthalmol* 1968;80:166–170.

Pigmentary Glaucoma

Campbell DG. Pigmentary dispersion and glaucoma: a new theory. *Arch Ophthalmol* 1979;97:1667–1672.

Fine B, Yanoff M, Scheie H. Pigmentary "glaucoma": a histologic study. *Trans Am Acad Ophthalmol Otolaryngol* 1978;78:314–325.

Farrar SM, Shields MB. Current concepts in pigmentary glaucoma. *Surv Ophthalmol* 1993;37:233–252.

Potash S, Tello C, Liebmann J, et al. Ultrasound biomicroscopy in pigment dispersion syndrome. *Ophthalmology* 1994;101:332–339.

Scheie HG, Cameron JD. Pigment dispersion syndrome: a clinical study. *Br J Ophthalmol* 1981;65:264–269.

Siddiqui Y, Ten Hulzen RD, Cameron JD, et al. What is the risk of developing pigmentary glaucoma from pigment dispersion syndrome? *Am J Ophthalmol* 2003;135:794–799.

Pseudoexfoliation

Schlotzer-Schrehardt U, Koca M, Naumann G, et al. Pseudoexfoliation syndrome. Ocular manifestation of a systemic disorder? *Arch Ophthalmol* 1992;110:1752–1756.

Schlotzer-Schrehardt U, Naumann GO. Trabecular meshwork in pseudoexfoliation syndrome with and without open-angle glaucoma. A morphometric, ultrastructural study. *Invest Ophthalmol Vis Sci* 1995;36:1750–1764.

Schlotzer-Schrehardt U, Pasutto F, Sommer P, et al. Genotype-correlated expression of lysyl oxidase-like 1 in ocular tissues of patients with pseudoexfoliation syndrome/glaucoma and normal patients. *Am J Pathol* 2008;173:1724–1735.

Streeten BW, Dark AJ. Pseudoexfoliation syndrome. In: Garner A, Klintworth GK, eds. *Pathobiology of Ocular Disease: A Dynamic approach*, 2nd ed., Part A. New York, NY: Marcel Dekker, 1994:591–629.

Streeten BW, Li Zy, Wallace RN, et al. Pseudoexfoliative fibrillopathy in visceral organs of a patient with pseudoexfoliation syndrome. *Arch Ophthalmol* 1992;110:1757–1762.

Other Secondary Glaucomas

Campbell DG, Simmons RJ, Grant WM. Ghost cells as a cause of glaucoma. *Am J Ophthalmol* 1976;81:441–450.

Campbell DG. Ghost cell glaucoma following trauma. *Ophthalmology* 1981;88:1151–1158.

Fenton RH, Zimmerman LE. Hemolytic glaucoma: an unusual case of acute, open-angle secondary glaucoma. *Arch Ophthalmol* 1963;70:236–239.

Knox DL. Glaucoma following syphilitic interstitial keratitis. *Arch Ophthalmol* 1961;66:18–25.

Lichter PR, Shaffer RN. Interstitial keratitis and glaucoma. *Am J Ophthalmol* 1969;68:241–248.

Matsuo T. Photoreceptor outer segments in aqueous humor: key to understanding a new syndrome. *Surv Ophthalmol* 1994;39:211–233.

Tumors and Glaucoma

Fineman MS, Eagle RC Jr, Shields JA, et al. Melanocytomalytic glaucoma in eyes with necrotic iris melanocytoma. *Ophthalmology* 1998;105:492–496.

Shields CL, Shields JA, Shields MB, et al. Prevalence and mechanisms of secondary intraocular pressure elevation in eyes with intraocular tumors. *Ophthalmology* 1987;94:839–846.

Teekhasaenee C, Ritch R, Rutnin U, et al. Glaucoma in oculodermal melanocytosis. *Ophthalmology* 1990;97:562–570.

Yanoff M. Glaucoma mechanisms in ocular malignant melanomas. *Am J Ophthalmol* 1970;70:898–904.

Yanoff M, Scheie HG. Melanomalytic glaucoma. *Arch Ophthalmol* 1970;84:471–473.

9 Retina

An outpost of the central nervous system (CNS), the retina is a colony of brain cells that is located in the periphery of the body where it is able to interact with and detect the rather narrow spectrum of electromagnetic radiation called visible light. Death, destruction, or loss of all or part of the retina renders the eye sightless. Visual loss due to the death of retinal cells is permanent and irrevocable, because, like brain cells, the cells of the retina are incapable of repair or regeneration. Retinal anatomy is discussed in detail in Chapter 1.

DEVELOPMENTAL ANOMALIES

Dysplasia of the retina is a characteristic manifestation of trisomy 13 and also occurs in the Walker-Warburg syndrome. Congenital nonattachment of the retina is a rare anomaly caused by faulty invagination of the optic vesicle. Congenital detachment of the retina causes leukocoria in male infants with X-linked Norrie disease, who also are deaf and mentally retarded. The retina lining a choroidal coloboma may be absent, hypoplastic, or dysplastic.

Aplasia of the fovea occurs in aniridia and albinism. Albinos also have a lightly pigmented albinotic fundus. Variants of oculocutaneous albinism are caused by recessively inherited mutations in four genes. Patients with OCA1a, the classic form of the so-called tyrosinase-negative oculocutuaneous albinism, have white hair, pink eyes, and pink irides that transilluminate vividly. OAC1a is caused by mutations in the tyrosinase gene on chromosome 11 (11q14-q21) that cause complete absence of tyrosinase enzyme activity. Some patients with less deleterious tyrosinase mutations (OCA1b) initially were classified as tyrosinase-positive albinos because they had some pigmentation. Temperature-sensitive tyrosinase mutations analogous to those responsible for the pigmented ears and limbs of Siamese cats cause peripheral pigmentation in some human albinos. Oculocutaneous albinism type 2 (OCA2) is another variant of tyrosinase-positive albinism that is very common in some African populations such as the Ibo of Nigeria, in whom the prevalence is 1/1,100. Affected patients have yellow hair and hazel irides. OCA2 is caused by mutations in the OCA2 or P gene on chromosome 15 (15q11.2-q12). OCA3 and OCA4 are caused by mutations in the genes for tyrosinase-related protein-1 (TYRP1) 9p23 and membrane-associated transporter protein (MATP), respectively. The Hermansky-Pudlak syndrome is common in Puerto Ricans who also have a bleeding diathesis and bruise easily. Parents of affected children have been wrongfully accused of child abuse. Albinos with the rare autosomal recessively inherited Chédiak-Higashi syndrome are subject to bacterial and fungal infection and a peculiar form of lymphoproliferation. They have abnormal leukocytes with giant lysosomes and macromelanosomes. The syndrome is caused by mutations in the lysosomal trafficking regulator gene (LYST) on chromosome 1 (1q42.1-q42.2).

Albinism may affect both the skin and eyes (oculocutaneous albinism) or the eyes primarily (ocular albinism). Ocular albinos typically present with decreased vision and nystagmus caused by foveal aplasia. Iris transillumination serves to identify ocular albinos, who have normal skin pigmentation and may have dark hair. Macromelanosomes are found in the retinal pigment epithelium (RPE) and skin in X-linked ocular albinism (Fig. 9-1). Skin biopsy occasionally is used to confirm the diagnosis. Although white female carriers of X-linked ocular albinism have normal vision, iris transillumination is present and ophthalmoscopy may disclose a "mud-spattered" appearance of the fundus caused by patchy depigmentation of the peripheral RPE. Most common, the X-linked or Nettleship-Falls type of ocular albinism is caused by mutations in the G-protein-coupled receptor 143 gene (GPR143) on the X chromosome (Xp22.3).

Congenital hypertrophy of the RPE (CHRPE) (Fig. 11-24A,B) and congenital grouped pigmentation of the RPE are characterized by increased pigmentation and hypertrophy of RPE cells (Fig. 11-24C,D). See Chapter 11 below.

Myelinated nerve fibers occur in about 1% of the population. Myelination of optic nerve axons normally terminates at the posterior margin of the lamina cribrosa. The patches of aberrant myelination of the nerve fiber layer (NFL) may or may not be contiguous with the optic disc. Myelinated nerve fibers produce a focal scotoma.

Congenital vascular abnormalities of the retina include retinal arteriovenous communication, cavernous hemangioma of the retina, Leber miliary retinal aneurysms, Coats disease (Fig. 12-18), and parafoveal telangiectsias. Retinal hemangioblastomas may occur sporadically or in association with Von Hippel–Lindau disease (Figs. 2-10 and 2-11).

A peripheral retinal fold called Lange fold occurs at the ora serrata in infant eyes. Lange fold does not occur *in vivo*; it is a fixation artifact caused by vitreous traction.

RETINAL HEMORRHAGES AND EXUDATES

The retinopathies that occur in a variety of systemic and ocular diseases actually are composed of six types of retinal hemorrhages and two types of retinal exudates that occur in varying constellations.

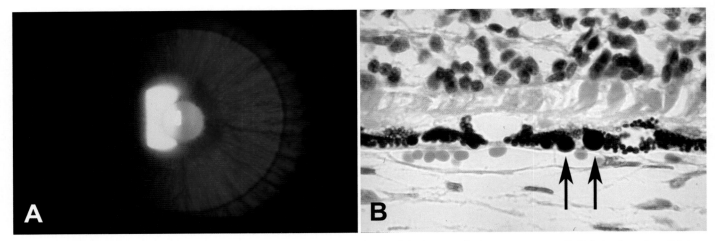

Fig. 9-1. Albinism. A. Transillumination of the iris discloses periphery of the lens and ciliary processes. **B.** X-linked ocular albinism. The RPE in postmortem eye contains large spherical macromelanosomes (*arrows*). (**B.** H&E ×250 [Microslide courtesy of Dr. W.R. Green, From Eagle RC Jr. Congenital, developmental and degenerative disorders of the iris and ciliary body. In: Albert DM, Jakobiec FA, eds. *Principles and Practice of Ophthalmology. Clinical Practice*, vol. 1. Philadelphia, PA: Saunders, 1993:367–389.])

The clinical appearance of retinal hemorrhages is determined by the location of blood in the retina (Fig. 9-2). Retinal hemorrhages are categorized as superficial (flame or splinter shaped), deep (blot and dot), sub-RPE, sub-internal limiting membrane (ILM), subhyaloid, and vitreous.

Splinter- or flame-shaped hemorrhages are located superficially in the inner NFL of the retina (Fig. 9-2A). The configuration and feathery margin of these hemorrhages are caused by tracking of the erythrocytes along the axons of the ganglion cells as they arch above and below the fovea. The pattern of hemorrhages can graphically highlight the arcuate distribution of the nerve fibers in patients who have numerous superficial hemorrhages, for instance, after a branch retinal vein occlusion.

Blot and dot hemorrhages occur in the deeper retinal layers where the axons are oriented perpendicular to the plane of Bruch membrane. Here, the extravasations of blood have a discrete localized configuration because the erythrocytes are corralled or fenced-in by the surrounding axons.

Scaphoid or boat-shaped hemorrhages are preretinal hemorrhages that have a fluid level caused by settling-out of the red cells. Two types of scaphoid hemorrhages are recognized histopathologically: sub-ILM and subhyaloid hemorrhages. True subhyaloid hemorrhages are common in patients with proliferative diabetic retinopathy, in whom blood collects between the ILM and the posterior face of the detached vitreous humor, which may be lined by a sheet of neovascularization (Fig. 9-2B). The term

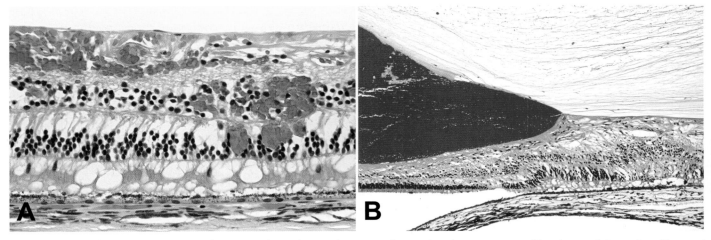

Fig. 9-2. Retinal hemorrhages. A. Flame or splinter hemorrhages are located in the inner nerve fiber layer of the retina. Blot and dot hemorrhages are located in the deeper retinal layers. **B.** Subhyaloid hemorrhage, proliferative diabetic retinopathy. Blood is located between the ILM and the posterior surface of the detached vitreous. (**A.** H&E ×100, **B.** H&E ×25)

hyaloid refers to the hyaloid body, another name for the vitreous humor. Sub-ILM hemorrhages are actually hemorrhagic detachments of the ILM. Blood is located between the NFL and the outer aspect of the ILM, the retina's single true basement membrane, which is secreted by the Müller cells. Occasionally, sub-ILM hemorrhages may be distinguished by the ophthalmoscopic observation of focal relucencies called Gunn dots on their inner surface. The latter correspond to focal concavities on the outer surface of the basement membrane that conform to the foot plates of the Müller cells.

Hemorrhagic detachment of the RPE often occurs in patients who have sub-RPE neovascular membranes. Sub-RPE hemorrhage is an important stage in the evolution of many disciform scars in age-related macular degeneration. Sub-RPE hemorrhages typically appear quite dark because blood is located beneath a layer of pigmented cells. They can be confused clinically with uveal malignant melanoma. However, in contrast to melanomas, sub-RPE hemorrhages block choroidal fluorescence and appear dark during intravenous fluorescein angiography.

Vitreous hemorrhage occurs when blood breaks through the hyaloid membrane into the substance of the formed vitreous. Blood in the formed vitreous can be quite persistent but gradually undergoes degeneration and assumes a characteristic yellow-ochre color. Nonresorbing vitreous hemorrhage is a common indication for vitrectomy, especially in patients with diabetes mellitus.

Retinal exudates and edema that occur in diabetes, hypertensive retinopathy, and other retinal vascular disorders reflect a breakdown in the **blood–retinal barrier** (Fig. 9-3A). The term blood–retinal barrier refers to structural modifications that protect the retina's delicate neural tissues from fluid overload and osmotic stress. The blood–retinal barrier is analogous to the blood–brain barrier in the CNS. The inner or intraretinal part of the blood–retinal barrier is composed of the tight junctions that join together the endothelial cells that line the retinal vessels. During fluorescein angiography, these impermeable intercellular junctions confine fluorescein dye within the lumens of healthy retinal vessels. The girdle of terminal bars that join the RPE cells near their apices forms the outer part of the blood–retinal barrier. The choriocapillaris, which supplies the avascular outer third of the retina, is composed of fenestrated capillaries that leak fluorescein dye profusely. The RPE serves as the barrier that protects the outer retina from an influx of fluid.

Incompetence of either the inner or the outer part of the blood–retinal barrier gives lipid- and protein-rich fluid access to the retinal parenchyma, leading to edema and exudate formation. Hard, yellow, and waxy exudates appear histopathologically as pools of eosinophilic proteinaceous fluid (Fig. 9-3B). **Hard exudates** usually are located in the outer plexiform layer, the watershed zone between the retina's dual blood supplies. In chronic cases, the exudates may be phagocytized by foamy macrophages called gitter cells.

Soft exudates or **cotton-wool spots** (Fig. 9-4) actually are not exudates in the true sense of the word. Cotton-wool spots represent focal areas in the NFL where the normal flow of axoplasm is blocked. This focal blockage of axoplasmic flow is thought to be a response to focal retinal ischemia and probably is caused by thrombosis of a precapillary arteriole. Cotton-wool spots are helpful clinical markers for retinal ischemia. They develop in the preproliferative phase of diabetic retinopathy and also are found

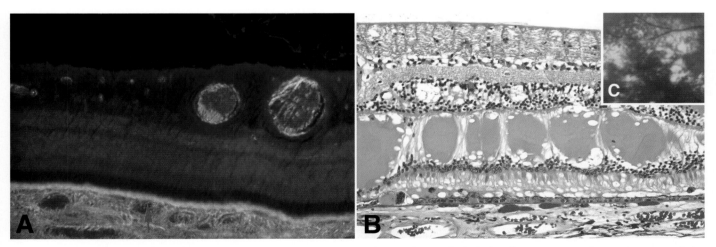

Fig. 9-3. A. Blood–retinal barrier. Tight junctions joining retinal vascular endothelial cells constitute the inner part of the blood–retinal barrier, which confines fluorescein dye within lumina of retinal vessels. Occluding junctions joining apices of RPE cells comprise outer part of barrier. Choriocapillaris is composed of leaky fenestrated capillaries. *Arrow* denotes yellow band of autofluorescent lipofuscin in RPE. (Freeze-dried preparation, fluorescent microscopy ×100) (From Eagle RC. Mechanisms of maculopathy. *Ophthalmology* 1984;91:613–625, Courtesy of *Ophthalmology*.) **B. Retinal hard exudates.** The pools of eosinophilic protein-rich fluid in the outer plexiform layer are hard exudates. Hard exudates typically occur in the OPL because that layer is the watershed zone between the retina's two blood supplies. **C. Inset** shows clinical appearance of hard exudates. (**B.** H&E ×100)

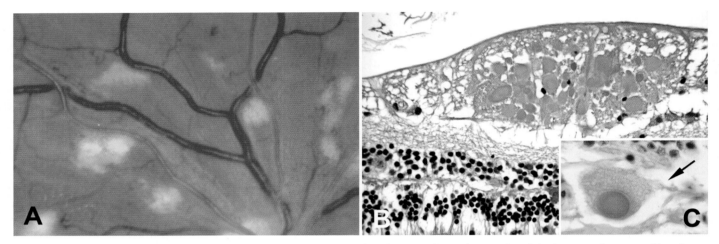

Fig. 9-4. Cotton-wool spots. A. Cotton-wool spots represent focal areas of axoplasmic flow blockage in the nerve fiber layer. They are a clinical marker for retinal ischemia. **B.** Histopathology of cotton-wool spot shows focus of dilated nerve fiber layer axons filled with eosinophilic axoplasm. Cytoid bodies with prominent eosinophilic nucleoids are evident. **C.** Cytoid body, cotton-wool spot. Eosinophilic staining distinguishes the nucleoid in the cytoid body from an actual nucleus. *Arrow* denotes axon entering the cytoid body. Cytoid bodies resemble cells but actually are focal areas of axonal swelling. (**B.** H&E ×100, **C.** H&E ×250)

in ischemic retinal vein occlusions and severe hypertensive retinopathy. Cotton-wool spots occur in relative isolation in patients who have HIV/AIDS or collagen vascular diseases such as systemic lupus erythematosus as a manifestation of intravascular immune complex deposition.

Histopathologic examination of a cotton-wool spot shows focal swelling of the NFL and cytoid bodies (Fig. 9-4B,C). Cytoid bodies are eosinophilic segments of ganglion cell axons ballooned by stagnant axoplasm. They are called cytoid because they superficially resemble cells. Some have a nucleoid composed of aggregated organelles

that mimics a cellular nucleus but is eosinophilic rather than basophilic.

ANGIOID STREAKS

Angioid streaks are linear structures seen on ophthalmoscopy that radiate from the optic disc in an *angioid* or vessellike fashion (Fig. 9-5). Histopathology has shown that angioid streaks correspond to breaks in Bruch membrane (Fig. 9-5B). Angioid streaks tend to develop in patients

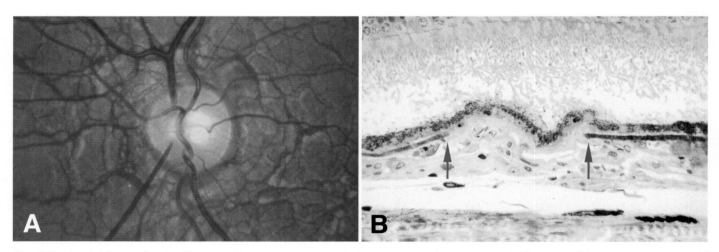

Fig. 9-5. Angioid streaks. A. The gray linear structures radiating the optic disc in an *angioid* or vessellike pattern are angioid streaks. They occur in several systemic disorders marked by massive calcification of Bruch membrane. **B.** *Arrows* denote margins of break in Bruch membrane. Heavily calcified Bruch membrane appears as a thick dark band beneath the RPE. The RPE is intact overlying the break in Bruch membrane. The patient had sickle cell anemia. (Toluidine blue ×150; From Jampol LM, Acheson R, Eagle RC Jr, et al. Calcification of Bruch membrane in angioid streaks with homozygous sickle cell disease. *Arch Ophthalmol* 1987;105:93–98, Copyright 1987, American Medical Association.)

who have certain systemic disorders marked by massive calcification of Bruch membrane. Such diseases include pseudoxanthoma elasticum, Paget disease of bone, and some cases of sickle hemoglobinopathy. Calcification may impart an egg shelllike fragility to Bruch membrane predisposing to fracture. The RPE usually is intact overlying the breaks in Bruch membrane. Sub-RPE neovascularization can complicate angioid streaks and actually is a major cause of visual loss in affected patients. Unfortunately, when sub-RPE membranes develop, they generally involve the region of the macula for reasons unknown. This fact implies that the development of subretinal neovascularization requires more than a break in Bruch membrane.

RETINAL ARTERY AND ARTERIOLAR OCCLUSIONS

Interruption of the vascular supply to the inner two thirds of the retina causes ischemic infarction and coagulative necrosis of its cells. The sequelae of central or branch retinal artery occlusion are evident histopathologically as inner ischemic retinal atrophy (Fig. 9-6). All of the cells nourished by capillaries derived from the central retinal artery are affected in inner ischemic retinal atrophy, including the nerve fiber and ganglion cell layers, the inner plexiform layer, and most of the inner nuclear layer. The outer part of the inner nuclear layer usually persists because its cells are sustained by diffusion from the choriocapillaris. In a long-standing case, the inner retinal layers are paucicellular and have a glassy, hyalinized appearance. Gliosis of the NFL is not observed because the fibrous astrocytes and other accessory glial cells that cause NFL gliosis in

chronic glaucoma perish in the retinal ictus. The additional involvement of the IPL and the inner part of the INL serves to differentiate inner ischemic retinal atrophy from glaucomatous retinal atrophy. Only the retinal ganglion cells and their axons that constitute the NFL and optic nerve are atrophic in glaucomatous retinal atrophy.

In the acute stages of **central retinal artery occlusion** (CRAO), the retina shows edema, cellular dissolution, and nuclear fragmentation or pyknosis. Clinically, the normally transparent retina is marked by milky-white opacification (Fig. 9-7). A macular cherry red spot is present because the cells comprising the floor of the foveola remain viable, and therefore transparent, because they are supplied by the choriocapillaris. Although the foveal photoreceptors persist, central vision is lost because other cells in the neural pathway are destroyed. Retinal hemorrhages usually are not seen.

Occlusion of the central retinal artery produces a "ministroke" of the entire retina. Only part of the retina is infarcted in hemiretinal or branch retinal arteriolar occlusions (Fig. 9-6B). Most branch artery occlusions are caused by emboli that lodge at the bifurcation of an arteriole.

CRAO is usually a disease of elderly individuals who are often atherosclerotic, hypertensive, and diabetic. Central or branch retinal artery occlusion in a young individual should suggest the possibility of a primary cardiac tumor such as a myxoma, vasculitis, or the presence of anticardiolipin (lupus anticoagulant) antibodies. Most CRAOs result from thrombosis or embolization. Thrombosis usually occurs within the optic nerve head and is related to atherosclerosis at this site. Atherosclerosis does not develop in retinal arterioles because those vessels lack a distinct muscularis.

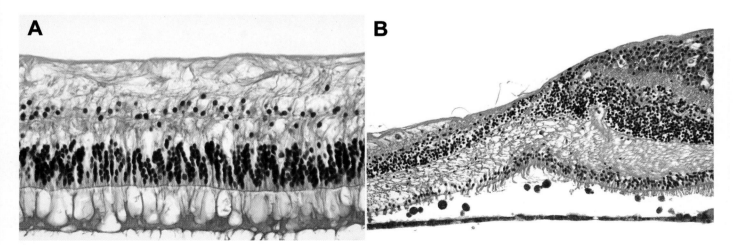

Fig. 9-6. A. Inner ischemic retinal atrophy, retinal artery occlusion. All inner retinal layers supplied by the central retinal artery are atrophic, including the nerve fiber and ganglion cell layers, the inner plexiform layer and most of the inner nuclear layer. No gliosis is present. The inner plexiform and inner nuclear layers are spared in glaucomatous retinal atrophy. **B. Branch retinal artery occlusion, fovea.** The fovea is seen centrally. The layers of the perfused parafoveal retina at right are well preserved. In contrast, the part of the retina supplied by the obstructed vessel (**at left**) shows marked inner ischemic atrophy. Photoreceptor atrophy was caused by a shallow detachment of the macula. (**A.** H&E ×100. **B.** H&E ×50)

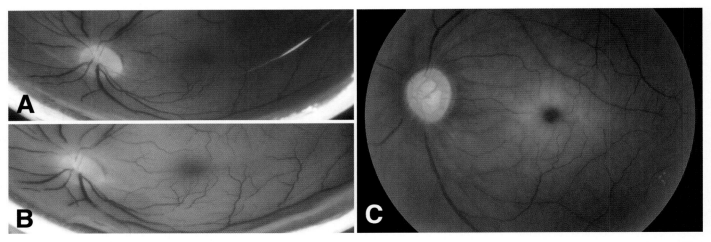

Fig. 9-7. Retinal opacification. A. The retina of freshly enucleated unfixed eye is transparent. **B.** Fixation causes retinal opacification (below). Cellular death caused by ischemia causes similar retinal opacification after CRAO. **C.** Central retinal artery occlusion. Foveola appears as cherry red spot in opacified, infarcted retina.

About 60% of retinal emboli are glistening crystals of cholesterol called Hollenhorst plaques, and about 11% are aggregates of platelets and fibrin. Most are shed from the surface of ulcerating atherosclerotic plaques in the internal carotid artery. Calcific emboli originating in the heart are less common.

GIANT CELL ARTERITIS

Giant cell arteritis is an important treatable condition that must be ruled out in any elderly patient who has retinal artery occlusion or ischemic optic neuropathy. The erythrocyte sedimentation rate is typically elevated in affected individuals, who also may have thrombocytosis and elevated levels of C-reactive protein. Expedient temporal artery biopsy is performed to confirm the diagnosis. Patients who

have giant cell arteritis classically have a history of malaise, weight loss, and muscle aches (polymyalgia rheumatica) and may complain of headache and painful mastication due to jaw claudication. Severely inflamed temporal arteries may be elevated, tender, and cordlike. Biopsy surgery may be relatively bloodless if the arteritis is severe.

An affected segment of artery appears firm, thickened, and opacified grossly. Histopathology discloses compromise or even occlusion of the vascular lumen and chronic inflammation within the thickened arterial wall (Fig. 9-8). The chronic granulomatous inflammatory infiltrate should contain epithelioid histiocytes, but giant cells *are not* particularly common in most positive biopsies, and are unnecessary for the diagnosis. Inflammation can affect all layers of the artery, but classically is concentrated in the vicinity of the internal elastic lamina, which almost invariably shows severe dissolution and segmental loss. Fibrosis and scarring are often seen

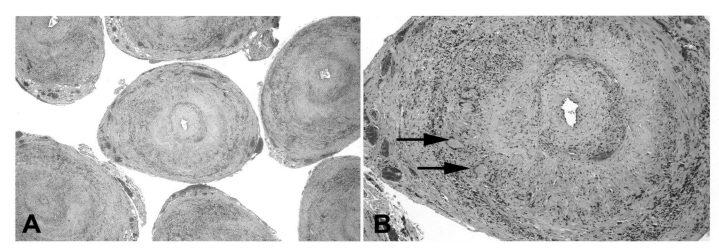

Fig. 9-8. Giant cell arteritis, temporal artery biopsy. A. The lumina of the chronically inflamed artery are largely occluded. No skip lesion are present. **B.** *Arrows* denote giant cells within chronic inflammatory infiltrate that includes epithelioid histiocytes and lymphocytes. There is extensive destruction of the lamina and the muscularis and fibrosis of the adventitia. Giant cell arteritis is an important cause of artery occlusion and ischemic optic neuropathy in elderly patients. (**A.** H&E ×10, **B.** H&E ×25)

in the adventitial connective tissue. Signs of old or "healed" giant cell arteritis, for example, in a patient who has received chronic corticosteroid therapy, include focal atrophy or destruction of the muscularis, extensive segmental destruction of the internal elastic lamina, and perivascular scarring. "Skip lesions" (uninflamed segments in a positive biopsy) do occur but are relatively rare. Hence, the biopsied segment of artery should be at least 2 cm long. Bilateral biopsy may be considered if the initial biopsy is negative and clinical suspicion is high, but the yield is quite low.

Prompt diagnosis of giant cell arteritis is critical because bilateral blindness can develop rapidly in untreated cases. High-dose systemic corticosteroid therapy should be instituted immediately if giant cell arteritis is suspected. The temporal artery is biopsied to confirm the diagnosis histopathologically because systemic steroids can have severe side effects in elderly patients.

RETINAL VENOUS OCCLUSION

Occlusion of the central retinal vein or one of its major branches produces hemorrhagic infarction of the retina. The terms "blood and thunder fundus" or "squashed tomato sign" that have been applied clinically to this retinopathy reflect the plethora of deep and superficial retinal hemorrhages that develop after venous occlusion (Fig. 9-9A).

Most retinal venous occlusions involve branches of the central retinal vein, typically (70%) the superotemporal branch vein. Venous occlusions tend to occur in men who are older than age 50 years and have diabetes mellitus, hypertension, and arteriosclerosis. Local intraocular conditions that predispose to venous occlusion include elevated intraocular pressure, papilledema, and large drusen of the optic disc. Many central retinal vein occlusions are thought to be related to arteriosclerosis of the central retinal artery, which shares a common adventitial sheath with the central retinal vein within the lamina cribrosa of the optic nerve (Fig. 9-9B). The sclerotic arteriole compresses the vein within the adventitial sheath causing turbulence in the lumen of the vein, which damages the vascular endothelium and predisposes to venous thrombosis.

The early stages of a retinal venous occlusion are characterized histopathologically by diffuse and cystoid edema of the macula. The hemorrhagic retina contains numerous deep, superficial, and full-thickness retinal hemorrhages. Preretinal hemorrhages are found in some cases, and in rare instances, blood may extend into the subretinal space causing hemorrhagic retinal detachment. Other findings include shallow serous retinal detachment and papilledema. If severe ischemia and capillary nonperfusion are present, focal retinal necrosis and cotton-wool spots are noted. Cotton-wool spots are an important clinical marker for the ischemic variant of central retinal vein occlusion (CRVO).

In chronic retinal venous occlusive disease, histopathology discloses disorganization of retinal architecture and marked gliosis. The retina often contains macrophages laden with golden brown hemosiderin pigment from blood breakdown, and the retina and other epithelial structures may stain positively for iron (hemosiderosis). Inner ischemic retinal atrophy may be present if the venous occlusion is ischemic. Most eyes requiring enucleation have painful neovascular glaucoma (NVG).

Secondary closed-angle glaucoma caused by iris neovascularization (rubeosis iridis) develops in about 20% of untreated patients who have ischemic CRVOs (Fig. 8-10). Profound visual loss, cotton-wool spots, and severe nonperfusion of the retinal capillary bed disclosed by fluorescein angiography are clinical signs of ischemic vein occlusion. This type of glaucoma has been called "90-day glaucoma,"

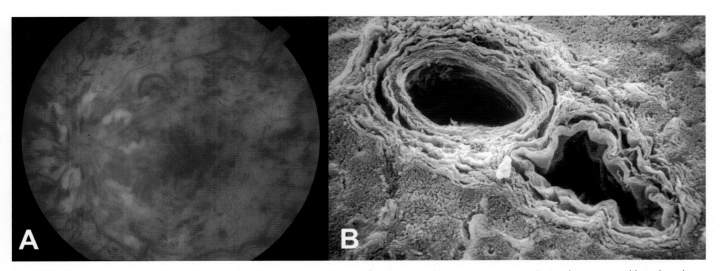

Fig. 9-9. Central retinal vein occlusion. A. Many deep and superficial hemorrhages are present. Retinal veins are dilated and tortuous. Cotton-wool spots surrounding swollen optic nerve indicate ischemia. **B.** Central retinal artery and vein. Common adventitial sheath (*yellow*) surrounds central retinal artery (*red*) and vein (*blue*) in transverse section of optic nerve. Sclerosis of the artery is a factor in the pathogenesis of many cases of CRVO. (**B.** False-colorized SEM ×320)

reflecting its fairly rapid onset. In the past, most of these blind, painful glaucomatous eyes were enucleated. Today, modern therapies including panretinal photocoagulation and tube shunts have dramatically diminished the number of eyes enucleated after CRVO.

HYPERTENSIVE RETINOPATHY

The retinopathy that develops in patients with severe systemic hypertension is caused by vascular incompetence and breakdown of the blood–retinal barrier. Acute severe elevation of blood pressure causes retinal arteriolar narrowing and focal vasospasm. If elevated blood pressure levels and vasospasm persist chronically, the muscular and endothelial coats of the vessels eventually become necrotic. Histopathologic studies have revealed changes in the endothelial lining, necrosis of the smooth muscle, and insudation of fibrin-rich plasma in the vessel wall. The endothelial damage causes vascular incompetence with resultant retinal edema, exudation, and occasionally even serous retinal detachment. Small exudates called *edema residues* may form a stellate pattern around the fovea (macular star figure). This pattern of exudation is governed by the radial orientation of the photoreceptor axons (Henle fibers) in the perifoveal outer plexiform layer (OPL). In the early days of ophthalmoscopy, severe hypertensive retinopathy with a macular star figure was often called hyperalbuminuric retinitis, reflecting the common association between severe hypertension and renal failure. Retinal hemorrhages and papilledema are additional manifestations of hypertensive retinopathy. Retinal hemorrhages are relatively common and occur in the disorder's early stages. Optic disc edema marks the fourth and final stage of hypertensive retinopathy, is an important clinical marker for malignant hypertension and potential encephalopathy, and an indication for aggressive antihypertensive therapy as well. Fibrinoid necrosis caused by the insudation and accumulation of plasma proteins in vessel walls may affect retinal and choroidal vessels. Occlusion of small, damaged vessels also occurs, causing microinfarctions of the NFL (cotton-wool spots), and occasionally, infarctions of larger areas of retina. Focal choroidal infarction with pigmentary change may be evident clinically as Elschnig spots and Siegrist streaks. These were considered to be grave prognostic signs before effective antihypertensive therapy became available. Retinal macroaneurysms occasionally develop in hypertensive patients.

RETINAL ARTERIOSCLEROSIS

Chronic low-grade hypertension induces fibrosis in the walls of retinal arterioles, a process called retinal arteriolarsclerosis (Fig. 9-10). Histopathologically, the sclerotic retinal vessels are encompassed by a thick mantle of collagenous connective tissue. The term "onion skin" is often applied to this change.

Like the surrounding neurosensory retina, the walls of healthy retinal vessels normally are transparent. What one observes ophthalmoscopically as retinal vessels actually are the columns of pigmented erythrocytes filling the lumina of the vessels. The progressive accumulation of connective tissue in the vessel walls of patients with retinal arteriosclerosis gradually obscures the blood column, widening the light reflex and imparting an orange or coppery hue to the arterioles (Fig. 9-10A). Eventually, if the process is prolonged and severe, perivascular fibrosis may totally hide the blood column, and the vessels will appear as white lines or *silver wires*. Arteriovenous crossing defects (*a-v nicking*) result when the opaque walls of thickened arterioles obscure part of the underlying venules. In advanced cases, there may be deflection or banking of the retinal vein.

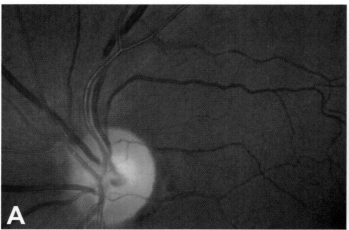 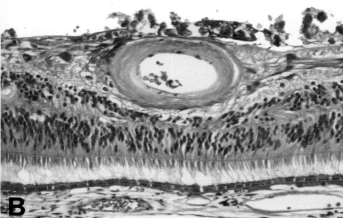

Fig. 9-10. Retinal arteriolarsclerosis. A. Fundus photo shows copper-hued sclerotic arterioles and A-V crossing defects. **B.** Thick mantle of collagenous connective tissue surrounds sclerotic vessel. Blue staining with Masson trichrome (below) confirms the presence of collagen. (**B.** Masson trichrome ×100)

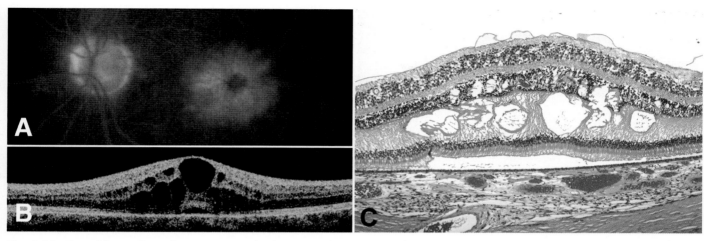

Fig. 9-11. Cystoid macular edema. A. IVFA discloses petalloid pattern of intraretinal cystoid edema in fovea. **B.** OCT graphically shows cysts and retinal thickening. **C.** Large cystoid spaces filled with granular proteinaceous fluid are seen in the outer plexiform and inner nuclear layers. Thickened retina is detached artifactitiously. (**C.** H&E ×50)

CYSTOID MACULAR EDEMA

Cystoid macular edema (CME) is characterized by the accumulation of serous fluid in cystoid spaces in the parenchyma of the perifoveal retina (Fig. 9-11). The intraretinal cysts have a characteristic petalloid appearance on intravenous fluorescein angiography, and are disclosed by optical coherence tomography (OCT). This pattern undoubtedly reflects the radial orientation of the Henle fibers in the perifoveal OPL. Fine has suggested that CME initially may begin as intracellular edema in Müller cells. Cystoid spaces presumably form as a consequence of cellular death in the milieu of chronic edema. Histopathologically, the cystoid spaces appear relatively empty or contain scant amounts of granular or fibrinous material. The latter serves to distinguish them from hard exudates, which are usually pools of eosinophilic hyaline material.

Inflammatory mediators such as prostaglandins that are made in the anterior segment are responsible for some cases of CME. The dramatic response of CME to antivascular endothelial growth factor therapy indicates that vascular endothelial growth factor (VEGF) also plays an important pathogenic role. Vitreous traction on the macula has been incriminated in other instances. Visual loss due to CME may be the presenting clinical manifestation of peripheral lesions including tumors or peripheral uveitis (pars planitis). CME is an important complication of ocular surgery. The association of CME with cataract surgery is called the Irvine-Gass syndrome. A relatively high incidence of CME occurred in patients who had iris-supported intraocular lenses (IOLs) implanted after intracapsular cataract surgery. The IOL probably stimulated prostaglandin production by the iris, and complete removal of the lens allowed the inflammatory mediator to readily diffuse to the posterior segment. CME can complicate any severe chronic ocular inflammatory disorder. Visual loss may respond to medical therapy in early cases.

AGE-RELATED MACULOPATHY (AMD, AGE-RELATED MACULAR DEGENERATION, ARMD)

Age-related maculopathy (AMD) or age-related macular degeneration (ARMD) is the leading cause of irreversible blindness in people 50 years of age or older in the developed world. (Legal blindness generally is defined as a best-corrected visual acuity of 20/200 or 6/60.) AMD causes loss of central vision because it involves the fovea, the specialized part of the retina used for high-resolution color vision (Figs. 9-12–9-14). Although affected patients have trouble reading and recognizing faces, they retain their peripheral vision and are able to ambulate. Anxious patients may be assured that they will never go totally blind. (This in not entirely true, however, since patients receiving anticoagulant therapy occasionally develop massive hemorrhagic retinal detachment.)

There are atrophic or *dry* and exudative or *wet* forms of AMD. The simultaneous or sequential development of *dry* and *wet* changes in a single patient suggests that both are variants of a clinical and pathologic spectrum. **Dry or atrophic macular degeneration** is characterized by atrophy and death of subfoveal RPE, which leads to photoreceptor degeneration, outer retinal atrophy, and involution of the choriocapillaris (Fig. 9-13).

Yellowish white subretinal deposits called drusen are clinical hallmarks of AMD (Figs. 9-14A and 9-15). Drusen are focal deposits of extracellular debris located between the basal lamina of the RPE and the inner collagenous layer of Bruch membrane. The composition of drusen is complex. Constituents are numerous and include neutral lipids, unesterified cholesterol, carbohydrates, vitronectin, C-reactive protein, apolipoprotein E, and a variety of proteins involved in inflammation such as amyloid-beta, immunoglobulin light chains, factor X, complement factor H, C5, and the C5b complex.

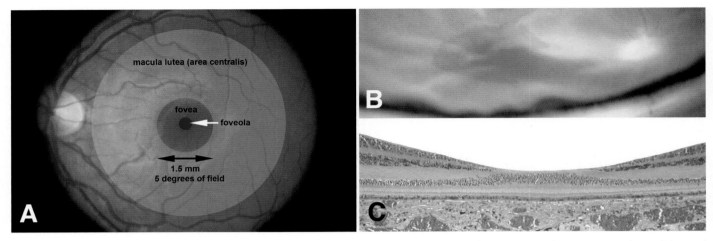

Fig. 9-12. A. The "macula." The foveola is located in the center of the 1.5-mm-wide fovea or pit. The area centralis is delimited by the temporal vascular arcades. The imprecise term macula (from macula lutea, "yellow spot") is often applied clinically to this region. **B.** Irregular yellow spot of carotenoid xanthophyll pigment that encompasses the fovea is readily seen in opacified retina after fixation. **C.** Retina comprising foveal floor consists only of photoreceptors, outer nuclear layer, and part of outer plexiform layer. (**C.** H&E ×25)

Several varieties of drusen are recognized clinically, and a number of somewhat confusing and occasionally conflicting classification schemes based on histopathologic and ultrastructural features have been proposed. **Hard or cuticular drusen** are most abundant and are found throughout the retina. They are discrete, round or globular mounds of homogeneous, deeply periodic acid-Schiff (PAS)-positive hyaline material (Fig. 9-15A,B). Soft drusen are found only in the region of the macula and are strongly associated with AMD. **Soft drusen** typically comprise loose amorphous material called membranous debris. Their contents may be liquefied and often is lost during histologic processing. Soft drusen are often associated with diffuse deposits of extracellular matrix material called basal laminar deposits. Basal laminar deposits play an extremely

important role in the pathogenesis of AMD, especially the severe exudative type, which is complicated by the formation of subretinal neovascular membranes and disciform scar formation.

Basal laminar deposits appear light microscopically as extensive plaques or layers of "soft" granular eosinophilic material that elevate the atrophic RPE from the inner surface of Bruch membrane (Fig. 9-15C). Transmission electron microscopy has shown that such deposits are located between the plasma membrane and the basement membrane of the RPE and are composed of extracellular matrix material rich in "curly collagen" or 1,000 Å banded basement membrane material. Basal laminar deposits adhere loosely to Bruch membrane, predisposing to RPE detachments and tears. The deposits theoretically

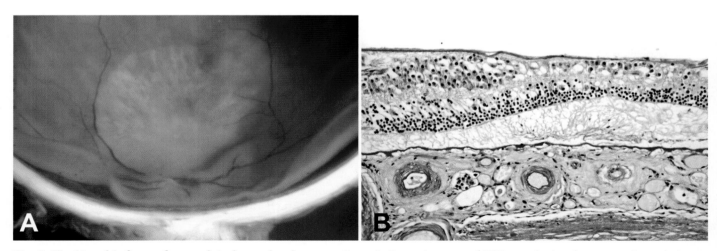

Fig. 9-13. Atrophic form of age-related macular degeneration. A. Extensive area of RPE atrophy involves posterior pole in eye removed from a nonagenarian with a long history of blindness who underwent enucleation for invasive mucoepidermoid carcinoma. Window defect reveals choroidal vessels. **B.** Corresponding histopathology shows total loss of RPE, photoreceptors, and outer nuclear layer. Outer retina is fused to Bruch membrane, which is thickened and PAS positive. The choriocapillaris has undergone involution. (**B.** PAS ×50)

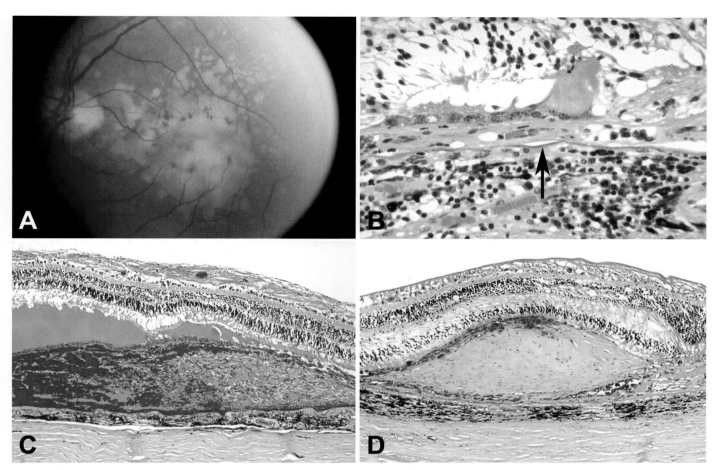

Fig. 9-14. Exudative form of age-related macular degeneration. A. Large confluent soft drusen blanket posterior retina. **B.** Subretinal neovascular membrane. A thin layer of fibrous tissue containing capillaries elevates the atrophic RPE from the inner surface of Bruch membrane. The atrophic outer retina shows extensive photoreceptor loss. Bruch membrane (*arrow*) is fractured and focally calcified. The choroid contains an incidental focus of chronic inflammatory cells. **C.** The retinal pigment epithelium is detached by blood and vascularized connective tissue. A collagenous disciform scar is forming on the inner surface of Bruch membrane as the hemorrhagic RPE detachment undergoes organization. **D.** Disciform scar. Mound of collagen incorporating RPE and vessels elevates fovea. Severe photoreceptor atrophy is present. (**B.** H&E ×100, **C.** H&E ×25, **D.** H&E ×25)

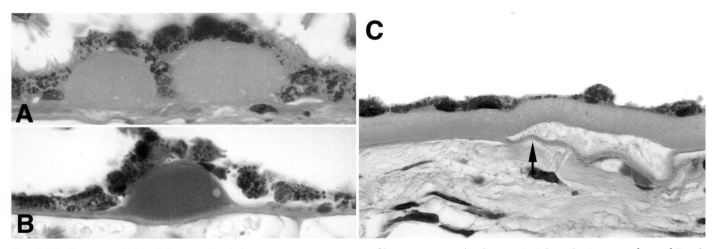

Fig. 9-15. Drusen. A. Hard drusen. Hard drusen are excrescences of homogeneous hyaline material on the inner surface of Bruch membrane that focally detach the RPE. **B.** Many hard drusen are intensely PAS positive. **C.** Basal laminar deposit (diffuse soft drusen). A thick band of abnormal basement membrane material elevates the retinal pigment epithelium off the inner surface of Bruch membrane. Part of the deposit has detached artifactitiously from Bruch membrane (*arrow*). The RPE cells are flattened and atrophic. Basal laminar deposits predispose to RPE detachment and age-related macular degeneration. (**A.** H&E ×250, **B.** PAS ×250, **C.** H&E ×250)

could interfere with biochemical modulation of the choriocapillaris by the RPE and also could provide a plane for sub-RPE neovascular invasion. A second less important variety of diffuse soft drusen called a basal linear deposit has been identified electron microscopically. Basal linear deposits are located within Bruch membrane external to the RPE basement membrane and are composed of multivesicular particles of lipoprotein, which are also the primary constituent of soft drusen. It is impossible to distinguish these two varieties of diffuse soft drusen with routine light microscopy.

Subretinal neovascular membranes characterize the exudative type of AMD (Fig. 9-14B). Angiogenic factors, most notably VEGF, stimulate the proliferation of the new vessels. Clinically, patients typically present with decreased visual acuity or distorted vision ("metamorphopsia"). Membranes appear as grayish patches on ophthalmoscopy, frequently with associated hemorrhage and overlying subretinal fluid. Intravenous fluorescein angiography is used to confirm the presence of neovascularization. OCT also can disclose the neovascular membranes but is used primarily to evaluate retinal thickness and cystoid edema and gauge response to anti-VEGF therapy. In the past, laser photocoagulation was used to obliterate the vessels. In recent years, however, laser therapy has been largely supplanted by the intravitreal injection of monoclonal antibodies or antibody fragments such as bevacizumab or ranibizumab that target VEGF. Such agents are highly efficacious in many cases, but they must be administered repeatedly by intravitreal injection at relatively frequent intervals. Neovascularization and its complications recur if therapy is stopped. Anti-VEGF therapy halts the progression of AMD and improves vision in many patients but does not address the underlying causes of the disease.

In untreated cases, the new vessels leak or bleed forming **serous and/or hemorrhagic detachments of the RPE** (Fig. 9-14C). When the RPE detaches, the plane of the detachment usually is between the inner surface of Bruch membrane and a basal laminar deposit, which detaches with the RPE. If new vessels have invaded a basal laminar deposit, they are apt to be sheared off during detachment, causing hemorrhagic detachment of the RPE. Fibrous disciform scar formation, the endstage of exudative AMD, may result from the organization of hemorrhagic RPE detachment. Histopathologically, mature scars are composed of mounds of dense collagenous connective tissue on the inner surface of Bruch membrane (Fig. 9-14D). The collagenous scar usually contains vessels and aggregates of RPE cells. The outer part of the overlying retina undergoes degeneration because the disciform scar is a solid retinal detachment that separates the photoreceptors from their usual source of nourishment. The collagenous part of the scar is derived in part from the fibroblastic component of the granulation tissue that invades and organizes the sub-RPE hemorrhage. The RPE also contributes to scar formation. RPE cells are able to produce large quantities of extracellular matrix material including drusenoid basement membrane material, collagen, and even bone.

Heredity plays a role in the susceptibility to AMD, but development of the disorder appears to depend on a complex interplay of genetic and environmental factors. Environmental risk factors include a history of smoking, white ethnicity, obesity, high dietary intake of vegetable fat, and low dietary intake of antioxidants and zinc. Other contributing factors appear to be photooxidative damage, the accumulation of lipofuscin and chromophores that accumulate within and damage RPE cells, accumulation of lipid in Bruch membrane that impedes its conductivity, and hypoxia caused by involution of choriocapillaris.

There is recent evidence that suggests that chronic inflammation may play an important role in the pathogenesis of AMD. Cellular remnants and debris from damaged RPE cells trapped between the RPE and Bruch membrane are thought to trigger local up-regulation of cytokines, acute phase reactants such as C-reactive protein, and inflammatory mediators causing activation of the complement cascade. The debris also may attract choroidal dendritic cells that function as antigen-presenting cells. Immunohistochemical studies have disclosed complement components C5 and complement attack complex C5b-9 in drusen and damaged RPE cells. This observation is quite important because patients who have a characteristic polymorphism in the gene for complement factor H (CFH) are at significantly greater risk for AMD. CFH encodes the major inhibitor of the complement alternative pathway.

Subretinal neovascular membranes also complicate other conditions such as angioid streaks. Idiopathic subretinal membranes occasionally occur in relatively young individuals without antecedent cause. **Ocular histoplasmosis syndrome** (OHS) typically affects patients from the Ohio Valley or other areas where histoplasmosis is endemic (Fig. 9-16). Histopathologically, the disciform scars found in patients with OHS resemble those seen in AMD but typically have a prominent infiltrate of lymphocytes in the underlying choroid (Fig. 9-16B). In addition to disciform macular scars, patients with OHS have peripapillary chorioretinal atrophy and multiple white "punched-out" chorioretinal scars (Fig. 9-16A). The latter also contain chronic inflammatory cells.

THE RETINAL PIGMENT EPITHELIUM

The RPE is vital to the health and survival of the overlying retina (Fig. 1-4). Responsible for most of the characteristic reddish brown color of the human fundus, the RPE absorbs excess light and prevents intraocular light scattering like the black coating on the inside of a camera. The RPE is also involved in the transport of fluid, nutrients, and vital metabolites to and from the outer retina, and

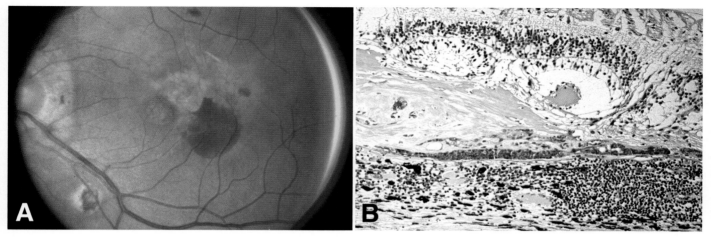

Fig. 9-16. Ocular histoplasmosis syndrome. A. Fundus photo shows triad of hemorrhagic disciform macular scar, peripapillary chorioretinal atrophy, and "punched-out" chorioretinal scars. **B.** Disciform scar, ocular histoplasmosis syndrome. A mound of connective tissue containing vessels and RPE cells rests on Bruch membrane and focally detaches the retina. The photoreceptors are atrophic. Chronic inflammation is seen in the underlying choroid. (**B.** H&E ×100)

the regeneration of the visual pigment rhodopsin. It also appears to play a major active role in retinal adherence by actively pumping fluid from the subretinal space. Finally, the RPE phagocytizes and digests the tips of millions of damaged and discarded photoreceptor outer segments every day.

STARGARDT DISEASE (FUNDUS FLAVIMACULATUS)

Striking RPE abnormalities occur in several inherited human retinal diseases including Stargardt disease or fundus flavimaculatus (Fig. 9-17). Affected patients lose vision in their teens from an atrophic type of macular degeneration caused by the death of the subfoveal RPE. The term fundus flavimaculatus, applied to this disorder by Franceschetti, literally means "yellow-spotted fundus" and refers to characteristic yellow pisciform spots at the level of the RPE disclosed by ophthalmoscopy. The fundus may have a vermilion hue, and a striking clinical abnormality called the dark choroid or the sign of choroidal silence is evident on intravenous fluorescein angiography. This obscuration of the normal choroidal pattern is caused by the massive accumulation of an abnormal lipofuscin-like lipopigment in the cytoplasm of the RPE cells. The surfeit of pigment absorbs excitatory blue wavelengths during angiography and makes the RPE intensely PAS positive (Fig. 9-17B,C). The RPE cells are taller than normal, and their nuclei are often displaced toward the apex of the cell. Scanning electron microscopy (SEM) has revealed markedly enlarged RPE cells, which are more numerous in the posterior part of the fundus (Fig. 9-17A). Groups of abnormal enlarged RPE cells surrounded by smaller relatively normal cells may be responsible for the yellow-flecked appearance of

the fundus. All of the RPE cells contain yellow-brown lipopigment, but the lipofuscin is hidden by a relatively normal complement of apical melanin in the smaller cells. The pisciform aggregates of larger cells appear yellow because these grossly abnormal cells are relatively amelanotic. Macrophages or detached, lipopigment-laden RPE in the subretinal space may also contribute to the flecked retinal appearance. The massive accumulation of pigment probably contributes to RPE dysfunction and death. The death of subfoveal RPE cells in turn leads to photoreceptor degeneration and atrophic macular degeneration.

Although Stargardt disease was long considered to be a classic disorder of the RPE, the striking retinal pigment epithelial abnormalities described above actually are secondary. Autosomal recessively inherited Stargardt disease is caused by mutations in the ABCA4 gene (1p21-p13), which is expressed exclusively in the outer segments of rod photoreceptors. The gene encodes a transmembrane protein that is involved in the clearance of all-trans-retinal aldehyde from the outer segment discs. ABCA4 mutations cause the accumulation of a toxic vitamin A derivate A2-E in the outer segments, which are phagocytized by the RPE. A2-E poisons the lysosomes in the RPE's phagolysosomal system, leading to the accumulation of large quantities of poorly digested rod outer segment (ROS) material as lipofuscin, which in turn causes dysfunction and "terminal constipation" of the cells. Teens who have homozygous mutations in the ABCR gene develop fundus flavimaculatus. Heterozygous mutations have been found in a small percentage of adults with the atrophic form of ARMD. The gene has also been implicated in a few cases of retinitis pigmentosa (RP) and cone-rod dystrophy.

Lipopigment accumulation may be a relatively stereotyped response of the RPE, because excessive amounts of RPE lipopigment have been found in several other disorders. One

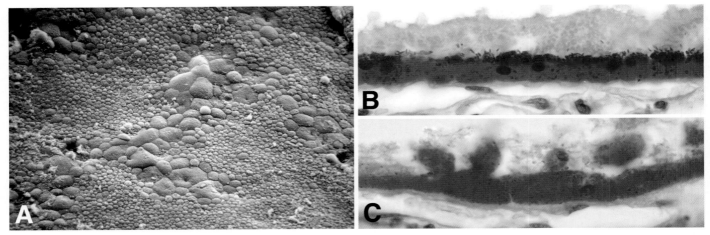

Fig. 9-17. Stargardt disease (fundus flavimaculatus). A. RPE abnormalities. False-colorized scanning electron micrograph shows aggregates of markedly enlarged RPE cells in posterior part of eye obtained postmortem from a patient with autosomal recessive fundus flavimaculatus. Hypothetically, the groups of larger cells may appear as yellow spots clinically because they have less apical melanin pigment than the surrounding smaller, more normal cells. **B.** RPE cells are packed with granules of PAS-positive material consistent with an abnormal form of lipofuscin. Nuclei in small peripheral RPE cells are displaced apically. **C.** Posterior RPE cells contain more lipofuscin and are abnormally large, amelanotic, and focally detached. The abnormal pigment in the RPE blocks normal choroidal fluorescence during intravenous fluorescein angiography, producing a dark choroid. The massive accumulation of lipofuscin is caused by a toxic vitamin A derivative contained in ingested photoreceptor outer segments. The ABCA4 gene is expressed only in rod outer segments. (**A.** False-colorized SEM ×120 [From Eagle RC et al. Retinal pigment epithelial abnormalities in fundus flavimaculatus: a light and electron microscopic study. *Ophthalmology* 1980;87:1189–1200. Courtesy of Ophthalmology], **B.** PAS ×250, **C.** PAS ×250)

of these hereditary disorders is **Best disease**. This macular dystrophy is also called vitelliform degeneration because a yellowish plaque resembling an egg yolk is observed in the macula in the early stages of the disorder. Visual loss develops when the egg "scrambles" and chorioretinal scarring develops. Although the early stage of Best disease has not been examined histopathologically, the egg yolk probably is composed of lipopigment. An abnormal electro-oculogram incriminates the RPE in Best disease. Best disease is caused by mutations in the bestrophin gene (BEST1) on chromosome 11q (11q13), which encodes a calcium-activated chloride channel. Some cases of adult-onset vitelliform macular degeneration have been linked to defects in the peripherin gene (PRPH2).

RETINITIS PIGMENTOSA

Retinitis pigmentosa includes a large, complex, and diverse group of inherited retinal disorders that have similar characteristic clinical features (Fig. 9-18). Patients with RP usually present with nyctalopia (night blindness) early in life. The electroretinogram typically reveals a marked diminution or total extinction of the retina's electrical responses. A ring-shaped area of blindness called a ring scotoma develops in the patient's equatorial visual field. As the disease progresses, this annular zone of blindness moves posteriorly, progressively encroaching on central vision and producing "tunnel vision."

Ophthalmoscopy discloses RPE atrophy and a characteristic segmental pattern of black intraretinal "bone spicule"

pigmentation arranged along retinal vessels (Fig. 9-18A). The retinal vessels are usually markedly narrowed, presumably reflecting the atrophic retina's diminished nutritional needs. Although the optic nerve classically displays "waxy pallor," the nerve does not appear to be especially atrophic histopathologically, and this clinical appearance probably is related to decreased vascularity. Macular edema, preretinal membrane formation, and optic disc drusen are also encountered. Patients frequently develop posterior subcapsular cataracts.

Histopathology shows variable degrees of photoreceptor degeneration that initially affects the rods and ultimately the cones (Fig. 9-18B). The outer nuclear layer comprising the photoreceptor cell nuclei also becomes atrophic. The extent of involvement depends on both the variant and stage of the disease. The RPE is usually relatively spared compared to the photoreceptors. Presumably, since it is no longer constrained by photoreceptor cell contact inhibition, the RPE proliferates and invades the atrophic retina and grows in the space around retinal vessels, forming perivascular cuffs of intensely pigmented, polarized cells that are evident clinically as bone spicule pigmentation (Fig. 9-18C). Electron microscopy has shown that the vascular endothelial cells adjacent to the translocated RPE cells are thin and fenestrated, resembling the choriocapillaris, and are separated from the RPE by an organized layer of extracellular matrix resembling Bruch membrane. The intense black pigmentation of the bone spicules is caused by numerous large round granules of intracytoplasmic melanin, which include macromelanosomes. This pattern of intraretinal pigmentation is not

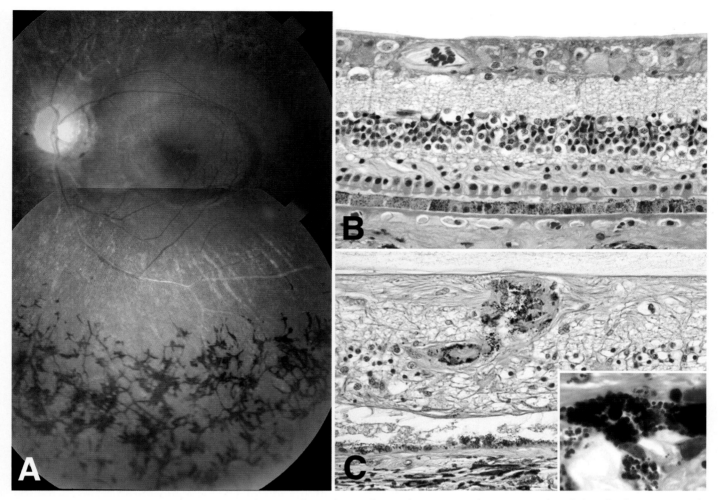

Fig. 9-18. Retinitis pigmentosa. A. Optic disc is pale and retinal vessels are severely attenuated and sheathed. Bone spicule pigmentation ensheaths atrophic vessels in peripheral retina. **B.** Autosomal dominant retinitis pigmentosa. Only an interrupted monolayer of cone nuclei persists as the outer nuclear layer in the posterior part of the retina. The inner segments of the residual cones are grossly abnormal and outer segments are not seen. The RPE and the inner retinal layers are well preserved. **C.** Retinitis pigmentosa, intraretinal pigmentation. Focus of bone spicule pigmentation comprises intraretinal perivascular proliferation of RPE cells. **Inset** shows macromelanosomes in hyperplastic RPE. (**B.** H&E ×100 [Case presented by Dr. David. G. Cogan, Verhoeff Society, 1989] **C.** H&E ×100; **inset**, H&E ×250)

specific for RP; identical findings including macromelanosomes are found in eyes with secondary pigmentary retinopathies related to long-standing retinal detachment. In the latter instance, photoreceptor atrophy caused by chronic retinal detachment presumably facilitates retinal invasion by the RPE.

The retina's response to a wide variety of molecular or enzymatic defects appears to be relatively limited and stereotyped. Nonsyndromic RP is associated with disparate defects in at least 45 genes. Rhodopsin (RHO), the first gene linked to RP, was identified by Dryja and coworkers in 1990. RHO mutations cause 15% to 20% of dominantly inherited cases of nonsydromic RP. Most are single amino acid (missense) mutations in the opsin part of the molecule. The most common RHO mutation is the substitution of histidine for the normal proline at position 23. This amino acid substitution is caused by a single nucleotide

transversion (C to A) in the triplet of nucleotides in the patient's DNA that code for amino acid 23. Detailed marker studies suggest that all families who have Pro-23-His autosomal dominant (AD) RP are descended from a single individual.

Additional RP genes encode other proteins involved in rod phototransduction, including the alpha and beta subunits of rod phosphodiesterase, the alpha and beta subunits of rod cGMP-gated channel, arrestin, and guanylate cyclase activating protein. Others encode cytoskeletal proteins such as peripherin/retinal degeneration slow (RDS) or proteins involved in cellular trafficking including retinitis pigmentosa GTPase regulator (RPGR). Mutations in RPGR account for 13% of cases of RP. Other RP genes are involved in photoreceptor differentiation, mRNA splicing, extracellular matrix composition, and other metabolic pathways. Although most RP genes are expressed in rod photoreceptors, a few are expressed in the RPE where they are involved in retinol metabolism or the phagocytosis of photoreceptor outer segments. Some RP genes have been implicated in other retinal dystrophies and degenerations.

Almost 40% of RP occurs sporadically in patients who have a negative family history. About 37% are autosomal recessively inherited, 20% autosomal dominantly inherited, and 4% are X-linked. The disease tends to be more severe and have an earlier onset in patients with X-linked RP. Autosomal dominantly inherited cases tend to have the most benign course. However, the severity of the disease measured by objective clinical and electrophysiologic criteria in a given kindred of AD RP appears to correlate well with the specific amino acid substitution found in that family, that is, whether the substituted amino acid occurs in the intradiskal, transmembrane, or cytoplasmic region of the ROS.

In 2010, the online database Online Mendelian Inheritance in Man included 289 articles dealing with different subtypes of nonsyndromic RP, genes and proteins incriminated in the pathogenesis of RP, and a variety of syndromes whose clinical manifestations include RP. Common syndromic variants of RP include Usher syndrome, in which typical RP is associated with neurosensory deafness and Bardet Biedl syndrome which comprises polydactyly, truncal obesity, hypogenitalism, and renal failure. Severe RP also accompanies renal failure in Senior-Loken syndrome. RP also occurs in certain dysmorphic syndromes and metabolic and neurologic diseases. Metabolic associations include abetalipoproteinemia or Bassen-Kornzweig syndrome, Bietti corneoretinal crystalline dystrophy, cystinosis, mucopolysaccharidoses, and Refsum disease. Bietti disease has microcrystalline deposits in the fundus and cornea and is caused by mutations in the CYP4V2 gene encoding cytochrome P450. Neurologic diseases with RP include neuronal ceroid lipofuscinosis or Batten disease, Joubert syndrome, autosomal dominant cerebellar ataxia type II, and Hallervorden-Spatz syndrome.

Leber congenital amaurosis (LCA) is the designation for a heterogenous group of autosomal recessive retinal dystrophies that cause congenital visual impairment in infants and children. LCA is caused by mutations in at least eight genes including CEP290, which is responsible for about one fifth of cases. Gene therapy has been used to successively treat Briard dogs and humans with LCA2 caused by mutations in RPE65, an RPE-specific isomerase involved in the regeneration of light-altered vitamin A molecules.

OTHER HERITABLE DISORDERS OF THE RETINA

In recent years, specific genetic defects have been discovered in a variety of retinal and vitreous disorders using the tools of molecular genetics. Ironically, few of these disorders have been examined histopathologically, or show relatively nonspecific findings. They include Oguchi disease (mutation in the arrestin or RHO-kinase genes involved in the shutoff of phototransduction), Sorsby pseudoinflammatory fundus dystrophy (mutation in gene on chromosome 22 encoding tissue inhibitor of metalloproteinase-3) (TIMP3), pattern or butterfly dystrophy (mutations in the RDS or photoreceptor peripherin gene (PRPH2) cause pattern dystrophy in some patients; others have RP-like picture), choroideremia (X-linked defect in the CHM gene that encodes for Rab escort protein-1 (REP1), which is involved in membrane trafficking), Norrie disease and X-linked variants of familial exudative vitreoretinopathy (defects in NDP gene encoding norrin), gyrate atrophy (autosomal recessive ornithine-delta-aminotransferase deficiency), Stickler syndrome (autosomal dominant mutation in COL2A1 for type II collagen), Kearns-Sayre and MERRF and MELAS syndromes (defects in mitochondrial DNA), and Stargardt disease (mutations in outer segment ABCA4 gene—see above). Autosomal dominant familial exudative vitreoretinopathy is caused by mutations in the frizzled-4 gene (FZD4) on chromosome 11q14 that encodes receptors for Wnt signaling proteins.

The retina and RPE are involved in a wide variety of heritable metabolic storage diseases including the systemic mucopolysaccharidoses, sphingolipidoses, mucolipidoses, neuronal ceroid lipofuscinoses, and disorders of glycoprotein degradation. Retinal pigmentary degeneration resembling RP occurs in patients with Hurler (MPS I-H), Scheie (MPS I-S), Hunter (MPS II), Sanfilipo (MPS III), and Morquio (MPS IV) syndromes. Accumulation of GM2 ganglioside in retinal ganglion cells opacifies the ganglion cell-rich perifoveal retina in infants with Tay-Sachs disease (GM2 gangliosidosis type I) who are deficient in hexosaminidase A (Fig. 9-19). This is evident clinically as a macular cherry red spot because ganglion cells are absent in the floor of the fovea (foveola), which remains transparent. Electron microscopy discloses multimembranous inclusions called zebra bodies within lysosomes. Macular cherry red spots also occur in Sandhoff disease and the Niemann-Pick group of diseases.

TOXIC RETINOPATHIES

The chronic administration of certain drugs can cause irreversible visual loss. Some of these chemical compounds are toxic to the RPE. Chloroquine and its hydroxy derivative plaquenil, antimalarial drugs used in the treatment of rheumatoid arthritis and lupus erythematosus, can cause a toxic maculopathy that has a characteristic "bull's-eye" appearance. These drugs have an affinity for melanin and are concentrated in the RPE. The macular degeneration appears to be dose related, and severe visual loss usually develops after patients have received many grams of the drug.

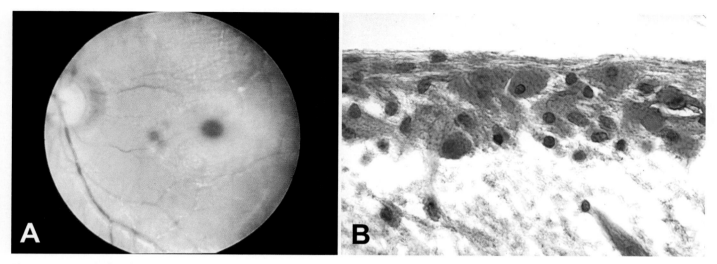

Fig. 9-19. Tay-Sachs disease. A. Foveal cherry red spot is caused by opacification of perifoveal retinal ganglion cells by GM-2 ganglioside. **B.** PAS-positive GM-2 ganglioside fills cytoplasm of retinal ganglion cells. (**B.** PAS ×250)

The chronic administration of high doses of phenothiazines, particularly thiorizadine or Mellaril, can cause extensive irreversible damage to the RPE and photoreceptors. NP27, a phenothiazine derivative, has been used experimentally as an RPE toxin.

Experimental studies suggest that high levels of the amino acid ornithine are toxic to the RPE. This toxicity appears to be the basis for the widespread chorioretinal atrophy that occurs in patients who have **gyrate atrophy**. At the molecular level, this rare autosomal recessively inherited disorder is caused by the absence or dysfunction of the mitochondrial matrix enzyme ornithine-delta-aminotransferase, which normally converts ornithine to glutamate. The gene is located on chromosome 10. Serum levels of ornithine are elevated 10- to 20-fold in patients with gyrate atrophy. Clinically, gyrate atrophy is characterized by widespread chorioretinal atrophy that blinds most patients by age 40 or 50 years.

PERIPHERAL RETINAL DEGENERATIONS

Peripheral chorioretinal degeneration (commonly called cobblestone or paving stone degeneration) occurs in more than one fourth of individuals over age 20 years and is more common in myopes. The lesions appear as yellow–white patches of chorioretinal atrophy that have scalloped, sharply demarcated borders, which often are pigmented (Fig. 9-20A). Cobblestone degeneration occurs most often in the inferotemporal retina and is separated from the ora serrata by a zone of normal retina. The patches appear white because the overlying sclera is bared by the severe atrophy of the RPE and choriocapillaris. Large choroidal vessels often persist, however. The pigmented border surrounding many lesions reflects hyperplasia of the adjacent RPE.

Histopathologically, the outer retina is welded to the inner surface of Bruch membrane, which is devoid of RPE (Fig. 9-20B). Replaced by gliosis, the rods and cones are absent in the area of chorioretinal adhesion and the underlying choriocapillaris is atrophic as well. Unlike lattice degeneration (see below), cobblestone degeneration does not predispose to retinal detachment. In fact, these peripheral chorioretinal scars are quite similar histopathologically to mature laser burns or cryotherapy scars used to treat retinal disorders. Both therapeutic modalities use thermal effects to induce chorioretinal scarring that firmly binds the outer retina to the denuded inner surface of Bruch membrane. One sees the typical pattern of outer ischemic retinal atrophy with loss of choriocapillaris, RPE, and outer retina. Retinal breaks do not form because there is no associated vitreoretinal traction. Markedly asymmetric involvement in patients with unilateral ocular ischemia suggests that cobblestone degeneration might be caused by choroidal vascular insufficiency.

Peripheral microcystoid degeneration is a ubiquitous, generally innocuous degeneration of the peripheral retina found in all adults older than 20 years. The condition is bilaterally symmetrical and most prominent temporally. Clinically or macroscopically, one sees a stippled pattern that corresponds to an array of interconnecting channels or lacunae in the peripheral retina just posterior to the ora serrata (Fig. 9-21A). Microscopically, the outer plexiform layer contains multiple cystoid spaces called Blessig-Iwanoff cysts, which are filled with hyaluronic acid and are separated by residual pillars of Müller cells (Fig. 9-21B,C). Zonular traction on the peripheral retina during accommodation may be a cause of peripheral microcystoid degeneration.

Typical degenerative retinoschisis, a split centered in the outer plexiform layer of the retina, is caused by coalescence of the cystoid spaces in peripheral microcystoid degeneration.

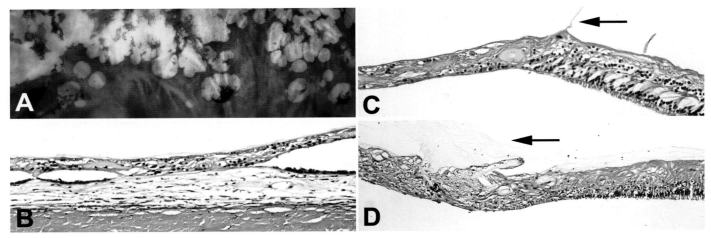

Fig. 9-20. Peripheral retinal degenerations. A. Peripheral chorioretinal atrophy (cobblestone or paving stone degeneration). Macrophoto (**A**) shows *yellow-white* patches of chorioretinal atrophy with scalloped, sharply demarcated borders. **B.** Atrophic outer retina is bound to denuded segment of Bruch membrane by firm chorioretinal adhesion. The peripheral retina is thin and atrophic. **C, D.** Lattice degeneration of the retina. The involved part of the retina (**at left**) is diffusely atrophic and disorganized. A sclerotic vessel is seen in (**C**) and an intraretinal focus of pigment in (**D**). *Arrows* denote vitreous strands attached to the margin of both lesions. Tractional retinal breaks caused by vitreoretinal traction predispose to retinal detachment in patients with lattice degeneration. Pools of liquefied vitreous typically are found overlying lattice lesions, and the internal limiting membrane of the retina is focally absent. (**A.** H&E ×50, **B.** H&E ×50, **C.** H&E ×50)

Degenerative or senile retinoschisis occurs in 1% of adults and usually is located inferotemporally. Although degenerative retinoschisis produces a localized scotoma (a focal area of blindness), the retinal split rarely progresses posteriorly and usually remains confined to the pre-equatorial retina. Rarely, retinal detachment can complicate retinoschisis if large holes develop in the outer layer of the retina.

A rarer variant of peripheral microcystoid degeneration called **reticular cystoid degeneration** is said to occur in about 18% of adults and is bilateral in 41%. Evident as a polygonal patch of delicate tunnels with a finely stippled appearance, reticular cystoid degeneration typically is located posterior to a patch of typical cystoid degeneration. The cysts are located in the NFL of the retina (Fig. 9-22A). Reticular cystoid degeneration may spawn a corresponding type of retinoschisis called reticular retinoschisis. The split in the retina occurs in the NFL.

Juvenile X-linked retinoschisis is an inherited disorder caused by mutations in the RS1 gene on the X chromosome (Xp22.2-p22.1).

When affected men present with decreased visual acuity in the first decade, ophthalmoscopy often discloses a curious stellate pattern of foveal schisis seen as a cartwheel pattern of radiating lines or folds surrounding the

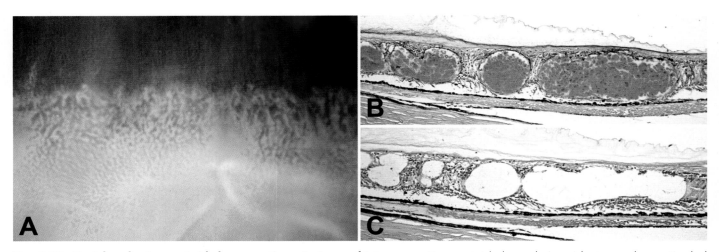

Fig. 9-21. Peripheral microcystoid degeneration. A. Array of interconnecting cystoid channels is evident grossly as stippled pattern in the peripheral retina bordering the ora serrata. Peripheral microcystoid degeneration is almost a universal finding in the peripheral retina after age 8 years. **B.** Cystoid spaces called Blessig-Iwanoff cysts are located in the mid-retina. The cysts contain acid mucosaccharide disclosed by colloidal iron stain. **C.** Pretreatment with hyaluronidase abolishes staining, confirming that material in cysts is hyaluronic acid. (**B.** Colloidal iron for AMP ×50, **C.** Colloidal iron for AMP after hyaluronidase digestion ×50)

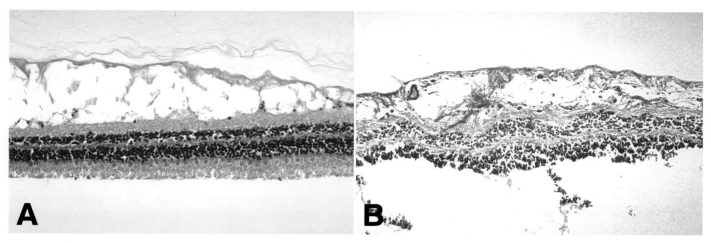

Fig. 9-22. A. Reticular cystoid degeneration. The cystoid spaces are located in the nerve fiber layer of the retina. Reticular cystoid degeneration always occurs posterior to a focus of typical peripheral microcystoid degeneration. It can evolve into reticular retinoschisis. **B. Juvenile X-linked retinoschisis.** The retinal split in this rare X-linked hereditary disorder is located in the nerve fiber layer. Many affected patients have a pattern of stellate folds in the macula. (**A.** H&E ×50, **B.** H&E ×50)

fovea. OCT shows that the cysts involve multiple layers of the inner retina, but they do not leak on fluorescein angiography. Peripheral retinoschisis typically occurs in the inferotemporal retina and can become quite extensive. The split develops in the superficial layers of the retina (Fig. 9-22B). Retinoschisin protein produced by the RS1 gene is believed to function in cellular adhesion in the development and maintenance of retinal architecture. In one study, electron microscopy disclosed an accumulation of amorphous PAS-positive material in the retina adjoining schisis cavities. The authors postulated that juvenile x-linked retinoschisis might be a disorder of Müller cells.

Lattice degeneration is a fairly common degenerative condition found in 6% to 11% of the population. Lattice degeneration is important because it predisposes to the development of rhegmatogenous retinal detachment, particularly in myopic patients. The vitreoretinal degeneration is characterized by the presence of oval areas of retinal thinning, which are sharply demarcated, circumferentially oriented, and located anterior to the equator in the vertical meridians of the eye. The term lattice degeneration is derived from a latticelike pattern of crisscrossing white lines (sclerotic vessels) that occur in relatively few (12%) lesions.

Histopathologically, lattice degeneration appears as a focal area of retinal thinning (Fig. 9-20C,D). The inner retinal layers are atrophic and the internal limiting membrane is absent. A pocket of liquefied vitreous overlies the discontinuity in the ILM. Firm vitreoretinal condensations, occasionally fortified by glial cell proliferation, adhere to the margins of the lattice lesions. Thick-walled vessels, which correlate with the white lattice lines seen clinically, are present. Hypertrophy, hyperplasia, and intraretinal RPE migration are seen in some cases. The retinal capillary bed is focally occluded.

The firm vitreoretinal adhesions to the margins of the patches of thin atrophic retina predispose to the development of tractional retinal breaks and rhegmatogenous retinal detachment. The tractional breaks typically develop at the posterior or lateral margins of the lesions, and patches of lattice degeneration are often found in the flaps of horseshoe breaks, or within small opercula extracted by vitreoretinal traction.

Pars plana cysts usually are innocuous, acquired degenerative lesions that occur in about one third of normal individuals over age 70 years (Fig. 9-23). Most are found incidentally during pathologic examination. Pars plana cysts are formed by detachment of the inner nonpigmented layer of ciliary epithelium from the outer pigmented layer. In normal individuals, the cysts contain an acidic glycosaminoglycan presumed to be hyaluronic acid because it is sensitive to digestion with the enzyme hyaluronidase (Fig. 9-23A,D,E, and F). Multiple pars plana cysts occur in patients with multiple myeloma or other dysproteinemic or hyperproteinemic disorders. Myeloma cysts contain Bence Jones or myeloma protein, which is precipitated by fixation and causes milky-white opacification of the cysts (Fig. 9-23B,C).

The temporal ora serrata is relatively smooth, while the nasal ora is marked by prominent dentate processes and oral bays. Small, yellow transparent jewellike nodules of calcification called ora pearls occasionally are found intraretinally within dentate processes. A meridional complex is an elongated dentate process that bridges the pars plana and attaches to a ciliary process anteriorly.

RETINAL DETACHMENT

Retinal detachment is a physical separation of the neurosensory retina from the RPE (the two layers derived, respectively, from the inner and outer layers of the embryonic

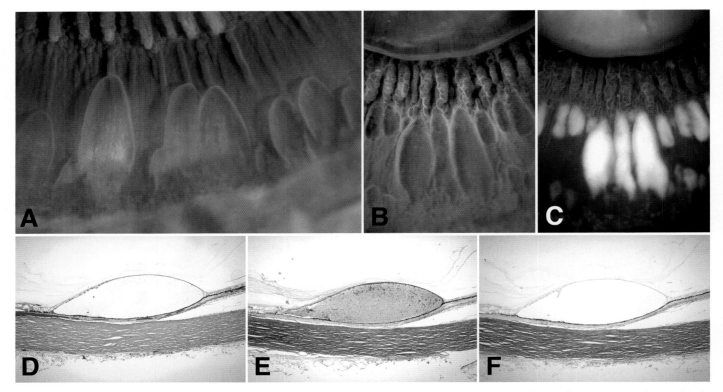

Fig. 9-23. Pars plana cysts. A. Cysts of the pars plana filled with hyaluronic acid occasionally are found in eyes from elderly patients. **D.** The inner nonpigmented layer of the ciliary epithelium has detached from the outer pigmented layer, which remains attached to the pars plana. **E.** Cyst contents stain blue with colloidal iron stain for acid mucopolysaccharide. **F.** Colloidal iron staining is abolished by pretreatment with hyaluronidase, confirming the presence of hyaluronic acid. **B.** Pars plana cysts, multiple myeloma. Multiple pars plana cysts in eye obtained postmortem from a patient with multiple myeloma are seen before (**B**) and after fixation (**C**). The cysts are clear *in vivo*. Fixation has precipitated the myeloma protein filling the cysts, causing milky-white opacification (**C**). (**D.** H&E ×10, **E.** Colloidal iron for AMP ×10, **F.** Colloidal iron for AMP after hyaluronidase digestion ×10)

neuroectodermal optic cup) (Fig. 9-24C). Although these two layers normally are closely apposed, they are not joined by intercellular connections, and a potential space called the subretinal space exists between the two. Fluid collects in this potential space in retinal detachment. The fluid prevents reapproximation and reattachment of the retina unless it resorbs or is drained. The physical separation deprives the outer, avascular part of the retina of its normal supply of oxygen and nutrients from the choroid, and also precludes vital interactions between the energy-intensive photoreceptors

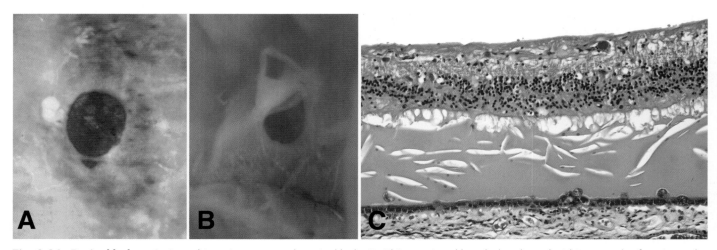

Fig. 9-24. Retinal holes. A. Atrophic retina surrounds retinal hole. **B.** This tractional break developed within a patch of perivascular lattice degeneration. **C.** Chronic retinal detachment. Eosinophilic proteinaceous fluid fills the subretinal space. The photoreceptors are totally absent and the outer nuclear layer is mildly atrophic. The RPE shows focal budding. The subretinal fluid contains cholesterol clefts. (**C.** H&E ×100)

and the RPE. These factors can lead rapidly to permanent visual loss from irreversible degeneration and atrophy of the rods and cones. Hence, vision may remain poor after a seemingly successful reattachment operation; that is, surgery can be a technical success, but a functional failure.

There are three basic categories of retinal detachment: rhegmatogenous, exudative, and tractional. **Rhegmatogenous retinal detachments** are caused by holes or breaks (rhegma = break) in the neurosensory retina that provide fluid (usually liquid vitreous) access to the subretinal space (Fig. 9-24A,B). Most retinal holes found in eyes with rhegmatogenous retinal detachment are tears caused by vitreoretinal traction. The vitreous humor's framework of type II collagen fibers is adherent to the ILM of the retina. Especially firm vitreoretinal adhesions occur at the vitreous base, which straddles the ora serrata, the circumference of the optic disc, around the fovea and along major retinal vessels.

The framework of vitreous humor frequently detaches from the posterior retina in elderly patients or in individuals who have diabetes or other retinal pathology. Anterior movement of the posteriorly detached vitreous caused by eye movements can exert traction on areas where the vitreous and retina remain firmly adherent, causing tears in the retina (that release the traction). Rhegmatogenous retinal detachment was a relatively common complication of intracapsular cataract extraction, in which the entire lens is removed within its capsule. Aphakic (no lens) retinal detachment after intracapsular surgery typically is caused by small horseshoe tears located at the posterior vitreous base. Hole formation is related to increased mobility of the posteriorly detached vitreous, which has been deprived of support anteriorly. The apices of horseshoe tears always point posteriorly, that is, the horse always walks toward the optic nerve. Posterior vitreous detachment and the mechanics of vitreoretinal traction are responsible for this characteristic orientation.

Rhegmatogenous retinal detachment is also relatively common in patients who are myopic and/or who have lattice degeneration of the retina. Several factors probably contribute to the development of retinal detachment in high myopia. Vitreous degeneration or syneresis is extremely common in myopic eyes. This is evident clinically to most affected persons as vitreous floaters. Most cases of myopia are caused by enlargement of the eye, which usually occurs as the refractive disorder develops toward the end of the first decade. Presumably, the vitreous framework degenerates as the sclera and retina "outgrow" the vitreous. Retinal stretching and attenuation in high myopes also contribute to retinal hole formation. Subretinal neovascularization, macular hemorrhage, and disciform scar formation can complicate pathologic high myopia. Stretching of Bruch membrane causes splits or ruptures, which are evident clinically as "lacquer cracks" or lightning figures. A central, circular, dark spot called a Förster-Fuchs spot may develop in the macula during the fourth or fifth decade in association with lacquer cracks. Blood pigment from choroidal hemorrhage and RPE proliferation probably contribute to this spot.

Trauma is another cause of rhegmatogenous retinal detachment. The retina can be torn by severe distortion of the globe during contusion injuries. Lengthy rips in the retina called giant tears can result. Giant tears are typically oriented parallel to the limbus and generally extend for 90 degrees or more. Contusion injuries also can avulse or physically disinsert the retina from its attachment to the ora serrata. The large peripheral gaps that result are called retinal dialyses. Most retinal dialyses affect the inferotemporal quadrant and occur in young emmetropes.

Tractional retinal detachments are caused by fibrous or fibrovascular vitreoretinal membranes that contract and mechanically pull off the retina (Fig. 9-25). Tractional

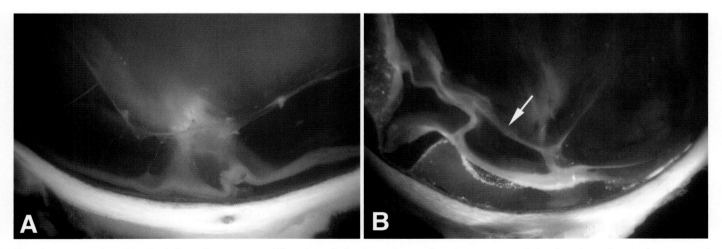

Fig. 9-25. Tractional retinal detachments, proliferative diabetic retinopathy. A. New vessels bridge the subretinal space and arborize on posterior face of the detached vitreous. The organized vitreous is exerting A-P traction on retina, causing focal retinal detachment. **B.** Fibrosis accentuates the posterior face of the organized and partially detached vitreous (*arrow*) which remains focally adherent to the retina. A-P traction lines are evident. Blood fills the subhyaloid space where the organized posterior hyaloid face bridges the retina. The formed vitreous contains blood. Gelatinous subretinal fluid detaches the posterior retina. The glistening white particles in the subretinal fluid are lipid histiocytes.

detachment of the posterior retina, which unfortunately often involves the macula, is a major complication of proliferative diabetic retinopathy. Vitreoretinal traction in diabetics is caused by the contraction of fibrovascular membranes. The neovascular component of such membranes originates within the retina and proliferates on the face of the posteriorly detached vitreous. The organization of vitreous hemorrhage also contributes to vitreoretinal membrane formation and traction. In the past, severe fibroplasia and organization of the vitreous in diabetics was termed *retinitis proliferans*. Tractional retinal detachment caused by vitreoretinal neovascularization also complicates sickle cell retinopathy and the retinopathy of prematurity.

Tractional retinal detachment can also follow severe trauma, especially perforating injuries of the globe. The retinal traction is caused by vitreoretinal bands formed by the ingrowth of fibrous scar tissue from the wound, or by the organization of tracks of hemorrhage in the vitreous. Removal of vitreous hemorrhage after severe injury can help to reduce the incidence of this complication.

Severe inflammatory and infectious conditions that stimulate organization of the vitreous are additional causes of tractional retinal detachment. A relatively high incidence of detachment complicates ocular toxocariasis, particularly the peripheral form of the disease. Retinal detachment is also a major problem in patients who have necrotizing retinitides such as cytomegalovirus retinitis or acute retinal necrosis (see Chapter 2).

Exudative retinal detachment is caused by the accumulation of fluid in the subretinal space. The subretinal fluid may derive from "leaky" vascular lesions in the retina but more typically is caused by choroidal infiltration by tumor or inflammation. Exudative retinal detachments are nonrhegmatogenous; careful clinical examination fails to disclose a hole in the neurosensory retina.

Exudative retinal detachments caused by leaky retinal lesions occur in patients who have Coats disease or retinal hemangioblastomas. Coats disease is discussed in Chapter 12. Retinal hemangioblastomas (commonly called retinal capillary hemangiomas) occur in isolation or may be a manifestation of autosomal dominantly inherited Von Hippel–Lindau disease (see Chapter 2).

Most primary or secondary choroidal tumors usually have some degree of associated exudative retinal detachment. Exudative detachment occurs in most patients who have choroidal malignant melanomas and is often the presenting manifestation of the tumor. Initially, fluid percolates into the space at the margins of the "solid detachment" formed by "tenting-up" and anterior displacement of the retina by the tumor. Degeneration or destruction of the RPE and choriocapillaris overlying the tumor may be additional contributory factors. Extensive exudative retinal detachment typically is found in eyes with carcinoma metastatic to the uvea. The location of the bulk of the subretinal fluid may shift with eye movements (shifting fluid). Exudative retinal detachment

is a major cause of visual loss in eyes with choroidal hemangiomas and ultimately can lead to loss of the eye if painful pupillary block glaucoma results. Treatment of these benign vascular tumors is often warranted to prevent this complication.

Exudative retinal detachment also complicates choroidal inflammatory disease, particularly disorders marked by extensive choroidal infiltration such as sympathetic uveitis or Vogt-Koyanagi-Harada disease. Exudative retinal detachment also complicates toxemia of pregnancy and oxygen toxicity.

TRUE AND ARTIFACTITIOUS RETINAL DETACHMENTS

Nearly all intact eyes that are fixed routinely by immersion in neutral buffered formalin have an artifactitious detachment of the retina. Several features serve to differentiate true and artifactitious retinal detachments histopathologically. True retinal detachments are characterized by eosinophilic proteinaceous fluid in the subretinal space (this is *not* present in all cases) and degeneration and atrophy of the photoreceptors, which can involve the outer nuclear layer in long-standing cases (Fig. 9-24C). On the contrary, if the retinal detachment is artifactual, the subretinal space is empty, the photoreceptors are well preserved, and ellipsoidal granules of RPE pigment remain attached to the tips of the outer segments.

SIGNS OF CHRONIC RETINAL DETACHMENT

Findings that indicate that a retinal detachment has persisted for a long time include budding, and papillary and pseudoadenomatous proliferation of the RPE. The RPE has a great capacity for reactive proliferation and migration, which under normal circumstances presumably is held in check by contact inhibition by healthy retinal photoreceptors. Retinal detachment removes this inhibition.

The RPE cells are capable of elaborating enormous quantities of extracellular matrix material including drusenoid basement membrane material, collagen, and even bone. Curious, large drusenlike structures with a central core of soft granular extracellular matrix material enveloped by RPE cells are occasionally found in eyes with long-standing retinal detachments (Fig. 9-26B,C). Osseous metaplasia of the RPE is almost invariably found in blind phthisic eyes with chronic retinal detachment. The intraocular bone is always located on the inner surface of Bruch membrane, and typically occurs at sites of traction near the ora serrata or the optic disc. The bone is mature lamellar bone and it often contains fatty marrow (Fig. 3-20B).

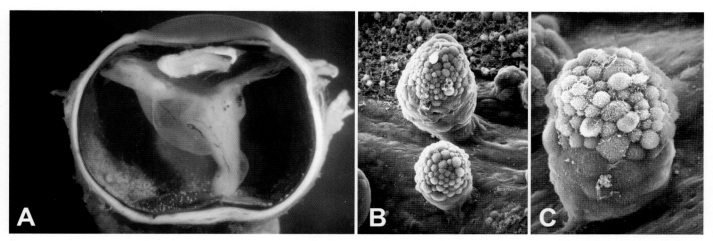

Fig. 9-26. Chronic retinal detachment. A. Long-standing retinal detachments typically have a funnel or morning glory configuration caused by proliferative vitreoretinopathy. Retinal macrocysts and large pedunculated drusen are indicators of chronicity. **B, C.** Large pedunculated drusenlike structures found in eye with long-standing retinal detachment are capped by plump RPE cells. Most of the RPE is flattened and atrophic. These curious structures were composed of soft drusenoid matrix material. (**B.** SEM ×160, **C.** SEM ×640)

Chronically detached retinas found in blind painful eyes typically have a funnel or "morning glory" configuration (Fig. 9-26A). This configuration reflects the end stage of proliferative vitreoretinopathy (PVR). It is caused by the growth of cells on both the inner and outer surfaces of the detached retina and on the posterior surface of the detached vitreous, which remains firmly attached to the vitreous base. The cellular constituents include RPE cells, glial cells, and myofibroblasts that migrate, proliferate, and elaborate extracellular matrix material and form fibrocellular membranes. Organization of the vitreous and contraction of this scar tissue exert traction on the inner part of the peripheral retina, drawing it centrally and permanently welding the retina into this floral configuration. Organization of the vitreous also forms cyclitic membranes, which bridge the vitreous cavity behind the lens. The cyclitic membranes exert traction on the vitreous base and detach the ciliary body. PVR is a major cause of inoperable retinal detachment or recurrent detachment after reattachment surgery. Fibrocellular membranes on its inner and outer surfaces bind adjacent parts of the retina together, forming fixed folds. Other findings in long-standing retinal detachment include gliosis and microcystic and macrocystic retinal degeneration.

THE OCULAR PATHOLOGY OF DIABETES MELLITUS

The ocular complications of diabetes mellitus are an important cause of acquired visual disability and blindness. In the United States, diabetic retinopathy is the leading cause of new cases of legal blindness between the ages of 20 and 74 years. Diabetic retinopathy occurs in patients with either type I (juvenile-onset or insulin-dependent) or type II (maturity-onset) diabetes mellitus. The prevalence of retinopathy is higher in patients with type I diabetes. Patients with juvenile diabetes also are at greater risk for developing proliferative retinopathy, probably because they generally have more severe hyperglycemia. Overall, however, a significant proportion of the disorder's blinding complications actually develops in patients with type II diabetes because adult-onset diabetes is more common. The prevalence of retinopathy in both groups is related to the duration of the disease. Retinopathy occurs in about 50% of patients who have had juvenile diabetes mellitus for 15 years. Strict control of blood sugar and glycosylated hemoglobin A1c appears to slow the progression of the disease.

Background, preproliferative and proliferative forms of diabetic retinopathy are recognized clinically. The initial stage of diabetic retinopathy called **background retinopathy** is marked by retinal edema, hemorrhages and exudates (see above), and capillary microaneurysms (Fig. 9-27A). The onset of many soft exudates or cotton-wool spots heralds progressive retinal ischemia as diabetic retinopathy enters the preproliferative phase. Retinal and vitreoretinal neovascularization occur in proliferative diabetic retinopathy (Fig. 9-28). Neovascularization predisposes to the blinding complications vitreous hemorrhage and tractional retinal detachment.

Diabetic retinopathy is the retinal manifestation of the generalized microangiopathy that occurs throughout the body in diabetes mellitus (Fig. 9-27). Breakdown of the blood–retinal barrier is one of the earliest functional lesions in diabetic eyes and contributes to the development of hemorrhages, exudates, and retinal edema. Retinal edema is an extremely important cause of visual loss in

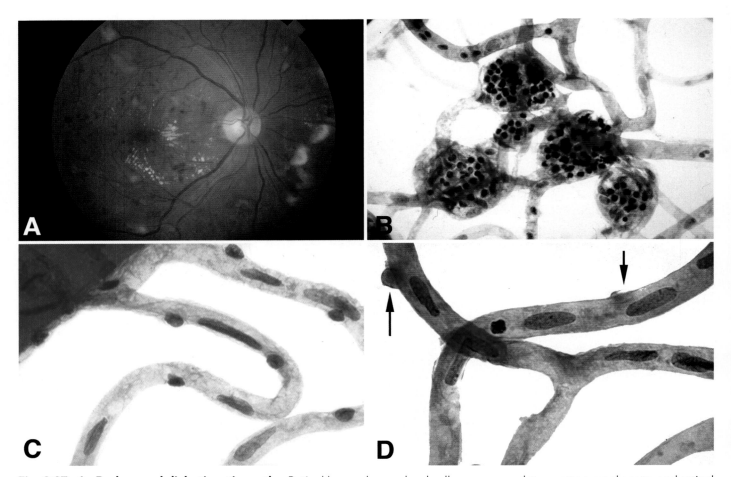

Fig. 9-27. A. Background diabetic retinopathy. Retinal hemorrhages, hard yellow waxy exudates, cotton-wool spots, and retinal edema are present. **B.** Diabetic microaneurysms, trypsin retinal digestion. **C.** Normal retinal capillaries, trypsin retinal digestion. Normal retinal capillaries are composed of approximately equal numbers of endothelial cells and pericytes. The nuclei of the endothelial cells are cigar shaped. The pericyte nuclei are round. The pericytes are embedded in the basement membrane of the capillary wall. **D.** Retinal capillaries in diabetes mellitus, trypsin retinal digestion. A preferential loss of pericytes occurs in the early stages of diabetic retinopathy, disturbing the normal 1:1 ratio between pericytes and endothelial cells. *Arrows* denote pericyte ghosts in the capillary basement membrane. Diabetic thickening of the basement membrane causes intense staining with PAS stain. (**B.** PAS ×100, **C.** PAS ×250, **D.** PAS ×250)

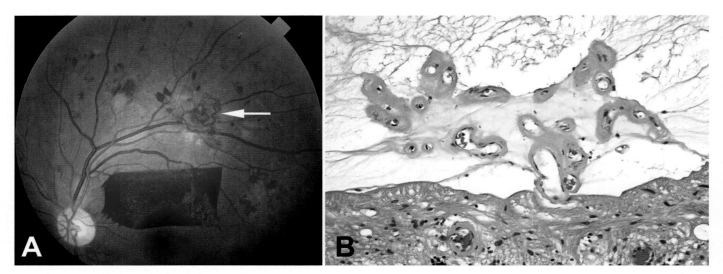

Fig. 9-28. A. Proliferative diabetic retinopathy. *Arrow* points to a large frond of vitreoretinal neovascularization above flat-topped subhyaloid hemorrhage. Fluorescein retinopathy disclosed extensive retinal capillary nonperfusion. **B.** Retinal neovascularization, PDR. A feeder vessel passes through the internal limiting membrane and enters the base of the neovascular frond. The new vessels are encompassed by collagen. (**B.** H&E ×100)

diabetic patients. The characteristic retinal vascular abnormalities of diabetic retinopathy can be demonstrated by the trypsin retinal digestion technique (Fig. 9-27B–D). Normal retinal capillaries are composed of endothelial cells, which form the lining of the capillary, and pericytes or mural cells, which reside in capsules in the perivascular basement membrane (Fig. 9 -27C). Pericytes have contractile properties that regulate capillary caliber and the flow within the retinal microcirculation. Normally, endothelial cells and pericytes occur in a one-to-one ratio. Pericytes are lost preferentially in the early stages of diabetic retinopathy (Fig. 9-27D). Pericyte loss appears to be directly related to hyperglycemia, which induces apoptosis.

Trypsin digestion of diabetic retinas also discloses capillary microaneurysms and generalized thickening of the capillary basement membranes evident as increased PAS-positive staining (Fig. 9-27B,D). Totally, acellular areas of the retinal capillary bed devoid of both endothelial cells and pericytes also are found. The latter correspond to areas of capillary nonperfusion seen on fluorescein angiography. Histopathologic examination of zones of capillary nonperfusion shows inner ischemic retinal atrophy.

Retinal capillary microaneurysms (Fig. 9-27B) are grape-like or spindle-shaped dilatations of retinal capillaries. Many microaneurysms appear quite cellular, suggesting that capillary endothelial cell proliferation may be involved in their formation. Weakening of the capillary wall secondary to focal pericyte loss may also contribute.

Retinal capillary pericyte loss has several important consequences. Retinal capillaries lose the ability to autoregulate, leading to changes in retinal blood flow. In addition, pericytes appear to have an inhibitory effect on vascular endothelial cell proliferation, which is mediated by TGF-β. Loss of this inhibitory effect may stimulate endothelial cell proliferation and neovascularization.

Neovascularization occurs in proliferative diabetic retinopathy and is a major factor in the pathogenesis of blinding complications such as vitreous hemorrhage and tractional retinal detachment (Figs. 9-25, 9-28, and 9-29). Neovascularization is stimulated by angiogenesis factors produced by the ischemic retina such as VEGF. VEGF is a potent angiogenesis factor and endothelial cell-specific mitogen whose synthesis is regulated by the level of oxygen in the cellular microenvironment. VEGF has been identified in ocular fluid from patients with active retinal and anterior segment neovascularization associated with several ocular diseases with retinal ischemia

Neovascularization begins in the retina where it is evident clinically as intraretinal microvascular abnormalities. The new vessels break through the ILM and grow on the inner surface of the retina (Fig. 9-28). Neovascularization cannot invade the formed vitreous, but it readily grows on the posterior face of the detached vitreous (Fig. 9-29). Neovascularization that originates on the optic disc typically grows into the conical posterior opening of Cloquet canal called the area of Martegiani. The neovascularization stimulates fibroplasia and vitreous fibrosis. Contraction of vitreoretinal membranes and progression of posterior vitreous detachment frequently tear the delicate new vessels, causing subhyaloid and vitreous hemorrhage. Organization of hemorrhage, in turn, engenders a vicious cycle of additional fibrosis, traction, and hemorrhage. Localized tractional detachment of the macula often occurs because the vitreous typically remains adherent to the temporal arcades of the major retinal vessels. The vascularized bridge of detached vitreous contracts, causing retinal-retinal traction (Fig. 9-25B). Antero-posterior traction also contributes to the retinal detachment (Fig. 9-25A).

Eyes with proliferative diabetic retinopathy are also prone to develop **neovascularization of the iris (NVI)** and **NVG** (Fig. 8-11). NVI is caused by the anterior diffusion of VEGF. NVI (initially called *rubeosis iridis diabetica*) may develop or progress markedly after intracapsular cataract extraction, which presumably removes a barrier to diffusion. Iris neovascularization usually starts near the pupillary border and in the angle.

The normal architecture of the iris is flattened and effaced by the fibrovascular membrane on its normally avascular anterior surface. Secondary closed-angle glaucoma results

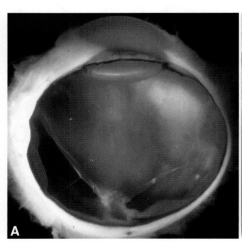
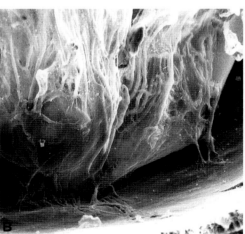

Fig. 9-29. Proliferative diabetic retinopathy. A. Eye obtained postmortem from patient with chronic type I diabetes mellitus has tractional detachment of posterior retina caused by vitreoretinal neovascularization. Detachment is seen at higher magnification in Figure 9-25A. **B.** Scanning electron microscopy discloses new vessels proliferating on scaffold of posteriorly detached vitreous. (**B.** SEM ×40)

when the formation of adhesions between the peripheral iris and the trabecular meshwork called peripheral anterior synechiae blocks aqueous outflow.

A rarer, more innocuous form of diabetic iridopathy called **lacy vacuolization of the iris pigment epithelium** occurs in some patients (Fig. 9-30B–D). Lacy vacuolization is marked by accumulation of glycogen in cystoid spaces within the iris pigment epithelium. The focal glycogenosis of the iris pigment epithelium is thought to be related to chronically elevated levels of blood glucose and may be analogous to accumulation of glycogen in the renal tubules called Armanni-Ebstein glycogen nephropathy. Transient pigmentation of aqueous humor observed intraoperatively in some diabetics may reflect pigment epithelial damage caused by lacy vacuolization. Lacy vacuolization may be evident during slit lamp biomicroscopy as a faint moth-eaten pattern of iris transillumination.

Basement membrane thickening occurs throughout the body in diabetic patients. Thickening of the basement membrane of the pigmented ciliary epithelium occurs in many diabetic eyes and is a helpful histologic marker for the disease (Fig. 9-30A). An analogous thickening of the glomerular basement membrane is found in the Kimmelstiel-Wilson form of diabetic nephropathy. Thickening of the corneal epithelial basement membrane can predispose to sheetlike desquamation of corneal epithelium during vitreoretinal surgery.

Cataracts also complicate diabetes mellitus. A specific form of diabetic cataract may be the presenting manifestation of the disease. Relatively rare, such cataracts probably are caused by the osmotic effect of sorbitol accumulation in the lens. Such opacities may be partially reversible if blood sugar levels are normalized. Diabetics also develop typical senile cataracts at an earlier age. Variable refractive errors in diabetics reflect changes in lens hydration caused by hyperglycemia. Patients usually become more myopic when their blood sugar is elevated.

Diabetics also are at increased risk for infection. One of the most serious infections that can complicate diabetes is mucormycosis. Poorly controlled diabetics who are acidotic are particularly at risk for infection by normally saprophytic fungi in the order *Mucorales*. The fungal infection begins in the paranasal sinuses and then invades the orbital tissues secondarily. Usually evident in routine sections stained with hematoxylin and eosin (H&E), the large nonseptate fungal hyphae typically invade vessels, producing thrombosis and necrosis (Fig. 14-5). Neural invasion is also common. In rare instances, diabetes mellitus may present with unilateral or even bilateral central retinal artery occlusion caused by mucormycosis.

SICKLE HEMOGLOBINOPATHY

Vitreoretinal neovascularization is a characteristic finding in patients who have sickle hemoglobinopathy, particularly hemoglobin SC disease. Occlusion of peripheral retinal vessels by sickled erythrocytes causes extensive capillary nonperfusion and inner ischemic atrophy of the peripheral retina, particularly the longer arc of the temporal retina. Neovascularization develops within the retina just behind the characteristically abrupt junction between its peripheral ischemic nonperfused and posterior perfused parts and then extends into the vitreous. The appearance of the neovascular fronds has been likened to that of the marine organism *Gorgonia flabellum*, the sea fan. The sea fans bleed causing vitreous hemorrhage. Vitreoretinal traction caused by organization of the vitreous blood produces holes in the retina that cause rhegmatogenous retinal detachment.

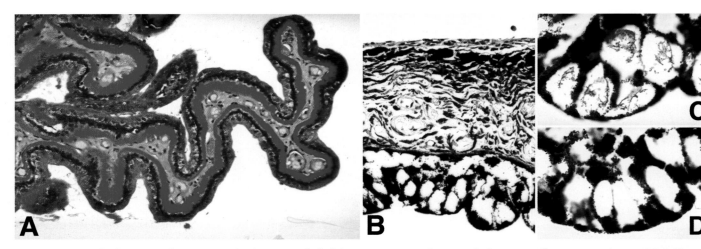

Fig. 9-30. A. Thickening of pigmented ciliary epithelial basement membrane, diabetes mellitus. Periodic acid-Schiff stain accentuates massive thickening of the basement membrane of pigmented pars plicata ciliary epithelium in eye from a relatively young diabetic patient. **B. Diabetic iridopathy.** A fibrovascular membrane flattens the anterior iridic surface. Multiple vacuoles impart a lacy appearance to the thickened iris pigment epithelium. **C.** The vacuoles are filled with PAS-positive granules of glycogen. **D.** Diastase digestion abolishes PAS staining, confirming that the material is glycogen. (**A.** PAS ×100, **B.** H&E ×50, **C.** PAS ×250, **D.** PAS after diastase digestion ×250)

Neovascularization is more likely to occur in patients with Hb SC disease because they are less anemic than patients with sickle cell anemia (Hb SS disease), and vascular occlusion is more apt to occur when the hematocrit is higher. Pigmented scars called black sunburst signs caused by chorioretinal hemorrhage are more common in patients with Hb SS disease. The partial resorption of hemorrhages in these patients is evident clinically as salmon patches. Angioid streaks also occur in a small number of patients with sickle hemoglobinopathy. It has been postulated that the deposition of iron in Bruch membrane somehow predisposes to massive calcification of Bruch membrane.

BIBLIOGRAPHY

General Reference

Green W. Pathology of the retina. In: Spencer W, ed. *Ophthalmic Pathology: An Atlas and Textbook*, vol. 2. Philadelphia, PA: WB Saunders, 1996:667–1331.

Albinism and Other Developmental Anomalies

Bergsma D, Kaiser-Kupfer M. A new form of albinism. *Am J Ophthalmol* 1974;77:837–844.

Blume R, Wolff S. The Chediak-Higashi syndrome: studies in four patients and a review of the literature. *Medicine* 1972;51:247–280.

Dessinioti C, Stratigos AJ, Rigopoulos D, et al. A review of genetic disorders of hypopigmentation: lessons learned from the biology of melanocytes. *Exp Dermatol* 2009;18:741–749.

Di Pietro SM, Dell'Angelica EC. The cell biology of Hermansky-Pudlak syndrome: recent advances. *Traffic* 2005;6:525–533.

Falls H. Sex-linked ocular albinism displaying typical fundus changes in the female heterozygote. *Am J Ophthalmol* 1951;34:41–50.

Garrod A. *Inborn Errors of Metabolism*. London, UK: Frowde, 1909.

Gronskov K, Ek J, Brondum-Nielsen K. Oculocutaneous albinism. *Orphanet J Rare Dis* 2007;2:43.

Hornyak TJ. The developmental biology of melanocytes and its application to understanding human congenital disorders of pigmentation. *Adv Dermatol* 2006;22:201–218.

Huizing M, Anikster Y, Gahl WA. Hermansky-Pudlak syndrome and Chediak-Higashi syndrome: disorders of vesicle formation and trafficking. *Thromb Haemost* 2001;86:233–245.

King R, Creel D, Cervenka J, et al. Albinism in Nigeria with delineation of a new recessive oculocutaneous type. *Clin Genet* 1980;17:259–270.

Kirkwood BJ. Albinism and its implications with vision. *Insight* 2009;34:13–16.

Messmer E, Font RL, Laqua H, et al. Cavernous hemangioma of the retina. Immunohistochemical and ultrastructural observations. *Arch Ophthalmol* 1984;102:413–418.

Mietz H, Green WR, Wolff SM, et al. Foveal hypoplasia in complete oculocutaneous albinism. A histopathologic study. *Retina* 1992;12:254–260.

Naumann GOH, Lerche W, Schroeder W. Foveola-Aplasie bei Tyrosinase-positivem oculocutanem Albinismus. *Graefes Arch Clin Exp Ophthalmol* 1976;200:39–50.

O'Donnell Fe Jr, Green WR, Fleischman JA, et al. X-linked ocular albinism in Blacks. Ocular albinism cum pigmento. *Arch Ophthalmol* 1978;96:1189–1192.

O'Donnell FJ, Hambrick GJ, Green W, et al. X-linked ocular albinism: an oculocutaneous macromelanosomal disorder. *Arch Ophthalmol* 1976;94:1883–1892.

O'Donnell FJ, King R, WR G, et al. Autosomal recessively inherited ocular albinism: A new form of ocular albinism affecting women as severely as men. *Arch Ophthalmol* 1978;96:1621–1625.

Oetting WS, Fryer JP, Shriram S, et al. Oculocutaneous albinism type 1: the last 100 years. *Pigment Cell Res* 2003;16:307–311.

Ray K, Chaki M, Sengupta M. Tyrosinase and ocular diseases: some novel thoughts on the molecular basis of oculocutaneous albinism type 1. *Prog Retin Eye Res* 2007;26:323–358.

Read AP; Newton VE. Waardenburg syndrome. *J Med Genet* 1997;34:656–665.

Russell-Eggitt I. Albinism. *Ophthalmol Clin North Am* 2001;14:533–546.

Scheinfeld NS. Syndromic albinism: a review of genetics and phenotypes. *Dermatol Online J* 2003;9:5.

Shiflett SL, Kaplan J, Ward DM. Chediak-Higashi Syndrome: a rare disorder of lysosomes and lysosome related organelles. *Pigment Cell Res* 2002;15:251–257.

Straatsma BR, Foos RY, Heckenlively J, et al. Myelinated retinal nerve fibers. *Am J Ophthalmol* 1981;91:25–38.

Straatsma BR, Foos RY, Heckenlively JR, et al. Myelinated retinal nerve fibers associated with ipsilateral myopia, amblyopia and nystagmus. *Am J Ophthalmol* 1979;88:506–510.

Tran T, Kaufman LM. The child's eye in systemic diseases. *Pediatr Clin North Am* 2003;50:241–258.

Wei ML. Hermansky-Pudlak syndrome: a disease of protein trafficking and organelle function. *Pigment Cell Res* 2006;19:19–42.

Wong L, O'Donnell FE Jr, Green WR. Giant pigment granules in the retinal pigment epithelium of a fetus with X-linked ocular albinism. *Ophthalmic Paediatr Genet* 1983;2:47–65.

Retinal Hemorrhages and Exudates

Ashton N. Pathological and ultrastructural aspect of the cotton-wool spots. *Proc R Soc Med* 1969;62:1271–1276.

Ashton N. Pathophysiology of retinal cotton-wool spots. *Br Med Bull* 1970;26:143–150.

Ashton N, Harry J. The pathology of cotton-wool spots and cytoid bodies in hypertensive retinopathy and other diseases. *Trans Ophthalmol Soc U K* 1963;83:91–114.

Cunha-Vaz JG. The blood-retinal barriers. *Doc Ophthalmol* 1976;41:287–327.

Duane TD, Osher RH, Green WR. White centered hemorrhages: their significance. *Ophthalmology* 1980;87:66–69.

Wolter JR. Pathology of a cotton-wool spot. *Am J Ophthalmol* 1959;48:473–485.

Wolter JR. Axonal enlargements in the nerve-fiber layer of the human retina. *Am J Ophthalmol* 1968;65:1–12.

Angioid Streaks

Dreyer R, Green WR. Pathology of angioid streaks. *Trans Pa Acad Ophthalmol Otolaryngol* 1978;31:158–167.

Jampol LM, Acheson R, Eagle RC Jr, et al. Calcification of Bruch's membrane in angioid streaks with homozygous sickle cell disease. *Arch Ophthalmol* 1987;105:93–98.

Retinal Artery Occlusion

Arruga J, Sanders MD. Ophthalmologic findings in 70 patients with evidence of retinal embolism. *Ophthalmology* 1982;89:1336–1347.

Ball CJ. Atheromatous embolism to the brain, retina, and choroid. *Arch Ophthalmol* 1966;76:690–695.

Brownstein S, Font RL, Alper MG. Atheromatous plaques of the retinal blood vessels. *Arch Ophthalmol* 1973;90:49–52.

Dahrling BE. The histopathology of early central retinal artery occlusion. *Arch Ophthalmol* 1965;73:506–510.

Fineman MS, Savino PJ, Federman JL, et al. Branch retinal artery occlusion as the initial sign of giant cell arteritis. *Am J Ophthalmol* 1996;122:428–430.

Jampol LM, Setogawa T, Rednam KR, et al. Talc retinopathy in primates. A model of ischemic retinopathy: I. Clinical studies. *Arch Ophthalmol* 1981;99:1273–1280.

Jampol LM, Wong AS, Albert DM. Atrial myxoma and central retinal artery occlusion. *Am J Ophthalmol* 1973;75:242–249.

Levine SR, Crofts JW, Lesser GR, et al. Visual symptoms associated with the presence of a lupus anticoagulant. *Ophthalmology* 1988;95:686–692.

McDonnell PJ, Moore GW, Miller NR, et el.Temporal arteritis. A clinicopathologic study. *Ophthalmology* 1986;93:518–530.

Mckibbin DW, Gott VL, Hutchins GM. Fatal cerebral atheromatous embolization after cardiopulmonary bypass. *J Thorac Cardiovasc Surg* 1976;71:741–745.

Penner R, Font RL. Retinal embolism from calcified vegetations of aortic valve. Spontaneous complications of rheumatic heart disease. *Arch Ophthalmol* 1969;81:565–568.

Pfaffenbach DD, Hollenhorst RW. Morbidity and survivorship of patients with embolic cholesterol crystals in the ocular fundus. *Trans Am Ophthalmol Soc* 1972;70:337–349.

Pulido JS, Ward LM, Fishman GA, et al. Antiphospholipid antibodies associated with retinal vascular disease. *Retina* 1987;7:215–218.

Wang FM, Henkind P. Visual system involvement in giant cell (temporal) arteritis. *Surv Ophthalmol* 1979;23:264–271.

Weyand CM. The Dunlop-Dottridge Lecture: the pathogenesis of giant cell arteritis. *J Rheumatol* 2000;27:517–522.

Weyand CM, Goronzy JJ. Pathogenic principles in giant cell arteritis. *Int J Cardiol* 2000;75(Suppl 1):S9–S15, discussion S17–S19.

Weyand CM, Goronzy JJ. Giant-cell arteritis and polymyalgia rheumatica. *Ann Intern Med* 2003;139:505–515.

Weyand CM, Goronzy JJ. Medium- and large-vessel vasculitis. *N Engl J Med* 2003;349:160–169.

Retinal Vein Occlusion

Frangieh GT, Green WR, Barraquer-Somer E, et al. Histopathologic study of nine branch retinal vein occlusions in eight eyes of seven patients. *Arch Ophthalmol* 1982;100:1132–1140.

Green WR, Chan CC, Hutchins GM, et al. Central retinal vein occlusion: a prospective histopathologic study of 29 eyes of 28 patients. *Trans Am Ophthalmol Soc* 1981;79:371–422.

Hayreh SS. Pathogenesis of occlusion of the central retinal vessels. *Am J Ophthalmol* 1971;72:998–1011.

Rothstein T. Bilateral retinal vein closure as the initial manifestation of polycythemia. *Am J Ophthalmol* 1972;74:256–260.

Hypertensive Retinopathy

Garner A, Ashton N. Pathogenesis of hypertensive retinopathy: a review. *J R Soc Med* 1979;72:362–365.

Garner A, Ashton N, Tripathi R, et al. Pathogenesis of hypertensive retinopathy. An experimental study in the monkey. *Br J Ophthalmol* 1975;59:3–44.

Hayreh SS, Servais GE, Virdi PS. Fundus lesions in malignant hypertension. VI. Hypertensive choroidopathy. *Ophthalmology* 1986;93:1383–1400.

Tso MO, Jampol LM. Pathophysiology of hypertensive retinopathy. *Ophthalmology* 1982;89:1132–1145.

Walsh JB. Hypertensive retinopathy. Description, classification, and prognosis. *Ophthalmology* 1982;89:1127–1131.

Age-Related Maculopathy

Allikmets R, Shroyer NF, Singh N, et al. Mutation of the Stargardt disease gene (ABCR) in age-related macular degeneration. *Science* 1997;277:1805–1807.

Anderson DH, Mullins RF, Hageman GS, et al. A role for local inflammation in the formation of drusen in the aging eye. *Am J Ophthalmol* 2002;134:411–431.

Bressler NM, Silva JC, Bressler SB, et al. Clinicopathologic correlation of drusen and retinal pigment epithelial abnormalities in age-related macular degeneration. *Retina* 1994;14:130–142.

Bressler SB, Silva JC, Bressler NM, et al. Clinicopathologic correlation of occult choroidal neovascularization in age-related macular degeneration. *Arch Ophthalmol* 1992;110:827–832.

Bynoe LA, Chang TS, Funata M, et al. Histopathologic examination of vascular patterns in subfoveal neovascular membranes. *Ophthalmology* 1994;101:1112–1117.

Curcio CA, Johnson M, Huang JD, et al. Aging, age-related macular degeneration, and the response-to-retention of apolipoprotein B-containing lipoproteins. *Prog Retin Eye Res* 2009;28:393–422.

el Baba F, Jarrett WHd, Harbin TS Jr, et al. Massive hemorrhage complicating age-related macular degeneration. Clinicopathologic correlation and role of anticoagulants. *Ophthalmology* 1986;93:1581–2592.

Gehrs KM, Anderson DH, Johnson LV, et al. Age-related macular degeneration–emerging pathogenetic and therapeutic concepts. *Ann Med* 2006;38:450–471.

Gorin MB, Breitner JC, De Jong PT, et al. The genetics of age-related macular degeneration. *Mol Vis* 1999;5:29.

Green WR. Clinicopathologic studies of treated choroidal neovascular membranes. A review and report of two cases. *Retina* 1991;11:328–356.

Green WR, Enger C. Age-related macular degeneration histopathologic studies. The 1992 Lorenz E. Zimmerman Lecture. *Ophthalmology* 1993;100:1519–1535.

Green WR, McDonnell PJ, Yeo JH. Pathologic features of senile macular degeneration. *Ophthalmology* 1985;92:615–627.

Grossniklaus HE, Hutchinson AK, Capone A Jr, et al. Clinicopathologic features of surgically excised choroidal neovascular membranes. *Ophthalmology* 1994;101:1099–1111.

Hageman GS, Anderson DH, Johnson LV, et al. A common haplotype in the complement regulatory gene factor H (HF1/CFH) predisposes individuals to age-related macular degeneration. *Proc Natl Acad Sci U S A* 2005;102:7227–7232.

Hageman GS, Mullins RF. Molecular composition of drusen as related to substructural phenotype. *Mol Vis* 1999;5:28.

Jager RD, Mieler WF, Miller JW. Age-related macular degeneration. *N Engl J Med* 2008;358:2606–2617.

Johnson LV, Anderson DH. Age-related macular degeneration and the extracellular matrix. *N Engl J Med* 2004;351:320–322.

Johnson LV, Leitner WP, Staples MK, et al. Complement activation and inflammatory processes in Drusen formation and age related macular degeneration. *Exp Eye Res* 2001;73:887–896.

Johnson LV, Ozaki S, Staples MK, et al. A potential role for immune complex pathogenesis in drusen formation. *Exp Eye Res* 2000;70:441–449.

Johnson PT, Betts KE, Radeke MJ, et al. Individuals homozygous for the age-related macular degeneration risk-conferring variant of complement factor H have elevated levels of CRP in the choroid. *Proc Natl Acad Sci U S A* 2006;103:17456–17461.

Johnson PT, Lewis GP, Talaga KC, et al. Drusen-associated degeneration in the retina. *Invest Ophthalmol Vis Sci* 2003;44:4481–4488.

Kenyon KR, Maumenee AE, Ryan SJ, et al. Diffuse drusen and associated complications. *Am J Ophthalmol* 1985;100:119–128.

Rudolf M, Clark ME, Chimento MF, et al. Prevalence and morphology of druse types in the macula and periphery of eyes with age-related maculopathy. *Invest Ophthalmol Vis Sci* 2008;49:1200–1209.

Rudolf M, Malek G, Messinger JD, et al. Sub-retinal drusenoid deposits in human retina: organization and composition. *Exp Eye Res* 2008;87:402–408.

Russell SR, Mullins RF, Schneider BL, et al. Location, substructure, and composition of basal laminar drusen compared with drusen associated with aging and age-related macular degeneration. *Am J Ophthalmol* 2000;129:205–214.

Spraul CW, Grossniklaus HE. Characteristics of Drusen and Bruch's membrane in postmortem eyes with age-related macular degeneration. *Arch Ophthalmol* 1997;115:267–273.

Spraul CW, Lang GE, Grossniklaus HE. Morphometric analysis of the choroid, Bruch's membrane, and retinal pigment epithelium in eyes with age-related macular degeneration [see comments]. *Invest Ophthalmol Vis Sci* 1996;37:2724–2735.

Other Macula Degenerations

Boozalis GT, Schachat AP, Green WR. Subretinal neovascularization from the retina in radiation retinopathy. *Retina* 1987;7:156–161.

Dastgheib K, Green WR. Granulomatous reaction to Bruch's membrane in age-related macular degeneration. *Arch Ophthalmol* 1994;112:813–818.

Grossniklaus HE, Green WR. Pathologic findings in pathologic myopia. *Retina* 1992;12:127–133.

Saxe SJ, Grossniklaus HE, Lopez PF, et al. Ultrastructural features of surgically excised subretinal neovascular membranes in the ocular histoplasmosis syndrome. *Arch Ophthalmol* 1993;111:88–95.

Toxic Maculopathies

Bernstein HN. Some iatrogenic ocular diseases from systemically administered drugs. *Int Ophthalmol Clin* 1970;10:553–587.

Henkind P, Rothfield NF. Ocular abnormalities in patients treated with synthetic antimalarial drugs. *N Engl J Med* 1963;269: 433–439.

Ramsey MS, Fine BS. Chloroquine toxicity in the human eye: histopathologic observations by electron microscopy. *Am J Ophthalmol* 1972;73:229–235.

Rosenthal AR, Kolb H, Bergsma D, et al. Chloroquine retinopathy in the rhesus monkey. *Invest Ophthalmol Vis Sci* 1978;17:1158–1175.

Smith RS, Berson EL. Acute toxic effects of chloroquine on the cat retina: ultrastructural changes. *Invest Ophthalmol Vis Sci* 1971;10:237–246.

Wetterholm DH, Winter FC. Histopathology of chloroquine retinal toxicity. *Arch Ophthalmol* 1964;71:82–87.

Macular Dystrophies

Allikmets R, Singh N, Sun H, et al. A photoreceptor cell-specific ATP-binding transporter gene (ABCR) is mutated in recessive Stargardt macular dystrophy. *Nat Genet* 1997;15:236–246.

Armstrong JD, Meyer D, Xu S, et al. Long-term follow-up of Stargardt's disease and fundus flavimaculatus. *Ophthalmology* 1998;105:448–457, discussion 457–448.

Boon CJ, Theelen T, Hoefsloot EH, et al. Clinical and molecular genetic analysis of best vitelliform macular dystrophy. *Retina* 2009;29:835–847.

Chong NH, Alexander RA, Gin T, et al. TIMP-3, collagen, and elastin immunohistochemistry and histopathology of Sorsby's fundus dystrophy. *Invest Ophthalmol Vis Sci* 2000;41:898–902.

Davidson AE, Millar ID, Urquhart JE, et al. Missense mutations in a retinal pigment epithelium protein, bestrophin-1, cause retinitis pigmentosa. *Am J Hum Genet* 2009;85:581–592.

Demirci FY, Gupta N, Radak AL, et al. Histopathologic study of X-linked cone-rod dystrophy (CORDX1) caused by a mutation in the RPGR exon ORF15. *Am J Ophthalmol* 2005;139:386–388.

Eagle RC, Lucier AC, Bernardino VB, et al. Retinal pigment epithelial abnormalities in fundus flavimaculatus: a light and electron microscopic study. *Ophthalmology* 1980;87:1189–1200.

Frangieh GT, Green WR, Fine SL. A histopathologic study of Best's macular dystrophy. *Arch Ophthalmol* 1982;100:1115–1121.

Guziewicz KE, Zangerl B, Lindauer SJ, et al. Bestrophin gene mutations cause canine multifocal retinopathy: a novel animal model for best disease. *Invest Ophthalmol Vis Sci* 2007;48: 1959–1967.

Klevering BJ, Deutman AF, Maugeri A, et al. The spectrum of retinal phenotypes caused by mutations in the ABCA4 gene. *Graefes Arch Clin Exp Ophthalmol* 2005;243:90–100.

Koenekoop RK. The gene for Stargardt disease, ABCA4, is a major retinal gene: a mini-review. *Ophthalmic Genet* 2003;24:75–80.

Lois N, Halfyard AS, Bird AC, et al. Fundus autofluorescence in Stargardt macular dystrophy-fundus flavimaculatus. *Am J Ophthalmol* 2004;138:55–63.

Lois N, Holder GE, Bunce C, et al. Phenotypic subtypes of Stargardt macular dystrophy-fundus flavimaculatus. *Arch Ophthalmol* 2001;119:359–369.

Lopez PF, Maumenee IH, de la Cruz Z, et al. Autosomal-dominant fundus flavimaculatus. Clinicopathologic correlation. *Ophthalmology* 1990;97:798–809.

O'Gorman S, Flaherty WA, Fishman GA, et al. Histopathologic findings in Best's vitelliform macular dystrophy. *Arch Ophthalmol* 1988;106:1261–1268.

Querques G, Regenbogen M, Quijano C, et al. High-definition optical coherence tomography features in vitelliform macular dystrophy. *Am J Ophthalmol* 2008;146:501–507.

Spaide RF, Noble K, Morgan A, et al. Vitelliform macular dystrophy. *Ophthalmology* 2006;113:1392–1400.

Weingeist TA, Kobrin JL, Watzke RC. Histopathology of Best's macular dystrophy. *Arch Ophthalmol* 1982;100:1108–1114.

Zhang K, Nguyen TH, Crandall A, et al. Genetic and molecular studies of macular dystrophies: recent developments. *Surv Ophthalmol* 1995;40:51–61.

Gyrate Atrophy

Kaiser-Kupfer MI, Valle D, Del Valle LA. A specific enzyme defect in gyrate atrophy. *Am J Ophthalmol* 1978;85:200–204.

Kuwabara T, Ishikawa Y, Kaiser-Kupfer MI. Experimental model of gyrate atrophy in animals. *Ophthalmology* 1981;88:331–334.

Wilson DJ, Weleber RG, Green WR. Ocular clinicopathologic study of gyrate atrophy. *Am J Ophthalmol* 1991;111:24–33.

Retinitis Pigmentosa

Drack AV, Traboulsi EI. Systemic associations of pigmentary retinopathy. *Int Ophthalmol Clin* 1991;31:35–59.

Dryja TP. Doyne Lecture. Rhodopsin and autosomal dominant retinitis pigmentosa. *Eye* 1992;6:1–10.

Dryja TP. Gene-based approach to human gene-phenotype correlations. *Proc Natl Acad Sci U S A* 1997;94:12117–12121.

Dryja TP, Hahn LB, Kajiwara K, et al. Dominant and digenic mutations in the peripherin/RDS and ROM1 genes in retinitis pigmentosa. *Invest Ophthalmol Vis Sci* 1997;38:1972–1982.

Dryja TP, Li T. Molecular genetics of retinitis pigmentosa. *Hum Mol Genet* 1995;4:1739–1743.

Dryja TP, McGee TL, Hahn LB, et al. Mutations within the rhodopsin gene in patients with autosomal dominant retinitis pigmentosa. *N Engl J Med* 1990;323:1302–1307.

Fingert JH, Oh K, Chung M, et al. Association of a novel mutation in the retinol dehydrogenase 12 (RDH12) gene with autosomal dominant retinitis pigmentosa. *Arch Ophthalmol* 2008;126:1301–1307.

Hartong DT, Berson EL, Dryja TP. Retinitis pigmentosa. *Lancet* 2006;368:1795–1809.

Huang SH, Pittler SJ, Huang X, et al. Autosomal recessive retinitis pigmentosa caused by mutations in the alpha subunit of rod cGMP phosphodiesterase. *Nat Genet* 1995;11:468–471.

Li ZY, Possin DE, Milam AH. Histopathology of bone spicule pigmentation in retinitis pigmentosa. *Ophthalmology* 1995;102:805–816.

Luckenbach MW, Green WR, Miller NR, et al. Ocular clinico-pathologic correlation of Hallervorden-Spatz syndrome with acanthocytosis and pigmentary retinopathy. *Am J Ophthalmol* 1983;95:369–382.

Sandberg MA, Weigel-DiFranco C, Dryja TP, et al. Clinical expression correlates with location of rhodopsin mutation in dominant retinitis pigmentosa. *Invest Ophthalmol Vis Sci* 1995;36:1934–1942.

Sippel KC, DeStefano JD, Berson EL, et al. Evaluation of the human arrestin gene in patients with retinitis pigmentosa and stationary night blindness. *Invest Ophthalmol Vis Sci* 1998;39:665–670.

Choroideremia

Cameron JD, Fine BS, Shapiro I. Histopathologic observations in choroideremia with emphasis on vascular changes of the uveal tract. *Ophthalmology* 1987;94:187–196.

MacDonald IM, Chen MH, Addison DJ, et al. Histopathology of the retinal pigment epithelium of a female carrier of choroideremia. *Can J Ophthalmol* 1997;32:329–333.

Rodrigues MM, Ballintine EJ, Wiggert BN, et al. Choroideremia: a clinical, electron microscopic, and biochemical report. *Ophthalmology* 1984;91:873–883.

Seabra MC, Brown MS, Goldstein JL. Retinal degeneration in choroideremia: deficiency of rab geranylgeranyl transferase. *Science* 1993;259:377–381.

Other Heritable Disorders

Bergsma DR Jr, Chen CJ. The Mizuo phenomenon in Oguchi disease. *Arch Ophthalmol* 1997;115:560–561.

Bensaoula T, Shibuya H, Katz ML, et al. Histopathologic and immunocytochemical analysis of the retina and ocular tissues in Batten disease. *Ophthalmology* 2000;107:1746–1753.

Carrero-Valenzuela RD, Klein ML, Weleber RG, et al. Sorsby fundus dystrophy. A family with the Ser181Cys mutation of the tissue inhibitor of metalloproteinases 3. *Arch Ophthalmol* 1996;114:737–738.

Dryja TP. Molecular genetics of Oguchi disease, fundus albipunctatus, and other forms of stationary night blindness: LVII Edward Jackson Memorial Lecture. *Am J Ophthalmol* 2000;130:547–563.

Edwards AO. Clinical features of the congenital vitreoretinopathies. *Eye (Lond)* 2008;22:1233–1242.

Fishman GA, Roberts MF, Derlacki DJ, et al. Novel mutations in the cellular retinaldehyde-binding protein gene (RLBP1) associated with retinitis punctata albescens: evidence of interfamilial genetic heterogeneity and fundus changes in heterozygotes. *Arch Ophthalmol* 2004;122:70–75.

Jacobson SG, Aleman TS, Cideciyan AV, et al. Identifying photoreceptors in blind eyes caused by RPE65 mutations: prerequisite for human gene therapy success. *Proc Natl Acad Sci U S A* 2005;102:6177–6182.

Jacobson SG, Cideciyan AV, Aleman TS, et al. Leber congenital amaurosis caused by an RPGRIP1 mutation shows treatment potential. *Ophthalmology* 2007;114:895–898.

Nakazawa M, Wada Y, Fuchs S, et al. Oguchi disease: phenotypic characteristics of patients with the frequent 1147delA mutation in the arrestin gene. *Retina* 1997;17:17–22.

Nichols BE, Drack AV, Vandenburgh K, et al. A 2 base pair deletion in the RDS gene associated with butterfly-shaped pigment dystrophy of the fovea. *Hum Mol Genet* 1993;2:601–603.

Shastry BS, Hejtmancik JF, Trese MT. Identification of novel missense mutations in the Norrie disease gene associated with one X-linked and four sporadic cases of familial exudative vitreoretinopathy. *Hum Mutat* 1997;9:396–401.

Sieving PA, Boskovich S, Bingham E, et al. Sorsby's fundus dystrophy in a family with a Ser-181-CVS mutation in the TIMP-3 gene: poor outcome after laser photocoagulation. *Trans Am Ophthalmol Soc* 1996;94:275–294.

Wong F, Goldberg MF, Hao Y. Identification of a nonsense mutation at codon 128 of the Norrie's disease gene in a male infant. *Arch Ophthalmol* 1993;111:1553–1557.

Peripheral Retinal Degenerations

Foos RY. Senile retinoschisis: relationship to cystoid degeneration. *Trans Am Acad Ophthalmol Otolaryngol* 1970;74:33–51.

Foos RY, Feman SS. Reticular cystoid degeneration of the peripheral retina. *Am J Ophthalmol* 1970;69:392–403.

O'Malley PF, Allen RA. Peripheral cystoid degeneration of the retina: incidence and distribution in 1,000 autopsy eyes. *Arch Ophthalmol* 1967;77:769–776.

O'Malley PF, Allen RA, Straatsma BR, et al. Pavingstone degeneration of the retina. *Arch Ophthalmol* 1965;73:169–182.

Straatsma BR, Foos RY. Typical and reticular degenerative retinoschisis. XXVI Francis I. Proctor memorial lecture. *Am J Ophthalmol* 1973;75:551–575.

Zimmerman LE, Spencer WH. The pathologic anatomy of retinoschisis: with a report of two cases diagnosed clinically as malignant melanoma. *Arch Ophthalmol* 1960;63:10–19.

Juvenile Retinoschisis

Condon GP, Brownstein S, Wang NS, et al. Congenital hereditary (juvenile X-linked) retinoschisis. Histopathologic and ultrastructural findings in three eyes. *Arch Ophthalmol* 1986;104:576–583.

Harris GS, Yeung J. Maculopathy of sex-linked juvenile retinoschisis. *Can J Ophthalmol* 1976;11:1–10.

Manschot WA. Pathology of hereditary juvenile retinoschisis. *Arch Ophthalmol* 1972;88:131–138.

Yanoff M, Kertesz Rahn E, Zimmerman LE. Histopathology of juvenile retinoschisis. *Arch Ophthalmol* 1968;79:49–53.

Lattice Degeneration

Straatsma BR, Allen RA. Lattice degeneration of the retina. *Trans Am Acad Ophthalmol Otolaryngol* 1962;66:600–613.

Streeten BW, Bert M. The retina surface in lattice degeneration of the retina. *Am J Ophthalmol* 1972;74:1201–1209.

Straatsma BR, Zeegan PD, Foos RY, et al. Lattice degeneration of the retina. *Trans Am Acad Ophthalmol Otolaryngol* 1974;78:87–113.

Pars Plana Cysts

Baker T, Spencer W. Ocular findings in multiple myeloma. *Arch Ophthalmol* 1974;91:110–113.

Gärtner J. Fine structure of pars plana cysts. *Am J Ophthalmol* 1972;73:971–984.

Johnson B. Proteinaceous cysts of the ciliary epithelium. II. Their occurrence in nonmyelomatous hypergammaglobulinemic conditions. *Arch Ophthalmol* 1970;84:171–175.

Johnson B, Storey J. Proteinaceous cysts of the ciliary epithelium. I. Their clear nature and immunoelectrophoretic analysis in a case of multiple myeloma. *Arch Ophthalmol* 1970;84:166–170.

Zimmerman L, Fine B. Production of hyaluronic acid by cysts and tumors of the ciliary body. *Arch Ophthalmol* 1964;72:365–379.

Diabetic Retinopathy

Aiello LP. Vascular endothelial growth factor. 20th-century mechanisms, 21st-century therapies. *Invest Ophthalmol Vis Sci* 1997;38:1647–1652.

Aiello LP, Avery RL, Arrigg PG, et al. Vascular endothelial growth factor in ocular fluid of patients with diabetic retinopathy and other retinal disorders. *N Engl J Med* 1994;331:1480–1487.

Cogan DG, Toussaint D, Kuwabara T. Retinal vascular patterns: IV. Diabetic retinopathy. *Arch Ophthalmol* 1961;66:366–378.

D'Amore PA. Mechanisms of retinal and choroidal neovascularization. *Invest Ophthalmol Vis Sci* 1994;35:3974–3979.

DCCT Research Group. The effect of intensive treatment of diabetes in the development and progression of long-term complications in insulin-dependent diabetes. *N Engl J Med* 1993;329:977–986.

Engerman RL, Kern TS. Experimental galactosemia produces diabetic-like retinopathy. *Diabetes* 1984;33:97–100.

Fine BS, Berkow JW, Helfgott JA. Diabetic lacy vacuolization of the iris pigment epithelium. *Am J Ophthalmol* 1970;69:197–200.

Gabbay KH. The sorbitol pathway and the complications of diabetes mellitus. *N Engl J Med* 1973;288:831–836.

Jampol LM, Ebroon DA, Goldbaum MH. Peripheral proliferative retinopathies: an update on angiogenesis, etiologies and management. *Surv Ophthalmol* 1994;38:519–540.

Kador PF, Akagi Y, Takahashi Y, et al. Prevention of retinal vessel changes associated with diabetic retinopathy in galactose-fed dogs by aldose reductase inhibitors. *Arch Ophthalmol* 1990;108:1301–1309.

Klein R, Klein BEK, Moss SE, et al. The Wisconsin epidemologic study of diabetic retinopathy. III. Prevalence and risk of diabetic retinopathy when age of diagnosis is 30 or more years. *Arch Ophthalmol* 1984;102:527–532.

Kuwabara T, Cogan DG. Studies of retinal vascular patterns: I. Normal architecture. *Arch Ophthalmol* 1960;64:904–911.

Yanoff M, Fine BS, Berkow JW. Diabetic lacy vacuolization of iris pigment epithelium. *Am J Ophthalmol* 1970;69:201–210.

Yanoff M. Diabetic retinopathy. *N Engl J Med* 1966;274:1344–1349.

Sickle Retinopathy

Eagle RC Jr, Yanoff M, Fine BS. Hemoglobin SC retinopathy and fat emboli to the eye: a light and electron microscopical study. *Arch Ophthalmol* 1974;92:28–32.

Goldberg MF. Classification and pathogenesis of proliferative sickle retinopathy. *Am J Ophthalmol* 1971;71:649–665.

Romayananda N, Goldberg MF, Green WR. Histopathology of sickle cell retinopathy. *Trans Am Acad Ophthalmol Otolaryngol* 1973;77:652–676.

Macular Holes

Frangieh GT, Green WR, Engel HM. A histopathologic study of macular cysts and holes. *Retina* 1981;1:311–336.

Gass JD. Idiopathic senile macular hole. Its early stages and pathogenesis. *Arch Ophthalmol* 1988;106:629–639.

Gass JD. Reappraisal of biomicroscopic classification of stages of development of a macular hole. *Am J Ophthalmol* 1995;119:752–759.

Yooh HS, Brooks HL Jr, Capone A Jr, et al. Ultrastructural features of tissue removed during idiopathic macular hole. *Am J Ophthalmol* 1996;122:67–75.

Retinal Detachment and Proliferative Vitreoretinopathy

Aaberg TM. Management of anterior and posterior proliferative vitreoretinopathy. XLV. Edward Jackson memorial lecture. *Am J Ophthalmol* 1988;106:519–532.

Elner SG, Elner VM, Diaz-Rohena R, et al. Anterior proliferative vitreoretinopathy. Clinicopathologic, light microscopic, and ultrastructural findings. *Ophthalmology* 1988;95:1349–1357.

Elner SG, Elner VM, Freeman HM, et al. The pathology of anterior (peripheral) proliferative vitreoretinopathy. *Trans Am Ophthalmol Soc* 1988;86:330–353.

Lean JS, Stern WH, Irvine AR, et al. Classification of proliferative vitreoretinopathy used in the silicone study. The Silicone Study Group. *Ophthalmology* 1989;96:765–771.

Lewis H, Aaberg TM, Abrams GW, et al. Subretinal membranes in proliferative vitreoretinopathy. *Ophthalmology* 1989;96:1403–1414.

Lewis H, Burke JM, Abrams GW, et al. Perisilicone proliferation after vitrectomy for proliferative vitreoretinopathy. *Ophthalmology* 1988;95:583–591.

Lopez PF, Grossniklaus HE, Aaberg TM, et al. Pathogenetic mechanisms in anterior proliferative vitreoretinopathy. *Am J Ophthalmol* 1992;114:257–279.

Machemer R. Proliferative vitreoretinopathy (PVR): a personal account of its pathogenesis and treatment. Proctor lecture. *Invest Ophthalmol Vis Sci* 1988;29:1771–1783.

Machemer R, Aaberg TM, Freeman HM, et al. An updated classification of retinal detachment with proliferative vitreoretinopathy. *Am J Ophthalmol* 1991;112:159–165.

Mazure A, Grierson I. In vitro studies of the contractility of cell types involved in proliferative vitreoretinopathy. *Invest Ophthalmol Vis Sci* 1992;33:3407–3416.

Schwartz D, de la Cruz ZC, Green WR, et al. Proliferative vitreoretinopathy. Ultrastructural study of 20 retroretinal membranes removed by vitreous surgery. *Retina* 1988;8:275–281.

Wiedemann P, Weller M. The pathophysiology of proliferative vitreoretinopathy. *Acta Ophthalmol Suppl* 1988;189:3–15.

Wilkes SR, Mansour AM, Green WR. Proliferative vitreoretinopathy. Histopathology of retroretinal membranes. *Retina* 1987;7:94–101.

10 Vitreous

INTRODUCTION

The transparent gelatinous vitreous humor fills most of the interior of the eye. The most delicate connective tissue in the body, the vitreous humor is composed of a framework of thin, randomly oriented, unbranched fibrils of type II collagen and is rich in hyaluronic acid, an extremely large, negatively charged, hydrophilic polysaccharide. Hyaluronic acid is named after the hyaloid body, an older term for the vitreous humor (both *hyaloid* and *vitreous* mean *glassy*).

The collagenous framework of the vitreous humor adheres to the internal limiting membrane (ILM) of the retina, the periphery of the optic disc, and most firmly to the 2-mm wide vitreous base that straddles the ora serrata. The anterior attachment of the vitreous is particularly firm. Relatively severe trauma that typically disrupts the ciliary epithelium is required to detach or avulse the vitreous humor from the vitreous base. In contrast, the posterior attachments of the vitreous are tenuous. **Posterior vitreous detachment** affects many individuals after age 55 years and is found in more than 60% of the population in the eighth decade (Fig. 10-1). Patients usually complain of the abrupt onset of floaters and occasionally light flashes that signify vitreoretinal traction. The peripapillary condensation of the vitreous framework may be evident clinically or macroscopically after detachment as a Weiss ring (Fig. 10-1B).

The vitreous humor contributes to visual loss in two basic ways. First, the vitreous framework serves as a growth scaffold for cellular proliferation, and resultant **vitreoretinal traction** plays an important role in the pathogenesis of many retinal detachments. Second, under pathologic conditions, the transparent medium may be opacified by the accumulation of a variety of materials including blood, acute or chronic inflammatory cells, tumor cells, iridescent particles, and amyloid.

Vitreoretinal adhesions and traction cause retinal holes or breaks that predispose to rhegmatogenous retinal detachment. New blood vessels, cells, and fibrous tissue also proliferate on exposed surfaces of the vitreous framework. Tractional retinal detachment is caused by subsequent organization and contraction of the vitreous. The organization of vitreous hemorrhage or inflammation also stimulates vitreous traction.

Detachment of the vitreous and retina exposes new surfaces that can serve as a substrate for cellular growth. The contraction of delicate glial membranes on the inner retinal surface causes sinuous folds in the ILM (surface wrinkling or cellophane retinopathy) that distort vision (Fig. 10-2). Proliferation of myofibroblasts, retinal pigment epithelial (RPE) cells, and glial cells forms fibrocellular membranes on retinal surfaces exposed by retinal detachment. These membranes can bind the detached retina into a folded mass that may be impossible to reattach surgically. Analogous cellular proliferation can also occur on the detached posterior face of the vitreous, inducing fibrosis. Somewhat analogous to "in vivo tissue culture," this process is called **proliferative vitreoretinopathy (PVR)** or **massive periretinal proliferation (MPP)**. PVR is an important cause

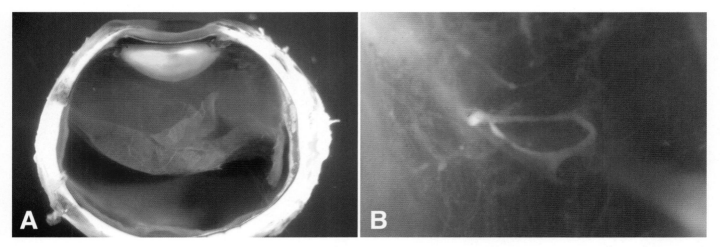

Fig. 10-1. Posterior vitreous detachment. A. Mild opacification by protein accentuates the vitreous. The vitreous framework has detached from the inner retina posteriorly. It remains attached to the anterior vitreous base that straddles the ora serrata. The attachment there is very strong. The anterior chamber is flat, and part of the retina is shallowly detached by a gelatinous exudate rich in lipid. **B.** Weiss ring, posterior vitreous detachment. The white ring represents the peripapillary condensation of the vitreous framework, which has separated from the optic disc during a posterior vitreous detachment.

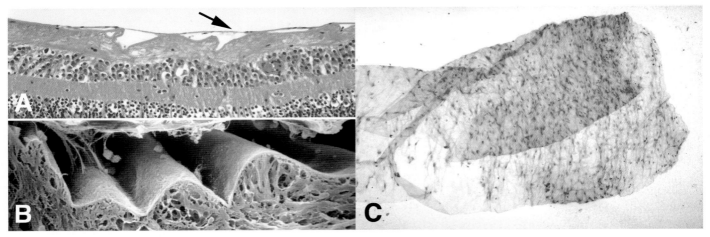

Fig. 10-2. Epiretinal gliosis (surface wrinkling retinopathy). A. *Arrow* denotes delicate membrane of glial cells on inner retinal surface after posterior vitreous detachment. Contraction of the membrane has caused folds in the internal limiting membrane (ILM). **B.** SEM shows folds in ILM. Glial membrane has partially detached. **C.** Vitreoretinal membrane in vitrectomy specimen. Presumed glial cells form a subconfluent membrane on the surface of a condensed sheet of vitreous. The cells have bland spindled nuclei. The indication for vitrectomy was macular pucker. (**A.** H&E ×100, **B.** SEM ×640, **C.** Millipore filter preparation, H&E ×50)

of inoperable retinal detachment, or recurrent detachment after reattachment surgery (Fig. 10-3).

Blood is the substance that opacifies the vitreous most frequently. Common sources of vitreous hemorrhage include trauma, proliferative diabetic retinopathy, and other disorders with vitreoretinal neovascularization, tractional retinal tears, and posterior vitreous detachment. Rarer causes include intraocular tumors, exudative age-related maculopathy, and subarachnoid hemorrhage (Terson syndrome).

Persistent vitreous hemorrhage is a major indication for vitreous surgery. Blood and other opacities in the vitreous are removed by a surgical procedure called vitrectomy that employs miniaturized cutting and aspiration instruments, intraocular illuminators, and laser photocoagulators, which

are inserted through small incisions in the pars plana. The excised vitreous is replaced with saline, which is introduced through an infusion port.

Vitrectomy specimens can be processed using a variety of cytologic techniques including cytocentrifugation, liquid-based monolayer cytology, or Millipore filtration. If particulates are numerous, the fluid can be centrifuged and the pellet embedded in paraffin as a cell block for histology. The latter is particularly helpful if specimen evaluation requires special stains for microorganisms or immunohistochemistry.

Microscopic examination of vitrectomy specimens from patients with chronic **vitreous hemorrhage** discloses blood and blood breakdown products including erythroclasts or erythrocyte ghost cells, hemoglobin spherules, and

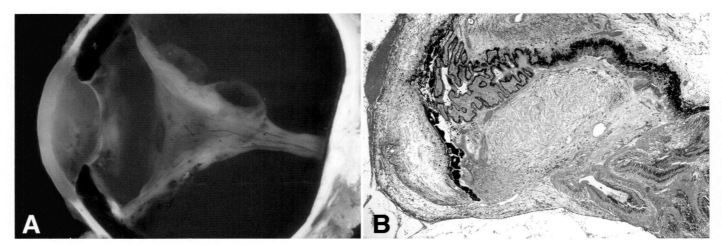

Fig. 10-3. Anterior variant of proliferative vitreoretinopathy (PVR). A. Chronic retinal detachment with macrocysts persists after vitrectomy. PVR membrane extends anteriorly from inner retinal surface to cover ciliary body and iris. Traction draws iris posteriorly. **B.** Fibrosis of residual vitreous overlying ciliary body exerts traction on retina and produces anterior loop retinal detachment. Iris is drawn posteriorly. (**B.** H&E ×10)

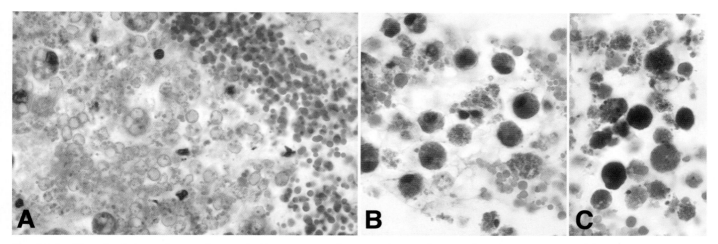

Fig. 10-4. Chronic vitreous hemorrhage. A. Numerous erythrocyte ghost cells or erythroclasts are seen below. Ghost cells are the empty cell membranes of erythrocytes that have lost their hemoglobin-rich cytoplasm. The eosinophilic bodies above are hemoglobin spherules. Macrophages that have ingested ghost cells and other blood breakdown products also are present. **B.** Hemosiderin-laden macrophages, chronic vitreous hemorrhage. The yellow-brown pigment in the macrophages is the blood breakdown product hemosiderin. **C.** The pigment in some of the macrophages in this chronic vitreous hemorrhage stains positively (blue) for iron. Many large hemoglobin spherules are present. (**A.** H&E ×250, **B.** H&E ×250, **C.** Perl stain for iron, ×250)

macrophages laden with ghost cells and golden-brown granules of the blood pigment hemosiderin (Fig. 10-4). In very chronic cases, the blood breakdown products occasionally stimulate a granulomatous inflammatory foreign body response. Hemoglobin spherules may be quite large if the vitreous blood originates from the choroid. Clinically and macroscopically, chronic vitreous hemorrhage typically is yellow-ochre in color and may appear as an "ochre membrane" (Fig. 4-1A). If the anterior face of the vitreous is ruptured, ghost cells and hemosiderin-laden macrophages may enter the anterior chamber and block the trabecular meshwork, causing secondary open-angle glaucoma (ghost cell or hemolytic glaucoma) (Fig. 8-14B).

The vitreous is rapidly opacified by an intense influx of polymorphonuclear leukocytes and macrophages in acute purulent endophthalmitis (Fig. 3-12). A vitreous abscess composed of polys forms in neglected cases or virulent infections. Some of the inflammatory cells in a **vitreous abscess** may be arranged in a linear fashion, reflecting the alignment of the cells along the fibrils of the collagenous vitreous framework. A large solitary vitreous abscess characterizes bacterial endophthalmitis. Fungal endophthalmitis, which generally is a more indolent infection, typically is marked by the presence of multiple smaller vitreous microabscesses (Fig. 3-13). Digestive enzymes released from degenerating polys in a vitreous abscess can cause extensive necrosis of intraocular tissues including retinal destruction (Fig. 3-12B). Vitrectomy is used tosurgically "drain" the vitreous abscess in some patients with endophthalmitis. If vitrectomy is not performed, the vitreous abscess may be organized by an ingrowth of granulation tissue from the ciliary body and choroid. Eventually, a dense collagenous scar elaborated by fibroblasts and metaplastic RPE cells fills the vitreous cavity.

Remnants of the embryonic hyaloid vascular system are seen by patients as innocuous vitreous opacities called **floaters** or *muscae volitantes* ("flying flies"). Patients frequently complain that they see a spot like a moving insect in their peripheral visual field that darts away when they move their eyes. Floaters are especially prevalent in myopes and are caused by syneresis or degeneration of the vitreous framework in the enlarging myopic eye. When light flashes accompany floaters, vitreoretinal traction is present and retinal holes must be excluded by a careful and expedient ophthalmoscopic examination.

Iridescent particles accumulate in the vitreous humor in two disorders: asteroid hyalosis (AH) and synchysis scintillans. **Asteroid hyalosis** (Benson disease) is relatively common, occurring in about 2% of the population (Fig. 10-5). AH was once called asteroid hyalitis, but the name was changed when it became apparent that the disorder is degenerative and not inflammatory in nature. Ironically, histopathologic examination occasionally discloses asteroid bodies enveloped by foreign body giant cells.

Clinical examination with the slit lamp biomicroscope or ophthalmoscope discloses a starry array of white iridescent particles in the vitreous (Fig. 10-5A). The asteroid bodies are firmly attached to the vitreous framework; they move with the vitreous and do not sink to the bottom of the eye (Fig. 10-5D). The iridescent particles are tiny spherules of calcium hydroxyapatite and are not calcium soap as was previously reported. The spherules stain gray with hematoxylin and eosin (H&E), are moderately periodic acid-Schiff (PAS) positive, and show a positive histochemical reaction for calcium (Fig. 10-5B). They display a vivid "Maltese cross" pattern of birefringence on polarization microscopy (Fig. 10-5C).

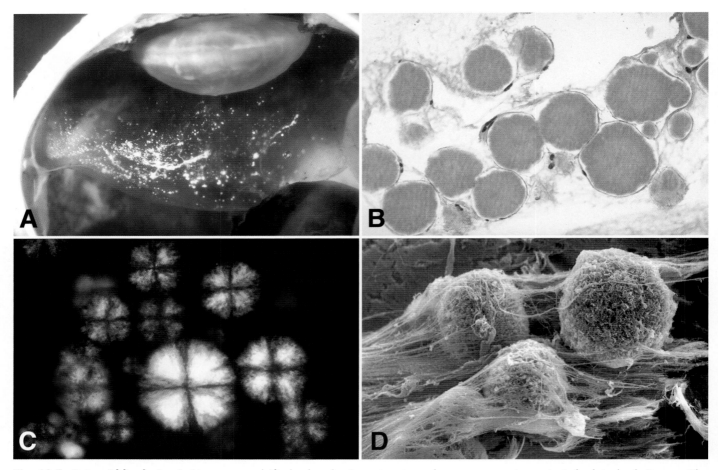

Fig. 10-5. Asteroid hyalosis. A. Numerous calcified spherules impart a starry sky appearance to posteriorly detached vitreous. The asteroid hyalosis was an incidental finding in an eye enucleated for uveal melanoma. **B.** Asteroid bodies appear as grayish blue spherules in routine H&E sections. They are attached to the vitreous framework. **C.** Intact asteroid bodies in vitrectomy specimen show characteristic Maltese cross pattern of birefringence during polarization microscopy. **D.** Scanning electron microscopy (SEM) shows attachment of asteroid bodies to vitreous fibrils. (**B.** H&E ×250, **C.** Millipore filter preparation, H&E with crossed polarizers ×250, **D.** SEM ×640)

How and why the spherules form remains uncertain. A large autopsy cohort study of AH and its systemic associations found no statistically significant correlation between AH and diabetes mellitus. AH was strongly correlated with age and inversely correlated with posterior vitreous detachment.

Synchisis scintillans is an exceedingly rare disorder marked by the accumulation of sparkling crystals of cholesterol in the vitreous (Fig. 10-6). Synchisis scintillans is said to occur bilaterally in young patients who are blind from a chronic degenerative disorder. Although intraocular cholesterol (cholesterolosis bulbi) is not that uncommon, involvement of the vitreous is quite unusual. Cholesterol crystals typically are found in the subretinal fluid of chronic exudative detachments caused by retinal vascular abnormalities (e.g., Coats disease, diabetes, or radiation retinopathy), or less often in the anterior chamber. Blood breakdown is a major source of intraocular cholesterol. Erythrocyte cell membranes are an excellent source of lipid. The cholesterol crystals in synchisis scintillans are not attached to the vitreous framework, and they sink to a dependent position when the eye is at rest.

The first therapeutic vitrectomy was performed for **vitreous amyloidosis** (Fig. 10-7). This rare form of vitreous opacification occurs in patients who have several types of primary familial amyloidosis (familial amyloidotic

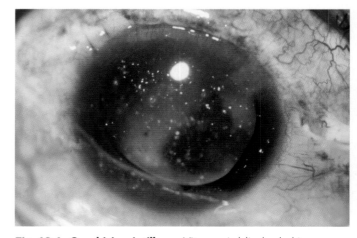

Fig. 10-6. Synchisis scintillans. Vitreous in blind aphakic eye contains blood and glistening polychromatic crystals of cholesterol.

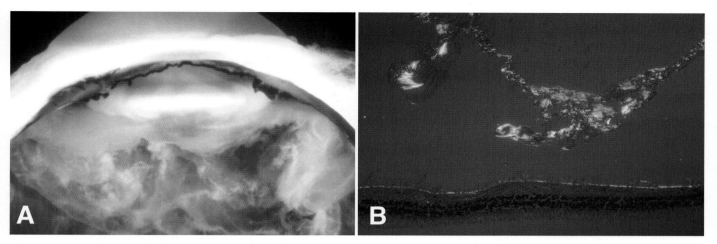

Fig. 10-7. Vitreous amyloidosis. A. Amyloid composed of mutant transport protein transthyretin opacifies the vitreous in eye obtained postmortem from a patient with the Indiana (SER 84) type of hereditary amyloidosis. A vitrectomy has been performed previously. **B.** Amyloid in detached vitreous shows apple-green birefringence during polarization microscopy. Amyloid also lines the inner retinal surface. (**A.** Specimen submitted by Dr. Merrill Benson, Indianapolis, Indiana. **B.** Congo red with crossed polarizers ×25)

polyneuropathy) caused by autosomal recessively inherited allelic missense mutations in the transthyretin (TTR) gene encoding transthyretin, a plasma transport protein for thyroxine and retinol (vitamin A). Many patients who present with vitreous involvement are elderly women who have the Portuguese variant of familial amyloidosis caused by substitution of methionine for valine at codon 30. The family history is typically negative, and vitreous amyloidosis is often the initial manifestation of the disease.

VITREOUS INVOLVEMENT BY TUMOR CELLS

Tumors cells can infiltrate or seed the vitreous humor. A form of primary central nervous system (CNS) **lymphoma** characteristically involves the vitreous and presents with vitreous floaters or visual loss due to vitreous cells. Primary lymphoma of the CNS and retina should be suspected in elderly patients who have chronic vitritis that does not respond to therapy. Although most cases affect elderly patients, the disease also occurs in younger individuals who are immunosuppressed. Vitreous lymphoma is bilateral in 60% to 90% of cases but may be quite asymmetric or seemingly unilateral at onset. Approximately 80% of patients with primary vitreous lymphoma develop CNS lymphoma and most die from CNS disease. Hence, imaging studies and spinal fluid examination are mandatory to exclude CNS involvement. The eye is involved before the CNS in 50% to 80% of cases. Many CNS lesions occur in the frontal lobe and cause behavioral changes or dementia. Most cases of vitreous lymphoma are high-grade, aggressive B-cell non-Hodgkin lymphomas that have a poor

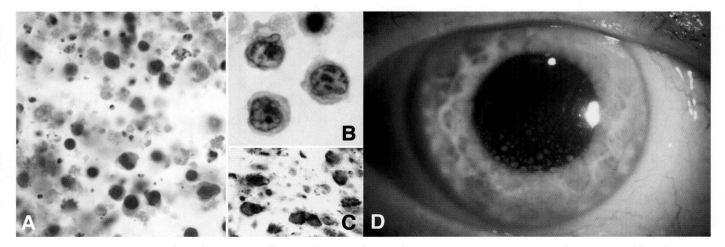

Fig. 10-8. Primary vitreous lymphoma. A. Infiltrate obtained during diagnostic vitrectomy contains large atypical lymphocytes, necrotic lymphoid cells, and nuclear debris. **B.** Large lymphoma cells have prominent nucleoli, and folds and protrusions of nuclear membrane. **C.** Positive immunoreactivity of cells for CD20 confirms B-cell lineage of lymphoma cells. **D.** Patients with vitreous lymphoma may have large keratic precipitates. (**A.** Millipore filter, H&E ×250, **B.** H&E ×400, **C.** IHC for CD20 ×100)

prognosis. These are subtyped as diffuse large B-cell lymphomas and probably are derived from early post-germinal center B cells.

In addition to the vitreous, the lymphoma cells infiltrate the retina and typically collect between Bruch membrane and the retinal pigment epithelium, forming solid yellowish RPE detachments. Cytologic examination of diagnostic vitrectomy specimens typically reveals a highly cellular and extensively necrotic infiltrate that contains atypical lymphocytes with prominent nucleoli and protrusions of the nuclear membrane, as well as tumors that are totally necrotic or undergoing apoptosis (Fig. 10-8). Immunophenotypic analysis by flow cytometry or immunohistochemistry can help to confirm the diagnosis when cytologic findings are subtle. Enzyme-linked immunosorbent assays of interleukin levels in ocular fluids also can support the diagnosis. Malignant B cells often express high levels of IL-10, while inflammatory cells produce IL-6. A ratio of IL-10 to IL-6 >1.0 suggests that a patient has a B-cell lymphoma.

The vitreous usually is spared when disseminated, non-CNS, visceral lymphomas involve the eye secondarily. Such lymphomas usually involve the uvea. Many patients who undergo diagnostic vitrectomy to exclude primary virteous lymphoma actually are found to have a form of granulomatous vitritis termed idiopathic senile vitritis. Cytologically, the latter lacks necrosis and contains a mixture of well-differentiated lymphocytes and epithelioid histiocytes with a spindled or dendritiform configuration. Careful cytologic screening and follow-up are warranted in such cases, however, because vitreous lymphoma occasionally presents with chronic inflammation.

Uveitis and vitritis occur rarely in patients with **Whipple disease**, who may also have CNS signs. PAS-positive macrophages filled with bacterial cell walls and degenerating

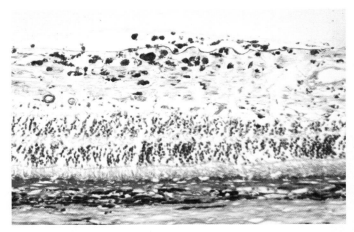

Fig. 10-9. Whipple disease. PAS-positive macrophages that have phagocytized *Tropheryma whippelii* bacteria infiltrate in the inner retina and cortical vitreous. (PAS ×250; Courtesy of Dr. Ramon L. Font, Houston, Texas.)

Tropheryma whippelii bacteria comprise the retinal and vitreal infiltrate in Whipple disease (Fig. 10-9). Endophytic or diffuse infiltrating retinoblastomas often cause vitreous seeding (Fig. 10-10A–C). Vitreous seeding by retinoblastoma is an important factor in the failure of eye-sparing therapy. The presence of vitreous seeds places eyes in higher risk categories in the international classification of retinoblastoma.

Although the choroid is the most common site of **metastasis from cutaneous melanoma**, vitreous metastasis can occur, and occasionally occurs in isolation (Fig. 10-10D,E). In one report, 6 of the 17 patients who had metastatic cutaneous melanoma to the vitreous had only vitreous involvement.

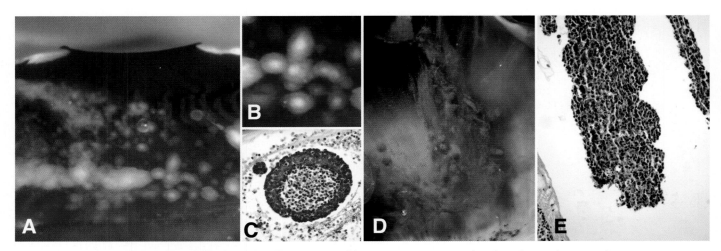

Fig. 10-10. Vitreous involvement by tumor cells. A. Retinoblastoma, vitreous seeds. The white spheres in the anterior vitreous are seeds of retinoblastoma shed by an endophytic tumor in the posterior segment. **B.** Some seeds have a white center reflecting central necrosis. **C.** Histopathology of seed shows central focus of necrotic cells enveloped by viable retinoblastoma. **D.** Vitreous involvement by metastatic cutaneous melanoma. Sheets and nodules of pigment infiltrate vitreous. **E.** Posterior vitreous contains aggregates of melanoma cells. (**C.** H&E ×100, **E.** H&E ×100)

BIBLIOGRAPHY

General References

Brucker AJ, Michels RG, Green WR. Pars plana vitrectomy in the management of blood-induced glaucoma with vitreous hemorrhage. *Ann Ophthalmol* 1978;10:1427–1437.

Chess J, Sebag J, Tolentino FI, et al. Pathologic processing of vitrectomy specimens: a comparison of findings with celloidin bag and cytocentrifugation of 102 vitrectomy specimens. *Ophthalmology* 1983;90:1560–1564.

Eagle RC Jr. Specimen handling in the ophthalmic pathology laboratory. In: Grossniklaus HE, Margo CE, eds. *Advances in Ophthalmic Pathology. Ophthalmol Clin North Am* 1995;8:1–15.

Eagle RC Jr. The pathology of vitrectomy specimens. In: Cohen EJ, ed. *The Year Book of Ophthalmology.* Mosby, 1996:353–368.

Engel H, de la Cruz ZC, Jiminiz-Abalihin LD, et al. Cytopreparatory techniques for eye fluid specimens obtained by vitrectomy. *Acta Cytol* 1982;26:551–560.

Engel HM, Green WR, Michels RG, et al. Diagnostic vitrectomy. *Retina* 1981;1:121–149.

Green WR. Diagnostic cytopathology of ocular fluid specimens. *Ophthalmology* 1984;91:726–749.

Spencer WH. The vitreous. In: Spencer WH, ed. *Ophthalmic Pathology: An Atlas and Textbook*, 3rd ed. Philadelphia, PA: WB Saunders, 1985:548–588.

Streeten BAW, Wilson DJ. Disorders of the vitreous. In: Garner A, Klintworth GK, eds. *Pathobiology of Ocular Disease: A Dynamic Approach*, 2nd ed, Part A. New York, NY: Marcel Dekker, 1994:701–742.

Posterior Vitreous Detachment

Foos RY. Posterior vitreous detachment. *Trans Am Acad Ophthalmol Otolaryngol* 1972;76:480–497.

Foos RY, Kreiger AE, Forsythe AB, et al. Posterior vitreous detachment in diabetic subjects. *Ophthalmology* 1980;87:122–128.

Foos RY, Wheeler NC. Vitreoretinal juncture synchysis senilis and posterior vitreous detachment. *Ophthalmology* 1982;89:1502–1512.

Linder B. Acute posterior vitreous detachment and its retinal complications. A clinical biomicroscopic study. *Acta Ophthalmol Suppl* 1966;87:1–108.

Vitreoretinal Membranes and Proliferative Vitreoretinopathy

Clarkson JG, Green WR, Massof D. A histopathologic review of 168 cases of preretinal membrane. *Am J Ophthalmol* 1977;84:1–17.

Elner SG, Elner VM, Diaz-Rohena R, et al. Anterior proliferative vitreoretinopathy. Clinicopathologic, light microscopic, and ultrastructural findings. *Ophthalmology* 1988;95:1349–1357.

Elner SG, Elner VM, Freeman HM, et al. The pathology of anterior (peripheral) proliferative vitreoretinopathy. *Trans Am Ophthalmol Soc* 1988;86:330–353.

Kampik A, Kenyon KR, Michels RG, et al. Epiretinal and vitreous membranes: a comparative study of 56 cases. *Arch Ophthalmol* 1981;99:1445–1453.

Lopez PF, Grossniklaus HE, Aaberg TM, et al. Pathogenetic mechanisms in anterior proliferative vitreoretinopathy. *Am J Ophthalmol* 1992;114:257–279.

Machemer R, Aaberg TM, Freeman HM, et al. An updated classification of retinal detachment with proliferative vitreoretinopathy. *Am J Ophthalmol* 1991;112:159–165.

Michels RG. A clinical and histopathologic study of epiretinal membranes affecting the macula and removed by vitreous surgery. *Trans Am Ophthalmol Soc* 1980;80:580–656.

Peczon BD, Wolfe JK, Gipson IK, et al. Characterization of membranes removed during open-sky vitrectomy. *Invest Ophthalmol Vis Sci* 1983;24:1382–1389.

Schwartz D, de la Cruz ZC, Green WR, et al. Proliferative vitreoretinopathy. Ultrastructural study of 20 retroretinal membranes removed by vitreous surgery. *Retina* 1988;8:275–281.

Wilkes SR, Mansour AM, Green WR. Proliferative vitreoretinopathy. Histopathology of retroretinal membranes. *Retina* 1987;7:94–101.

Vitreous Hemorrhage

Campbell DG. Ghost cell glaucoma following trauma. *Ophthalmology* 1981;88:1151–1158.

Campbell DG, Simmons RJ, Grant WM. Ghost cells as a cause of glaucoma. *Am J Ophthalmol* 1976;81:441–450.

Grossniklaus HE, Frank E, Fahri DC, et al. Hemoglobin spherulosis in the vitreous cavity. *Arch Ophthalmol* 1988;106:961–962.

Meredith TA, Gordon PA. Pars plana vitrectomy for severe penetrating injury with posterior segment involvement. *Am J Ophthalmol* 1987;103:549–554.

Ryan SJ. Penetrating ocular trauma and pars plana vitrectomy. *Trans New Orleans Acad Ophthalmol* 1983;31:129–136.

Spraul CW, Grossniklaus HE. Vitreous hemorrhage. *Surv Ophthalmol* 1997;42:3–39.

Asteroid Hyalosis

Bergren RL, Brown GC, Duker JS. Prevalence and association of asteroid hyalosis with systemic diseases. *Am J Ophthalmol* 1991;111:289–293.

Eagle RC, Yanoff M. Cholesterolosis of the anterior chamber. *Albrecht von Graefe's Arch Ophthalmol* 1975;193:121–134.

Fawzi AA, Vo B, Kriwanek R, et al. Asteroid hyalosis in an autopsy population: The University of California at Los Angeles (UCLA) experience. *Arch Ophthalmol* 2005;123:486–490.

Miller H, Miller B, Rabinowitz H, et al. Asteroid bodies—an ultrastructural study. *Invest Ophthalmol Vis Sci* 1983;24:133–136.

Renaldo DP. Pars plana vitrectomy for asteroid hyalosis. *Retina* 1981;1:252–254.

Streeten BW. Vitreous asteroid bodies. Ultrastructural characteristics and composition. *Arch Ophthalmol* 1982;100:969–975.

Topilow HW, Kenyon KR, Takahashi M, et al. Asteroid hyalosis. Biomicroscopy, ultrastructure, and composition. *Arch Ophthalmol* 1982;100:964–968.

Vitreous Amyloidosis

Benson MD. Hereditary amyloidosis—disease entity and clinical model. *Hosp Pract* 1988;23:165–172, 177, 181.

Ciulla TA, Tolentino F, Morrow JF, et al. Vitreous amyloidosis in familial amyloidotic polyneuropathy. Report of a case with the Val30Met transthyretin mutation. *Surv Ophthalmol* 1995;40:197–206.

Doft BH, Machemer R, Skinner M, et al. Pars plana vitrectomy for vitreous amyloidosis. *Ophthalmology* 1987;94:607–611.

Sandgren O, Holmgren G, Lundgren E. Vitreous amyloidosis associated with homozygosity for the transthyretin methionine-30 gene. *Arch Ophthalmol* 1990;108:1584–1586.

Vitreous Lymphoma

Barr CC, Green WR, Payne JW, et al. Intraocular reticulum cell sarcoma. Clinical pathological study of 4 cases and review of the literature. *Surv Ophthalmol* 1975;19:224–239.

Carroll DM, Franklin RM. Vitreous biopsy in uveitis of unknown cause. *Retina* 1981;1:245–251.

Chan CC. Molecular pathology of primary intraocular lymphoma. *Trans Am Ophthalmol Soc* 2003;101:275–292.

Chan CC, Buggage RR, Nussenblatt RB. Intraocular lymphoma. *Curr Opin Ophthalmol* 2002;13:411–418.

Chan CC, Wallace DJ. Intraocular lymphoma: update on diagnosis and management. *Cancer Control* 2004;11:285–295.

Chan CC, Whitcup SM, Solomon D, et al. Interleukin-10 in the vitreous of patients with primary intraocular lymphoma. *Am J Ophthalmol* 1995;120:671–673.

Char DH, Ljung B-M, Miller T, et al. Primary intraocular lymphoma (ocular reticulum cell sarcoma), diagnosis and management. *Opthalmology* 1988;95:625–630.

Coupland SE, Damato B. Understanding intraocular lymphomas. *Clin Experiment Ophthalmol* 2008;36:564–578.

Coupland SE, Heimann H, Bechrakis NE. Primary intraocular lymphoma: a review of the clinical, histopathological and molecular biological features. *Graefes Arch Clin Exp Ophthalmol* 2004;242:901–913.

Dean JM, Novak MA, Chan CC, et al. Tumor detachments of the retinal pigment epithelium in ocular/central nervous system lymphoma. *Retina* 1996;16:47–56.

Freeman LN, Schachat AP, Knox DL, et al. Clinical features, laboratory investigations, and survival in ocular reticulum cell sarcoma. *Ophthalmology* 1987;94:1631–1639.

Rankin GA, Jakobiec FA, Hidayat AA. Intraocular lymphoproliferations simulating uveitis. In: Albert DM, Jakobiec FA, eds. *Principles and Practice of Ophthalmology: Clinical Practice*, vol. 1. Philadelphia, PA: WB Saunders, 1994:524–548.

Vogel MH, Font RL, Zimmerman LE, et al. Reticulum cell sarcoma of the retina and uvea. Report of six cases and review of the literature. *Am J Ophthalmol* 1968;66:205–215.

Whitcup SM, de Smet MD, Rubin BI, et al. Intraocular lymphoma: clinical and histopathologic diagnosis. *Ophthalmology* 1993;100:1399–1406.

Whipple's Disease

Avila MP, Jalkh AE, Feldman E, et al. Manifestations of Whipple's disease in the posterior segment of the eye. *Arch Ophthalmol* 1984;102:384–390.

Durant WJ, Flood T, Goldberg MF, et al. Vitrectomy and Whipple's disease. *Arch Ophthalmol* 1984;102:848–851.

Font RL, Rao NA, Issarescu S, et al. Ocular involvement in Whipple's disease: light and electron microscopic observations. *Arch Ophthalmol* 1978;96:1431–1436.

Knox DL, Green WR, Troncoso JC, et al. Cerebral ocular Whipple's disease: a 62-year odyssey from death to diagnosis. *Neurology* 1995;45:617–625.

Rickman LS, Freeman WR, Green WR, et al. Uveitis caused by Tropheryma whippelii (Whipple's bacillus). *N Engl J Med* 1995;332:390–392.

Selsky EJ, Knox DL, Maumenee AE, et al. Ocular involvement in Whipple's disease. *Retina* 1984;4:103–106.

11

Intraocular Tumors in Adults

MELANOCYTIC TUMORS OF THE UVEAL TRACT

Introduction

In adults, most intraocular tumors arise from, or involve the uveal tract, the eye's middle coat composed of the stroma of the iris, ciliary body, and choroid. The uvea tract is highly vascular and pigmented. The pigment is contained within the cytoplasm of dendritic uveal melanocytes, which are derived embryologically from the neural crest (Fig. 11-1). A similar number of uveal melanocytes are present in lightly and heavily pigmented eyes. Increasing intensity of uveal pigmentation (and eye color) is caused by a corresponding increase in the size and number of melanin pigment granules or melanosomes in the cytoplasm of the melanocytes. The pigment may protect against the development of uveal tumors, because uveal malignant melanoma occurs most often in patients with blue eyes and is rare in heavily pigmented individuals.

The choroidal vessels occasionally undergo hamartomatous proliferation forming hemangiomas, and the rich vascular supply of the posterior choroid explains that region's predilection for blood-borne metastases.

NEVI

Uveal nevi are benign melanocytic neoplasms that are incapable of metastasis. Nevi, which occur in 5% of adults, are the most common intraocular tumor. Most choroidal nevi typically appear as flat or minimally elevated patches of increased choroidal pigmentation that measure 1 to 2 mm in diameter and are <2 mm in thickness (Fig. 11-2A). They may be pigmented or amelanotic, and they often have an irregular or feathery border. Drusen often develop on the surface of nevi with time. Most nevi are stationary lesions that do not change on serial observation. However, nevi occasionally do undergo malignant transformation into malignant melanoma; the rate of malignant transformation is estimated to be only 1/10,000 to 15,000 per year.

It may be difficult to differentiate between a choroidal nevus and a small malignant melanoma clinically. The observation of tumor growth may be the only clinical criterion that is helpful in this regard. Clinical factors that suggest that a pigmented lesion will grow and probably is a melanoma include the presence of symptoms, subretinal fluid and orange pigment, tumor thickness >2 mm, and contact of the posterior margin of the lesion with the optic disc. A small melanocytic lesion of the choroid with none of these factors has a 3% risk of growth into melanoma at 5 years and most likely represents a choroidal nevus. Tumors that display one factor have a 38% risk of growth, and those with two or more factors show growth in over 50% of cases. Most tumors with two or more risk factors probably represent small choroidal melanomas, and early treatment is generally indicated.

Uveal nevi are bland spindle cell tumors that comprise the benign end of the biologic spectrum of melanocytic neoplasms. Histopathologically, a compact infiltrate of

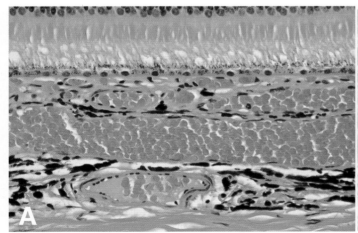
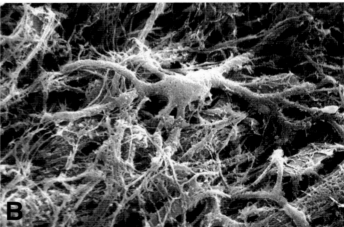

Fig. 11-1. A. Choroid. A. The choroid is the posterior part of the uveal tract. Its stroma contains dendritiform melanocytes and vessels. The latter include the choriocapillaris, which is located directly beneath Bruch membrane and the Sattler and Haller layers composed of progressively larger vessels. **B.** Scanning electron micrograph shows dendritic configuration of choroidal melanocyte. (**A.** H&E ×100, **B.** SEM ×1,250)

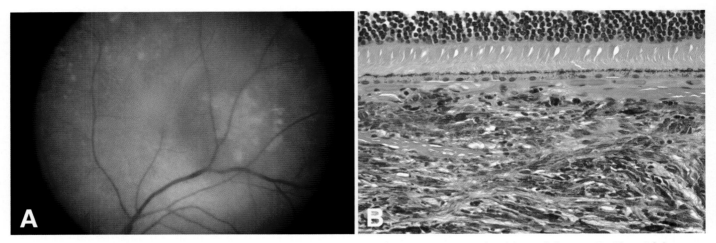

Fig. 11-2. Choroidal nevus. A. Small pigmented lesion presumed to be nevus remained stable on followup. **B. Choroidal nevus.** Choroid contains infiltrate of pigmented spindle cells with bland nuclei. The RPE and choriocapillaris are intact, and the overlying retina remains attached. (**B.** H&E ×100)

slender pigmented or nonpigmented spindle cells typically replaces the choroidal stroma (Fig. 11-2B). The nevus cells have bland oval or cigar-shaped nuclei that lack nucleoli or nuclear folds and have finely dispersed chromatin. Mitotic activity is absent. In some cases, the nevus cells are plump and dendritic in shape. Intranuclear cytoplasmic inclusions are common in some cases. Foamy balloon cells that appear to be undergoing lipoidal degeneration are found in 4% of nevi. Maximally pigmented, plump, polyhedral nevus cells comprise the magnocellular variant of nevus called melanocytoma (see below).

MELANOCYTOMA (MAGNOCELLULAR NEVUS)

A melanocytoma is a characteristic type of uveal nevus composed of plump polyhedral nevus cells filled with copious quantities of maximally pigmented cytoplasm. Melanocytomas have been called magnocellular nevi. In contrast to most nevi, melanocytoma may be relatively large and may be difficult to distinguish clinically from melanoma.

Melanocytomas classically involve the optic disc but can arise from any part of the uveal tract including the iris, choroid, or ciliary body. Clinically, they are intensely pigmented and often occur in young patients. Unlike melanoma, they do not have a predilection for whites; 37% to 50% of optic disc melanocytomas have been reported in African Americans.

Melanocytomas are so intensely pigmented that they appear black on routine microscopy. The copious cytoplasmic pigmentation typically obscures the nuclei of the melanocytoma cells requiring bleached sections for proper evaluation (Figs. 11-3D and 11-4). When bleached sections are examined, the tumor cells are found to have a low nuclear/cytoplasmic ratio and bland nuclei. Nucleoli usually are inconspicuous, but there are exceptions to the rule. Melanocytomas often undergo spontaneous necrosis and

typically contain pigment-laden macrophages. Extensive tumor necrosis typically is observed more often in a melanocytoma than a melanoma of comparable size, and totally necrotic melanocytomas occasionally are encountered. Melanophages released by partially necrotic iris melanocytomas can cause secondary melanocytomalytic glaucoma by physically obstructing the trabecular meshwork (Fig. 8-16). Transformation into malignant melanoma occurs rarely (1%–2%).

UVEAL MALIGNANT MELANOMA

Clinical Features

Worldwide, uveal melanoma is the most common primary malignant intraocular neoplasm in adults. Uveal melanoma is the most common intraocular malignancy in the United States and Europe. Elsewhere, the pediatric retinal neoplasm retinoblastoma is more common. Uveal melanomas are relatively rare; about 1,800 tumors occur yearly in the United States. The annual age-adjusted incidence in the United States is about 6 cases per 1 million population.

Uveal melanomas arise from the dendritic melanocytes of the uvea, the middle pigmented and vascularized coat of the eye, which includes the iris, ciliary body, and the choroid (Fig. 11-1B). Choroidal melanomas are most common. Uveal melanoma affects both sexes equally. Although pediatric and even rare congenital cases have been reported, uveal melanoma generally occurs in older persons. The mean age of patients eligible for treatment in the Collaborative Ocular Melanoma Study (COMS) was 59 years. Less than 1% of cases occur in patients less than age 20 years. Older patients tend to have larger tumors and are more likely to die from their tumors after enucleation.

Race is an important predisposing factor for uveal melanoma. The tumor has a predilection for Europeans with lightly colored eyes. In the United States, the incidence of uveal melanoma in white patients is 8.5 times greater than the incidence

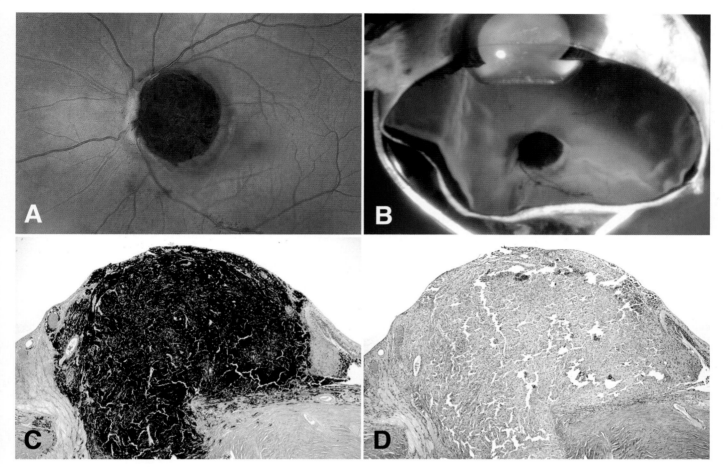

Fig. 11-3. Melanocytoma. A. Large, intensely pigmented melanocytoma of optic disc in African American woman was enucleated because patient complained of intractable pain and there was concern about malignant transformation. **B.** Pigmented mass protrudes from optic disc. **C.** Intensely pigmented tumor replaces parenchyma of optic disc. **D.** Bleached sections revealed no evidence of malignant transformation. (**C.** H&E ×25, **D.** Bleach ×25)

in African Americans. The tumor is also relatively uncommon in Latin America and Asia. The incidence of uveal melanoma in the United States is 15 times greater than that in Taiwan, that is, 6 per million versus 0.39 per million.

White patients who have congenital ocular or oculodermal melanocytosis (Nevus of Ota) (Fig. 5-26) are especially at risk to develop uveal malignant melanoma. The tumor is spawned by a diffuse nevus of the uvea, which is evident

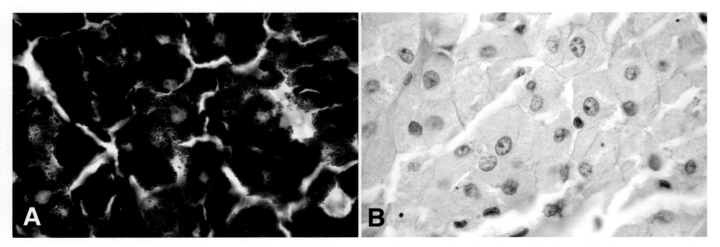

Fig. 11-4. Melanocytoma. A. Copious quantities of melanin pigment obscure nuclear details. **B.** Bleaching of melanin pigment discloses bland nuclei and low nuclear/cytoplasmic ratio consistent with benign magnocellular nevus. (**A.** H&E ×250, **B.** Bleach ×250)

clinically as hyperchromic heterochromia iridum. Affected patients often have slate-gray epibulbar pigmentation and a bluish discoloration of adnexal skin as well. It has been estimated that about one in 400 white patients with oculodermal melanocytosis will develop uveal melanoma in their lifetime. This risk is about 25 times greater than the risk in unaffected patients. Melanomas have developed in young patients with Ota nevus. Ocular and oculodermal melanocytosis are relatively common in Asians but do not appear to predispose them to melanoma.

As noted above, uveal melanomas occasionally arise from localized uveal nevi, but the estimated incidence of malignant transformation is quite low. Uveal melanoma has been reported in patients with neurofibromatosis type I and the dysplastic nevus or familial atypical mole-melanoma syndrome. Uveal melanoma can arise in patients who have a rare paraneoplastic syndrome called benign diffuse uveal melanocytic proliferation or BDUMP syndrome. The tumor's propensity for blue-eyed individuals and the inferior exposed part of the iris suggests that exposure to ultraviolet light could be a predisposing factor.

The clinical signs and symptoms of uveal malignant melanoma depend largely on the location of the tumor and the extent of the disease when the patient initially seeks medical attention. Most posterior uveal melanomas present with painless visual loss. Visual symptoms are caused most often by serous and/or solid detachment of the retina. Other mechanisms of visual loss include physical obscuration of the fovea by overhanging tumor, cystoid macular edema, cataracts caused by expanding ciliary body tumors, and rarely vitreous hemorrhage, which usually develops when tumors erode through the retina. Melanomas occasionally are found in asymptomatic patients during routine ophthalmologic examinations. Iris melanomas may present as an enlarging pigmented blemish or a change in eye color (heterochromia iridum) (Fig. 8-20). Other tumors present with unilateral glaucoma. Anterior

segment melanomas cause secondary glaucoma by directly seeding or infiltrating the aqueous outflow pathways. Posterior segment tumors usually cause secondary closed-angle glaucoma through a pupillary block mechanism or by stimulating iris neovascularization. Infarcted or extensively necrotic tumors can cause prominent inflammatory signs that can mimic orbital cellulitis. Advanced cases with extrascleral tumor extension into the orbit may present with ocular proptosis. Unsuspected melanomas occasionally are found when blind, painful, glaucomatous eyes with opaque media are examined pathologically. Before the advent of ultrasonography, as many as 10% of blind, painful eyes were said to harbor previously undiagnosed tumors. Care should be taken to exclude the presence of an occult tumor preoperatively if ocular evisceration is planned. Distant metastases usually are not evident when the tumor is first detected and treated.

Diagnosis

Many posterior uveal melanomas are diagnosed by direct ophthalmoscopic visualization of the tumor by experienced clinicians (Fig. 11-5). Adjunctive studies including A and B scan ultrasonography, intravenous fluorescein angiography (IVFA), and computed tomography or magnetic resonance imaging frequently are used to confirm the clinical impression and may be particularly important if the ocular media are opacified. Transvitreal fine needle aspiration biopsy (FNAB) performed under direct ophthalmoscopic visualization occasionally is performed if the diagnosis remains uncertain after routine tests, and choice of therapy requires an accurate diagnosis. Examples where FNAB might be used include the patient who has a history of breast cancer who presents with a solitary amelanotic choroidal tumor that could be a second primary amelanotic melanoma or the patient who is thought to have a choroidal metastasis but has no history of cancer.

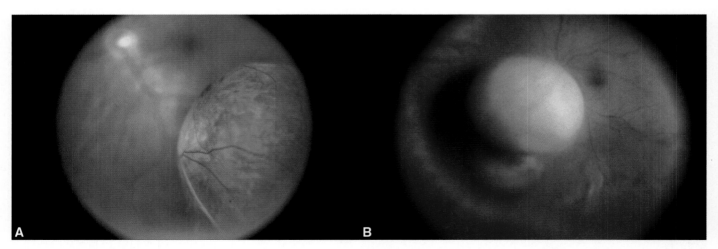

Fig. 11-5. Choroidal melanoma. A. Fundus photograph shows mushrooming head of pigmented choroidal tumor elevating inferotemporal retina. **B.** Tumor seen in wide angle photograph has broken through Bruch membrane and assumed characteristic mushroom or collar button configuration.

Gross Pathology

Melanomas initially arise in the uveal stroma. In early cases of choroidal melanoma, the profile of the sectioned tumor is oval or almond-shaped, and its tissue usually appears relatively cohesive after fixation (Fig. 11-6A). Although some melanomas diffusely infiltrate the uvea, most uveal melanomas are relatively well-circumscribed tumors with distinct margins. In many cases, the growing melanoma perforates Bruch membrane and enters the subretinal space where its apex typically assumes a spherical shape that often is likened to a mushroom or collar button (Figs. 11-5, 11-6B,D, and 11-7). If a choroidal tumor has a mushroom configuration, one can be reasonably certain that it is a uveal melanoma. There are exceptions to this rule, but they are exceedingly rare. Dilated blood vessels typically are found in the mushrooming head of the tumor (Fig. 11-7). The ruptured ends of Bruch membrane exert a compressive cinchlike effect on the waist of the tumor causing vascular congestion in its apex. Rupture of Bruch membrane was present in 87.7% of 1,527 large or medium sized

melanomas examined in the COMS study. Retinal invasion was present in nearly half (49.1%) and tumor cells were found in the vitreous body in one quarter. About 3% of melanomas diffusely thicken the choroid without forming an elevated mass. These diffuse melanomas usually are of mixed cell type, are more likely to infiltrate the sclera, and invade the optic nerve or orbit (Fig. 11-8D). Delayed diagnosis or misdiagnosis is common.

Choroidal melanomas are classified as *small, medium,* and *large* based on the tumor's largest basal diameter (LTD). Small choroidal melanomas measure ≤10 mm in LTD and appear as a focal discoid or oval area of choroidal thickening. Medium-sized melanomas measure 11 to 15 mm, and large tumors are more than 15 mm in largest basal tumor diameter.

Choroidal melanomas typically cause an exudative serous detachment of the overlying and adjacent retina. Large tumors may cause total retinal detachment (Figs. 11-6B,D and 11-7). The detached retina typically shows photoreceptor atrophy and microcystoid retinal degeneration. The retinal pigment epithelium (RPE) on the

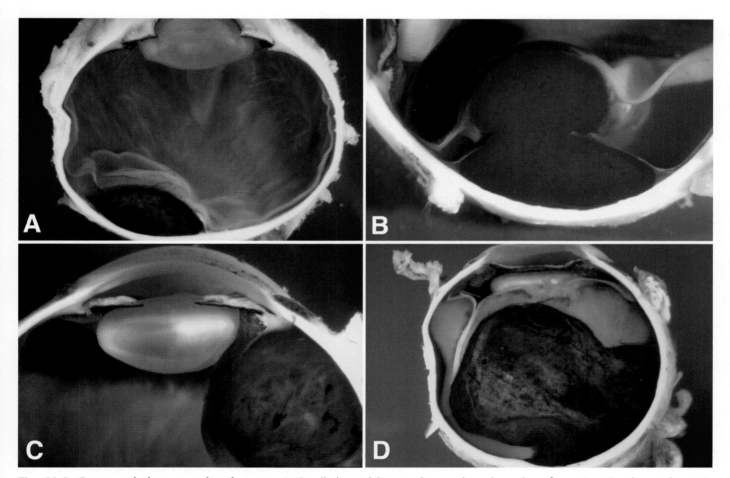

Fig. 11-6. Gross pathology, uveal melanoma. A. Small choroidal tumor has oval or almond configuration. Bruch membrane is intact. **B.** Heavily pigmented melanoma has arisen from the equatorial choroid and ruptured through Bruch membrane. The tumor has a characteristic mushroom or collar button configuration. Infiltration of the retina is seen at the tumor's apex. Posterior to the tumor, the retina is detached by serous fluid. **C.** Ciliary body melanoma. Heavily pigmented ciliary body tumor deforms and displaces lens. **D.** Large choroidal melanoma. Large, heavily pigmented mushroom-shaped melanoma has produced a total retinal detachment and secondary glaucoma.

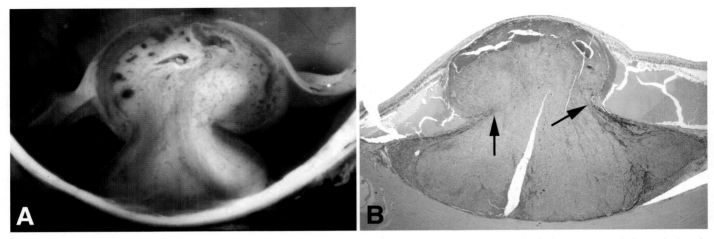

Fig. 11-7. A. Dilated vessels are present in mushrooming head of choroidal melanoma, which has ruptured through Bruch membrane. Scleral infiltration is present at the base of the tumor. The adjacent retina is detached, and the retina on the tumor's apex is severely atrophic. **B.** *Arrows* point to edge of rupture in Bruch membrane. Dilated vessels in mushrooming head of tumor are caused by the compressive cinchlike effect of the ends of Bruch membrane on the waist of the tumor. The retina is detached by serous fluid. (**B.** H&E ×5)

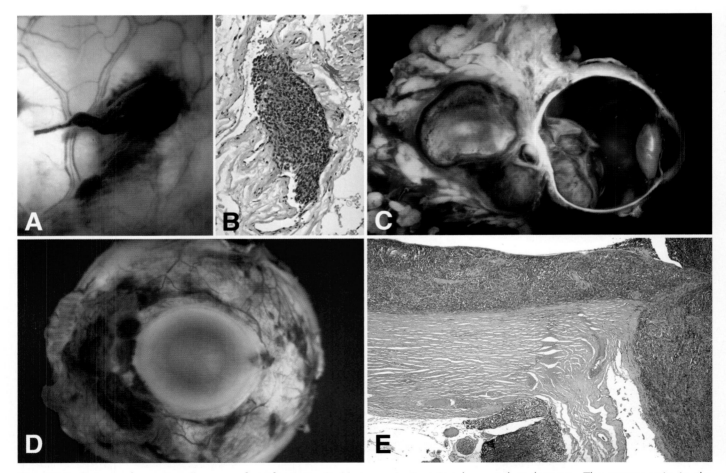

Fig. 11-8. Extraocular extension, uveal melanoma. A. Vortex vein invasion by uveal melanoma. The vortex vein in the macrophoto is massively distended by heavily pigmented tumor. **B.** Photomicrograph shows melanoma in the lumen of the vessel. **C. Massive posterior extrascleral extension**. Posterior choroidal melanoma has extended extrasclerally forming large pigmented orbital mass that dwarfs the intraocular tumor. Optic nerve invasion is present. The patient presented with ocular proptosis. **D. Anterior extraocular extension**. Ciliary body melanoma exited globe via anterior emissarial canals. **E. Diffuse choroidal melanoma**. Melanoma diffusely thickens choroid. Highly aggressive tumor has invaded optic nerve and grown through posterior emissarial canal forming juxtapapillary epibulbar mass. (**B.** H&E ×100, **E.** H&E ×25)

surface of the tumor undergoes atrophy and proliferation forming drusenoid material and occasionally a plaque of metaplastic fibrous tissue. Many tumors infiltrate the overlying retina. The melanoma may perforate the retina in exceptional cases, causing vitreous hemorrhage and tumor seeding of the vitreous and the inner retinal surface. Large tumors may totally fill the globe. Eventually, some melanomas extend extraocularly through the sclera and invade the orbit (Fig. 11-8C,E). Secondary glaucoma is often present in eyes with advanced or neglected tumors. Uveal melanomas vary markedly in their pigment content. Some tumors are totally amelanotic. Other maximally pigmented tumors appear jet-black grossly and must be bleached before they can be interpreted histopathologically. Varying degrees of pigmentation are typically found within a single tumor. The cut surface of some tumors has a marbleized appearance. Clumps of orange pigment are found on the surface of many melanomas (Fig. 11-9). The orange pigment comprises aggregates of macrophages that have ingested lipofuscin pigment and melanin from the damaged RPE (Fig. 11-9C,D). The pigment generally is thought to be a

clinical marker for an actively growing tumor and can be highlighted with fundus autofluorescence.

Ciliary body melanomas are less common than choroidal tumors and tend to have a more spherical shape (Fig. 11-6C). Ciliary body tumors may be larger when they are first detected because they remain hidden behind the iris and often remain asymptomatic because they cause late retinal detachment. Ciliary body melanomas can deform the crystalline lens and cause unilateral cataract. Occasionally, they can invade the anterior chamber and present with iris heterochromia and secondary glaucoma. The glaucoma is caused by seeding of the trabecular meshwork by tumor cells, or by circumferential tumor growth around the angle (*ring melanoma*).

Histopathology

The biologic spectrum of uveal melanoma cells comprises bland spindle A melanoma cells at one end and wildly anaplastic epithelioid cells at the other (Figs. 11-10 and 11-11). The term spindle cell is derived from

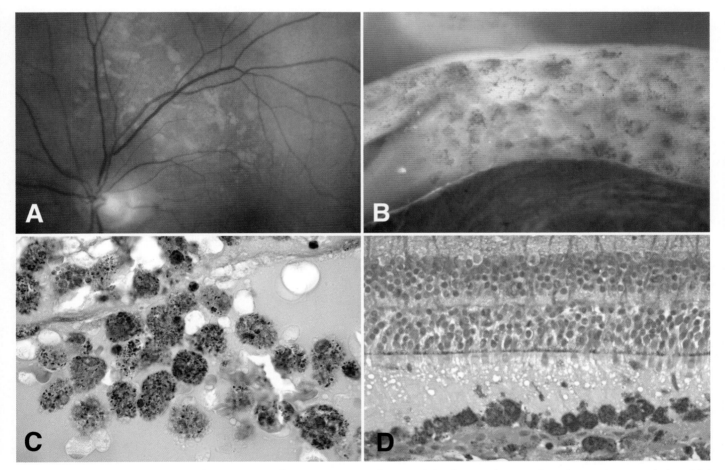

Fig. 11-9. Orange pigment. A. The presence of orange pigment is one of the factors that predicts that a pigmented choroidal lesion will grow and probably is a melanoma. **B.** Clumps of orange pigment adhere to posterior surface of detached retina overlying actively growing melanoma. **C.** Orange pigment is composed of aggregates of macrophages that have phagocytized lipofuscin and melanin pigment released by RPE cells that have been disrupted by an actively growing tumor. **D.** Macrophages that have ingested lipofuscin pigment are PAS-positive. (**C.** H&E ×250, **D.** PAS ×100)

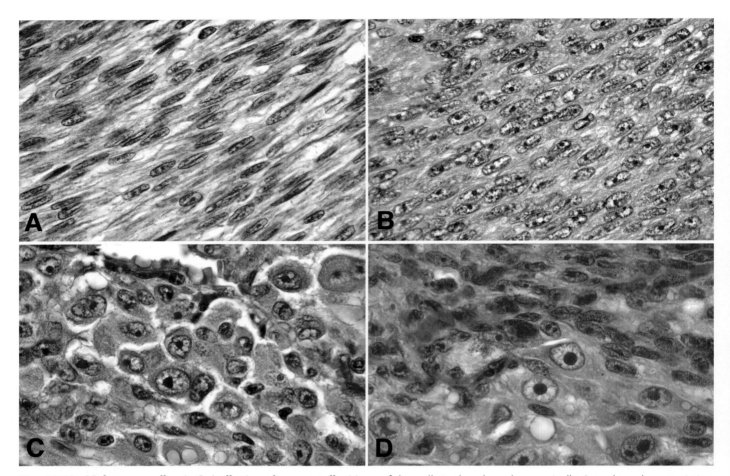

Fig. 11-10. Melanoma cells. A. Spindle A melanoma cells. Many of the cells in the photo have spindle A nuclear characteristics. The nuclei are bland slender and cigar-shaped and have finely dispersed chromatin and indistinct nucleoli. Longitudinal folds in the nuclear membrane are apparent microscopically as a chromatin stripe or line. The spindle cells form a syncytium with indistinct cytoplasmic borders. **B. Spindle B melanoma cells**. Most of the cells in this field are spindle B melanoma cells. They have oval nuclei and an obvious nucleolus. Compared to spindle A cells, their chromatin is more coarsely clumped. The spindle cells form a syncytium. **C. Epithelioid melanoma cells**. The cytoplasmic margins of these large, poorly cohesive epithelioid melanoma cells are easily discernible. Epithelioid cell nuclei are typically round and have peripheral margination of coarsely clumped chromatin. Epithelioid cells usually have prominent reddish purple nucleoli. They typically are polyhedral in shape and have copious amounts of cytoplasm. **D. Uveal melanoma, mixed cell type**. Mixed cell melanomas are composed of a mixture of spindle (above) and epithelioid cells (below). (**All figures** H&E ×250)

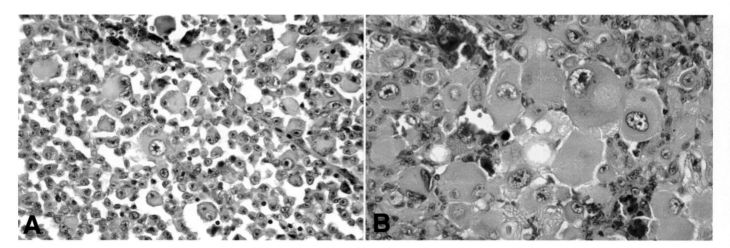

Fig. 11-11. A, B. Tumor giant cells, uveal melanoma. Tumor giant cells are highly anaplastic epithelioid cells. They are relatively rare, and their prognostic significance is uncertain. (**A.** H&E ×50, **B.** H&E ×100)

the fusiform or spindled configuration of the cells' cytoplasmic outline. Spindle cells are bipolar in shape and many have long tapering processes that occasionally are visible when individual pigmented cells are seen in a largely amelanotic tumor. Spindle cells grow in a syncytial fashion and form interweaving fascicles of parallel oriented cells (Fig. 11-10A,B). The cells can be pigmented or nonpigmented.

There are two types of spindle cells, spindle A and spindle B, which are distinguished by their nuclear characteristics. Spindle A nuclei are cigar-shaped and have finely dispersed chromatin (Fig. 11-10A). Many spindle A cells have a longitudinally-oriented chromatin stripe caused by a fold in the nuclear membrane. If a nucleolus is present, it usually is inconspicuous. The nuclei of spindle B cells tend to be plumper and more oval in shape and have coarser chromatin and distinct nucleoli (Fig. 11-10B).

Epithelioid melanoma cells comprise the poorly differentiated end of the cytologic spectrum. Uveal melanomas that contain epithelioid cells have a poorer prognosis. The term epithelioid, which means "epithelial-like," reflects the superficial resemblance of the tumor cells to simple epithelial cells. Epithelioid cells have abundant cytoplasm and are often polygonal in shape (Fig. 11-10C). They have distinct cytoplasmic margins, are poorly cohesive, and do not grow as a syncytium. The nuclei of epithelioid cells typically are round or oval in shape, and they often appear vesicular due to margination or clumping of chromatin along the inner side of the nuclear membrane. Epithelioid melanoma cells also have prominent nucleoli that are often large and reddish-purple in color. The large nucleoli are often visible at lower magnification. Variants of epithelioid cells include wildly anaplastic tumor giant cells (Fig. 11-11) and relatively uniform small epithelioid cells (Fig. 11-12A).

During histopathologic assessment, melanoma cells are classified by their nuclear characteristics. Spindle-shaped cells that have epithelioid nuclei occasionally are encountered; such cells are classified as epithelioid. In recent years, the term intermediate cell has been used more and more. Intermediate cells are cells that have nuclear characteristics that are intermediate between spindle B and epithelioid. For example, one might apply the term intermediate cell to a spindle B cell that has a nucleus that is somewhat large and has a fairly prominent nucleolus.

Occasionally, spindle cells in a uveal melanoma are arranged radially around vessels or perpendicular to fibrovascular septa (vasocentric pattern), or their nuclei form rows that resemble the Verocay bodies or the Antoni A pattern seen in Schwannoma (Verocay pattern). Melanomas are called fascicular if these patterns dominate (Fig. 11-13A). Fascicular melanoma was a separate category in Callender's initial classification that was dropped from McLean's 1983 modification.

Varying degrees of necrosis may be are found (Fig. 11-12B). Necrosis tends to be more prominent in rapidly growing high-grade tumors, or tumors that have had prior brachytherapy. The necrosis may be patchy and focal or may involve extensive parts, or even all of the tumor. Aggregates of melanophages typically are found in the necrotic areas. Total infarction of the tumor (and other intraocular structures) may occur in eyes with severe secondary closed-angle glaucoma. As mentioned above, melanocytoma is especially prone to spontaneous necrosis. The latter diagnosis should always be considered when a totally necrotic, heavily pigmented tumor is found.

Choroidal melanomas produce abnormalities in the overlying retinal pigment epithelial including atrophy,

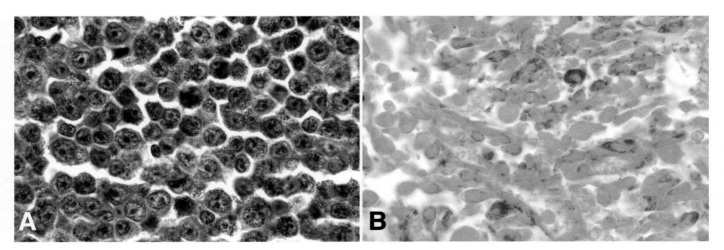

Fig. 11-12. A. Small epithelioid cells. Although these cells are relatively small, they are definitely epithelioid in character. They are polyhedral in shape and have distinct cytoplasmic outlines. The round or oval nuclei have prominent nucleoli. Clones of small epithelioid cells are encountered occasionally in uveal melanomas. **B. Necrotic uveal melanoma**. The cells of this necrotic melanoma are eosinophilic because they have lost their basophilic nuclear DNA. The cell type of a necrotic melanoma often can be ascertained if careful microscopy with an oil-immersion lens is performed. Necrotic uveal melanomas tend to behave clinically like mixed-cell type melanomas. (**A.** H&E ×250, **B.** H&E ×250)

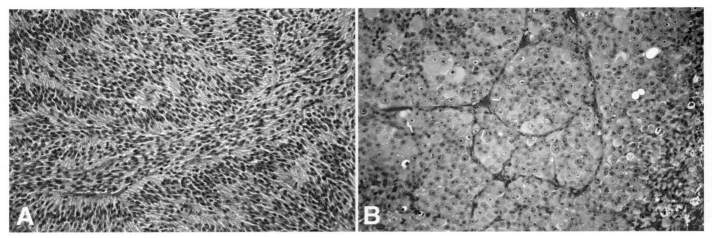

Fig. 11-13. A. Fascicular melanoma. The fascicular category of uveal melanoma has been removed from the modern revision of the Callender classification because cellular arrangement does not appear to affect prognosis. This amelanotic melanoma has a striking fascicular appearance. The nuclei of its constituent spindle cells form rows that resemble the Antoni A pattern seen in schwannoma. **B. Vascular mimicry patterns, uveal melanoma**. Fibrovascular septa divide parts of this predominantly epithelioid melanoma into roughly circular zones initially called vascular loops. Vascular networks are composed of adjacent vascular loops. Uveal melanomas that contain vascular mimicry patterns called loops and networks have a poorer prognosis. (**A.** H&E ×50, **B.** H&E ×50)

hyperplasia, and the formation of drusen and drusenoid material. The overlying retina often shows photoreceptor loss and may develop cystoid edema. The latter tends to be more common over slower growing lesions, especially choroidal hemangiomas. After Bruch membrane has ruptured, the vessels located in the mushrooming head of the tumor are often quite prominent, reflecting vascular stagnation caused by the compression at the waist of the tumor (Fig. 11-7). Aggregates of macrophages that have ingested periodic acid-Schiff (PAS)-positive lipofuscin pigment, and melanin from the damaged RPE can be found in the subretinal fluid (Fig. 11-9). These are evident ophthalmoscopically as clumps of orange pigment that serve as a clinical marker for an actively growing neoplasm.

Uveal melanomas are placed into four categories based on their cytology. Tumors composed entirely of spindle A cells or even blander nevus cells are classified as spindle cell nevi. Tumors composed of a mixture of malignant spindle A and spindle B cells are called spindle melanomas. Melanomas of mixed cell type contain a mixture of spindle and epithelioid melanoma cells (Fig. 11-10D). Some laboratories specify the predominant cell type found in a mixed cell melanoma, for example, reporting mixed cell, predominantly spindle if only a few epithelioid cells are present. Epithelioid melanomas are composed predominantly of epithelioid cells. They are relatively rare and have the poorest prognosis. Most medium and large-sized melanomas contain a mixture of spindle and epithelioid cells. About 86% of the posterior melanomas in the COMS histopathology study were classified as mixed cell type; 8% were of spindle cell type, and 5% were epithelioid. The association between cytology and mortality is known as the Callender classification (see section on prognostic factors below).

Prognostic Factors

About one half of patients with choroidal and ciliochoroidal malignant melanomas eventually die from their tumors. Because the eye and orbit lack lymphatics, uveal melanoma spreads via the blood stream. Hematogenous metastasis to the liver occurs most often; more than 90% of cases with metastatic melanoma have liver metastases, and they are the first metastases detected in 80% (Fig. 11-14). For this reason, liver enzymes and hepatic imaging are used clinically to monitor patients for recurrence. Other common sites of metastatic uveal melanoma include the lung (24%) and bone (16%). Multiple sites are found in 87%. Unfortunately, once distant metastases are manifest clinically, therapy generally is ineffective. More than 50% of patients who have metastatic uveal melanoma die within 1 year. In recent years, there has been an effort to identify prognostic factors that could identify patients at high risk for metastatic disease who hopefully might benefit from prophylactic chemo- or immunotherapy.

The association between the cytologic characteristics of uveal melanoma ("**cell type**") and mortality was initially reported in 1931 by Major George Russel Callender who examined a series of cases on file in the Registry of Ophthalmic Pathology at the Army Medical Museum in Washington, DC. Callender observed that melanomas were composed of two types of spindle cells that he designated spindle A and B and less differentiated epithelioid cells. He found that tumors that contained epithelioid cells had a poorer prognosis. Ian McLean et al. at the Armed Forces Institute of Pathology modified Callender's original classification in 1978.

The presence or absence of **epithelioid cells** is an extremely important prognostic factor in uveal melanoma.

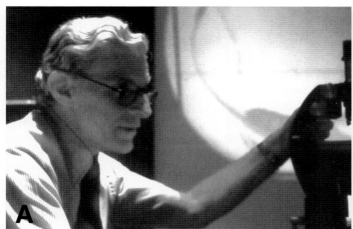
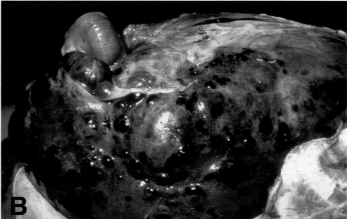

Fig. 11-14. A. Dr. Lorenz E. Zimmerman conducting ophthalmic pathology conference at the Armed Forces Institute of Pathology in Washington, DC circa 1978. A short time later "Zimm" formulated his hypothesis concerning the effect of enucleation on the dissemination of uveal melanoma. **B. Liver metastases, uveal melanoma.** Postmortem examination of patient who died from metastatic uveal melanoma shows massive replacement of liver by tumor. (Slide courtesy of Dr. Daniel M. Albert.)

McLean reviewed a series of 3,432 cases of malignant melanoma of the choroid and ciliary body on file in the *AFIP's Registry of Ophthalmic Pathology* and found that 56% were mixed cell tumors composed of a mixture of spindle and epithelioid cells. The 15-year mortality of patients with melanomas of mixed cell type was three times that of patients whose tumors were composed solely of spindle cells. Tumor size, measured as the largest tumor diameter (LTD), was also highly correlated with mortality.

Callender cell type as modified at the Armed Forces Institute of Pathology remains one of the most reliable prognosticators of mortality from uveal melanoma. Tumor mortality is greater if uveal melanomas contain epithelioid cells (epithelioid melanomas or mixed epithelioid/spindle cell type). The 5-year mortality of uveal melanomas that contain epithelioid cells is 42%. At 15 years, death from metastatic melanoma increases to 63%. The prognosis of spindle cell tumors is much better; 90% survive 5 years and 72% survive 15 years. Although rare fatal spindle A melanomas have been reported, most tumors composed entirely of spindle A cells are thought to be benign spindle cell nevi.

Cell type remains one of prognostic mainstays of surgical pathologists because assessment is relatively rapid and requires no special stains or equipment. However, determination of cell type is highly subjective and diagnostic accuracy of can vary with the expertise and experience of the pathologist. A masked study showed that even experienced ophthalmic pathologists disagree about their classification of individual tumor cells. Secondly, melanoma cells constitute a continuous biologic spectrum that includes extremely bland spindle A melanoma cells at one end and highly anaplastic epithelioid cells at the other. Despite this, only three categories—spindle, mixed or epithelioid—are available for the classification of a given tumor, and tumors in a single category, for example, mixed cell type, can vary significantly in their apparent degree of differentiation.

The limitations of the Callender classification prompted a search for more objective and reliable criteria for the histopathologic assessment of the malignant potential of uveal melanomas. Gamel et al. showed that certain **nucleolar parameters**, most notably the inverse of the standard deviation of the area of the nucleolus, were useful predictors of death from metastatic melanoma. Gamel's laboratory subsequently developed another simpler objective method of nucleolar assessment based on the measurement of the ten largest nucleoli. Although these techniques more accurately predicted survival after enucleation using morphologic data contained within routine histologic slides, they were not widely adopted because they were labor-intensive and relatively time-consuming and required special expertise and equipment.

Other attempts to make the assessment of cell type more objective and quantitative include counting the number of epithelioid cells and intermediate cells in 40 high power fields. The mitotic activity of uveal melanoma is routinely assessed by counting the number of mitotic figures in 40 high power fields.

Tumor size is another important prognostic factor. Large melanomas have a poorer prognosis than medium and small-sized melanomas. Tumor size generally is recorded as the largest tumor diameter or LTD measured at the base. The 5-year survival of small (<10 mm), medium (10–15 mm), and large (>15 mm) melanomas are 86%, 66%, and 56%, respectively. These survival rates drop to 76%, 51%, and 41% at 10 years and 70%, 43%, and 35% at 15 years. Smaller melanomas are more likely to be spindle cell tumors.

Certain **extracellular matrix patterns** within uveal melanomas that initially were termed microvascular patterns have been shown to be prognostic indicators for death from metastatic melanoma. The so-called vascular loops and networks composed of back-to-back loops encircling microdomains of tumor are the vascular mimicry patterns that are strongly associated with death from metastatic melanoma (Fig. 11-13B). The term vasculogenic mimicry looping matrix patterns has been applied to these patterns in recent publications.

Other prognostic factors, which have been shown by multivariant statistical analysis to be less important, include mitotic activity, extraocular tumor extension (Fig. 11-8), necrosis, pigmentation, anterior location, and lymphocytic infiltration. Paradoxically, the prognosis of heavily pigmented tumors may be slightly poorer.

Ocular pathologists routinely assess the mitotic activity of uveal melanoma by counting the number of **mitotic figures** in 40 high power ("high dry") microscopic fields. Forty fields are counted because most uveal melanomas contain relatively few mitoses, that is, only five or ten per 40 HPF. Not unexpectedly, patients whose tumors have more mitoses have a poorer prognosis.

About 8% of 1,527 enucleated globes with uveal melanoma evaluated in the COMS had some degree of **extrascleral extension** on histopathologic examination. Although direct scleral infiltration occurs in some cases, melanomas typically extend out of the eye through the emissarial canals of vessels and nerves in the sclera, or via the lumina of the vortex veins (Fig. 11-8). Unlike retinoblastoma, uveal melanoma rarely invades the optic nerve. Coupland and Damato found that extraocular spread correlates with increased mortality because it is associated with increased tumor malignancy and, in the case of posterior tumors, more advanced disease.

The presence of **tumor infiltrating lymphocytes** is associated with decreased survival. De la Cruz et al examined 1,078 cases of uveal melanoma with known survival and found that 12.4% harbored 100 or more lymphocytes per 20 high-power (×400) microscopic fields. The survival rate at 15 years was 36.7% for patients in the high lymphocytic group and 69.6% for patients in the low lymphocytic group. This seemingly counterintuitive observation is explained by the fact that extraocular dissemination of tumor cells is a requisite for stimulation of a T lymphocyte-mediated immune response.

Uveal melanomas harbor recurrent nonrandom **chromosomal abnormalities** that include monosomy 3, trisomy 8, and structural or numerical abnormalities of chromosome 6. Loss of chromosome 3 and gains in chromosome 8 are associated with metastatic death. Monosomy 3 has been shown to be a significant predictor of poor prognosis in uveal melanoma. In one study, 57% of patients with monosomy 3 had developed metastases at 3 years, compared to none of the patients wth disomy 3. Chromosomal 3 abnormalities have been identified using a variety of techniques including fluorescence *in situ* hybridization and DNA amplification and microsatellite assay. Increasingly used in recent years, chromosomal analysis enables clinicians to reassure patients with a good prognosis and identifies high-risk patients who need intensive systemic screening.

Microarray analysis has also been used to assess **gene expression profiling** in primary uveal melanoma.

Harbour et al. showed that uveal melanomas naturally cluster into two groups based on their gene expression signature. This gene expression–based classification appears to accurately predict metastatic death. Class I melanomas are low-grade and do not metastasize. In contrast, patients who have class 2 tumors are at high risk for metastases. Class II tumors have a primitive neural/ectodermal stem cell–like phenotype and are more likely to contain epithelioid cells, looping extracellular matrix patterns and monosomy 3. They are characterized by down-regulation of neural crest and melanocyte-specific genes and up-regulation of epithelial genes. Molecular classification based on gene expression profiling of the primary tumor has been reported to be superior to monosomy 3 and clinicopathologic prognostic factors for predicting metastasis in uveal melanoma. The technique is commercially available.

IRIS NEVUS AND MELANOMA

Most melanocytic lesions of the iris are benign nevi or low-grade spindle cell tumors (Figs. 11-15 and 11-16). About half of the adult population has small nonprogressive iris nevi called freckles (Fig. 11-15). Larger pigmented iris lesions initially should be observed for growth. Only 6.5% will enlarge during a 5-year observation period. Clinical features that suggest that a pigmented iris tumor is a melanoma include large size, documented growth, elevated intraocular pressure, hyphema, and tumor vascularity. The mean age of patients with iris melanomas is about 10 years younger (age 43 years) than the age of patients with posterior segment melanomas. The prognosis of iris melanoma is also relatively favorable compared to tumors of the posterior segment. Shields studied 169 patients with histologically confirmed iris melanoma and found that distant metastases developed in 5% at 10 years follow-up. The relatively small size of most iris melanomas probably is a major factor in their good prognosis.

Diffuse iris melanomas that cause hyperchromic heterochromia iridis and secondary glaucoma are a rare but clinically important group of iris tumors (Fig. 8-19). Many diffuse iris melanomas are higher grade tumors that contain epithelioid cells, which are poorly cohesive and prone to aqueous dispersal. Patients are often misdiagnosed clinically and undergo filtering surgery for glaucoma. The latter invariably fails and puts patients at greater risk for extraocular extension and metastasis. Pigmented tumors of the iris pigment epithelium are exceedingly rare (Fig. 11-17).

Treatment

Current therapy for uveal melanoma is unsatisfactory in many cases. Although metastatic disease typically is not evident clinically when the patient presents to the ophthalmologist, it currently is believed that many uveal melanomas continuously shed tumor cells into the circulation

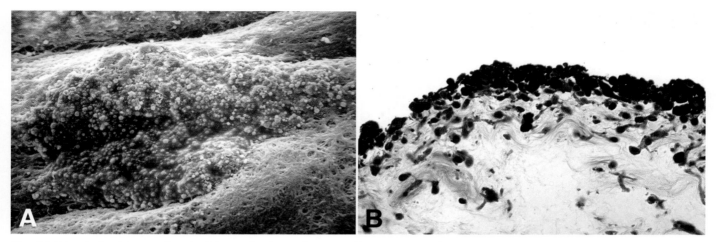

Fig. 11-15. Iris freckle. A. Sharply delimited colony of nevus cells in scanning electron micrograph is located anterior to the plane of the surrounding iris stroma. Round cellular processes decorate surface of nevus. **B.** Iris freckles are small nonprogressive nevi that occur in nearly half the adult population. Their constituent cells have rounded cellular processes that are densely packed with large melanosomes. (**A.** False-colorized scanning electron micrograph ×160 [Modified from Eagle RC Jr. Congenital, developmental and degenerative disorders of the iris and ciliary body. In Albert DM, Jakobiec FA, eds. *Principles and Practice of Ophthalmology. Clinical Practice*, vol. 1. Philadelphia, PA: Saunders, 1993:367–389], **B.** Epon section, PD ×100)

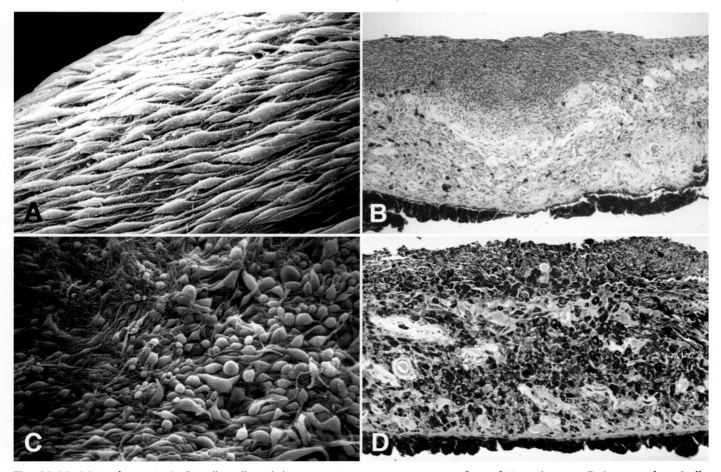

Fig. 11-16. Iris melanoma. A. Spindle cells with long tapering processes cover surface of iris melanoma. **B. Low-grade spindle cell melanoma of the iris.** Moderately pigmented spindle cells infiltrate and thicken stroma and form plaque on anterior iridic surface. The nuclei of the tumor cells are quite bland. **C. Mixed cell melanoma of iris.** Scanning electron microscopy discloses bizarrely pleomorphic cells presumed to be epithelioid cells on surface of tumor. **D. Mixed cell melanoma of iris.** The heavily pigmented tumor is composed of a mixture of spindle and epithelioid melanoma cells. The epithelioid cells in the stroma are distinguished by their round cytoplasmic profiles and round nuclei with prominent nucleoli. The tumor cells form a plaque on the anterior surface of the iris. (**A.** SEM ×640, **B.** H&E ×50, **C.** SEM ×320 [Modified from Eagle RC Jr. Iris pigmentation and pigmented lesion: an ultrastructural study. *Trans Am Ophthalmol Soc* 1989;87:581–687], **D.** H&E ×50)

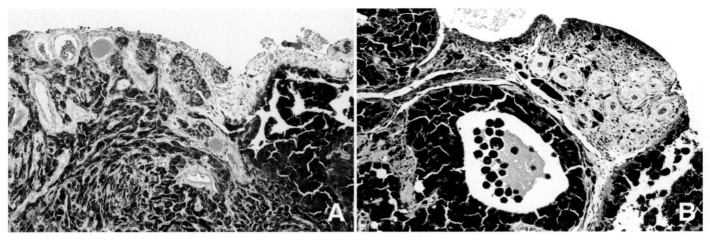

Fig. 11-17. Adenoma of iris pigment epithelium. A. Cords and sheets of intensely pigmented epithelial cells comprise rare iris tumor. **B.** Islands of heavily pigmented iris pigment epithelial cells erode through iris and invade anterior chamber. (**A.** H&E ×50, **B.** H&E ×100)

and that systemic micrometastases are present several years before the tumor is treated. Therefore, in many instances, the ophthalmologist merely achieves local control. What he or she does ultimately has little effect on systemic spread or surivival. To make matters worse, current chemotherapeutic regimens have little effect on metastatic uveal melanoma; more than 50% of patients die within 1 year.

Local tumor control is achieved in the majority of cases by enucleation or radiotherapy, typically plaque brachytherapy. The latter treatment employs radioactive plaques composed of radioisotopes such as iodine-125. The plaques are surgically affixed to the sclera external to uveal tumors and left in place for period of time calculated to deliver a lethal dose of radiation to the tumor. Radiation therapy with beams of protons or helium ions is performed at a few centers. Larger tumors or tumors that have caused secondary glaucoma generally are enucleated. Medium sized tumors can be treated with brachytherapy. The COMS showed that the mortality rates after I-125 plaque therapy and enucleation are similar. Another arm of the COMS study showed that pre-enucleation external beam radiotherapy of large choroidal melanomas does not improve survival. The COMS study also shed doubt on Zimmerman's hypothesis that enucleation of an eye containing a malignant melanoma might accelerate the dissemination of tumor cells (Fig. 11-14).

Although plaque brachytherapy conserves eyes, radiation retinopathy or papillopathy occurs commonly leading to loss of useful vision. Almost half of treated eyes have 20/200 vision 3 years after therapy. Some smaller tumors can be locally resected by partial lamellar sclerouvectomy. Today, this technique generally is performed on iridociliary tumors. Small relatively thin tumors of the posterior choroid can be treated with transpupillary thermotherapy (TTT), an infrared diode laser therapy that kills tumors cells by slowly heating them. A sandwich technique combining TTT and plaque brachytherapy has been used to prevent

tumor recurrence from cells sheltered in scleral canals at the base of a tumor. Endoresection of uveal melanoma has been investigated in some centers.

If a pigmented lesion of the iris is thought to be a melanoma based on documented growth or other clinical factors, it can be locally excised by iridectomy, or by iridocyclectomy if there is focal angle and ciliary body involvement. Enucleation is often necessary when an iris melanoma has caused glaucoma or is unresectable. Enucleation also may be done after histopathologic examination has shown that a previously resected tumor is a high-grade lesion. Plaque brachytherapy occasionally is used to treat unresectable iris melanomas.

THE DIFFERENTIAL DIAGNOSIS OF UVEAL MELANOMA

The differential diagnosis of posterior uveal malignant melanoma includes other benign and malignant neoplasms such as melanocytic nevi, choroidal hemangioma, and metastases from distant nonocular primary neoplasms. The list includes other rare primary intraocular neoplasms that arise in the uveal stroma such as schwannoma, leiomyoma, hemangiopericytoma, and adenomas and adenocarcinomas of the RPE and the pigmented and nonpigmented ciliary epithelium that typically are situated on its inner surface. Nonneoplastic conditions that can simulate posterior uveal melanoma and other intraocular neoplasms include vascular and hemorrhagic lesions, Inflammatory and infectious conditions, and a variety of miscellaneous disorders. Age-related maculopathy and peripheral exudative hemorrhagic chorioretinopathy ("peripheral disciform") are important vascular lesions. Inflammatory causes include nodular posterior scleritis, uveal effusion syndrome, and granulomas. Many of these simulating conditions are beautifully illustrated in Shields' Atlas and Textbook of Intraocular Tumors.

CHOROIDAL HEMANGIOMA

Choroidal hemangiomas are benign vascular hamartomas composed of relatively large, thin-walled vascular channels lined by endothelial cells. Choroidal hemangiomas occur sporadically, or in association with the Sturge-Weber syndrome (encephalotrigeminal angiomatosis). Sporadic cases appear as discrete orange-red tumefactions (Fig. 11-18). In contrast, the hemangiomas in patients with Sturge-Weber syndrome typically are diffuse lesions that obscure normal choroidal landmarks and impart a tomato-ketchup appearance to the fundus on ophthalmoscopy (Fig. 2-12). Both types of hemangiomas frequently have an associated serous detachment of the neurosensory retina that involves the fovea. Hemangiomas can produce visual loss if they are located beneath the fovea and induce hyperopia, or if they produce a retinal detachment.

Based on the size of their vascular channels, choroidal hemangiomas have been classified as cavernous, capillary, or mixed. In contrast to cavernous hemangiomas in the orbit, choroidal hemangiomas have relatively little stroma and lack the thick fibrous septa found in orbital lesions (Fig. 11-18B). The individual vascular channels almost appear to abut each other. Solitary tumors have clearly demarcated pushing margins that compress adjacent melanocytes and choroidal lamellae. Patients with Sturge-Weber syndrome have a diffuse angiomatosis that involves more than half of the choroid and shows intermixture of engorged preexisting vessels with the vascular tumor.

In addition to causing exudative retinal detachment, choroidal hemangiomas often produce secondary changes in adjacent ocular structures such as photoreceptor degeneration and cystoid retinal edema that can progress to retinoschisis. Varying degrees of retinal pigment epithelial hyperplasia and metaplasia may be present; in rare instances, circumscribed hemangiomas may be capped by dense plaques of fibrous metaplasia or even bone.

Although choroidal hemangiomas are benign neoplasms, they can prove "fatal" to the eye. Chronic retinal detachment and cystoid retinal edema can cause loss of vision, and the eye, as well, can be lost to secondary closed angle glaucoma caused by iris neovascularization or pupillary block induced by anterior displacement of the lens-iris diaphragm by a high bullous exudative retinal detachment. About three quarters of eyes with the diffuse hemangiomas of Sturge-Weber syndrome have glaucoma. In addition to papillary block, glaucoma mechanisms include iris neovascularization, maldevelopment of the angle, and elevation of episcleral venous pressure related to associated epibulbar vascular hamartomatous changes.

IVFA is often helpful in differentiating circumscribed choroidal hemangiomas from melanomas or metastases. IVFA typically shows lacy hyperfluorescence of vessels in the tumor in the prearterial phase and diffuse late staining of the mass. Late cystoid edema within the overlying retina may be prominent. Indocyanine green angiography shows early filling and a characteristic "washout" of hyperfluorescence in the later frames.

A scan ultrasonography shows high internal reflectivity within the tumor, and B scan shows a placoid or round choroidal mass that is acoustically solid. Hemangiomas appear acoustically solid on B-scan ultrasonography because their constituent vascular channels form multiple acoustic interfaces. Uveal melanomas usually show acoustic hollowness. A highly reflective cap may be present on the surface of hemangiomas with fibrous or osseous metaplasia. Magnetic resonance imaging shows a choroidal hemangioma to be hyperintense to the vitreous on T1-weighted images and isointense to vitreous on T2-weighted images.

Treatment of the benign vascular hamartoma is designed to preserve the eye by controlling exudative retinal detachment. Treatment modalities include delimiting laser photocoagulation, low-dose plaque radiotherapy, lens sparing external beam radiotherapy, TTT, and photodynamic

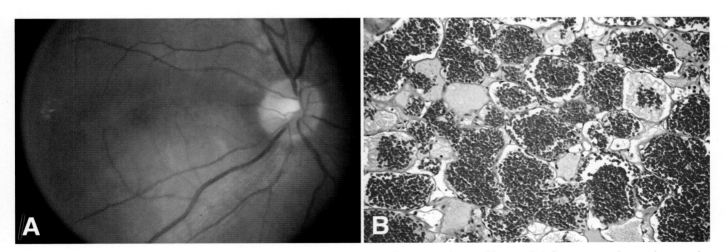

Fig. 11-18. A. Sporadic choroidal hemangioma. Discrete orange-red tumor is located beneath inferotemporal vascular arcade. The patient did not have Sturge-Weber syndrome. **B.** Benign vascular tumor in choroid is composed of large thin walled vessels with little intervening stroma. (**B.** H&E ×50)

therapy using verteporfin. Visual prognosis is guarded, however. More than 60% of patients have poor visual acuity 10 years after treatment despite successful control of associated subretinal fluid.

Uveal Metastases

Although ocular oncologists see many more patients with uveal melanoma, metastatic cancer to the eye probably is the most common malignant intraocular neoplasm. It has been estimated that 4% of patients dying from all types of carcinoma have ocular metastases, more than 12 times the incidence of uveal melanoma. Most of these secondary ocular tumors occur in terminally ill patients, however, and few are detected clinically or referred to ophthalmologists.

Most of the solid tumors that metastasize to the uvea are carcinomas; sarcomas rarely metastasize to the eye. Although any part of the eye may be involved by metastatic tumor, the uveal tract, especially the posterior part of the choroid, is affected most often (Fig. 11-19A). A retrospective review of 520 eyes with uveal metastases in 420 patients evaluated by the Oncology Service at the Wills Eye Hospital during a 20-year period showed that 88% of 950 metastatic foci involved the choroid. Most of the choroidal metastases involved the macula (12%) or the region between the macula and the equator (80%). The posterior choroid is affected most often because its blood supply is greater. Metastases to the retina, vitreous and optic disc are relatively uncommon.

Choroidal metastases typical appear as yellow or creamy-yellow, nummular, sessile dome- or plateau-shaped masses (Fig. 11-19A). Uveal metastases may be solitary or multiple and occasionally involve both eyes. Two or more separate foci of metastatic tumor are found in about 30% of affected eyes. Visual loss usually is caused by an associated exudative retinal detachment, which typically has shifting subretinal fluid. Metastases often are creamy-yellow in

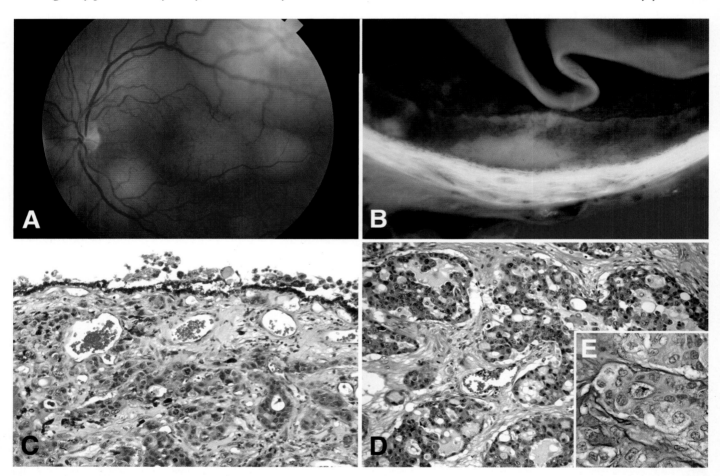

Fig. 11-19. Carcinoma metastatic to choroid. A. The posterior pole contains multiple nodules of amelanotic tumor. The patient was known to have metastatic mammary carcinoma. **B.** Lung carcinoma metastatic to the choroid. Metastatic tumor diffusely thickens the choroid. Bruch membrane is intact. The retina is detached and the RPE is focally disrupted. The apparent pigmentation of the cut surface of the extensively necrotic tumor was caused by dispersal of uveal pigment. **C.** Choroidal metastasis, lung carcinoma. Nests and islands of metastatic pulmonary adenocarcinoma infiltrate the choroidal stroma. The tumor forms glands and is producing mucin. The detached retina is not seen. Uveal metastasis may herald an occult lung cancer. **D.** Mucin-secreting adenocarcinoma metastatic to choroid. Tumor forms glandlike structures and contains large quantities of mucin. **E.** Alcian blue stain discloses presence of mucin in tumor. (**A.** Photo courtesy of Dr. Carol L.Shields, Wills Eye Institute, **C.** H&E ×50, **D.** H&E ×50, **E.** Alcian blue ×100)

color but may be hemorrhagic or can appear partially pigmented if necrosis has dispersed uveal pigment or the primary tumor is a cutaneous melanoma. Metastases from carcinoid tumors, thyroid carcinoma or renal cell carcinomas may be orange in color. Cutaneous melanoma often seeds the vitreous with pigmented cells (Fig. 10-10C, D).

Breast and lung carcinomas are responsible for more than two thirds of uveal metastases. Nearly half (47%) of the 420 patients reported by Shields et al. had breast carcinoma and about one fifth (21%) had lung cancer. Other primary tumors included gastrointestinal (4%), kidney (2%), skin (2%), prostate (2%), and other cancers (4%). Overall, about one third of patients who present with uveal metastases have no prior history of cancer. Systemic evaluation fails to disclose a primary tumor in half of these patients. About 35% of occult primary tumors spawing uveal metastases are lung carcinomas and 7% breast carcinomas. Women with metastases from breast carcinoma usually have a prior history of the disease. In contrast, metastasis is often the presenting manifestation of an occult lung cancer; less than half of the patients with metastatic lung cancer to the uvea were known to have cancer when the ocular diagnosis was made. Metastatic lung cancer is more common in men.

The prognosis of patients with uveal metastasis generally is quite poor; the mean survival has been reported to be approximately 9 to 10 months. Today, relatively few eyes with metastatic carcinoma are accessioned by ophthalmic pathology laboratories because the diagnosis is made clinically and most eyes are treated with radiotherapy and/or chemotherapy. Relief of pain is a major indication for enucleation of eyes with advanced disease. Plaque brachytherapy is advantageous compared to external beam radiotherapy because it can be delivered over a relatively short period of the patient's limited remaining life span.

The diagnosis of intraocular metastasis usually is made by slit lamp biomicroscopy and ophthalmoscopy in a patient who has been carefully questioned about a past medical history of cancer. Ancillary techniques such as IVFA and ultrasonography often can assist in making the diagnosis. Metastases generally begin to show

hyperfluorescence in the late venous phase of fluorescein angiography, somewhat later than most melanomas or hemangiomas. Metastases have many acoustical interfaces because they are composed of nests, cords, and islands of tumor cells surrounded by stroma. Hence, they show high internal reflectivity on A scan ultrasonography and appear acoustically solid in B scan, characteristics they share with hemangiomas. When routine studies give equivocal results, cytopathologic examination of material obtained by FNAB may establish the diagnosis.

The macroscopic appearance of eyes with uveal metastases is somewhat variable. In most instances, the uveal tract is diffusely thickened by an infiltrate of white, pink, or yellow tissue (Fig. 11-19B). Metastases occasionally have a multinodular growth pattern, and some larger lesions may be oval in configuration. Some lesions may be hemorrhagic and cavitary. Bruch membrane almost always remains intact. Although there are exceedingly rare exceptions to the rule, one generally can conclude that a mushroom-shaped tumor of the choroid is a malignant melanoma.

Microscopically, the uveal stroma is infiltrated by nests, cords, and islands of tumor cells whose general appearance and arrangement is dependent on the identity of the primary neoplasm (Fig. 11-19C,D). Most of the breast and lung tumors that metastasize to the eye are mucous-secreting adenocarcinomas. In such cases, special stains such as alcian blue, PAS, or mucicarmine are used to demonstrate the presence of intracytoplasmic mucin (Fig. 11-19E).

In recent years, immunohistochemical (IHC) stains are used to confirm the diagnosis and occasionally can identify the site of the occult primary tumor that has spawned the metastasis (Fig. 11-20). Carcinomas are distinguished by positive immunoreactivity for epithelial markers such as cytokeratins and epithelial membrane antigen. Most melanomas stain with S-100 protein and vimentin and a variety of other melanocytic markers including so-called melanoma specific antigen HMB-45, Melan A and microphthalmia transcription factor (MITF). The panel of IHC stains used to evaluate metastases often includes cytokeratins 7 and 20 (CK7 and CK20). Breast and lung carcinomas typically are CK7 positive and CK20 negative,

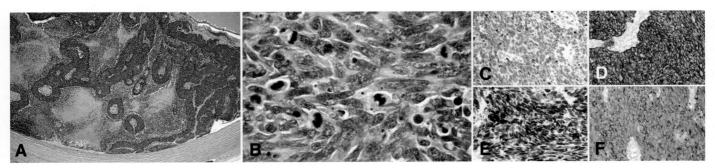

Fig 11-20. Small cell pulmonary carcinoma metastatic to choroid. A. Choroid metastasis shows extensive necrosis and perivascular growth pattern reminiscent of retinoblastoma. **B.** Mitotically active, undifferentiated tumor cells have scant cytoplasm. **C.** Negative immunoreactivity for melanocytic markers excludes melanoma. **D.** Carcinoma cells express cytokeratin. **E.** Ki-67 proliferation index is >90%. **F.** Tumor cells are immunoreactive for neuroendocrine marker synaptophysin. (**A.** H&E ×10, **B.** H&E ×250, **C.** IHC for melan A ×250, **D.** IHC for CAM 5.2, **E.** IHC for Ki-67 [MIB-1], **F.** IHC for Synaptophysin)

compared to colorectal carcinoma, which is CK20 positive and CK7 negative. Specific markers such as gross cystic disease fluid protein 15 (GCDFP-15) or BRST-2, a monoclonal antibody against the same protein, can confirm that a tumor is metastatic breast carcinoma (Fig. 16-7B). Breast metastases also are evaluated for estrogen and progesterone receptors and the HER2/neu gene product (Fig. 16-7C,D). The latter markers provide prognostic information regarding response to therapy. Lung cancers are often immunoreactive for TTF-1. Neuroendocrine carcinomas such as small cell lung carcinoma and carcinoid tumors stain for some cytokeratins and for neuroendocrine markers neuron specific enolase (NSE) and chromogranin (Fig. 11-20). Other primary tumors that often can be identified in a fairly convincing manner include thyroid carcinoma, renal cell carcinoma, and prostate carcinoma.

IHC is particularly helpful in the assessment of the small amount of tissue typically obtained by FNAB when the major clinical differential diagnosis includes melanoma and a metastasis. Immunocytologic assessment generally includes one or more melanoma markers such as S-100 protein, Melan A, MITF or HMB-45, and a carcinoma marker such as CAM 5.2, which reacts with cytokeratin 8, or a cytokeratin "cocktail" such as AE1/AE3, which reacts with a wide spectrum of high and low molecular weight cytokeratins.

OTHER INTRAOCULAR TUMORS

Primary intraocular tumors occasionally arise from the neuroepithelial layers of the eye. These include rare adenomas and adenocarcinomas of the iris pigment epithelium, the pigmented and nonpigmented ciliary epithelia, and RPE. These tumors also have been termed epitheliomas and malignant epitheliomas. Primary neoplasms of the RPE are exceedingly rare. This is somewhat surprising since the RPE readily undergoes reactive hyperplasia and metaplasia forming extensive amounts of fibrous tissue and even bone. Although they occasionally are amelanotic, **RPE tumors** classically are jet black in color and have abruptly elevated margins (Fig. 11-21). They are located on the inner surface of the

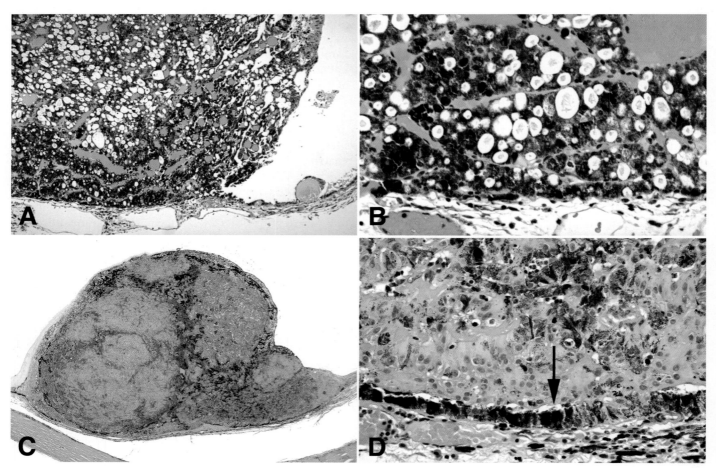

Fig. 11-21. RPE tumors. A. RPE Adenoma. Heavily pigmented, highly vascular tumor arises abruptly from the RPE. The tumor is located on the inner surface of Bruch membrane and does not involve the choroidal stroma. It contains many small cystoid spaces. **B.** The adenoma contains bands and islands of cells and small cystoid spaces that contain granular eosinophilic material. **C.** Low-grade RPE carcinoma arising from CHRPE. Tumor rests on inner surface of Bruch membrane and perforates retina. Varying degrss of pigmentation are present. **D.** *Arrow* denotes thick layer of heavily pigmented RPE consistent with residual CHRPE at base of tumor. Extracellular matrix material separates bands and islands of tumor cells, which vary in pigment content. Rare mitoses were present. Tumor was observed to arise from preexisting CHRPE clinically. (**A.** H&E ×50, **B.** H&E ×100, **C.** H&E ×10, **D.** H&E ×100)

choroid and frequently perforate the overlying retina, which shows intrareretinal lipid, exudation and dilated vessels. Histopathologically, tumors arising from the anterior part of the RPE often have a vacuolated pattern similar to adenomas of the pigmented ciliary epithelium (Fig. 11-21A,B). The cells comprising tumors of the posterior RPE are often arranged in linear strands and may form tubules or pseudoglands. The cells typically rest on prominent PAS-positive connective-tissue septa. Nuclear atypia, mitotic activity and a locally invasive growth pattern serve to distinguish RPE carcinomas from adenomas. RPE carcinomas may show an infiltrative growth pattern but do not metastasize. Epipapillary RPE adenoma may simulate optic disc melanocytoma.

Ciliary epithelial tumors (Figs. 11-22 and 11-23) can be predominantly pigmented or nonpigmented. Small pseudoadenomatous proliferations of the nonpigmented ciliary epithelium called Fuchs' or coronal adenomas are a common incidental finding in elderly eyes (Fig. 11-22). The cytoplasm of many pigmented ciliary epithelial tumors contains multiple small cystoid spaces. Nonpigmented tumors are white or yellowish-white in color and often produce focal cataract or lens dislocation. Many contain pools of hyaluronic acid, which can be extensive in some cases. In contrast to melanomas, which affect the uveal stroma, ciliary epithelial tumors arise from the epithelium lining on the inner surface of the ciliary body and often do not invade its stroma. The cells rest on connective tissue septa and form nests, cords, and islands. Local resection usually is curative. Although most ciliary epithelial tumors are benign, malignant variants have been reported. Invasion, mitotic activity, and nuclear pleomorphism are signs of malignancy. Pleomorphic adenocarcinomas of the nonpigmented ciliary epithelium (NPCE) typically are found in phthisical eyes in adults. In such cases, extraocular extension appears to be a requisite for metastatic spread. Fatalities have been associated with extraocular extension.

Congenital Hypertrophy of the RPE (CHRPE) appears ophthalmoscopically as a flat, round or oval pigmented spot (Fig. 11-24). The lesions are surrounded by a depigmented halo and usually develop depigmented lacunae with time. CHRPE occasionally was confused with melanoma before the advent of the modern binocular indirect ophthalmoscope. Microscopy discloses patches of tall RPE cells packed with large round melanosomes (Fig. 11-24B). Within lacunae, the atrophic outer retina adheres to the denuded inner surface of Bruch membrane. Although CHRPE originally was considered to be stationary, some lesions have been documented to grow by serial photography. Recently, Shields has reported that CHRPE rarely may give rise to solid tumors. Histopathology (Fig. 11-21C,D) showed that one of these lesions was a low-grade adenocarcinoma of the RPE.

Congenital grouped pigmentation ("bear tracks") is a variant of CHRPE (Fig. 11-24C,D). Multiple bilateral pigmented RPE lesions that bear a superficial resemblance to CHRPE recently have been reported to be an ocular marker for the heritable cancer diathesis Gardner syndrome (familial adenomatous polyposis with extracolonic manifestations).

Leiomyomas are rare nonpigmented ciliary body tumors that usually affect young women. Most are situated in the supraciliary space, and they characteristically transmit light during transillumination. Compared to melanomas, leiomyomas are paucicellular and their cells have fibrillar eosinophilic cytoplasm (Fig. 11-25). Positive immunoreactivity for smooth muscle actin and other muscle markers serves to differentiate leiomyoma from uveal melanoma and from rare **peripheral nerve sheath tumors** (schwannoma) (Fig. 11-26), which also are paucicellular. The latter distinction is important because some leiomyomas have a distinctly neural appearance on routine light microscopy. The term mesectodermal leiomyoma has been applied to such tumors, emphasizing the derivation of intraocular smooth muscle from neural crest.

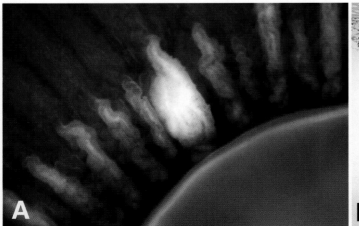
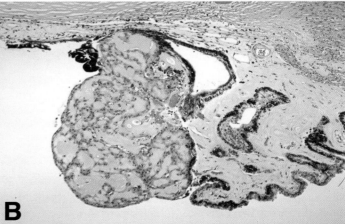

Fig. 11-22. Fuchs (coronal) adenoma. A. Miniature tumor appears grossly as an enlarged, white ciliary process. **B.** Adenoma is composed of hyperplastic nonpigmented ciliary epithelium surrounding acellular stroma of amorphous eosinophilic extracellular matrix material. (**B.** H&E ×50)

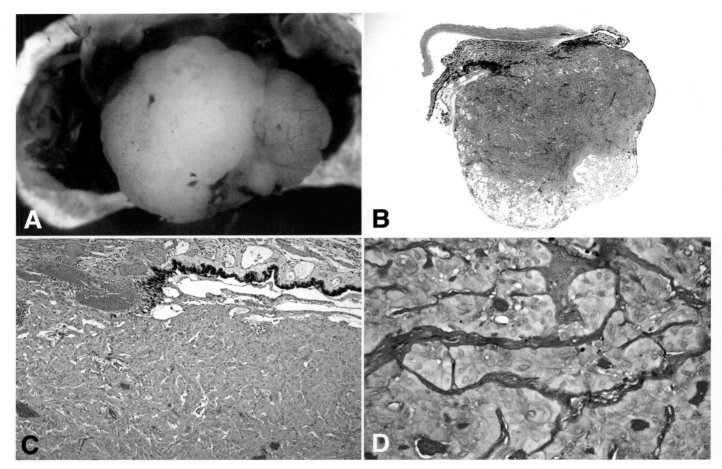

Fig. 11-23. Ciliary epithelial neoplasms. A. Adenoma of nonpigmented ciliary epithelium arises from inner surface of pars plicata. Tumor was locally resected. **B.** Nonpigmented ciliary epithelial tumor rests on inner surface of ciliary body and does not involve its stroma. Apical part of tumor contains clear vacuoles of hyaluronic acid. **C.** Benign adenoma arises from ciliary epithelium on inner surface of pars plicata. It is composed of cords and bands of nonpigmented ciliary epithelial cells. **D.** PAS-positive septa separate bands of nonpigmented ciliary epithelial cells. (**B.** H&E ×10, **C.** H&E ×50, **D.** PAS ×100)

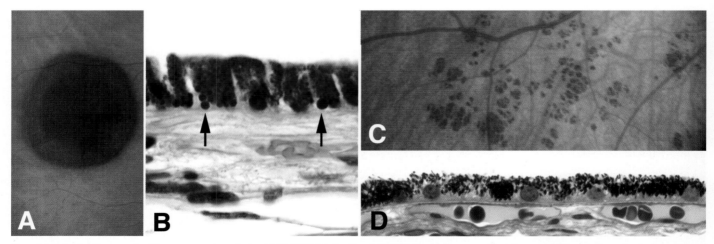

Fig. 11-24. A. Congenital hypertrophy of the RPE (CHRPE). Oval CHRPE lacks lacunae. **B.** Histopathology of similar lesion shows tall hypertrophic RPE cells filled with pigment. *Arrows* denote large round macromelanosomes. **C.** Congenital grouped pigmentation of the RPE ("bear tracks"). Clinical photo shows numerous flat, well demarcated pigmented lesions that have been likened to animal tracks. **D.** Corresponding photomicrograph shows increased numbers of ellipsoidal melanin granules filling the cytoplasm of the RPE cells. In normal RPE cells, melanosomes are confined to the apical cytoplasm. (**B.** H&E ×250, **D.** Toluidine blue ×250)

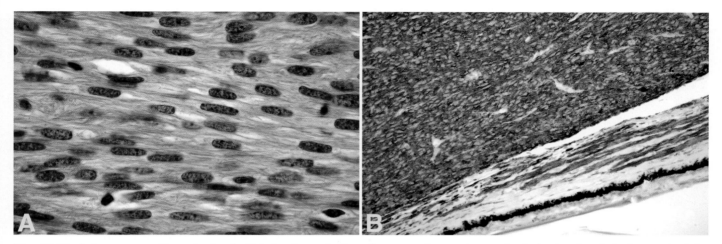

Fig. 11-25. Leiomyoma, ciliary body. A. This benign spindle cell tumor of smooth muscle derivation is relatively paucicellular compared to an amelanotic spindle cell melanoma. The spindle cells have bland nuclei and finely fibrillar cytoplasm. **B.** IHC stain for smooth muscle actin is strongly positive. Ciliary muscle (below) serves as normal internal control. Some uveal leiomyomas have a distinctly neural appearance. (**A.** H&E ×250, **B.** IHC for SMA ×50)

Choroidal osteoma or osseous choristoma is another rare primary uveal tumor that chiefly affects young women (Fig. 11-27). These interesting lesions are often bilateral and peripapillary in their location. Choroidal osteoma appears clinically as a yellow-orange placoid tumor with sharply defined scalloped margins. The bone in osseous choristomas is located within the choroid, not on its inner surface like the osseous metaplasia of the RPE found in phthisical eyes. Osteomas may be confused ophthalmoscopically with metastases but are easily distinguished either by ultrasonography, which shows a highly reflective plaque that persists at lower sensitivity or by computed tomography that reveals a plaque with bone density. Serum calcium, phosphorus, and alkaline phosphatase levels usually are normal.

Iris pigment epithelial cysts are easily confused clinically with anterior uveal malignant melanomas because they are heavily pigmented and may cause focal shallowing of the anterior chamber. Histopathologically, these cysts are composed of polarized iris pigment epithelium that is one or more layers thick. The lumen contains clear fluid.

Primary lymphomas of the uvea were initially thought to be reactive lymphoid hyperplasias. Immunophenotypic studies indicate that they are low-grade lymphomas of mucosa associated lymphoid tissue (MALT) (Fig. 11-28). The uveal stroma may be affected in the late stages of a systemic lymphoma or by leukemia. Primary central nervous system (CNS) lymphoma involves the vitreous and retina but generally spares the uveal tract. Visceral lymphoma rarely involves the vitreous secondarily.

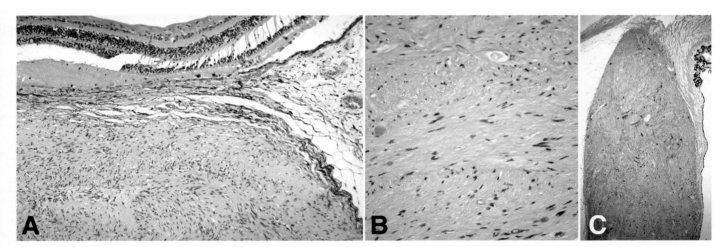

Fig. 11-26. Benign peripheral nerve sheath tumor, choroid. A. The cytology of this bland, paucicellular choroidal tumor is consistent with a Schwannoma. **B.** Another example is paucicellular. **C.** Tumor is immunoreactive for S-100 protein but did not stain with melanoma markers. Schwannomas are exceeding rare intraocular tumors that are often impossible to distinguish from melanoma clinically. IHC stains are necessary to confirm the diagnosis. (**A.** H&E ×50, **B.** H&E ×100, **C.** IHC for S-100 protein ×25)

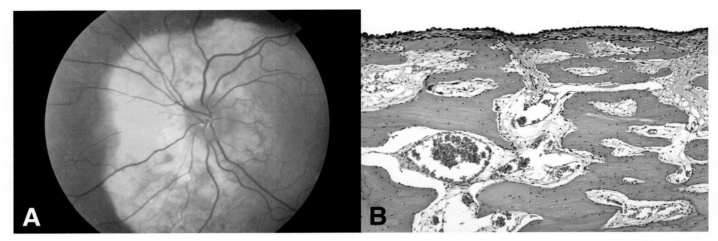

Fig. 11-27. Choroidal osteoma. A. Yellow-orange peripapillary tumor found in young woman has characteristic scalloped margins. **B.** Choroidal osteomas are composed of irregular spicules of bone that are surrounded by an areolar stroma containing large vascular channels. The bone is found within the choroid, deep to Bruch membrane, choriocapillaris, and an intact layer of RPE. The intrachoroidal location of the bone distinguishes choroidal osteoma from the bone formed by osseous metaplasia of the RPE in blind phthisical eyes. Metaplastic bone typically is located on the inner surface of Bruch membrane. (**B.** H&E ×50)

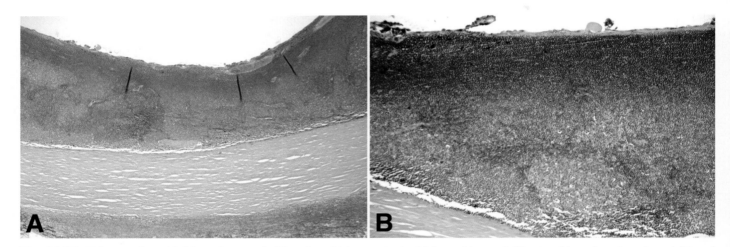

Fig. 11-28. Primary choroidal lymphoma. A. The choroid is massively thickened by an infiltrate of lymphocytes. An additional focus of lymphoid cells is present on the epibulbar surface of the eye. Previously called reactive lymphoid hyperplasia of the uvea, such tumors are now thought to be low-grade MALT lymphomas. **B.** Infiltrate is composed of well-differentiated lymphocytes. A few germinal centers are present. They are often found in MALT lymphomas. (**A.** H&E ×25, **B.** H&E ×50)

BIBLIOGRAPHY

Nevi

Augsburger JJ, Schroeder RP, Territo C, et al. Clinical parameters predictive of enlargement of melanocytic choroidal lesions. *Br J Ophthalmol* 1989;73:911–917.

Eagle RC Jr. Iris pigmentation and pigmented lesions: an ultrastructural study. *Trans Am Ophthalmol Soc* 1988;86:581–687.

Gass JD. Problems in the differential diagnosis of choroidal nevi and malignant melanomas. The XXXIII Edward Jackson Memorial Lecture. *Am J Ophthalmol* 1977;83:299–323.

Naumann G. Pigmented nevi of the choroid and ciliary bodies. A clinical and histopathological study. *Adv Ophthalmol* 1970;23: 187–272.

Naumann G, Yanoff M, Zimmerman LE. Histogenesis of malignant melanomas of the uvea: I. Histopathologic characteristics of nevi of the choroid and ciliary body. *Arch Ophthalmol* 1966;76: 784–796.

Shields CL, Cater J, Shields JA, et al. Combination of clinical factors predictive of growth of small choroidal melanocytic tumors. *Arch Ophthalmol* 2000;118:360–364.

Shields CL, Demirci H, Materin MA, et al. Clinical factors in the identification of small choroidal melanoma. *Can J Ophthalmol* 2004;39:351–357.

Sumich P, Mitchell P, Wang JJ. Choroidal nevi in a white population: The Blue Mountains Eye Study. *Arch Ophthalmol* 1998;116:645–650.

Melanocytoma

Apple DJ, Craythorn JM, Reidy JJ, et al. Malignant transformation of an optic nerve melanocytoma. *Can J Ophthalmol* 1984;19:320–325.

Bhorade AM, Edward DP, Goldstein DA. Ciliary body melanocytoma with anterior segment pigment dispersion and elevated intraocular pressure. *J Glaucoma* 1999;8:129–133.

Cogan DG. Discussion of Melanocytoma. In: Boniuk M, ed. *Ocular and Adnexal Tumors: New and Controversial Aspects.* St. Louis, MO: Mosby, 1964:385.

De Potter P, Shields CL, Eagle RC Jr, et al. Malignant melanoma of the optic nerve. *Arch Ophthalmol* 1996;114:608–612.

Fineman MS, Eagle RC Jr, Shields JA, et al. Melanocytomalytic glaucoma in eyes with necrotic iris melanocytoma. *Ophthalmology* 1998;105:492–496.

Frangieh GT, el Baba F, Traboulsi EI, et al. Melanocytoma of the ciliary body: presentation of four cases and review of nineteen reports. *Surv Ophthalmol* 1985;29:328–324.

Joffe L, Shields JA, Osher RH, et al. Clinical and follow-up studies of melanocytomas of the optic disc. *Ophthalmology* 1979;86:1067–1083.

Juarez CP, Tso MO. An ultrastructural study of melanocytomas (magnocellular nevi) of the optic disk and uvea. *Am J Ophthalmol* 1980;90:48–62.

LoRusso FJ, Boniuk M, Font RL. Melanocytoma (magnocellular nevus) of the ciliary body: report of 10 cases and review of the literature. *Ophthalmology* 2000;107:795–800.

Mansour AM, Zimmerman LE, La Piana FG, et al. Clinicopathologic findings in a growing optic nerve melanocytoma. *Br J Ophthalmol* 1989;73:410–415.

Osher RH, Shields JA, Layman PR. Pupillary and visual field evaluation in patients with melanocytoma of the optic disc. *Arch Ophthalmol* 1979;97:1096–1099.

Shields JA, Augsburger JJ, Bernardino V Jr, et al. Melanocytoma of the ciliary body and iris. *Am J Ophthalmol* 1980;89:632–635.

Shields JA, Demirci H, Mashayekhi A, et al. Melanocytoma of optic disc in 115 cases: The 2004 Samuel Johnson Memorial Lecture, part 1. *Ophthalmology* 2004;111:1739–1746.

Shields JA, Demirci H, Mashayekhi A, et al. Melanocytoma of the optic disk: a review. *Surv Ophthalmol* 2006;51:93–104.

Shields JA, Eagle RC Jr, Shields CL, et al. Pigmented adenoma of the optic nerve head simulating a melanocytoma. *Ophthalmology* 1992;99:1705–1708.

Shields JA, Shields CL, Eagle RC Jr, et al. Malignant melanoma associated with melanocytoma of the optic disc. *Ophthalmology* 1990;97:225–230.

Shields JA, Shields CL, Eagle RC Jr, et al. Malignant melanoma arising from a large uveal melanocytoma in a patient with oculodermal melanocytosis. *Arch Ophthalmol* 2000;118:990–993.

Shields JA, Shields CL, Eagle RC Jr, et al. Central retinal vascular obstruction secondary to melanocytoma of the optic disc. *Arch Ophthalmol* 2001;119:129–133.

Teichmann KD, Karcioglu ZA. Melanocytoma of the iris with rapidly developing secondary glaucoma. *Surv Ophthalmol* 1995;40:136–144.

Zimmerman LE. Melanocytes, melanocytic nevi and melanocytomas. *Invest Ophthalmol Vis Sci* 1965;4:11–41.

Zimmerman LE, Garron LK. Melanocytoma of the optic disk. *Int Ophthalmol Clin* 1962;2:431–440.

Uveal Melanoma—Epidemiology and Predisposing Features

Albert DM, Chang MA, Lamping K, et al. The dysplastic nevus syndrome. A pedigree with primary malignant melanomas of the choroid and skin. *Ophthalmology* 1985;92:1728–1734.

Albert DM, Lahav M, Packer S, et al. Histogenesis of malignant melanomas of the uvea. Occurrence of nevus-like structures in experimental choroidal tumors. *Arch Ophthalmol* 1974;92:318–323.

Albert DM, Robinson NL, Fulton AB, et al. Epidemiological investigation of increased incidence of choroidal melanoma in a single population of chemical workers. *Int Ophthalmol Clin* 1980;20:71–92.

Antle CM, Damji KF, White VA, et al. Uveal malignant melanoma and optic nerve glioma in von Recklinghausen's neurofibromatosis. *Br J Ophthalmol* 1990;74:502–504.

Bacin F, Kemeny JL, D'Hermies F, et al: Malignant melanoma of the choroid associated with neurofibromatosis. *J Fr Ophtalmol* 1993;16:184–190.

Balmaceda CM, Fetell MR, O'Brien JL, et al. Nevus of Ota and leptomeningeal melanocytic lesions. *Neurology* 1993;43:381–386.

Barr CC, Zimmerman LE, Curtin VT, et al. Bilateral diffuse melanocytic uveal tumors associated with systemic malignant neoplasms. A recently recognized syndrome. *Arch Ophthalmol* 1982;100:249–255.

Bordon AF, Wray ML, Belfort R, et al. Choroidal malignant melanoma in association with oculodermal melanocytosis in a black patient. *Br J Ophthalmol* 1995;79:191–192.

Broadway D, Lang S, Harper J, et al. Congenital malignant melanoma of the eye. *Cancer* 1991;67:2642–2652.

Diener-West M, Earle JD, Fine SL, et al. The COMS randomized trial of iodine 125 brachytherapy for choroidal melanoma: II. Characteristics of patients enrolled and not enrolled. COMS Report No. 17. *Arch Ophthalmol* 2001;119:951–965.

Dutton JJ, Anderson RL, Schelper RL, et al. Orbital malignant melanoma and oculodermal melanocytosis: report of two cases and review of the literature. *Ophthalmology* 1984;91:497–507.

Gass JD, Gieser RG, Wilkinson CP, et al. Bilateral diffuse uveal melanocytic proliferation in patients with occult carcinoma. *Arch Ophthalmol* 1990;108:527–533.

Gass JD, Glatzer RJ. Acquired pigmentation simulating Peutz-Jeghers syndrome: initial manifestation of diffuse uveal melanocytic proliferation. *Br J Ophthalmol* 1991;75:693–695.

Gonder JR, Shields JA, Albert DM, et al. Uveal malignant melanoma associated with ocular and oculodermal melanocytosis. *Ophthalmology* 1982;89:953–960.

Gunduz K, Shields JA, Shields CL, et al. Choroidal melanoma in a 14-year-old patient with ocular melanocytosis. *Arch Ophthalmol* 1998;116:1112–1114.

Holly EA, Aston DA, Char DH, et al. Uveal melanoma in relation to ultraviolet light exposure and host factors. *Cancer Res* 1990;50:5773–5777.

Honavar SG, Singh AD, Shields CL, et al. Iris melanoma in a patient with neurofibromatosis. *Surv Ophthalmol* 2000;45:231–236.

Lee SB, Au Eong KG, Saw SM, et al. Eye cancer incidence in Singapore. *Br J Ophthalmol* 2000;84:767–770.

Leung AK, Kao CP, Cho HY, et al. Scleral melanocytosis and oculodermal melanocytosis (nevus of Ota) in Chinese children. *J Pediatr* 2000;137:581–584.

Margo CE, McLean IW. Malignant melanoma of the choroid and ciliary body in black patients. *Arch Ophthalmol* 1984;102:77–79.

Margo CE, Mulla Z, Billiris K. Incidence of surgically treated uveal melanoma by race and ethnicity. *Ophthalmology* 1998;105:1087–1090.

Nik NA, Glew WB, Zimmerman LE. Malignant melanoma of the choroid in the nevus of Ota of a black patient. *Arch Ophthalmol* 1982;100:1641–1643.

Rehany U, Rumelt S. Iridocorneal melanoma associated with type 1 neurofibromatosis: a clinicopathologic study. *Ophthalmology* 1999;106:614–618.

Rice CD, Brown HH. Primary orbital melanoma associated with orbital melanocytosis. *Arch Ophthalmol* 1990;108:1130–1134.

Rodriguez-Sains RS. Ocular findings in patients with dysplastic nevus syndrome. *Ophthalmology* 1986;93:661–665.

Sang DN, Albert DM, Sober AJ, et al. Nevus of Ota with contralateral cerebral melanoma. *Arch Ophthalmol* 1977;95:1820–1824.

Shields JA, Shields CL. *Intraocular Tumors: An Atlas and Textbook.* Philadelphia, PA: Lippincott Williams & Wilkins, 2008.

Shields CL, Shields JA, Milite J, et al. Uveal melanoma in teenagers and children. A report of 40 cases. *Ophthalmology* 1991;98:1662–1666.

Singh AD, De Potter P, Fijal BA, et al. Lifetime prevalence of uveal melanoma in white patients with oculo(dermal) melanocytosis. *Ophthalmology* 1998;105:195–198.

Singh AD, Shields CL, Shields JA, et al. Uveal melanoma in young patients. *Arch Ophthalmol* 2000;118:918–923.

Singh AD, Shields JA, Eagle RC, et al. Iris melanoma in a ten-year-old boy with familial atypical mole-melanoma (FAM-M) syndrome. *Ophthalmic Genet* 1994;15:145–149.

Singh AD, Wang MX, Donoso LA, et al. Genetic aspects of uveal melanoma: a brief review. *Semin Oncol* 1996;23:768–772.

Ticho BH, Tso MO, Kishi S. Diffuse iris nevus in oculodermal melanocytosis: a light and electron microscopic study. *J Pediatr Ophthalmol Strabismus* 1989;26:244–250.

Vajdic CM, Kricker A, Giblin M, et al. Eye color and cutaneous nevi predict risk of ocular melanoma in Australia. *Int J Cancer* 2001;92:906–912.

Wells CG, Bradford RH, Fish GE, et al. Choroidal melanomas in American Indians. COMS Group. Collaborative Ocular Melanoma Study. *Arch Ophthalmol* 1996;114:1017–1018.

Wilkes TD, Uthman EO, Thornton CN, et al. Malignant melanoma of the orbit in a black patient with ocular melanocytosis. *Arch Ophthalmol* 1984;102:904–906.

Uveal Melanoma—Clinical Features

Augsburger JJ, Shields JA, Folberg R, et al. Fine needle aspiration biopsy in the diagnosis of intraocular cancer. Cytologic-histologic correlations. *Ophthalmology* 1985;92:39–49.

Eagle RC Jr, Brucker AJ. Choroidal melanoma with retinal perforation and vitreous hemorrhage: a scanning electron microscopic study. *Jpn J Ophthalmol* 1983;27:512–521.

Eagle RC Jr, Grossniklaus HE, Syed N, et al. Inadvertent evisceration of eyes containing uveal melanoma. *Arch Ophthalmol* 2009;127:141–145.

Eagle RC Jr, Shields JA. Pseudoretinitis pigmentosa secondary to preretinal malignant melanoma cells. *Retina* 1982;2:51–55.

Eskelin S, Pyrhonen S, Summanen P, et al. Tumor doubling times in metastatic malignant melanoma of the uvea: tumor progression before and after treatment. *Ophthalmology* 2000;107: 1443–1449.

Font RL, Zimmerman LE, Armaly MF. The nature of the orange pigment over a choroidal melanoma. Histochemical and electron microscopical observations. *Arch Ophthalmol* 1974;91:359–362.

Fuchs E. *Sarcom des Uvealtractus*. Wien: Wilhelm Braumüller, 1882.

Shields CL, Bianciotto C, Pirondini C, et al. Autofluorescence of orange pigment overlying small choroidal melanoma. *Retina* 2007;27:1107–1111.

Shields CL, Santos MC, Shields JA, et al. Extraocular extension of unrecognized choroidal melanoma simulating a primary optic nerve tumor: report of two cases. *Ophthalmology* 1999;106:1349–1352.

Shields CL, Shields JA, Shields MB, et al. Prevalence and mechanisms of secondary intraocular pressure elevation in eyes with intraocular tumors. *Ophthalmology* 1987;94:839–846.

Shields CL, Shields JA, Yarian DL, et al. Intracranial extension of choroidal melanoma via the optic nerve. *Br J Ophthalmol* 1987;71:172–176.

Shields JA, Rodrigues MM, Sarin LK, et al. Lipofuscin pigment over benign and malignant choroidal tumors. *Trans Am Acad Ophthalmol Otolaryngol* 1976;81:871–881.

Shields JA, Shields CL. Massive orbital extension of posterior uveal melanomas. *Ophthal Plast Reconstr Surg* 1991;7:238–251.

Shields JA, Shields CL, Ehya H, et al. Fine-needle aspiration biopsy of suspected intraocular tumors. The 1992 Urwick Lecture. *Ophthalmology* 1993;100:1677–1684.

Yanoff M. Glaucoma mechanisms in ocular malignant melanomas. *Am J Ophthalmol* 1970;70:898–904.

Zimmerman LE. Problems in the diagnosis of malignant melanoma of the choroid and ciliary body. The 1972 Arthur J. Bedell Lecture. *Am J Ophthalmol* 1973;75:917–929.

Zimmerman LE, McLean IW. Metastatic disease from untreated uveal melanomas. *Am J Ophthalmol* 1979;88:524–534.

Uveal Melanoma—Pathology

Callender G. Malignant melanotic tumors of the eye: a study of histologic types in 111 cases. *Trans Am Acad Ophthalmol Otolaryngol* 1931;36:131–142.

Connolly BP, Regillo CD, Eagle RC Jr, et al. The histopathologic effects of transpupillary thermotherapy in human eyes. *Ophthalmology* 2003;110:415–420.

Damato BE, Foulds WS. Tumour-associated retinal pigment epitheliopathy. *Eye* 1990;4:382–387.

Font RL, Spaulding AG, Zimmerman LE. Diffuse melanoma of the uveal tract. A Clinicopathologic report of 54 cases. *Trans Am Acad Ophthalmol Otolaryngol* 1968;72:877–895.

Green WR. The uveal tract. In: Spencer W, ed. *Ophthalmic Pathology: An Atlas and Textbook*, vol. 3. Philadelphia, PA: WB Saunders, 1996.

Histopathologic characteristics of uveal melanomas in eyes enucleated from the Collaborative Ocular Melanoma Study: COMS report no. 6. *Am J Ophthalmol* 1998;125:745–766.

Lois N, Shields CL, Shields JA, et al. Cavitary melanoma of the ciliary body. A study of eight cases. *Ophthalmology* 1998;105: 1091–1098.

McLean IW, Foster WD, Zimmerman LE, et al. Modifications of Callender's classification of uveal melanoma at the Armed Forces Institute of Pathology. *Am J Ophthalmol* 1983;96:502–509.

Shields CL, Shields JA, De Potter P, et al. Diffuse choroidal melanoma. Clinical features predictive of metastasis. *Arch Ophthalmol* 1996;114:956–963.

Shields CL, Shields JA, Perez N, et al. Primary transpupillary thermotherapy for small choroidal melanoma in 256 consecutive cases: outcomes and limitations. *Ophthalmology* 2002;109:225–234.

Smith LT, Irvine AR. Diagnostic significance of orange pigment accumulation over choroidal tumors. *Mod Probl Ophthalmol* 1974;12:536–543.

Iris Melanoma

Demirci H, Shields CL, Shields JA, et al. Diffuse iris melanoma: a report of 25 cases. *Ophthalmology* 2002;109:1553–1560.

Grossniklaus H, Brown RH, Stulting RD, et al. Iris melanoma seeding through a trabeculectomy site. *Arch Ophthalmol* 1990;108:1287–1290.

Harbour JW, Augsburger JJ, Eagle RC Jr. Initial management and follow-up of melanocytic iris tumors. *Ophthalmology* 1995;102:1987–1993.

Jakobiec FA, Silbert G. Are most iris "melanomas" really nevi? A clinicopathologic study of 189 lesions. *Arch Ophthalmol* 1981;99:2117–2132.

Reese AB, Mund ML, Iwamoto T. Tapioca melanoma of the iris: 1. Clinical and light microscopy studies. *Am J Ophthalmol* 1972;74:840–850.

Rones B, Zimmerman LE. The production of heterochromia and glaucoma by diffuse malignant melanoma of the iris. *Trans Am Acad Ophthalmol Otolaryngol* 1957;61:447–463.

Shields CL, Shields JA, Materin M, et al. Iris melanoma. Risk factors for metastasis in 169 consecutive patients. *Ophthalmology* 2001; 108:172–178.

Territo C, Shields CL, Shields JA, et al. Natural course of melanocytic tumors of the iris. *Ophthalmology* 1988;95:1251–1255.

Uveal Melanoma—Prognostic Features

Al-Jamal RT, Kivela T. KI-67 immunopositivity in choroidal and ciliary body melanoma with respect to nucleolar diameter and other prognostic factors. *Curr Eye Res* 2006;31:57–67.

Anastassiou G, Schilling H, Djakovic S, et al. Expression of VLA-2, VLA-3, and alpha(v) integrin receptors in uveal melanoma: association with microvascular architecture of the tumour and prognostic value. *Br J Ophthalmol* 2000;84:899–902.

Anastassiou G, Schilling H, Stang A, et al. Expression of the cell adhesion molecules ICAM-1, VCAM-1 and NCAM in uveal melanoma: a clinicopathological study. *Oncology* 2000;58:83–88.

Assessment of metastatic disease status at death in 435 patients with large choroidal melanoma in the Collaborative Ocular Melanoma Study (COMS): COMS report no. 15. *Arch Ophthalmol* 2001;119:670–676.

Bechrakis NE, Sehu KW, Lee WR, et al. Transformation of cell type in uveal melanomas: a quantitative histologic analysis. *Arch Ophthalmol* 2000;118:1406–1412.

Blom DJ, Luyten GP, Mooy C, et al. Human leukocyte antigen class I expression. Marker of poor prognosis in uveal melanoma. *Invest Ophthalmol Vis Sci* 1997;38:1865–1872.

Chana JS, Wilson GD, Cree IA, et al. c-myc, p53, and Bcl-2 expression and clinical outcome in uveal melanoma. *Br J Ophthalmol* 1999;83:110–114.

Chang SH, Worley LA, Onken MD, et al. Prognostic biomarkers in uveal melanoma: evidence for a stem cell-like phenotype associated with metastasis. *Melanoma Res* 2008;18:191–200.

Chowers I, Amer R, Pe'er J. The correlation among different immunostaining evaluation methods for the assessment of proliferative activity in uveal melanoma. *Curr Eye Res* 2002;25:369–372.

Coleman DJ, Rondeau MJ, Silverman RH, et al. Correlation of microcirculation architecture with ultrasound backscatter parameters of uveal melanoma. *Eur J Ophthalmol* 1995;5:96–106.

Coleman K, Baak JP, van Diest PJ, et al. DNA ploidy status in 84 ocular melanomas: a study of DNA quantitation in ocular melanomas by flow cytometry and automatic and interactive static image analysis. *Hum Pathol* 1995;26:99–105.

Coupland SE, Anastassiou G, Stang A, et al. The prognostic value of cyclin D1, p53, and MDM2 protein expression in uveal melanoma. *J Pathol* 2000;191:120–126.

Coupland SE, Bechrakis N, Schuler A, et al. Expression patterns of cyclin D1 and related proteins regulating G1-S phase transition in uveal melanoma and retinoblastoma. *Br J Ophthalmol* 1998;82:961–970.

Coupland SE, Campbell I, Damato B. Routes of extraocular extension of uveal melanoma: risk factors and influence on survival probability. *Ophthalmology* 2008;115:1778–1785.

Cree IA. Cell cycle and melanoma—two different tumours from the same cell type [Editorial; comment]. *J Pathol* 2000;191: 112–114.

Damato B, Coupland SE. Translating uveal melanoma cytogenetics into clinical care. *Arch Ophthalmol* 2009;127:423–429.

Damato B, Duke C, Coupland SE, et al. Cytogenetics of uveal melanoma: a 7-year clinical experience. *Ophthalmology* 2007;114:1925–1931.

de la Cruz PO Jr, Specht CS, McLean IW. Lymphocytic infiltration in uveal malignant melanoma. *Cancer* 1990;65:112–115.

De Vries TJ, Mooy CM, Van Balken MR, et al. Components of the plasminogen activation system in uveal melanoma—a clinico-pathological study. *J Pathol* 1995;175:59–67.

Ehlers JP, Harbour JW. NBS1 expression as a prognostic marker in uveal melanoma. *Clin Cancer Res* 2005;11:1849–1853.

Elavathil LJ, LeRiche J, Rootman J, et al. Prognostic value of DNA ploidy as assessed with flow cytometry in uveal melanoma. *Can J Ophthalmol* 1995;30:360–365.

Folberg R, Pe'er J, Gruman LM, et al. The morphologic characteristics of tumor blood vessels as a marker of tumor progression in primary human uveal melanoma: a matched case-control study. *Hum Pathol* 1992;23:1298–1305.

Folberg R, Rummelt V, Parys-Van Ginderdeuren R, et al. The prognostic value of tumor blood vessel morphology in primary uveal melanoma. *Ophthalmology* 1993;100:1389–1398.

Fuchs U, Kivela T, Summanen P, et al. An immunohistochemical and prognostic analysis of cytokeratin expression in malignant uveal melanoma. *Am J Pathol* 1992;141:169–181.

Gamel JW, Greenberg RA, McLean IW, et al. A clinically useful method for combining gross and microscopic measurements to select high-risk patients after enucleation for ciliochoroidal melanoma. *Cancer* 1986;57:1341–1344.

Gamel JW, McCurdy JB, McLean IW. A comparison of prognostic covariates for uveal melanoma. *Invest Ophthalmol Vis Sci* 1992;33:1919–1922.

Gamel JW, McLean IW. Quantitative analysis of the Callender classification of uveal melanoma cells. *Arch Ophthalmol* 1977;95: 686–691.

Gamel JW, McLean IW. Computerized histopathologic assessment of malignant potential: III. Refinements of measurement and data analysis. *Anal Quant Cytol* 1984;6:37–44.

Gamel JW, McLean IW, Foster WD, et al. Uveal melanomas: correlation of cytologic features with prognosis. *Cancer* 1978;41:1897–1901.

Gamel JW, McLean IW, Greenberg RA, et al. Computerized histologic assessment of malignant potential: a method for determining the prognosis of uveal melanomas. *Hum Pathol* 1982;13:893–897.

Ghazvini S, Kroll S, Char DH, et al. Comparative analysis of proliferating cell nuclear antigen, bromodeoxyuridine, and mitotic index in uveal melanoma. *Invest Ophthalmol Vis Sci* 1995;36:2762–2767.

Harbour JW. Eye cancer: Unique insights into oncogenesis: The Cogan Lecture. *Invest Ophthalmol Vis Sci* 2006;47:1736–1745.

Harbour JW. Molecular prognostic testing in uveal melanoma: has it finally come of age? *Arch Ophthalmol* 2007;125:1122–1123.

Hendrix MJ, Seftor EA, Seftor RE, et al. Biologic determinants of uveal melanoma metastatic phenotype: role of intermediate filaments as predictive markers. *Lab Invest* 1998;78:153–163.

Hendrix MJ, Seftor EA, Seftor RE, et al. Regulation of uveal melanoma interconverted phenotype by hepatocyte growth factor/scatter factor (HGF/SF). *Am J Pathol* 1998;152:855–863.

Hodge WG, Duclos AJ, Rocha G, et al. DNA index and S phase fraction in uveal malignant melanomas. *Br J Ophthalmol* 1995;79:521–526.

Huntington A, Haugan P, Gamel J, et al. A simple cytologic method for predicting the malignant potential of intraocular melanoma. *Pathol Res Pract* 1989;185:631–634.

Jager MJ, Volker-Dieben HJ, de Wolff-Rouendaal D, et al. Possible relation between HLA and ABO type and prognosis of uveal melanoma. *Doc Ophthalmol* 1992;82:43–47.

Jensen OA. Malignant melanomas of the human uvea: 25-year follow-up of cases in Denmark, 1943–1952. *Acta Ophthalmol (Copenh)* 1982;60:161–182.

Kantelip B, Albuisson E, Bacin F, et al. Intratumoral blood pools and prognosis of malignant uveal melanoma treated with enucleation. *Ophtalmologie* 1989;3:49–52.

Karlsson M, Boeryd B, Carstensen J, et al. Correlations of Ki-67 and PCNA to DNA ploidy, S-phase fraction and survival in uveal melanoma. *Eur J Cancer* 1996;32A:357–362.

Kilic E, van Gils W, Lodder E, et al. Clinical and cytogenetic analyses in uveal melanoma. *Invest Ophthalmol Vis Sci* 2006;47:3703–3707.

Kishore K, Ghazvini S, Char DH, et al. p53 gene and cell cycling in uveal melanoma. *Am J Ophthalmol* 1996;121:561–567.

Lattman J, Kroll S, Char DH, et al. Cell cycling and prognosis in uveal melanoma. *Clin Cancer Res* 1995;1:41–47.

Lawry J, Currie Z, Smith MO, et al. The correlation between cell surface markers and clinical features in choroidal malignant melanomas. *Eye* 1999;13:301–308.

Makitie T, Summanen P, Tarkkanen A, et al. Microvascular loops and networks as prognostic indicators in choroidal and ciliary body melanomas. *J Natl Cancer Inst* 1999;91:359–367.

Maniotis AJ, Folberg R, Hess A, et al. Vascular channel formation by human melanoma cells in vivo and in vitro: vasculogenic mimicry. *Am J Pathol* 1999;155:739–752.

Marcus DM, Minkovitz JB, Wardwell SD, et al. The value of nucleolar organizer regions in uveal melanoma. The Collaborative Ocular Melanoma Study Group. *Am J Ophthalmol* 1990;110:527–534.

McCurdy J, Gamel J, McLean I. A simple, efficient, and reproducible method for estimating the malignant potential of uveal melanoma from routine H & E slides. *Pathol Res Pract* 1991;187:1025–1027.

McLean IW, Foster WD, Zimmerman LE. Uveal melanoma: location, size, cell type, and enucleation as risk factors in metastasis. *Hum Pathol* 1982;13:123–132.

McLean IW, Gamel JW. Prediction of metastasis of uveal melanoma: comparison of morphometric determination of nucleolar size and spectrophotometric determination of DNA. *Invest Ophthalmol Vis Sci* 1988;29:507–511.

McLean IW, Keefe KS, Burnier MN. Uveal melanoma. Comparison of the prognostic value of fibrovascular loops, mean of the ten largest nucleoli, cell type, and tumor size. *Ophthalmology* 1997;104:777–780.

McLean IW, Sibug ME, Becker RL, et al. Uveal melanoma: the importance of large nucleoli in predicting patient outcome—an automated image analysis study. *Cancer* 1997;79:982–988.

McLean IW, Zimmerman LE, Evans RM. Reappraisal of Callender's spindle, a type of malignant melanoma of choroid and ciliary body. *Am J Ophthalmol* 1978;86:557–564.

Meecham WJ, Char DH. DNA content abnormalities and prognosis in uveal melanoma. *Arch Ophthalmol* 1986;104:1626–1629.

Mehaffey MG, Folberg R, Meyer M, et al. Relative importance of quantifying area and vascular patterns in uveal melanomas. *Am J Ophthalmol* 1997;123:798–809.

Mehaffey MG, Gardner LM, Folberg R. Distribution of prognostically important vascular patterns across multiple levels in ciliary body and choroidal melanomas. *Am J Ophthalmol* 1998;126:373–378.

Mera M. AgNOR values in Callender histopathological types of malignant uveal melanomas. *Rom J Morphol Embryol* 1995;41:125–128.

Merbs SL, Sidransky D. Analysis of p16 (CDKN2/MTS-1/INK4A) alterations in primary sporadic uveal melanoma. *Invest Ophthalmol Vis Sci* 1999;40:779–783.

Monique H, Hurks H, Metzelaar-Blok JA, et al. Expression of epidermal growth factor receptor: risk factor in uveal melanoma. *Invest Ophthalmol Vis Sci* 2000;41:2023–2027.

Mooy C, Vissers K, Luyten G, et al. DNA flow cytometry in uveal melanoma: the effect of pre-enucleation irradiation. *Br J Ophthalmol* 1995;79:174–177.

Mooy CM, De Jong PT. Prognostic parameters in uveal melanoma: a review. *Surv Ophthalmol* 1996;41:215–228.

Mooy CM, Luyten GP, de Jong PT, et al. Immunohistochemical and prognostic analysis of apoptosis and proliferation in uveal melanoma. *Am J Pathol* 1995;147:1097–1104.

Mueller AJ, Folberg R, Freeman WR, et al. Evaluation of the human choroidal melanoma rabbit model for studying microcirculation patterns with confocal ICG and histology. *Exp Eye Res* 1999;68:671–678.

Mueller AJ, Freeman WR, Schaller UC, et al. Complex microcirculation patterns detected by confocal indocyanine green angiography predict time to growth of small choroidal melanocytic tumors: MuSIC Report II. *Ophthalmology* 2002;109:2207–2214.

Onken MD, Ehlers JP, Worley LA, et al. Functional gene expression analysis uncovers phenotypic switch in aggressive uveal melanomas. *Cancer Res* 2006;66:4602–4609.

Onken MD, Worley LA, Ehlers JP, et al. Gene expression profiling in uveal melanoma reveals two molecular classes and predicts metastatic death. *Cancer Res* 2004;64:7205–7209.

Pe'er J, Gnessin H, Shargal Y, et al. PC-10 immunostaining of proliferating cell nuclear antigen in posterior uveal melanoma. Enucleation versus enucleation postirradiation groups. *Ophthalmology* 1994;101:56–62.

Pe'er J, Rummelt V, Mawn L, et al. Mean of the ten largest nucleoli, microcirculation architecture, and prognosis of ciliochoroidal melanomas. *Ophthalmology* 1994;101:1227–1235.

Prescher G, Bornfeld N, Hirche H, et al. Prognostic implications of monosomy 3 in uveal melanoma. *Lancet* 1996;347:1222–1225.

Rennie IG, Rees RC, Parsons MA, et al. Estimation of DNA content in uveal melanomas by flow cytometry. *Eye* 1989;3:611–617.

Richardson RP, Lawry L, Rees RC, et al. DNA index and % S phase fraction in posterior uveal melanoma: a 5 year prospective study of fresh tissue using flow cytometry. *Eye* 1997;11:629–634.

Royds JA, Sharrard RM, Parsons MA, et al. C-myc oncogene expression in ocular melanomas. *Graefes Arch Clin Exp Ophthalmol* 1992;230:366–371.

Rummelt V, Folberg R, Rummelt C, et al. Microcirculation architecture of melanocytic nevi and malignant melanomas of the ciliary body and choroid. A comparative histopathologic and ultrastructural study. *Ophthalmology* 1994;101:718–727.

Rummelt V, Folberg R, Woolson RF, et al. Relation between the microcirculation architecture and the aggressive behavior of ciliary body melanomas. *Ophthalmology* 1995;102:844–851.

Seddon JM, Polivogianis L, Hsieh CC, et al. Death from uveal melanoma. Number of epithelioid cells and inverse SD of nucleolar area as prognostic factors. *Arch Ophthalmol* 1987;105:801–806.

Seregard S, Spångberg B, Juul C, et al. Prognostic accuracy of the mean of the largest nucleoli, vascular patterns, and PC-10 in posterior uveal melanoma. *Ophthalmology* 1998;105:485–491.

Shields CL, Ganguly A, Materin MA, et al. Chromosome 3 analysis of uveal melanoma using fine-needle aspiration biopsy at the time of plaque radiotherapy in 140 consecutive cases: The Deborah Iverson, MD, Lectureship. *Arch Ophthalmol* 2007;125:1017–1024.

Silverman RH, Folberg R, Boldt HC, et al. Correlation of ultrasound parameter imaging with microcirculatory patterns in uveal melanomas. *Ultrasound Med Biol* 1997;23:573–581.

Singh AD, Damato B, Howard P, et al. Uveal melanoma: genetic aspects. *Ophthalmol Clin North Am* 2005;18:85–97.

Singh AD, Rennie IG, Kivela T, et al. The Zimmerman-McLean-Foster hypothesis: 25 years later. *Br J Ophthalmol* 2004;88:962–967.

Sisley K, Rennie IG, Parsons MA, et al. Abnormalities of chromosomes 3 and 8 in posterior uveal melanoma correlate with prognosis. *Genes Chromosomes Cancer* 1997;19:22–28.

Staibano S, Orabona P, Mezza E, et al. Morphometric analysis of AgNORs in uveal malignant melanoma [see comments]. *Anal Quant Cytol Histol* 1998;20:483–492.

Tschentscher F, Husing J, Holter T, et al. Tumor classification based on gene expression profiling shows that uveal melanomas with and without monosomy 3 represent two distinct entities. *Cancer Res* 2003;63:2578–2584.

Vaisanen A, Kallioinen M, von Dickhoff K, et al. Matrix metalloproteinase-2 (MMP-2) immunoreactive protein—a new prognostic marker in uveal melanoma? *J Pathol* 1999;188:56–62.

Weichselbaum RR, Zakov ZN, Albert DM, et al. New findings in the chromosome 13 long-arm deletion syndrome and retinoblastoma. *Ophthalmology* 1979;86:1191–1201.

Whelchel JC, Farah SE, McLean IW, et al. Immunohistochemistry of infiltrating lymphocytes in uveal malignant melanoma. *Invest Ophthalmol Vis Sci* 1993;34:2603–2606.

White VA, Chambers JD, Courtright PD, et al. Correlation of cytogenetic abnormalities with the outcome of patients with uveal melanoma. *Cancer* 1998;83:354–359.

Worley LA, Long MD, Onken MD, et al. Micro-RNAs associated with metastasis in uveal melanoma identified by multiplexed microarray profiling. *Melanoma Res* 2008;18:184–190.

Worley LA, Onken MD, Person E, et al. Transcriptomic versus chromosomal prognostic markers and clinical outcome in uveal melanoma. *Clin Cancer Res* 2007;13:1466–1471.

Zimmerman LE, McLean IW, Foster WD. Does enucleation of the eye containing a malignant melanoma prevent or accelerate the dissemination of tumour cells. *Br J Ophthalmol* 1978;62:420–425.

Zuidervaart W, van der Velden PA, Hurks MH, et al. Gene expression profiling identifies tumour markers potentially playing a role in uveal melanoma development. *Br J Cancer* 2003;89:1914–1919.

Uveal Melanoma—Treatment

Char DH, Kroll SM, Castro J. Ten-Year follow-up of helium ion therapy for uveal melanoma. *Am J Ophthalmol* 1998;125:81–89.

Damato B. Treatment of primary intraocular melanoma. *Expert Rev Anticancer Ther* 2006;6:493–506.

Damato B, Kacperek A, Chopra M, et al. Proton beam radiotherapy of iris melanoma. *Int J Radiat Oncol Biol Phys* 2005;63:109–115.

Diener-West M, Earle JD, Fine SL, et al. The COMS randomized trial of iodine 125 brachytherapy for choroidal melanoma: III. Initial mortality findings. COMS Report No. 18. *Arch Ophthalmol* 2001;119:969–982.

Gragoudas ES. Long-term results after proton irradiation of uveal melanomas. The 1996 Jules Gonin Lecture of the Retinal Research Foundation. *Graefes Arch Clin Exp Ophthalmol* 1997;235:265–267.

Gunduz K, Shields CL, Shields JA, et al. Radiation retinopathy following plaque radiotherapy for posterior uveal melanoma. *Arch Ophthalmol* 1999;117:609–614.

Incidence of cataract and outcomes after cataract surgery in the first 5 years after iodine 125 brachytherapy in the Collaborative Ocular Melanoma Study: COMS Report No. 27. *Ophthalmology* 2007;114:1363–1371.

Melia BM, Abramson DH, Albert DM, et al. Collaborative Ocular Melanoma Study (COMS) randomized trial of I-125 brachytherapy for medium choroidal melanoma: I. Visual acuity after 3 years. COMS report no. 16. *Ophthalmology* 2001;108:348–366.

Shields CL, Cater J, Shields JA, et al. Combined plaque radiotherapy and transpupillary thermotherapy for choroidal melanoma: tumor control and treatment complications in 270 consecutive patients. *Arch Ophthalmol* 2002;120:933–940.

Shields CL, Naseripour M, Shields JA, et al. Custom-designed plaque radiotherapy for nonresectable iris melanoma in 38 patients: tumor control and ocular complications. *Am J Ophthalmol* 2003;135:648–656.

Shields CL, Shields JA, De Potter P, et al. Plaque radiotherapy for the management of uveal metastasis. *Arch Ophthalmol* 1997;115:203–209.

Shields CL, Shields JA, Gunduz K, et al. Radiation therapy for uveal malignant melanoma. *Ophthalmic Surg Lasers* 1998;29:397–409.

Shields JA, Shields CL, De Potter P, et al. Diagnosis and treatment of uveal melanoma. *Semin Oncol* 1996;23:763–767.

The Collaborative Ocular Melanoma Study (COMS) randomized trial of pre-enucleation radiation of large choroidal melanoma: II. Initial mortality findings: COMS report no. 10. *Am J Ophthalmol* 1998;125:779–796.

Choroidal Metastases

Augsburger JJ, Shields JA. Fine needle aspiration biopsy of solid intraocular tumors: indications, instrumentation and techniques. *Ophthalmic Surg* 1984;15:34–40.

Dabbs DJ, Silverman JF. Immunohistochemical workup of metastatic carcinoma of unknown primary. *Pathol Case Rev* 2001;6:146–153.

Demirci H, Shields CL, Chao AN, et al. Uveal metastasis from breast cancer in 264 patients. *Am J Ophthalmol* 2003;136:264–271.

Eagle RC Jr. Immunohistochemistry in diagnostic ophthalmic pathology: a review. *Clin Experiment Ophthalmol* 2008;36:675–688.

Eagle RC Jr, Ehya H, Shields JA, et al. Choroidal metastasis as the initial manifestation of a pigmented neuroendocrine tumor. *Arch Ophthalmol* 2000;118:841–845.

ElSheikh TM, Silverman JF. Differential diagnosis of metastatic tumors. In: Silverberg SG DR, Frable WJ, LiVolsi VA, et al., eds. *Silverberg's Principles and Practice of Surgical Pathology and Cytopathology*, vol. 1. Philadelphia, PA: Churchill Livingston/Elsevier, 2006.

Ferry AP, Font RL. Carcinoma metastatic to the eye and orbit: I. A clinicopathologic study of 227 cases. *Arch Ophthalmol* 1974;92:276–286.

Font RL, Naumann G, Zimmerman LE. Primary malignant melanoma of the skin metastatic to the eye and orbit. Report of ten cases and a review of the literature. *Am J Ophthalmol* 1967;63:738–744.

Freedman MI, Folk JC. Metastatic tumors to the eye and orbit. Patient survival and clinical characteristics. *Arch Ophthalmol* 1987;105:1215–1219.

Gunduz K, Shields JA, Shields CL, et al. Cutaneous melanoma metastatic to the vitreous cavity. *Ophthalmology* 1998;105:600–605.

Gunduz K, Shields JA, Shields JA, et al. Lung carcinoma metastatic to the vitreous cavity. *Retina* 1998;18:285–286.

Leys AM, Van Eyck LM, Nuttin BJ, et al. Metastatic carcinoma to the retina. Clinicopathologic findings in two cases. *Arch Ophthalmol* 1990;108:1448–1452.

Liu Q, Teh M, Ito K, et al. CDX2 expression is progressively decreased in human gastric intestinal metaplasia, dysplasia and cancer. *Mod Pathol* 2007;20:1286–1297.

Nelson CC, Hertzberg BS, Klintworth GK. A histopathologic study of 716 unselected eyes in patients with cancer at the time of death. *Am J Ophthalmol* 1983;95:788–793.

Ormsby AH, Snow JL, Su WP, et al. Diagnostic histochemistry of cutaneous breast carcinoma: a statistical analysis of the utility of gross cystic disease fluid protein-15 and estrogen receptor protein. *J Am Acad Dermatol* 1995;32:711–716.

Robertson DM, Wilkinson CP, Murray JL, et al. Metastatic tumor to the retina and vitreous cavity from primary melanoma of the skin: treatment with systemic and subconjunctival chemotherapy. *Ophthalmology* 1981;88:1296–1301.

Shields CL, Shields JA, Gross NE, et al. Survey of 520 eyes with uveal metastases. *Ophthalmology* 1997;104:1265–1276.

Shields JA, Shields CL, Brown GC, et al. Mushroom-shaped choroidal metastasis simulating a choroidal melanoma. *Retina* 2002;22:810–813.

Shields JA, Shields CL, Kiratli H, et al. Metastatic tumors to the iris in 40 patients. *Am J Ophthalmol* 1995;119:422–430.

Shields JA, Shields CL, Singh AD. Metastatic neoplasms in the optic disc: The 1999 Bjerrum Lecture: Part 2. *Arch Ophthalmol* 2000;118:217–224.

Spraul CW, Martin DF, Hagler WS, et al. Cytology of metastatic cutaneous melanoma to the vitreous and retina. *Retina* 1996;16:328–332.

Traina A, Agostara B, Marasa L, et al. HER2/neu expression in relation to clinicopathologic features of breast carcinoma patients. *Ann N Y Acad Sci* 2006;1089:159–167.

Young SE, Cruciger M, Lukeman J. Metastatic carcinoma to the retina: Case report. *Ophthalmology* 1979;86:1350–1354.

Leukemia

Brown GC, Shields JA, Augsburger JJ, et al. Leukemic optic neuropathy. *Arch Ophthalmol* 1981;3:111–116.

Currie JN, Lessell S, Lessell IM, et al. Optic neuropathy in chronic lymphocytic leukemia. *Arch Ophthalmol* 1988;106:654–660.

Kincaid MC, Green WR. Ocular and orbital involvement in leukemia. *Surv Ophthalmol* 1983;27:211–232.

Leonardy NJ, Rupani M, Dent G, et al. Analysis of 135 autopsy eyes for ocular involvement in leukemia. *Am J Ophthalmol* 1990;109:436–444.

Rosenthal AR. Ocular manifestations of leukemia. a review. *Ophthalmology* 1983;90:899–905.

Wallace RT, Shields JA, Shields CL, et al. Leukemic infiltration of the optic nerve. *Arch Ophthalmol* 1991;109:1027.

Ocular Lymphoma

Brodsky MC, Casteel H, Barber LD, et al. Bilateral iris tumors in an immunosuppressed child. *Surv Ophthalmol* 1991;36:217–222.

Chan CC. Molecular pathology of primary intraocular lymphoma. *Trans Am Ophthalmol Soc* 2003;101:275–292.

Chan CC, Buggage RR, Nussenblatt RB. Intraocular lymphoma. *Curr Opin Ophthalmol* 2002;13:411–418.

Chan CC, Wallace DJ. Intraocular lymphoma: update on diagnosis and management. *Cancer Control* 2004;11:285–295.

Chan CC, Whitcup SM, Solomon D, et al. Interleukin-10 in the vitreous of patients with primary intraocular lymphoma. *Am J Ophthalmol* 1995;120:671–673.

Chatzistefanou K, Markomichelakis NN, Christen W, et al. Characteristics of uveitis presenting for the first time in the elderly. *Ophthalmology* 1998;105:347–352.

Cho AS, Holland GN, Glasgow BJ, et al. Ocular involvement in patients with posttransplant lymphoproliferative disorder. *Arch Ophthalmol* 119:183–189 2001.

Cockerham GC, Hidayat AA, Bijwaard KE, et al. Re-evaluation of "reactive lymphoid hyperplasia of the uvea": an immunohistochemical and molecular analysis of 10 cases. *Ophthalmology* 2000;107:151–158.

Coupland SE, Damato B. Lymphomas involving the eye and the ocular adnexa. *Curr Opin Ophthalmol* 2006;17:523–531.

Coupland SE, Damato B. Understanding intraocular lymphomas. *Clin Experiment Ophthalmol* 2008;36:564–578.

Coupland SE, Heimann H, Bechrakis NE. Primary intraocular lymphoma: a review of the clinical, histopathological and molecular biological features. *Graefes Arch Clin Exp Ophthalmol* 2004;242:901–913.

Durant WJ, Flood T, Goldberg MF, et al. Vitrectomy and Whipple's disease. *Arch Ophthalmol* 1984;102:848–851.

Freeman LN, Schachat AP, Knox DL, et al. Clinical features, laboratory investigations, and survival in ocular reticulum cell sarcoma. *Ophthalmology* 1987;94:1631–1639.

Holz FG, Boehmer HV, Mechtersheimer G, et al. Uveal non-Hodgkin's lymphoma with epibulbar extension simulating choroidal effusion syndrome. *Retina* 1999;19:343–346.

O'Hara M, Lloyd WC III, Scribbick FW, et al. Latent intracellular Epstein-Barr virus DNA demonstrated in ocular posttransplant lymphoproliferative disorder mimicking granulomatous uveitis with iris nodules in a child. *J AAPOS* 2001;5:62–63.

Ryan SJ, Zimmerman LE, King FM. Reactive lymphoid hyperplasia. An unusual form of intraocular pseudotumor. *Trans Am Acad Ophthalmol Otolaryngol* 1972;76:652–671.

Selsky EJ, Knox DL, Maumenee AE, et al. Ocular involvement in Whipple's disease. *Retina* 1984;4:103–106.

Whitcup SM, de Smet MD, Rubin BI, et al. Intraocular lymphoma. Clinical and histopathologic diagnosis. *Ophthalmology* 1993;100:1399–1406.

Histiocytic Lesions

Angell LK, Burton TC. Posterior choroidal involvement in Letterer-Siwe disease. *J Pediatr Ophthalmol Strabismus* 1978;15:79–81.

DeBarge LR, Chan CC, Greenberg SC, et al. Chorioretinal, iris, and ciliary body infiltration by juvenile xanthogranuloma masquerading as uveitis. *Surv Ophthalmol* 1994;39:65–71.

Mittelman D, Apple DJ, Goldberg MF. Ocular involvement in Letterer-Siwe disease. *Am J Ophthalmol* 1973;75:261–265.

Shields JA, Eagle RC Jr, Shields CL, et al. Iris juvenile xanthogranuloma studied by immunohistochemistry and flow cytometry. *Ophthalmic Surg Lasers* 1997;28:140–144.

Leiomyoma and Hemangiopericytoma

Gengler C, Guillou L. Solitary fibrous tumour and haemangiopericytoma: evolution of a concept. *Histopathology* 2006;48:63–74.

Jakobiec FA, Font RL, Tso MO, et al. Mesectodermal leiomyoma of the ciliary body: a tumor of presumed neural crest origin. *Cancer* 1977;39:2102–2113.

Papale JJ, Frederick AR, Albert DM. Intraocular hemangiopericytoma. *Arch Ophthalmol* 1983;101:1409–1411.

Shields JA, Shields CL, Eagle RC Jr. Mesectodermal leiomyoma of the ciliary body managed by partial lamellar iridocyclochoroidectomy. *Ophthalmology* 1989;96:1369–1376.

Shields JA, Shields CL, Eagle RC Jr, et al. Observations on seven cases of intraocular leiomyoma. The 1993 Byron Demorest Lecture. *Arch Ophthalmol* 1994;112:521–528.

Toth J, Kerenyi AA, Suveges II, et al. Leiomyoma of the ciliary body and hemangiopericytoma of the choroid. *Pathol Oncol Res* 1996;2:89–93.

Hemangioma

Arevalo JF, Shields CL, Shields JA, et al. Circumscribed choroidal hemangioma: characteristic features with indocyanine green videoangiography. *Ophthalmology* 2000;107:344–350.

Madreperla SA. Choroidal hemangioma treated with photodynamic therapy using verteporfin. *Arch Ophthalmol* 2001;119:1606–1610.

Mashayekhi A, Shields CL. Circumscribed choroidal hemangioma. *Curr Opin Ophthalmol* 2003;14:142–149.

Phelps CD. The pathogenesis of glaucoma in Sturge-Weber syndrome. *Ophthalmology* 1978;85:276–286.

Shields CL, Honavar SG, Shields JA, et al. Circumscribed choroidal hemangioma: clinical manifestations and factors predictive of visual outcome in 200 consecutive cases. *Ophthalmology* 2001;108:2237–2248.

Shields JA, Shields CL, Eagle RC Jr. Cavernous hemangioma of the iris. *Arch Ophthalmol* 2008;126:1602–1603.

Shields JA, Shields CL, Materin MA, et al. Changing concepts in management of circumscribed choroidal hemangioma: The 2003 J. Howard Stokes Lecture, Part 1. *Ophthalmic Surg Lasers Imaging* 2004;35:383–394.

Shields JA, Stephens RF, Eagle RC Jr, et al. Progressive enlargement of a circumscribed choroidal hemangioma. A clinicopathologic correlation. *Arch Ophthalmol* 1992;110:1276–1278.

Witschel H, Font RL. Hemangioma of the choroid. A clinicopathologic study of 71 cases and a review of the literature. *Surv Ophthalmol* 1976;20:415–431.

Retinal Hemangioblastoma and VHL

Chan CC, Collins AB, Chew EY, et al. Molecular pathology of eyes with von Hippel-Lindau (VHL) disease: a review. *Retina* 2007;27:1–7.

Chew EY. Ocular manifestations of von Hippel-Lindau disease: clinical and genetic investigations. *Trans Am Ophthalmol Soc* 2005;103:495–511.

Couch V, Lindor NM, Karnes PS, et al. von Hippel-Lindau disease. *Mayo Clin Proc* 2000;75:265–272.

Decker HJ, Weidt EJ, Brieger J. The von Hippel-Lindau tumor suppressor gene. A rare and intriguing disease opening new insight into basic mechanisms of carcinogenesis. *Cancer Genet Cytogenet* 1997;93:74–83.

Friedrich CA. Von Hippel-Lindau syndrome. A pleomorphic condition. *Cancer* 1999;86(11 Suppl):2478–2482.

Singh A, Shields J, Shields C. Solitary retinal capillary hemangioma: hereditary (von Hippel-Lindau disease) or nonhereditary? *Arch Ophthalmol* 2001;119:232–234.

Singh AD, Nouri M, Shields CL, et al. Retinal capillary hemangioma: a comparison of sporadic cases and cases associated with von Hippel-Lindau disease. *Ophthalmology* 2001;108:1907–1911.

Vasoproliferative Tumor

Cohen VM, Shields CL, Demirci H, et al. Iodine I 125 plaque radiotherapy for vasoproliferative tumors of the retina in 30 eyes. *Arch Ophthalmol* 2008;126:1245–1251.

Heimann H, Bornfeld N, Vij O, et al. Vasoproliferative tumours of the retina. *Br J Ophthalmol* 2000;84:1162–1169.

Hiscott P, Mudhar H. Is vasoproliferative tumour (reactive retinal glioangiosis) part of the spectrum of proliferative vitreoretinopathy? *Eye* 2009;23:1851–1858.

Irvine F, O'Donnell N, Kemp E, et al. Retinal vasoproliferative tumors: surgical management and histological findings. *Arch Ophthalmol* 2000;118:563–569.

Li HK, Shields JA, Shields CL, et al. Retinal vasoproliferative tumour as the initial manifestation of retinitis pigmentosa. *Clin Experiment Ophthalmol* 2008;36:895–897.

Murthy R, Honavar SG. Secondary vasoproliferative retinal tumor associated with Usher syndrome type 1. *J Aapos* 2009;13:97–98.

Shields CL, Shields JA, Barrett J, et al. Vasoproliferative tumors of the ocular fundus. Classification and clinical manifestations in 103 patients. *Arch Ophthalmol* 1995;113:615–623.

Smeets MH, Mooy CM, Baarsma GS, et al. Histopathology of a vasoproliferative tumor of the ocular fundus. *Retina* 1998;18:470–472.

Peripheral Nerve Sheath Tumors

Fan JT, Campbell RJ, Robertson DM. A survey of intraocular schwannoma with a case report. *Can J Ophthalmol* 1995;30:37–41.

Matsuo T, Notohara K. Choroidal schwannoma: immunohistochemical and electron-microscopic study. *Ophthalmologica* 2000;214:156–160.

Shields JA, Font RL, Eagle RC Jr, et al. Melanotic schwannoma of the choroid. Immunohistochemistry and electron microscopic observations. *Ophthalmology* 1994;101:843–849.

Shields JA, Hamada A, Shields CL, et al. Ciliochoroidal nerve sheath tumor simulating a malignant melanoma. *Retina* 1997;17:459–460.

Shields JA, Sanborn GE, Kurz GH, et al. Benign peripheral nerve tumor of the choroid: a clinicopathologic correlation and review of the literature. *Ophthalmology* 1981;88:1322–1329.

Smith PA, Damato BE, Ko MK, et al. Anterior uveal neurilemmoma–a rare neoplasm simulating malignant melanoma. *Br J Ophthalmol* 1987;71:34–40.

Woog JJ, Albert DM, Craft J, et al. Choroidal ganglioneuroma in neurofibromatosis. *Graefes Arch Clin Exp Ophthalmol* 1983;220:25–31.

Medulloepithelioma in Adults

Broughton WL, Zimmerman LE. A clinicopathologic study of 56 cases of intraocular medulloepithelioma. *Am J Ophthalmol* 1978;85:407–418.

Carrillo R, Streeten BW. Malignant teratoid medulloepithelioma in an adult. *Arch Ophthalmol* 1979;97:695–699.

Floyd BB, Minckler DS, Valentin L. Intraocular medulloepithelioma in a 79-year-old man. *Ophthalmology* 1982;89:1088–1094.

Husain SE, Husain N, Boniuk M, et al. Malignant nonteratoid medulloepithelioma of the ciliary body in an adult. *Ophthalmology* 1998;105:596–599.

Litricin O, Latkovic Z. Malignant teratoid medulloepithelioma in an adult. *Ophthalmologica* 1985;191:17–21.

Shields JA, Eagle RC Jr, Shields CL, et al. Congenital neoplasms of the nonpigmented ciliary epithelium (medulloepithelioma). *Ophthalmology* 1996;103:1998–2006.

Wilson ME, McClatchey SK, Zimmerman LE. Rhabdomyosarcoma of the ciliary body. *Ophthalmology* 1990;97:1484–1488.

Astrocytic Tumors

Eagle RC Jr, Shields JA, Shields CL, et al. Hamartomas of the iris and ciliary epithelium in tuberous sclerosis complex. *Arch Ophthalmol* 2000;118:711–715.

Gunduz K, Eagle RC Jr, Shields CL, et al Invasive giant cell astrocytoma of the retina in a patient with tuberous sclerosis. *Ophthalmology* 1999;106:639–642.

Margo CE, Barletta JP, Staman JA. Giant cell astrocytoma of the retina in tuberous sclerosis. *Retina* 1993;13:155–159.

Shields JA, Eagle RC Jr, Shields CL, et al. Aggressive retinal astrocytomas in four patients with tuberous sclerosis complex. *Trans Am Ophthalmol Soc* 2004;102:139–147.

Ulbright TM, Fulling KH, Helveston EM. Astrocytic tumors of the retina. Differentiation of sporadic tumors from phakomatosis-associated tumors. *Arch Pathol Lab Med* 1984;108:160–163.

Tumors of the Iris and Ciliary Epithelium

Bateman JB, Foos RY. Coronal adenomas. *Arch Ophthalmol* 1979;97:2379–2384.

Brown HH, Glasgow BJ, Foos RY. Ultrastructural and immunohistochemical features of coronal adenomas. *Am J Ophthalmol* 1991;112:34–40.

Dryja TP, Albert DM, Horns D. Adenocarcinoma arising from the epithelium of the ciliary body. *Ophthalmology* 1981;88:1290–1292.

Dryja TP, Zakov ZN, Albert DM. Adenocarcinoma arising from the epithelium of the iris and ciliary body. *Int Ophthalmol Clin* 1980;20:177–190.

Grossniklaus HE, Lim JI. Adenoma of the nonpigmented ciliary epithelium. *Retina* 1994;14:452–456.

Grossniklaus HE, Zimmerman LE, Kachmer ML. Pleomorphic adenocarcinoma of the ciliary body. Immunohistochemical and electron microscopic features. *Ophthalmology* 1990;97:763–798.

Laver NM, Hidayat AA, Croxatto JO. Pleomorphic adenocarcinomas of the ciliary epithelium. Immunohistochemical and ultrastructural features of 12 cases. *Ophthalmology* 1999;106:103–110.

Lieb WE, Shields JA, Eagle RC Jr, et al. Cystic adenoma of the pigmented ciliary epithelium. Clinical, pathologic, and immunohistopathologic findings. *Ophthalmology* 1990;97:1489–1493.

Rodrigues M, Hidayat A, Karesh J. Pleomorphic adenocarcinoma of ciliary epithelium simulating an epibulbar tumor. *Am J Ophthalmol* 1988;106:595–600.

Shields JA, Eagle RC Jr, Shields CL. Adenoma of nonpigmented ciliary epithelium with smooth muscle differentiation. *Arch Ophthalmol* 1999;117:117–119.

Shields JA, Eagle RC Jr, Shields CL, et al. Acquired neoplasms of the nonpigmented ciliary epithelium (adenoma and adenocarcinoma). *Ophthalmology* 1996;103:2007–2016.

Shields JA, Shields CL, Mercado G, et al. Adenoma of the iris pigment epithelium: a report of 20 cases: The 1998 Pan-American Lecture. *Arch Ophthalmol* 1999;117:736–741.

Streeten BW, McGraw JL. Tumor of the ciliary pigment epithelium. *Am J Ophthalmol* 1972;74:420–429.

Tumors of the Retinal Pigment Epithelial

Edelstein C, Shields CL, Shields JA, et al. Presumed adenocarcinoma of the retinal pigment epithelium in a blind eye with a staphyloma. *Arch Ophthalmol* 1998;116:525–528.

Kasner L, Traboulsi EI, Delacruz Z, et al. A histopathologic study of the pigmented fundus lesions in familial adenomatous polyposis. *Retina* 1992;12:35–42.

Lieb WE, Shields JA, Eagle RC Jr, et al. Cystic adenoma of the pigmented ciliary epithelium. Clinical, pathologic, and immunohistopathologic findings. *Ophthalmology* 1990;97:1489–1493.

Lloyd WC III, Eagle RC Jr, Shields JA, et al. Congenital hypertrophy of the retinal pigment epithelium. Electron microscopic and morphometric observations. *Ophthalmology* 1990;97:1052–1060.

Loeffler KU, Kivelä T, Borgman H, et al. Malignant tumor of the retinal pigment epithelium with extraocular extension in a phthisical eye. *Graefes Arch Clin Expl Ophthalmol* 1996;234:70–75.

Regillo CD, Eagle RC Jr, Shields JA, et al. Histopathologic findings in congenital grouped pigmentation of the retina. *Ophthalmology* 1993;100:400–405.

Shields CL, Mashayekhi A, Ho T, et al. Solitary congenital hypertrophy of the retinal pigment epithelium: clinical features and frequency of enlargement in 330 patients. *Ophthalmology* 2003;110:1968–1976.

Shields JA, Shields CL, Eagle RC Jr, et al. Adenocarcinoma arising from congenital hypertrophy of retinal pigment epithelium. *Arch Ophthalmol* 2001;119:597–602.

Shields JA, Shields CL, Gunduz K, et al. Neoplasms of the retinal pigment epithelium: The 1998 Albert Ruedemann, Sr, memorial lecture, Part 2. *Arch Ophthalmol* 1999;117:601–608.

Shields JA, Shields CL, Singh AD. Acquired tumors arising from congenital hypertrophy of the retinal pigment epithelium. *Arch Ophthalmol* 118:637–641 2000.

Sommacal A, Campbell RJ, Helbig H. Adenocarcinoma of the retinal pigment epithelium. *Arch Ophthalmol* 2003;121:1481–1483.

Traboulsi EI, Apostolides J, Giardiello FM, et al. Pigmented ocular fundus lesions and APC mutations in familial adenomatous polyposis. *Ophthalmic Genet* 1996;17:167–174.

Traboulsi EI, Murphy SF, de la Cruz ZC, et al. A clinicopathologic study of the eyes in familial adenomatous polyposis with extracolonic manifestations (Gardner's syndrome). *Am J Ophthalmol* 1990;110:550–561.

Choroidal Osteoma and Sclerochoroidal Calcification

Buettner H. Spontaneous involution of a choroidal osteoma. *Arch Ophthalmol* 1990;108:1517–1518.

Gupta R, Hu V, Reynolds T, et al. Sclerochoroidal calcification associated with Gitelman syndrome and calcium pyrophosphate dihydrate deposition. *J Clin Pathol* 2005;58:1334–1335.

Honavar SG, Shields CL, Demirci H, et al. Sclerochoroidal calcification: clinical manifestations and systemic associations. *Arch Ophthalmol* 2001;119:833–840.

Noble KG. Bilateral choroidal osteoma in three siblings. *Am J Ophthalmol* 1990;109:656–660.

Schachat AP, Robertson DM, Mieler WF, et al. Sclerochoroidal calcification. *Arch Ophthalmol* 1992;110:196–199.

Shields CL, Perez B, Materin MA, et al. Optical coherence tomography of choroidal osteoma in 22 cases: evidence for photoreceptor atrophy over the decalcified portion of the tumor. *Ophthalmology* 2007;114:e53–e58.

Shields CL, Shields JA, Augsburger JJ. Choroidal osteoma. *Surv Ophthalmol* 1988;33:17–27.

Shields CL, Sun H, Demirci H, et al. Factors predictive of tumor growth, tumor decalcification, choroidal neovascularization, and visual outcome in 74 eyes with choroidal osteoma. *Arch Ophthalmol* 2005;123:1658–1666.

Shields JA, Shields CL. CME review: sclerochoroidal calcification: The 2001 Harold Gifford Lecture. *Retina* 2002;22:251–261.

Shields JA, Shields CL, de Potter P, et al. Progressive enlargement of a choroidal osteoma. *Arch Ophthalmol* 1995;113:819–820.

Shields JA, Shields CL, Ellis J, et al. Bilateral choroidal osteoma associated with bilateral total blindness. *Retina* 1996;16:445–447.

Sivalingam A, Shields CL, Shields JA, et al. Idiopathic sclerochoroidal calcification. *Ophthalmology* 1991;98:720–724.

Sun H, Demirci H, Shields CL, et al. Sclerochoroidal calcification in a patient with classic Bartter's syndrome. *Am J Ophthalmol* 2005;139:365–366.

Trimble SN, Schatz H, Schneider GB. Spontaneous decalcification of a choroidal osteoma. *Ophthalmology* 1988;95:631–634.

Trimble SN, Schatz H. Decalcification of a choroidal osteoma. *Br J Ophthalmol* 1991;75:61–63.

Williams AT, Font RL, Van Dyk HJ, et al. Osseous choristoma of the choroid simulating a choroidal melanoma. Association with a positive 32P test. *Arch Ophthalmol* 1978;96:1874–1877.

12

Retinoblastoma and Simulating Lesions

Retinoblastoma is the most common intraocular tumor of childhood. In Asia, Africa, and South America, where uveal melanoma is relatively rare, it probably is the most common primary intraocular tumor. Retinoblastoma is relatively rare; only 300 cases occur yearly in the United States. The incidence has been estimated to be 1 in 15,000 to 1 in 34,000 births. All races and both sexes are affected equally, and the tumor has no predilection for either the right or left eye. The mean age at diagnosis is 18 months, and about 90% of cases are diagnosed before 3 years of age. Rare cases in older children and adults are often misdiagnosed.

CLINICAL PRESENTATION

In the United States and Europe, about 90% of patients present with leukocoria, an abnormal, typically white pupillary reflex that has been fancifully likened to the tapetal light reflex of the cat (amaurotic cat's-eye reflex) (Fig. 12-1). The white pupillary reflex is caused by tumor in the vitreous cavity (endophytic tumors) or the detached retina (exophytic tumors). Strabismus occurs in about one third of cases. For this reason, careful ophthalmoscopy should be performed on all children with strabismus to exclude retinoblastoma or some other significant retinal pathology. Rarer presentations include neovascular glaucoma (NVG), which may cause secondary buphthalmos and iris heterochromia. Some eyes with endophytic or diffuse infultrative retinoblastomas develop pseudohyppyons of tumor

cells in the anterior chamber. Aseptic orbital cellulitis caused by servere NVG that induces intraocular necrosis is another pseudoinflammatory presentation. Patients in underdeveloped countries often present in the late stages of the disease with proptosis or an orbital mass caused by extraocular extension of the tumor (Fig. 12-2). Exceptional cases of clinically manifest congenital retinoblastoma have been reported. These present with a massive hyphema and an enlarged ectatic cornea that spontaneously perforates. It has been estimated that half of retinoblastomas actually may be present at birth but are inapparent clinically.

GROSS PATHOLOGY AND GROWTH PATTERNS

Macroscopically, retinoblastoma has a white encephaloid or brainlike appearance, which is not surprising since the tumor arises from the retina, a peripheral colony of brain cells (Fig. 12-3). Lighter flecks of calcification or necrotic tumor usually are evident grossly in the tumor. Necrotic retinoblastomas found in infants with aseptic orbital cellulitis typically have a blood-tinged, orange, or soupy, grayish necrotic appearance.

Tumors with endophytic, exophytic, mixed or indeterminate, and diffuse infiltrating growth patterns occur. **Endophytic retinoblastomas** arise from the inner layers of the retina, which remains attached. The tumor invades the vitreous cavity and can seed the anterior chamber (Fig. 12-3A,B). A pseudohypopyon of tumor cells can

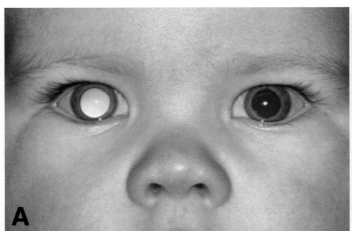
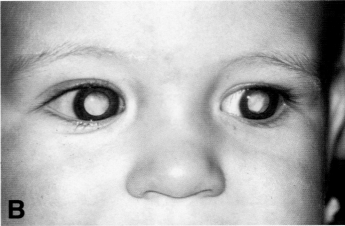

Fig. 12-1. A. Leukocoria. Unilateral sporadic retinoblastoma. About 90% of patients with retinoblastoma in the United States present with a white pupillary reflex. **B. Bilateral leukocoria, familial retinoblastoma.** Bilateral tumors occur in about two thirds of patients with familial retinoblastoma. The presence of bilateral tumors indicates that the affected patient is a carrier of familial retinoblastoma who can transmit the tumor to progeny. (Photos courtesy of Dr. Jerry A. Shields, Wills Eye Hospital.)

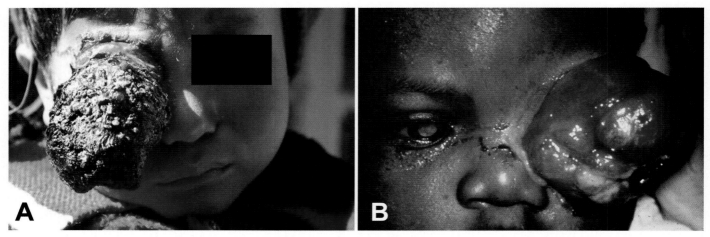

Fig. 12-2. A. Tibetan child with massive orbital involvement by retinoblastoma. Children in underdeveloped countries who have little access to medical care often present with in the late stages of the disease with proptosis or an orbital mass. **B. Neglected case of bilateral retinoblastoma from the United States.** Tumor fills left orbit. Leukocoria heralds a large tumor in the fellow eye. (From Zimmerman LE. Retinoblastoma, including a report of illustrative cases. *Med Ann Dist Columb* 1969;38:366–374.)

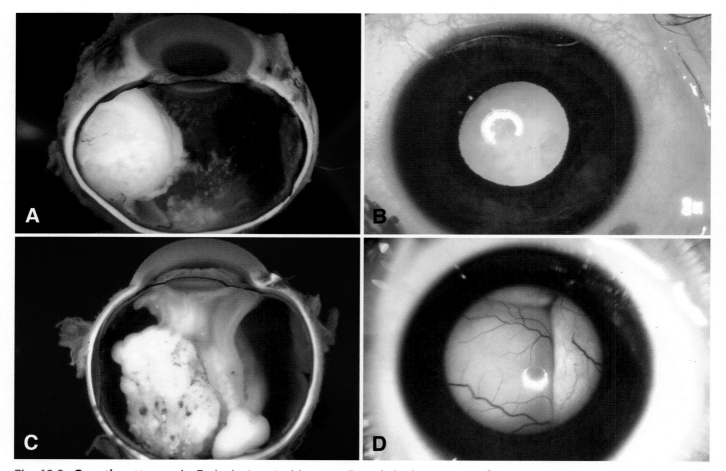

Fig. 12-3. Growth patterns. A. Endophytic retinoblastoma. Encephaloid tumor arises from inner retina, which remains attached. Extensive vitreous seeding is present. **B.** Leukocoria is caused by tumor in vitreous cavity. **C. Exophytic retinoblastoma.** Exophytic retinoblastomas arise from the outer layers of the retina and cause retinal detachment. Macrophoto of enucleated eye with exophytic retinoblastoma shows encephaloid tumor in subretinal space and total bullous retinal detachment, which adheres to the back of the lens. The lens-iris diaphragm is displaced anteriorly causing secondary closure of the angle. **D.** Retinal vessels are visible behind lens in eyes with exophytic retinoblastoma.

develop if there is extensive seeding of the anterior chamber. Hence, endophytic tumors can be confused with primary inflammatory disorders such as toxocariasis, mycotic endophthalmitis, or granulomatous uveitis.

Exophytic retinoblastomas arise from the outer layers of the retina and cause retinal detachment (Fig. 12-3B,C). The detached retina is often highly elevated, and its vessels are visible behind the lens on clinical examination. Exophytic retinoblastomas are usually confused clinically with simulating lesions such as Coats disease that cause an exudative retinal detachment. Totally endo- or exophytic retinoblastomas are actually relatively uncommon; most tumors have a mixed endophytic-exophytic or indeterminate growth pattern. About 1.4% of retinoblastomas diffusely thicken the retina without forming a distinct mass (Fig. 12-4). This rare **diffuse infiltrating growth pattern** usually is found in older children (mean age 6 years) who typically present with pseudoinflammatory signs and invariably have unilateral sporadic tumors. During gross or histopathologic examination, it is nearly impossible to distinguish multifocal primary lesions spawned by germline mutations from secondary tumors that result from tumor seeding.

HISTOPATHOLOGY

Under low magnification, retinoblastoma appears as a basophilic mass with pink and purple foci that arises from and destroys the retina and fills part or all of the vitreous cavity (Fig. 12-5). The basophilic areas are composed of viable retinoblastoma cells. The poorly differentiated neuroblastic cells appear blue because they have intensely basophilic nuclei and scanty cytoplasm (Fig. 12-5A). Numerous mitoses and fragments of apoptotic nuclear debris usually are present. Retinoblastoma grows rapidly and has a marked propensity to outgrow its blood supply and undergo spontaneous coagulative necrosis. This usually occurs when the proliferating cells have extended about 90 to 110 μm away

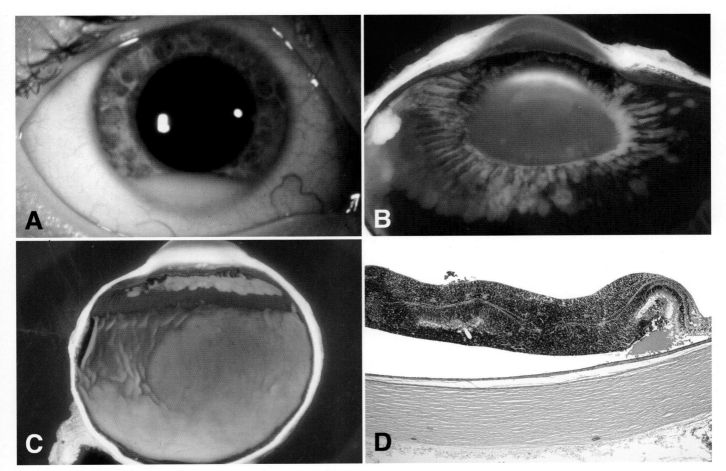

Fig. 12-4. Diffuse infiltrating retinoblastoma. A. Pseudohypopyon. Layered deposit of tumor cells in quiet eye was presenting manifestation of diffuse infiltrating retinoblastoma in older child. **B.** Infiltration of zonule by tumor occurs in many eyes with diffuse infiltrating tumors. **C.** The neoplasm diffusely infiltrates, thickens, and opacifies part of the retina but does not form a distinct mass. Tumor is present on the pars plana. The unilateral sporadic tumor was found in a 7-year-old boy who presented with anterior chamber seeding. **D.** The tumor diffusely infiltrates and thickens the retina but does not form a distinct mass. Calcification is absent. (**D.** H&E ×10)

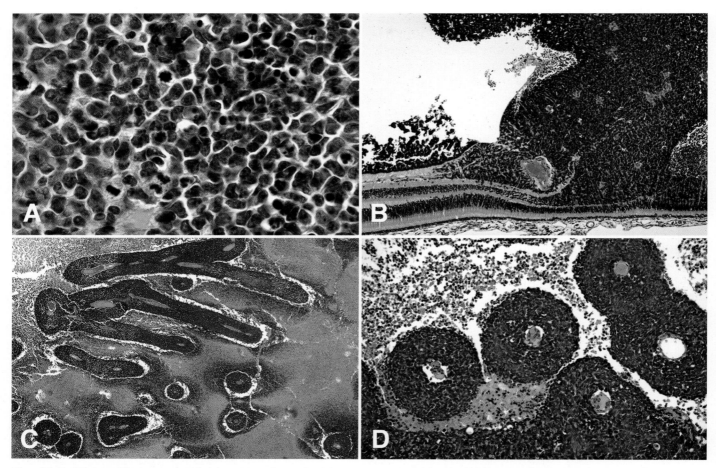

Fig. 12-5. Histopathology. A. Viable parts of a retinoblastoma appear blue in H&E stained sections because the tumor is composed of poorly differentiated neuroblastic cells that have scanty cytoplasm and prominent basophilic nuclei. Mitoses and apoptotic cells are common. **B. Endophytic retinoblastoma.** This poorly differentiated basophilic neoplasm arises from and destroys the retina. The retina remains attached as the endophytic tumor invades the vitreous cavity. Rosettes are not seen. **C.** Low magnification photomicrograph of retinoblastoma showing basophilic areas of viable tumor and eosinophilic zones of necrosis. The viable cells form characteristic sleeves and cuffs around vessels. **D.** Perivascular cuffs of tumor cells. Retinoblastoma typically outgrows its blood supply and undergoes necrosis. The necrotic cells become eosinophilic because they lose their nuclear DNA. Necrosis generally occurs when its cells have grown approximately 90 to 100 μm away from a vessel. The persistent viable cells form basophilic sleeves and cuffs around vessels. (**A.** H&E ×250, **B.** H&E ×50, **C.** H&E ×10, **D.** H&E ×50)

from a blood vessel (Fig. 12-5D). The necrotic tumor cells lose their basophilic nuclear DNA and become pink or eosinophilic. The residual viable cells typically form cuffs or sleeves around vessels, imparting a multilobulated or papillary appearance to some tumors (Fig. 12-5C,D). These perivascular cuffs were called pseudorosettes by some in the past. Foci of dystrophic calcification develop in the necrotic parts of the tumor in many cases (Fig. 12-6). Histopathologically, the calcific foci appear reddish purple in hematoxylin and eosin sections, and the presence of calcium can be confirmed by the von Kossa or alizarin red stains. Electron microscopy suggests that calcification probably begins in the mitochondria of necrotic cells. Clinically, the demonstration of calcification by ultrasonography or computed tomography can help to differentiate retinoblastoma from other simulating lesions.

Intensely basophilic deposits of DNA released from necrotic tumor cells are another characteristic histopathologic feature of retinoblastoma (Fig. 12-7). DNA deposition generally is found in eyes with extensively necrotic tumors. Typically, the DNA deposits surround retinal or iris vessels or are found in the trabecular meshwork or in basement membranes such as the lens capsule or the internal limiting membrane of the retina.

Retinoblastoma cells often collect on the inner surface of the Bruch membrane, causing focal retinal pigment epithelium (RPE) detachments. Such sub-RPE deposits of tumor cells do not constitute choroidal invasion. During histopathologic examination, care must be taken to distinguish artifactual contamination of the choroid (and epibulbar tissues) from true invasion. The presence of a mixture of viable and necrotic cells is one feature that serves to identify

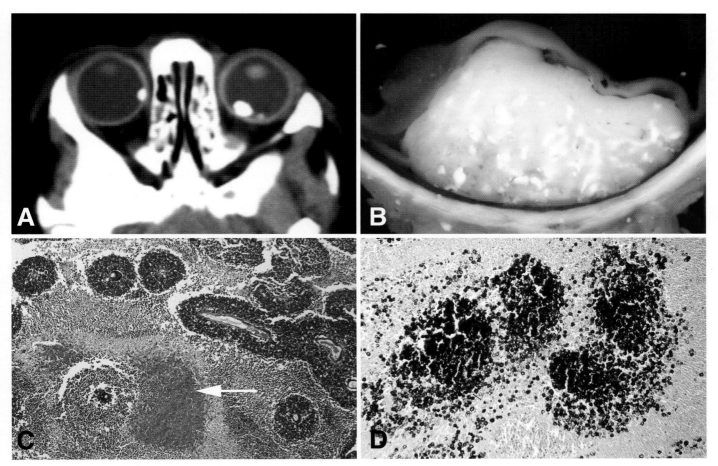

Fig. 12-6. Calcification. A. CT scan shows foci of residual calcified tumor in both eyes after chemoreduction therapy. **B.** Calcium and necrosis are evident grossly as lighter flecks in tumor. **C.** Dystrophic calcification develops in necrotic parts of tumor. The calcific foci appear purple in H&E stained sections (*arrow*). **D.** Calcified nuclei of tumor cells stain positively with von Kossa stain for calcium. (**A.** Photo courtesy of Carol L. Shields, MD, Wills Eye Institute. **C.** H&E ×25, **D.** von Kossa ×100)

artifactual seeding. Foci of extramedullary hematopoiesis also can be confused with uveal invasion in rare instances.

More than 40% of eyes enucleated for retinoblastoma have iris neovascularization, which may produce NVG, iris heterochromia, and even secondary buphthalmos. NVG is almost three times more common in eyes with high-risk features such as massive choroidal invasion or retrolaminar optic nerve invasion.

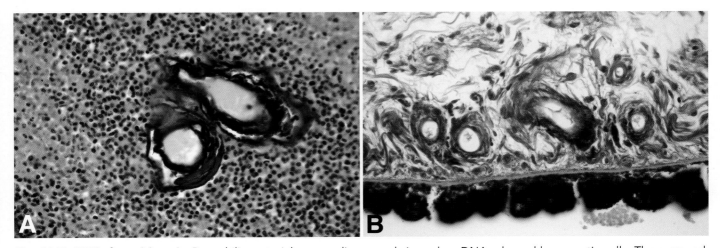

Fig. 12-7. DNA deposition. A. Basophilic material surrounding vessels is nuclear DNA released by necrotic cells. The surrounding tumor cells are necrotic. **B.** DNA deposition in iris stroma. DNA also may deposit in the ILM and the wall of the Schlemm canal. (**A.** H&E ×100, **B.** H&E ×100)

TUMOR DIFFERENTIATION: ROSETTES AND FLEURETTES

Varying degrees of retinal differentiation occur in retinoblastoma. This is evident as Homer Wright and Flexner-Wintersteiner rosettes and photoreceptor differentiation (fleurettes) as well (Figs. 12-8 and 12-9). **Flexner-Wintersteiner rosettes** represent an early attempt at retinal differentiation. Histologically, these rosettes are composed of a ring of cuboidal cells surrounding a central lumen (Fig. 12-8B). The lumen, which corresponds to the subretinal space, contains hyaluronidase-resistant acid mucopolysaccharide (AMP) similar to photoreceptor matrix AMP. The cells surrounding the lumen are joined near their apices by intercellular connections (zonulae adherentes), analogous to the external limiting membrane of the retina. Cilia, which exhibit the 9 + 0 pattern of microtubular doublets found in the central nervous system, project into the lumen. Cilia are hypothesized to be the precursor of photoreceptor outer segments. Although highly characteristic of retinoblastoma, Flexner-Wintersteiner rosettes are not pathognomonic because they do occur in malignant medulloepitheliomas and some pineal tumors.

Homer Wright rosettes (named after James Homer Wright) indicate neuroblastic differentiation (Fig. 12-8A). They lack a central lumen, and their constituent cells encompass a central tangle of neural filaments. Wright rosettes are relatively nonspecific. They also occur in neuroblastoma and are a characteristic feature of cerebellar medulloblastoma.

Retinoblastoma tends to become less well-differentiated with age. Numerous Flexner-Wintersteiner rosettes typically are found in eyes enucleated from younger infants, while tumors in older children tend to be poorly differentiated.

A recent study found that the mean age at enucleation for tumors with many rosettes was 10.4 months; for moderate rosettes, 18.3 months; for sparse rosettes, 20.4 months; and for poorly differentiated tumors, 33.9 months. These differences were statistically significant. The presence of many Flexner-Wintersteiner rosettes in a tumor may have prognostic significance. In one series, patients who had moderately well-differentiated tumors that contained abundant Flexner-Wintersteiner rosettes had about a sixfold better prognosis than those whose tumors lacked rosettes.

About 15% to 20% of retinoblastomas harbor very well-differentiated foci of actual **photoreceptor differentiation** (Fig. 12-9). Such areas contain aggregates of neoplastic photoreceptors called **fleurettes** by Ts'o, Zimmerman, and Fine, who described them in 1970. Photoreceptor differentiation typically is found in areas of viable tumor that appear relatively eosinophilic and paucicellular compared to adjacent undifferentiated retinoblastoma on low-magnification microscopy of H&E stained sections (Fig. 12-8A). The term "fleurette" denotes a bouquetlike arrangement of cytologically benign cells joined by a series of zonulae adherentes comprising a short segment of neoplastic external limiting membrane. Neoplastic photoreceptor inner segments evident as bulbous eosinophilic processes form the "flowers" of the bouquet (Fig. 12-8B). Electron microscopy has disclosed stacks of cellular membranes representing early outer segment differentiation in some cases. The demonstration and characterization of photoreceptor differentiation firmly established that retinoblastoma was not a retinal glioma and affirmed that the adoption of the name retinoblastoma by the American Ophthalmological Society in 1926 at Frederick Verhoeff's suggestion was indeed appropriate.

A retinal tumor composed entirely of photoreceptor differentiation is now thought to be a benign variant of

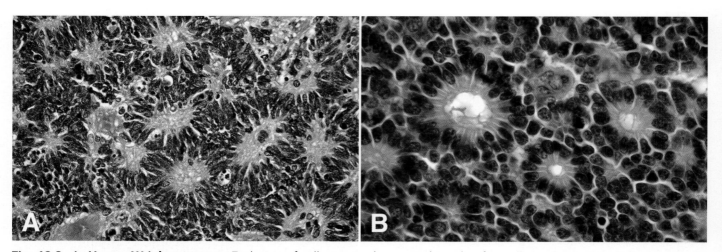

Fig. 12-8. A. Homer Wright rosettes. Each ring of cells surrounds a central tangle of neural processes. A central lumen is not present. Homer Wright rosettes are indicative of neuroblastic differentiation. They are the least differentiated form of rosette found in retinoblastoma and also occur in other tumors such as neuroblastoma. **B. Flexner-Wintersteiner rosettes.** Flexner-Wintersteiner rosettes represent differentiation toward primitive retina. The central lumen corresponds to the subretinal space. The tumor cells surrounding the lumen are joined near their apices by cellular connections that are analogous to the external limiting membrane. (**A.** H&E ×250, **B.** H&E ×250)

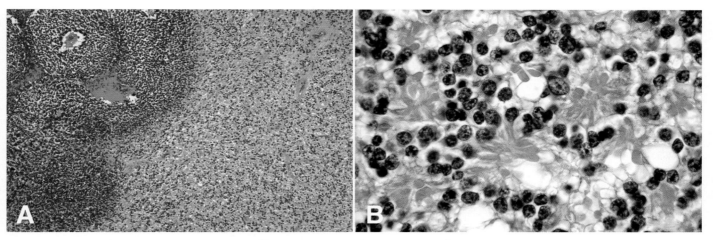

Fig. 12-9. Retinoblastoma, photoreceptor differentiation. A. Photoreceptor differentiation typically is found in an area of viable tumor that appears relatively eosinophilic compared to poorly differentiated retinoblastoma. **B.** Neoplastic photoreceptors typically form bouquets of pink "flowers" called fleurettes. The inner segments of the neoplastic photoreceptors appear as bulbous eosinophilic processes that often are aligned along a segment of neoplastic external limiting membrane. The nuclei are bland and mitoses and necrosis are not evident. Tumors composed entirely of fleurettes are considered to be benign variants of retinoblastoma called retinomas or retinocytomas. (**B.** H&E ×250)

retinoblastoma called a **retinoma or retinocytoma.** The cells comprising retinoma/retinocytoma are quite bland compared to those of retinoblastoma with a low nuclear cytoplasmic ratio, finely dispersed chromatin, and no apoptosis, mitoses, or necrosis. Calcification is found but occurs in viable parts of the tumor.

Retinomas or retinocytomas initially were thought to represent spontaneously regressed retinoblastomas on clinical grounds because they resemble retinoblastomas that have regressed after radiation therapy (Fig. 12-10A). They have a translucent "fish flesh" appearance, contain

abundant calcification that has been likened to cottage cheese, and are surrounded by a ring of RPE depigmentation. Retinomas/retinocytomas generally are small tumors that are found in eyes that retain useful vision. They may be found incidentally or are discovered in a parent or sibling when the detection of retinoblastoma in a child prompts examination of other family members. Retinocytomas are relatively resistant to radiation, as are other benign tumors. Therefore, it is not surprising that foci of photoreceptor differentiation are found more often in eyes that are enucleated after external-beam radiotherapy or chemotherapy.

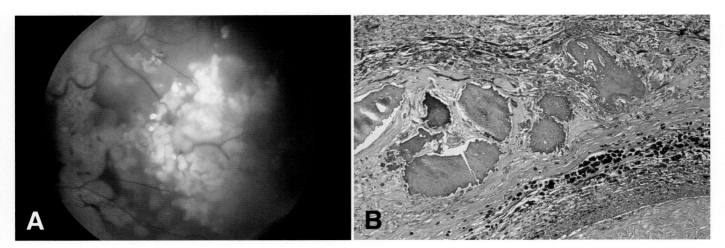

Fig. 12-10. A. Retinocytoma. The tumor has a translucent "fish flesh" appearance and contains large amounts of calcification that has been likened to cottage cheese. An annulus of RPE depigmentation typically surrounds the tumor. The tumor shown here was detected at a preschool vision screening and was observed unchanged for several years before undergoing malignant transformation. (From Eagle RC Jr, et al. Malignant transformation of spontaneously regressed retinoblastoma, retinoma/retinocytoma variant. *Ophthalmology* 1989;96:1389–1395. Courtesy of Ophthalmology.) **B. Spontaneously regressed retinoblastoma, phthisical eye.** Basophilic foci of necrotic calcified tumor cells are the only remnants of retinoblastoma in this phthisical eye. The calcified tumor is encased by scar tissue that contains strands of hyperplastic RPE. The choroid is scarred and shows evidence of necrosis. (**B.** H&E ×25)

There is evidence that retinoma/retinocytoma is a precursor of retinoblastoma. Rare cases of clinically documented malignant transformation have been reported, and photoreceptor differentiaton has been observed repeatedly at the base of endophytic retinoblastomas in enucleated eyes. Based on the results of molecular genetic studies, Dimaras recently has redefined retinoma as a precancerous lesion characterized by the loss of function of both copies of the RB1 gene, but lacking the additional genomic changes characteristic of retinoblastoma.

NATURAL HISTORY AND PROGNOSTIC FACTORS

Retinoblastoma is a highly malignant neoplasm that grows relentlessly and is invariably fatal if untreated. The tumor arises from the retina and invades the vitreous cavity and/ or the subretinal space. Tumor cells eventually breach the Bruch membrane and invade the choroidal stroma (Fig. 12-11A–D). Choroidal vessels serve as a major route for distant hematogenous dissemination, and massive **choroidal invasion** is an indication for adjuvant chemotherapy in many centers. Involvement of the anterior chamber, iris stromal, and trabecular meshwork also are thought to affect prognosis adversely, but the actual magnitude of this effect is uncertain. Of 297 previously untreated eyes enucleated for retinoblastoma at the Wills Eye Institute, 16.5% were found to have uveal invasion, which was classified as massive (>3 mm in diameter) in about half.

Retinoblastoma has a marked proclivity to invade the optic nerve, and **optic nerve invasion** is an extremely important prognostic factor (Fig. 12-11C,D). The tumor can travel along the optic nerve to the brain, or malignant cells may be dispersed along the neuraxis if they gain access to the cerebrospinal fluid. Of the 297 untreated eyes in the

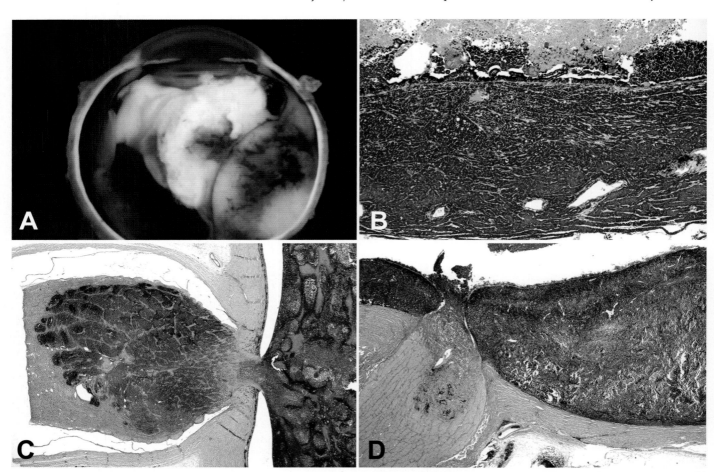

Fig. 12-11. High-risk histopathologic findings. A. Retinoblastomas, massive choroidal invasion. The right half of the choroid is massively thickened by invasive retinoblastoma. The area of choroidal invasion contains foci of hemorrhage. Careful examination disclosed no extraocular extension. The patient developed metastases after the parents declined prophylactic chemotherapy. **B. Retinoblastoma, massive choroidal invasion.** The entire thickness of the choroid is replaced by a basophilic infiltrate of poorly differentiated, viable retinoblastoma cells. Massive choroidal invasion recently has been defined as a full-thickness infiltrate >3 mm in diameter. **C. Retinoblastoma, optic nerve invasion.** There is massive replacement of the retrolaminar parenchyma of the optic nerve by basophilic tumor. Tumor is seen in close proximity to the cut surface of the nerve. A cross section of nerve containing the true surgical margin was excised and submitted for sections before the eye was opened. Equivalent to extraocular extension, retrolaminar optic nerve invasion is an indication for adjuvant chemotherapy in many centers. **D.** Eye with concurrent massive choroidal invasion and retrolaminar invasion of optic nerve. Multiple high-risk features often occur together. (**B.** H&E ×50, **C.** H&E ×25, **D.** H&E ×10)

Wills Eye Institute series, 38.7% had some degree of optic nerve invasion. Retrolaminar optic nerve invasion, an important indication for adjuvant chemotherapy, was present in about 10.4%. Mortality rates correlate directly with the depth of optic nerve invasion. In one series, 10% died if there was superficial invasion of the nerve head only (grade I) and 29% if the tumor reached and invaded the lamina cribrosa (stage II). Mortality rose to 42% when there was retrolaminar invasion (grade III) and 78% when the tumor extended to the surgical margin (grade IV). Hence, surgeons should try to obtain as long a segment of optic nerve as possible when enucleating an eye that is known or suspected to harbor retinoblastoma. In addition, enucleation should not be performed by an inexperienced surgeon.

After retinoblastoma has filled the globe and destroyed its contents, it extends extraocularly. Anteriorly, the tumor extends through the aqueous outflow pathways, preexisting emissarial canals, or perforations in the cornea. Posterior segment tumors that have invaded the choroid can extend extraocularly through emissarial canals or can invade the orbit by directly infiltrating and destroying the sclera. Secondary buphthalmos and staphylomas caused by secondary glaucoma can facilitate extrascleral extension. Secondary closed-angle glaucoma caused by pupillary block or iris neovascularization is relatively common in eyes with retinoblastoma. About 43% of eyes enucleated for retinoblastoma have iris neovascularization and 26% have NVG. In addition, NVG is much more common in eyes with high-risk histopathologic features.

Retinoblastoma typically metastasizes hematogenously to lungs, bones, brain, and other organs. Cervical and preauricular adenopathy can develop when tumors with extensive anterior segment involvement gain access to lymphatics in the conjunctival stroma. Lymphatics are not present in the orbit. Metastatic disease usually becomes evident within 1 or 2 years after therapy. Late metastasis is so rare in retinoblastoma that it should raise the possibility of a second independent primary tumor such as pineoblastoma.

Retinoblastoma occasionally undergoes spontaneous regression. A typical bona fide example of spontaneous regression is a phthisical eye that contains foci of calcified retinoblastoma cells. Both the tumor regression and phthisis bulbi probably are caused by extensive ischemic necrosis in an eye with severe NVG (Fig. 12-10B). Many lesions that previously were thought to be spontaneously regressed tumors actually are retinomas or retinocytomas.

MOLECULAR GENETICS AND THE RETINOBLASTOMA ONCOGENE

Retinoblastoma is a hereditary cancer: 5% to 10% of the tumors are inherited in what appears to be a classic Mendelian autosomal dominant trait; carriers transmit the tumor to one half of their offspring (Fig. 12-12B). Bilaterality is a characteristic feature of heritable retinoblastomas. Bilateral tumors occur in about 60% of patients who have germline mutations in the RB1 gene. The average age of patients with familial retinoblastoma is about 1 year. A germline mutation should be suspected when retinoblastoma is found in a very young infant.

The great majority of retinoblastomas (85%) are sporadic tumors that arise in patients with a negative family history (Fig. 12-12A). About 75% of these sporadic tumors are caused by somatic mutations in retinal cells. Sporadic retinoblastomas caused by somatic mutations are invariably unilateral, unifocal tumors that cannot be passed-on to progeny, and they tend to occur in older infants (mean age 2 years). The remaining 25% of sporadic cases are caused by germline mutations and represent new familial cases that are transmissible.

A small number (<5%) of retinoblastomas occur in infants who have a variety of congenital anomalies and are found to have deletions in the long arm of chromosome 13 that are evident in karyotypic analysis. In addition to

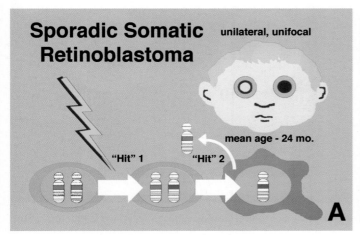
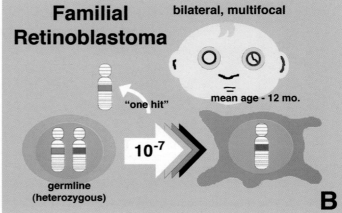

Fig. 12-12. **A. Sporadic somatic retinoblastoma.** Retinoblastomas caused by sporadic somatic mutations are most common. They are always unilateral and typically occur at about age 2 years. **B.** Familial retinoblastomas typically are bilateral and multifocal. They occur earlier than tumors caused by sporadic somatic mutations because only a single "hit" or gene inactivation is required.

retinoblastoma, the 13Q- deletion syndrome comprises severe mental retardation and other anomalies including microcephaly, hypertelorism, ptosis, micrognathia, deformed low-set ears, a wide nasal bridge, cardiac anomalies, anal atresia, microphthalmia, colobomas, and cataracts. The association of retinoblastoma with the 13Q-syndrome initially suggested that the retinoblastoma gene was located on chromosome 13.

The paradigmatic human recessive oncogene or tumor suppressor gene, the retinoblastoma or RB1 gene is located in the 14 band of the Q or long arm of chromosome 13 (13q14). The RB1 gene is 180,388 base pairs in length, and its protein product pRB comprises 928 amino acids. pRB is abundant in the nucleus, where it is involved in control of the cell cycle. During the G1 or resting phase of the cell cycle, pRB is bound to transcription factors such as E2F. Phosphorylation of pRB causes release of E2F. Uncomplexed E2F, in turn, activates a variety of other genes and transcription factors that are important in the initiation of DNA synthesis (S phase). Absence of pRB causes continual cell division and lack of terminal differentiation.

The RB protein is phosphorylated by cyclin D2 and its cyclin-dependent kinase (cdk) partner. Certain oncoviruses cause tumors by synthesizing proteins (e.g., adenoviral protein E1A and SV40 large T protein) that bind to pRB and inactivate it.

Classically, the Rb1 gene is thought to cause cancer when its protein product is absent or dysfunctional (Fig. 12-13). Healthy persons have two normal or wild-type Rb1 genes (Fig. 12-13A). Both alleles of the Rb1 gene are absent or inactivated in the retinoblastoma cells. Carriers of familial retinoblastoma are heterozygous for the Rb1 gene. Although the pRB produced by a heterozygote's single functional gene is sufficient to inhibit tumorigenesis, heterozygotes are at substantial risk to develop retinoblastoma. Although retinoblastoma appears to be inherited clinically as an autosomal dominant trait, the gene is recessive at a molecular level (Fig. 12-14).

The genotype of a child with familial retinoblastoma includes one functional copy of the Rb1 gene (Fig. 12-13B). The second copy of the gene is mutated and encodes dysfunctional RB protein or it may be absent. Retinoblastoma

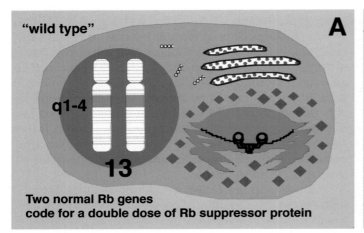

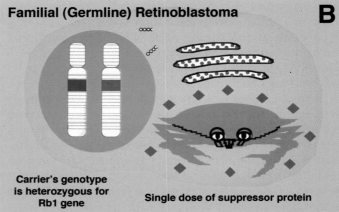

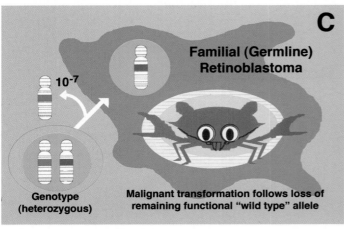

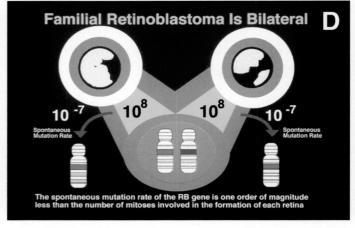

Fig. 12-13. The retinoblastoma gene. A. Normal individuals have two copies of the retinoblastoma gene, which is located on the long arm of chromosome 13. The gene encodes Rb protein that suppresses tumor formation. **B.** Patients with familial retinoblastoma are heterozygous for the retinoblastoma gene. **C.** Retinoblastoma develops when both copies of the retinoblastoma gene in a retinal cell are lost or inactivated. **D.** The spontaneous mutation rate of the Rb gene is less that the number of mitoses required for the formation of each retina. This is the basis for bilateral and multifocal tumors in heterozygous carriers.

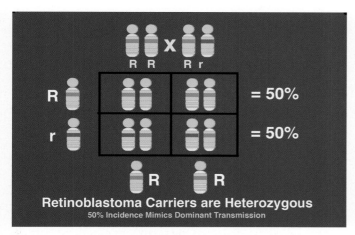

Fig. 12-14. Familial retinoblastoma appears to be an autosomal dominant trait, but the gene actually is recessive at the molecular level.

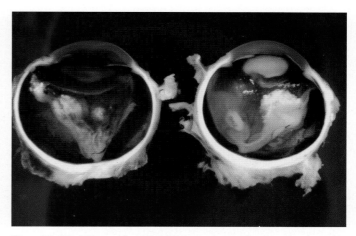

Fig. 12-15. Bilateral retinoblastoma. Both eyes had to be enucleated after therapy failed to control the tumors. Bilateral involvement indicates that the patient has a potentially transmissible germ-line mutation in the Rb gene.

develops when the solitary remaining wild-type gene is lost or inactivated, by chance, in a cell within the developing retina (Fig. 12-13C). Cytogenetic mechanisms responsible for gene inactivation (and resultant homozygosity for the recessive allele) include chromosomal loss or deletion, somatic recombination, and point mutation. The spontaneous mutation rate of the normal wild-type Rb1 gene is 1 in 10 million or greater. It is estimated that 100 million mitoses occur during the growth and development of each retina. Hence, it is highly probable that the second functional copy of the Rb1 gene will be lost or inactivated in at least one retinal cell in a carrier with a heterozygous genotype. Furthermore, it is equally probable that gene inactivation and tumorigenesis will occur in both eyes (Fig. 12-13D).

Immune surveillance appears to arrest some tumors, despite the appropriate additional mutations. This probably is responsible, in part, for the incomplete penetrance of the Rb1 gene, which is estimated to be approximately 80% (in other words, there is an 80% chance that one tumor will develop in one eye). A few families with low-penetrance retinoblastoma have been reported. They have reduced levels of wild-type RB protein or mutant RB protein that retains partial activity.

About one third of patients with retinoblastoma have bilateral tumors (Figs. 12-1B and 12-15). The sporadic occurrence of bilateral tumors indicates that the affected patient has a germline mutation and is capable of transmitting the disease to one half of his or her offspring. Unfortunately, the opposite is not true. As a result of incomplete penetrance and expressivity, 10% to 15% of unilateral, sporadic retinoblastomas are caused by potentially transmissible, germline mutations. Statistics used for genetic counseling (Table 12-1) reflect both the effect of gene penetrance and the proportion of familial, chromosomal deletion, and sporadic somatic and germline retinoblastomas in the population.

Molecular genetics readily explains several hitherto puzzling clinical features of retinoblastoma. For example,

retinoblastoma is predominantly a tumor of early childhood. Although rare adult cases have been reported, the mean age at diagnosis is 18 months and the tumor is extremely rare after age 4 years. Cytogenetic misadventures that cause gene inactivation generally occur during cellular division. Most mitotic activity in the retina actually ceases before birth, making neoplastic transformation in older persons highly unlikely. Retinoblastomas caused by germline mutations typically develop at an earlier age than retinoblastomas caused by sporadic somatic mutations (mean age 12 months vs. 23 months), presumably because only a single Rb1 gene allele, rather than two, must be inactivated. Knudson graphically compared the ages of patients who had unilateral and bilateral tumors with the logarithm of the proportion in each group as yet undiagnosed. His results led him to postulate that two separate events or "hits" are necessary for the development of sporadic retinoblastomas ("two-hit hypothesis"). The curve for bilateral, hereditary tumors is a simple exponential relation, consistent with a single gene inactivation or "hit" superimposed on the inherited genotypic defect.

TABLE 12-1	Genetic Counseling: Risk That Subsequent Child Will Have Retinoblastoma
Unilateral Retinoblastoma	**%**
Affected parent with no affected children	3
Normal parents, one affected child	3
One affected parent, one affected child	30
Bilateral Retinoblastoma	
One affected parent, no affected child	40
Normal parents, one affected child	10
One affected parent, one affected child	50

Patients who are heterozygous carriers of familial retinoblastoma are predisposed to develop other malignant tumors. A survivor of bilateral retinoblastoma has a 20% to 50% chance of developing a second tumor within 20 years (Armed Forces Institute of Pathology series: 26% within 30 years). These secondary nonocular tumors include osteogenic and other soft tissue sarcomas, carcinomas of the upper respiratory passages, malignant melanomas, and carcinomas of the skin. Most second tumors occur within the field of irradiation many years after external-beam radiotherapy for intraocular retinoblastoma. However, a 500-fold increase in the incidence of osteogenic sarcoma in the nonirradiated femur has been reported.

Some of the most interesting secondary nonocular neoplasms that develop in patients with germline mutations are tumors of the pineal gland or parasellar region that resemble ectopic retinoblastomas. This association between pinealoma (also termed pineoblastoma) and bilateral hereditary retinoblastoma has been termed "trilateral retinoblastoma." The pineal gland, which serves as a "third eye" in some primitive reptiles, shares antigenic determinants with the retina and exhibits transient photoreceptor differentiation in the neonatal rat. Photoreceptor differentiation has been identified in human pineal tumors.

The Rb1 gene has been implicated as a contributing factor in a variety of other systemic malignancies, including breast, lung, and bladder cancer. This is not surprising, considering the Rb1 gene's fundamental role in control of the cell cycle.

Recent molecular genetic studies suggest that the initial concepts outlined above concerning the Rb1 tumor suppressor gene and its role in the pathogenesis of retinoblastoma are an oversimplification. Dimaras recently has shown that both copies of the Rb1 gene are inactivated and Rb protein is absent in retinoma/retinocytoma, which is now considered to be a benign precursor lesion of retinoblastoma. Additional mutations are necessary for malignant transformation of retinoma into retinoblastoma. The retinoblastoma gene plays an important role in the regulation of cellular division in all cells in the body, yet only retinoblastoma, a relatively rare neoplasm that affects a small population of highly differentiated cells, results from the inactivation of both copies of the RB1 gene. The highly retinal-specific predisposition imposed by mutations in the RB1 gene is hypothesized to result from the specific pattern of expression of other genes in the unidentified cell of origin in the developing human retina rather than RB1.

THE CLASSIFICATION AND TREATMENT OF RETINBLASTOMA

There are several staging systems for retinoblastoma. The older Reese-Ellsworth classification has prognostic significance for retention of an eye, maintenance of sight, and the control of local disease; but is complicated; and recently has become less useful because it is based on the response to external beam radiotherapy, a treatment modality that has fallen out of favor and is now used infrequently. The newer International Classification of Retinoblastoma (ICRB) is a relatively simple, practical classification based on clinical findings that was designed primarily to evaluate the potential response to modern therapy including chemoreduction. The International Classification includes five stages A through E. Tumors with localized subretinal seeds are placed in group C and more diffuse seeding in group D. Group E tumors general require enucleation. They fill more than 50% of the globe or have opaque media, NVG, or high risk features such as postlaminar optic nerve invasion, significant choroidal invasion, and invasion of the anterior chamber, sclera, or orbit.

A detailed discussion of the treatment of retinoblastoma is beyond the scope of this chapter. A number of reports dealing with modern treatment modalities are referenced below. In short, there have been major changes in the treatment of retinoblastoma in developed countries in recent years. A concerted effort has been made to avoid the use of external beam radiotherapy, which leads to disfiguring facial deformities and predisposes retinoblastoma gene carriers to secondary malignant neoplasms in the field of radiation such as soft tissue sarcomas. Instead, many infants with retinoblastoma, particularly those with germline mutations and bilateral tumors are being treated with chemotherapy. In many instances, chemotherapy is used to shrink tumors so they are amenable to additional treatment or "consolidation" with local therapeutic agents such as cryotherapy, infrared laser transpupillary thermotherapy, or radioactive plaque brachyradiotherapy. Called chemoreduction, this form of chemotherapy is used most commonly in the treatment of bilateral retinoblastoma. Many eyes with unilateral retinoblastoma are still enucleated. A few centers are treating retinoblastoma by direct infusion of chemotherapy into the ophthalmic artery. This controversial experimental technique directly targets the tumor and may decrease complications of systemic chemotherapy.

In developed countries, retinoblastoma is one of the great success stories of pediatric ocular oncology. At some centers, survival rates from the primary tumor approach 100%, and secondary tumors are now the primary cause of death. Unfortunately, this is not the case in underdeveloped countries, where patients frequently present with advanced stages of the disease and therapy generally is palliative (Fig. 12-2).

THE DIFFERENTIAL DIAGNOSIS OF RETINOBLASTOMA

Retinoblastoma must be differentiated clinically from a variety of benign childhood disorders that cause leukocoria. The three most common conditions that are confused with retinoblastoma are ocular toxocariasis, persistent hyperplastic primary vitreous (PHPV), and Coats disease (see Table 12-2).

TABLE 12-2	The Differential Diagnosis of Retinoblastoma			
Lesion	Unilateral	Bilateral	Age	Comments
Retinoblastoma	X	X	Mean 18 mo	Calcification on imaging; pseudoinflammatory presentations
Toxocariasis	X	—	6–11 y	Contact with puppies; eosinophilic abscess, serial sections to disclose worm fragment, negative ELISA excludes
PHPV/PFV	X	—	Present at birth	Microphthalmic eye with retrolental fibrovascular plaque, inwardly drawn ciliary processes, iris shunts and other persistent fetal vessels
Coats disease	X	Rare	18 mo to 18 y, peak end of 1st decade	2/3 men, abnormal leaky retinal vessels (Leber's miliary aneurysms), bullous RD with lipid-rich subretinal fluid, massive exudation; bilateral cases my have fascioscapulohumeral muscular dystrophy
Retinopathy of prematurity	—	X	In early infancy, but not congenital	Premature infants, supplemental oxygen therapy
Incontinentia pigmenti (Bloch-Sulzberger)	—	X	Infancy	Perinatal bullous eruption with eosinophilia, whorled skin pigmentation develops, nonperfusion of periphery, X-linked dominent – lethal in men, NEMO gene, eotaxin
Norrie disease	—	X	Congenital	Men, X-linked recessive, bilateral pseudogliomas caused by detachment of dysplastic retina, deafess, mental retardation, Norrin gene (plays role in other disorders)
Medullepithelioma	X	—	4 y (rare—adults)	"diktyoma," benign and malignant, teratoid and nontertoid, teratoid tumors contain cartilage, muscle brain
Retinal dysplasia	X	—	Congenital	Microphthalmia, most have trisomy 13
Astrocytic hamartoma of tuberous sclerosis complex (TSC)		X		Tuberous sclerosis complex, family history, seizure disorder, retinal lesion easily confused with early retinoblastoma (RB) Rare progressive giant cell astrocytomas
Other				Colobomas, congenital cataract, myelinated nerve fibers, retinal detachment, vitreous hemorrhage, trauma, endogenous endophthalmitis

TOXOCARIASIS

Ocular toxocariasis, particularly the nematode endophthalmitis form of the disorder, is the most common inflammatory disease that simulates retinoblastoma (Fig. 12-16A). Ocular toxocariasis is a localized ocular manifestation of visceral larva migrans caused by second-stage larvae of the canine ascarid *Toxocara canis*. Ocular toxocariasis usually is unilateral and occurs in children toward the end of the first decade. Diffuse nematode endophthalmitis, retinal detachment, or an eosinophilic abscess located anteriorly in the vitreous can cause leukocoria. Subfoveal granulomas occasionally present with visual loss in eyes with clear media. Histopathology discloses necrotic larval fragments surrounded by granulomatous inflammation containing many eosinophils (Fig. 12-16A). Serial sections may be necessary to demonstrate the parasite in a presumptive eosinophilic abscess. Clinically, an ELISA test for Toxocara antigen excludes the diagnosis if it is negative. A positive ELISA test does not exclude retinoblastoma, however, because antibodies to *T. canis* are common in some populations.

Other inflammatory diseases that occasionally are misdiagnosed as retinoblastoma include endogneous endophthalmitis, congenital toxoplasmosis, cytomegalovirus retinitis, herpes simplex virus retinitis, and peripheral uveoretinitis.

PERSISTENT HYPERPLASTIC PRIMARY VITREOUS/PERSISTENT FETAL VASCULATURE (PHPV/PFV)

PHPV/PFV is an extremely common variety of pseudoretinoblastoma (Fig. 12-17). A congenital anomaly, PHPV/PFV is present at birth. Although exceptions have been reported, PHPV/PFV classically occurs in a microphthalmic eye

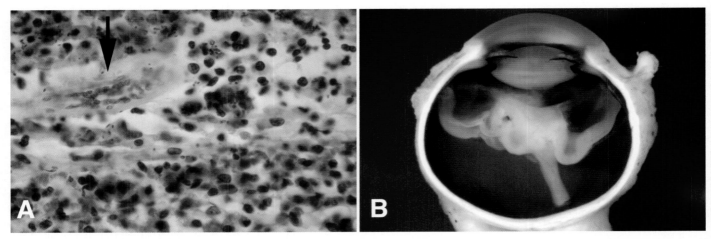

Fig. 12-16. A. Ocular toxocariasis. *Arrow* points to fragment of nematode in eosinophilic abscess. **B. Incontinentia pigmenti.** Enucleated eye has total retinal detachment caused by florid vitreoretinal neovascularization. Fellow eye had nonperfusion of the peripheral retina. Patient had characteristic dermal pigmentation. (**A.** H&E, ×100)

that has a shallow anterior chamber and a clear lens. The disorder usually is unilateral. Histopathologically, a plaque of fibrovascular tissue that resembles primary vitreous adheres to the posterior lens capsule, and the hyaloid artery is often patent. The tips of the ciliary processes typically adhere to the margins of the retrolenticular plaque. As the eye enlarges, the processes are drawn centrally and elongated. Visible behind the clear lens through a dilated pupil, these inwardly drawn ciliary processes are a helpful diagnostic sign (Fig. 12-17A). Abnormal shunt vessels often traverse the iridic surface, and other parts of the fetal vasculature may persist.

PHPV/PFV may occur in isolation or in association with other ocular abnormalities. It is a common finding in eyes with trisomy 13. Rare cases have been reported in

which both PHPV/PFV and retinoblastoma have occurred together, either ipsilaterally or contralaterally. The posterior lens capsule is interrupted in some cases. This occasionally leads to cataract formation and may allow mesenchymal tissue to invade the interior of the lens. Intraocular adipose tissue and even bone have been reported histopathologically. Approximately one fifth (10/47) of eyes with PHPV/PFV contain mature adipose tissue. Goldberg has suggested that PFV is a more appropriate term for this disorder, and many have adopted his new terminology.

Other congenital or developmental disorders occasionally confused with retinoblastoma include juvenile retinoschisis, dominant exudative vitreoretinopathy, congenital retinal fold, the morning-glory disc anomaly, and idiopathic retinal vascular hypoplasia.

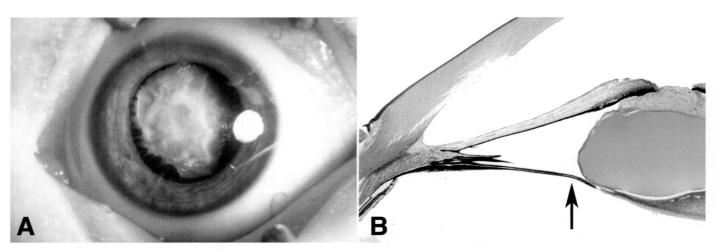

Fig. 12-17. Persistent hyperplastic primary vitreous. A. Inwardly drawn ciliary processes adhere to the margin of vascularized retrolental fibrous plaque. The lesion was present at birth and the affected eye was microphthalmic. **B.** Long attenuated ciliary process (*arrow*) attaches to margin of fibrous plaque on posterior surface of lens. An anterior subcapsular cataract also is present. (**B.** H&E ×5)

COATS DISEASE

Simulating lesions that produce retinal detachment are often confused with exophytic retinoblastoma. Coats disease is a classic example (Fig. 12-18). Coats disease is marked by an exudative retinal detachment caused by leakage of fluid from abnormal telangiectatic retinal vessels. Often called Leber miliary aneurysms, these fusiform or saccular "light bulb" venous dilatations tend to involve the temporal parafoveal quadrant of the retina and are especially common superotemporally. Intravenous fluorescein angiography typically discloses an area of capillary nonperfusion adjacent to the abnormal vessels. Some cases may present with decreased vision due to macular exudation.

Coats disease usually is unilateral, and two thirds of cases occur in boys. Although most cases are diagnosed in the second half of the first decade (age 4–10 years), the disease can affect children between 18 months and 18 years.

Macroscopically, enucleated eyes with Coats disease have a high bullous retinal detachment that typically abuts the back surface of the lens and ciliary body (Fig. 12-18A,B). The lens-iris diaphragm is displaced anteriorly, causing secondary closed-angle glaucoma via a pupillary block mechanism. The yellow, gelatinous subretinal fluid contains glistening crystals of cholesterol. In rare instances, the lipid-rich subretinal fluid has entered the anterior chamber through defects in the retina and anterior vitreous.

Histopathologically, parts of the inner retina contain an increased number of large telangiectatic vessels. The outer retinal layers are massively thickened by exudates, which appear as pools of eosinophilic material (Fig. 12-18C). The densely proteinaceous and lipid-rich subretinal fluid contains aggregates of foamy histiocytes and empty clefts that contained free, rhomboidal, crystals of cholesterol that were dissolved by lipid solvents during processing (Fig. 12-18D).

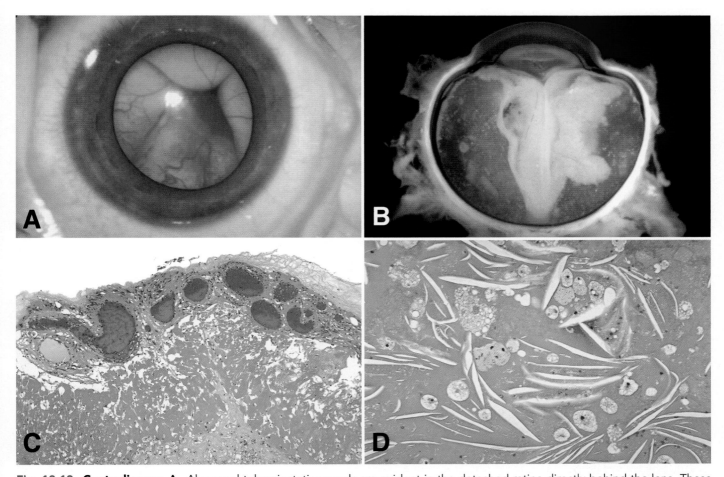

Fig. 12-18. Coats disease. A. Abnormal telangiectatic vessels are evident in the detached retina directly behind the lens. These leaky vessels have caused an exudative retinal detachment. The subretinal space contains yellowish fluid rich in lipid. Coats disease may simulate an exophytic retinoblastoma. **B.** The totally detached retina adheres to the back of the lens and the pars plana. The lens-iris diaphragm is displaced forward obliterating the anterior chamber and closing the angle. The yellow subretinal exudate contains cholesterol crystals and aggregates of lipid-laden histiocytes. The glaucomatous eye was enucleated because it was blind and painful and there was concern about a possible retinoblastoma. **C.** Many large abnormal retinal vessels are present. The outer two thirds of the retina is massively thickened by eosinophilic exudates. **D.** The eosinophilic, densely proteinaceous subretinal fluid contains slitlike cholesterol clefts and foamy histiocytes that have ingested lipid. (**C.** H&E ×50, **D.** H&E ×100)

A Coats disease–like picture may occur in patients who have fascioscapulohumeral muscular dystrophy caused by a partial deletion of chromosome 4q35. This association should be considered if both eyes are affected. It has been hypothesized that Coats disease may be caused by somatic mutations in the NDP gene that encodes norrin.

RETINOPATHY OF PREMATURITY

Organization or fibrosis of the vitreous (e.g., cyclitic membrane formation), which may lead to tractional retinal detachment, occurs in several conditions that simulate retinoblastoma, including retinopathy of prematurity (ROP) (Fig. 12-19). The term retrolental

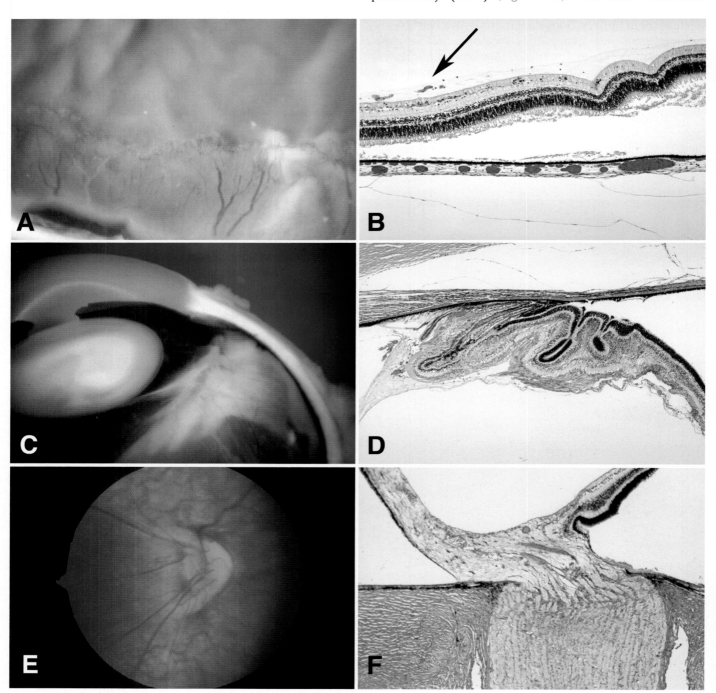

Fig. 12-19. Retinopathy of prematurity. A. Macrophoto shows band of vitreoretinal neovascularization bordering nonvascularized temporal periphery of retina. **B.** *Arrow* points to new vessels in photomicrograph. The peripheral part of the retina (**at right**) is avascular. **C.** Fibrovascular proliferation has led to the formation of a mass of folded retina in the temporal periphery behind the lens. The eye was obtained postmortem from a premature infant who had received supplemental oxygen. **D.** Photomicrograph shows folded retina comprising mass shown grossly in (**C**). **E.** Retinal traction causes dragging of optic disc. **F.** Disc is dragged temporally toward the mass of folded retina. (**B.** H&E ×25, **D.** H&E ×10, **F.** H&E ×10)

fibroplasia, originally applied to this largely iatrogenic disorder, emphasizes the causal role of vitreous organization in the tractional retinal detachment that complicates its final stages. ROP usually is bilateral and rarely is present at birth, two features it shares with retinoblastoma. ROP usually develops in premature infants who have received supplemental oxygen therapy. Infants born at a gestational age of <32 weeks or weighing less than 1,500 g at birth are at risk for developing ROP. However, occasional cases have been reported in full-term infants and in premature infants who did not receive oxygen therapy. Vascular proliferation and secondary vitreous fibrosis are thought to result from the effect of increased oxygen levels on the immature, incompletely vascularized retina. ROP typically arises in the temporal quadrant of the retina, because the temporal retina usually is not completely vascularized at term, especially in premature infants.

Experiments performed in newborn kittens suggest that excessive oxygen induces transient vasoconstriction, subsequent dilatation, and ultimately vaso-obliteration of immature retinal vessels. Retinal neovascularization may be a response of the vanguard of primitive, vasoformative spindle cells in the nonvascularized peripheral retina to elevated oxygen levels. In the early active stages of ROP, a band of glomeruloid capillaries proliferates at the junction between the peripheral nonperfused and the posterior perfused retina (Fig. 12-19A,B). The proliferating vessels break through the internal limiting membrane and invade the vitreous, inciting fibrosis and contraction. In the later cicatricial stages of ROP, the retina is folded on itself by the organized vitreous, forming a fibroneural mass that drags the macula and optic disc temporally (Fig. 12-19C–F). The end stage of the disease is marked by total retinal detachment, leukocoria, blindness, and phthisis bulbi.

RETINAL DETACHMENT

Retinal detachment in childhood can be confused with retinoblastoma, and vice versa. The possibility of an underlying retinoblastoma should always be considered when a child presents with retinal detachment and vitreous hemorrhage, even when a history of trauma is obtained. Appropriate preoperative studies (ultrasonography or computed tomography) are indicated. If vitrectomy is performed, the specimen should be submitted for cytologic examination. Clinicians must recall that retinoblastoma occasionally presents in older children who may have the diffuse infiltrative form of retinoblastoma. In addition, retinoblastoma or medulloepithelioma must be ruled out in any infant or child with NVG. NVG in a child is a neoplasm until proven otherwise. Finally, the ophthalmologist always should recall the association between retinal detachment and child abuse.

INCONTINENTIA PIGMENTI

Peripheral vascular abnormalities, which are believed to cause vitreoretinal neovascularization and secondary retinal detachment and leukocoria, occur in women who have incontinentia pigmenti or the Bloch-Sulzberger syndrome. This rare multisystem disorder has an X-linked dominant inheritance. Normal men die *in utero*, but the disorder has been reported in men with the Klinefelter syndrome (XXY) or XXY mosaicism. Affected female infants develop vesiculobullous skin lesions on the trunk and extremities at birth or shortly thereafter. The bullae contain many eosinophils, and systemic eosinophilia is often present. The term incontinentia pigmenti refers to the incontinence, or loss, of melanin from epidermal basal cells. The pigment collects in the dermis as free granules or as aggregates of melanophages. Clinically, the affected skin has a characteristic marbleized or whorllike pattern of pigmentation. Other manifestations of the syndrome include alopecia, dental anomalies (late dentition, absent, or misshapen teeth), and central nervous system abnormalities (seizures, mental retardation).

Ocular findings occur in approximately one third of patients and include strabismus (18.2%) and pseudoglioma caused by a retrolental mass of organized, chronically detached retina (15.4%). The latter probably is caused by vitreoretinal neovascularization spawned by peripheral retinal avascularity (Fig. 12-16B). Histopathologic examination, limited to "end-stage" eyes enucleated as possible retinoblastomas, have revealed relatively nonspecific findings.

Incontinentia pigmenti is caused by mutations in the NEMO/IKK gamma gene on Xq28, which interferes with NF-kappa B activation. The NEMO gene activates the eosinophil chemokine eotaxin. There is a single report of retinoblastoma arising in a patient with incontinentia pigmenti.

NORRIE DISEASE

Norrie disease, or the progressive oculoacousticocerebral degeneration of Norrie, is a rare, X-linked recessive heritable disorder characterized by bilateral leukocoria caused by retrolental masses of detached, malformed retina. Affected boys classically have a triad of blindness, deafness, and mental retardation. Apparent at birth or in early infancy, the ocular findings usually progress to phthisis bulbi. An identical disorder found in a Maltese kindred is called Episkopi blindness.

The Norrie disease gene NDP is located on the short arm of the X chromosome (Xp11.4). The gene's protein product norrin controls vascular development in the retina by binding to the Wnt receptor Frizzled4. Mutations in the norrin gene have been found in patients with other heritable retinal disorders including X-linked exudative vitreoretinopathy and may predispose some premature infants to develop severe ROP.

RETINAL DYSPLASIA AND TRISOMY 13

In the broadest sense, retinal dysplasia refers to an aberrant proliferation of the developing retina as branching tubules that communicate with the subretinal space. In routine histologic sections, such tubules appear as dysplastic rosettes. Variable in appearance, dysplastic rosettes generally are larger than the neoplastic Flexner-Wintersteiner rosettes of retinoblastoma and usually are composed of multiple retinal layers (Fig. 2-1C).

Retinal dysplasia and PHPV/PFV are characteristic ocular findings in trisomy 13; in fact, trisomy 13 was called retinal dysplasia before the chromosomal defect was identified. The multitude of systemic and ocular findings found in patients with trisomy 13 may include bilateral leukocoria. Rarely, retinal dysplasia occurs unilaterally in the congenitally malformed eyes of otherwise healthy persons.

MEDULLOEPITHELIOMA AND OTHER PEDIATRIC INTRAOCULAR TUMORS

Embryonal medulloepithelioma is the second most common intraocular tumor of childhood (Fig. 12-20). This rare intraocular neoplasm is thought to arise from congenital rests or anlagen of the embryonic medullary epithelium, which normally lines the forebrain and optic vesicle. Embryonal medulloepithelioma is also called diktyoma. Fuchs applied that term to an early case of the tumor that had an interlacing, netlike pattern of neuroepithelial cells, but the diktyomatous pattern is actually uncommon.

Embryonal medulloepithelioma presents most often with poor vision or blindness (39%), pain (30%), an iris or ciliary body mass (18%), or leukocoria (18%). In some cases, the tumor is an unexpected, incidental finding in an enucleated blind, painful eye. Unusual presentations include cataract, multiple translucent neoplastic cysts in the posterior or anterior chamber, and lens "colobomas" caused by segmental loss of zonular fibers. In some cases, the tumor stroma forms a diaphanous cyclitic membrane behind the lens. Although the average age at presentation is about 4 years, treatment often is delayed; thus, the median age at surgery and histopathologic diagnosis is 5 years.

Histopathologically, medulloepithelioma is composed of tubules, cords, and bands of polarized neuroectodermal cells that resemble neoplastic medullary epithelium (Fig. 12-20D). Although Homer Wright and Flexner-Wintersteiner rosettes can be observed within retinoblastoma-like foci in malignant medulloepitheliomas, most rosettes in medulloepithelioma are larger and are composed of multiple layers of elongated neuroepithelial cells, which closely resemble the embryonic ciliary epithelium. The lumina of the rosettes and slitlike structures formed by the polarized epithelium correspond to the subretinal space. The outer side is lined by a basement membrane analogous to the retina's internal limiting membrane. Tumors often contain pools of loose, mesenchymal stroma rich in hyaluronic acid (Fig. 12-20E). This "neoplastic vitreous" typically adheres to the side of the neuroepithelium that is lined by basement membrane.

Medulloepitheliomas are classified as benign or malignant and teratoid or nonteratoid. Teratoid medulloepitheliomas contain heteroplastic elements such as hyaline cartilage, rhabdomyoblasts, or brainlike tissue (Fig. 12-20A,B, and F). Slightly more than one third (37.5%) of tumors are teratoid. Two thirds of the medulloepitheliomas in the Broughton and Zimmerman series of 56 cases from the Armed Forces Institute of Pathology were malignant. Histologic criteria for malignancy include (a) areas of poorly differentiated neuroblastic cells resembling those of retinoblastoma, (b) pleomorphism and mitotic activity, (c) a sarcomatous appearance of the stroma, and (d) aggressive behavior evidenced by intraocular invasion of the uvea, cornea, sclera, or optic nerve, with or without extrascleral extension. Malignant medulloepitheliomas are more likely to be teratoid. Although typically a ciliary body tumor, medulloepithelioma occasionally arises from the retina or optic nerve. Direct intracranial invasion is responsible for most deaths and occurs in cases with extraocular extension and orbital spread. Enucleation is the treatment of choice because there is a high incidence of recurrence after local resection. Rare cases in adults have been reported.

ASTROCYTIC LESIONS

Other rare intraocular neoplasms that present in childhood may be confused with retinoblastoma clinically. These include astrocytomas and astrocytic hamartomas of the retina, and a reactive, nonneoplastic proliferation of retinal glial cells. The latter, termed massive gliosis, has a variety of causes, usually is unsuspected clinically, and is diagnosed histopathologically. Massive gliosis usually is found incidentally during the histopathologic examination of a blind and painful or phthisical eye.

Retinal astrocytic hamartomas or astrocytomas usually are found in patients with tuberous sclerosis complex or von Recklinghausen neurofibromatosis. Astrocytic lesions occur in more than 50% of cases of tuberous sclerosis complex. Most are small, slow-growing astrocytic hamartomas. These vary from small, semitranslucent plaques of the nerve fiber layer to elevated, partially calcified nodules. The accumulation of calcospherites often imparts a mulberry-like appearance to the nodules. Larger, progressive retinal tumors that resemble subependymal giant cell astrocytomas of the brain histopathologically occur rarely. These often affect the posterior retina and are readily confused with retinoblastoma clinically. The term giant drusen of the optic nerve has been applied to astrocytomas located in the prelaminar part of the disc.

Glioneuroma is an extremely rare anterior segment tumor that arises from the anterior lip of the optic cup;

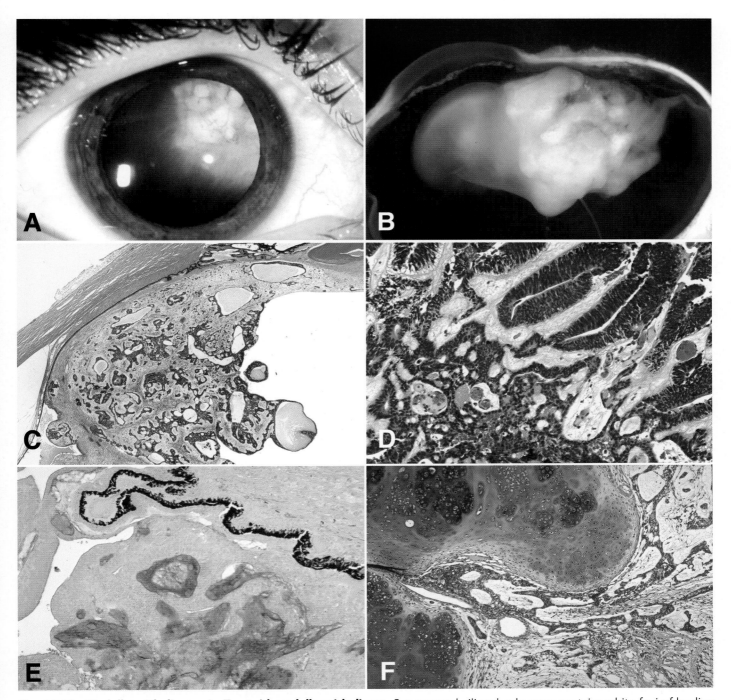

Fig. 12-20. Medulloepithelioma. A. Teratoid medulloepithelioma. Superonasal ciliary body mass contains white foci of hyaline cartilage. A delicate cyclitic membrane is present. (From Shields JA, et al. Fluorescein angiography and ultrasonography of malignant intraocular medulloepithelioma. *J Pediatr Ophthalmol Strabismus* 1996;33:193–196.) **B.** Macrophoto of ciliary body tumor shown in (**A**). **C.** Centered on the inner surface of the ciliary body, this medulloepithelioma is composed of cords of neuroepithelial cells resembling the primitive medullary epithelium. The epithelial elements are surrounded by loose stroma resembling embryonal mesenchyme. Several tumor cysts are present. A sheet of tumor extends anteriorly to envelop the lens at right. **D.** Nonteratoid medulloepithelioma contains thick bands of polarized neuroepithelium that resemble embryonic medullary epithelium. **E.** The tumor contains pools of vitreous-like material that stain vividly (*blue*) for AMP. Pretreatment with hyaluronidase abolishes the staining indicating that the mucin is hyaluronic acid, a major component of the vitreous humor. The medulloepithelioma rests on the inner surface of the ciliary epithelium above. **F.** Teratoid medulloepitheliomas contains heteroplastic elements including hyaline cartilage, striated muscle, rhabdomyoblasts, and brain. This tumor contains prominent lobules of neoplastic cartilage. Cords and ribbons of neuroepithelial cells are seen in the myxoid stroma at right. (**C.** H&E ×5, **D.** H&E ×50, **E.** Colloidal iron ×50, **F.** H&E ×25)

it actually may be a choristomatous malformation. Histopathologically, glioneuroma contains both glial and neuronal-like cells and has a brainlike appearance. In contrast to retinoblastoma that has invaded the anterior chamber, glioneuroma is a more distinct, cohesive mass.

A primitive neuroectodermal tumor of the retina with melanocytic differentiation has been reported. This "retinal melanoma" was misdiagnosed clinically as retinoblastoma.

OTHER SIMULATING LESIONS

Cataract, congenital corneal opacities, colobomas, and myelinated nerve fibers also are included in the differential diagnosis of retinoblastoma.

Although leukocoria caused by cataract should be obvious to the ophthalmologist, infants with retinoblastoma have undergone cataract surgery with fatal outcomes. Cataracts are rare in eyes with retinoblastoma. Most develop in eyes with extensive intraocular necrosis. Necrosis of the ciliary epithelium may also cause spontaneous dislocation of the lens in such eyes.

Corneal opacities or white pupillary reflexes caused by choroidal colobomas or myelinated nerve fibers understandably could confound the pediatrician or a general physician unskilled at ophthalmoscopy. Such lesions should be easily diagnosed by an ophthalmologist, however.

BIBLIOGRAPHY

Epidemiology

Abramson DH. Retinoblastoma incidence in the United States. *Arch Ophthalmol* 1990;108:1514.

al-Idrissi I, al-Kaff AS, Senft SH. Cumulative incidence of retinoblastoma in Riyadh, Saudi Arabia. *Ophthalmic Paediatr Genet* 1992;13:9–12.

BenEzra D, Chirambo MC. Incidence of retinoblastoma in Malawi. *J Pediatr Ophthalmol* 1976;13:340–343.

Berkow RL, Fleshman JK. Retinoblastoma in Navajo Indian children. *Am J Dis Child* 1983;137:137–138.

Devesa SS. The incidence of retinoblastoma. *Am J Ophthalmol* 1975;80:263–265.

Freedman J, Goldberg L. Incidence of retinoblastoma in the Bantu of South Africa. *Br J Ophthalmol* 1976;60:655–656.

Kock E, Naeser P. Retinoblastoma in Sweden 1958–1971. A clinical and histopathological study. *Acta Ophthalmol (Copenh)* 1979;57:344–350.

Mietz H, Hutton WL, Font RL. Unilateral retinoblastoma in an adult: report of a case and review of the literature. *Ophthalmology* 1997;104:43–47.

Orjuela MA, Titievsky L, Liu X, et al. Fruit and vegetable intake during pregnancy and risk for development of sporadic retinoblastoma. *Cancer Epidemiol Biomarkers Prev* 2005;14:1433–1440.

Shields JA, Michelson JB, Leonard BC, et al. Retinoblastoma in an eighteen-year-old male. *J Pediatr Ophthalmol* 1976;13:274–277.

Shields CL, Shields JA, Shah P. Retinoblastoma in older children. *Ophthalmology* 1991;98:395–399.

Tarkkanen A, Tuovinen E. Retinoblastoma in Finland 1912–1964. *Acta Ophthalmol (Copenh)* 1971;49:293–300.

Verhoeff FH. A retinoblastoma in a man aged forty-eight years. *Trans Am Ophthalmol Soc* 1929;27:176–188.

Clinical Features

Abramson DH, Frank CM, Susman M, et al. Presenting signs of retinoblastoma. *J Pediatr* 1998;132:505–508.

Abramson DH, Gombos DS. The topography of bilateral retinoblastoma lesions. *Retina* 1996;16:232–239.

Bhatnagar R, Vine AK. Diffuse infiltrating retinoblastoma. *Ophthalmology* 1991;98:1657–1661.

Byrnes GA, Shields CL, Shields JA, et al. Retinoblastoma presenting with spontaneous hyphema and dislocated lens. *J Pediatr Ophthalmol Strabismus* 1993;30:334–336.

Fontanesi J, Pratt C, Meyer D, et al. Asynchronous bilateral retinoblastoma: the St. Jude Children's Research Hospital experience. *Ophthalmic Genet* 1995;16:109–112.

Gallenga PE, Mancini A, Di Bastiano W, et al. Congenital retinoblastoma: appearance of calcifications during short-term follow-up. *Ophthalmologica* 1998;212(Suppl 1):61–64.

Morgan G. Diffuse infiltrating retinoblastoma. *Br J Ophthalmol* 1971;55:600–606.

Nicholson DH, Norton EW. Diffuse infiltrating retinoblastoma. *Trans Am Ophthalmol Soc* 1980;78:265–289.

Plotsky D, Quinn G, Eagle R Jr, et al. Congenital retinoblastoma: a case report. *J Pediatr Ophthalmol Strabismus* 1987;24:120–123.

Rubenfeld M, Abramson DH, Ellsworth RM, et al. Unilateral vs. bilateral retinoblastoma. Correlations between age at diagnosis and stage of ocular disease. *Ophthalmology* 1986;93:1016–1019.

Schofield PB. Diffuse infiltrating retinoblastoma. *Br J Ophthalmol* 1960;44:35–41.

Shields JA, Shields CL, Eagle RC, et al. Spontaneous pseudohypopyon secondary to diffuse infiltrating retinoblastoma. *Arch Ophthalmol* 1988;106:1301–1302.

Shields JA, Shields CL, Eagle RC, et al. Calcified intraocular abscess simulating retinoblastoma. *Am J Ophthalmol* 1992;114:227–229.

Shields JA, Shields CL, Eagle RC Jr, et al. Endogenous endophthalmitis simulating retinoblastoma. The 1993 David and Mary Seslen Endowment Lecture. *Retina* 1995;15:213–219.

Shields JA, Shields CL, Suvarnamani C, et al. Retinoblastoma manifesting as orbital cellulitis. *Am J Ophthalmol* 1991;112:442–449.

Spaulding G. Rubeosis iridis in retinoblastoma and pseudoglioma. *Trans Am Ophthalmol Soc* 1978;76:584–609.

Stafford WR, Yanoff M, Parnell BL. Retinoblastomas initially misdiagnosed as primary ocular inflammations. *Arch Ophthalmol* 1969;82:771–773.

Takahashi T, Tamura S, Inoue M, et al. Retinoblastoma in a 26-year-old adult. *Ophthalmology* 1983;90:179–183.

Verhoeff FH, Jackson E. Minutes of Proceedings, 62nd Annual Meeting. *Trans Am Ophthalmol Soc* 1926;24:38.

Walton DS, Grant WM. Retinoblastoma and iris neovascularization. *Am J Ophthalmol* 1968;65:598–599.

Yoshizumi MO, Thomas JV, Smith TR. Glaucoma-inducing mechanisms in eyes with retinoblastoma. *Arch Ophthalmol* 1978;96:105–110.

Zimmerman LE. Retinoblastoma, including a report of illustrative cases. *Med Ann Dist Columbia* 1969;38:366–374.

Histopathology and Ultrastructure

Albert DM, Craft J, Sang DN. Ultrastructure of retinoblastomas: transmission and scanning electron microscopy. In: Jakobiec FA, ed. *Ocular and Adnexal Tumors*. Birmingham, AL: Aesculapius, 1978:157–171.

Bunt AH, Tso MO. Feulgen-positive deposits in retinoblastoma. Incidence, composition, and ultrastructure. *Arch Ophthalmol* 1981;99:144–150.

Burnier MN, McLean IW, Zimmerman LE, et al. Retinoblastoma. The relationship of proliferating cells to blood vessels. *Invest Ophthalmol Vis Sci* 1990;31:2037–2040.

Datta BN. DNA coating of blood vessels in retinoblastomas. *Am J Clin Pathol* 1974;62:94–96.

Eagle RC Jr. High-risk features and tumor differentiation in retinoblastoma: a retrospective histopathologic study. *Arch Pathol Lab Med* 2009;133:1203–1209.

Kyritsis AP, Tsokos M, Triche TJ, et al. Retinoblastoma: a primitive tumor with multipotential characteristics. *Invest Ophthalmol Vis Sci* 1986;27:1760–1764.

Loeffler KU, McMenamin PG. An ultrastructural study of DNA precipitation in the anterior segment of eyes with retinoblastoma. *Ophthalmology* 1987;94:1160–1168.

Madhavan J, Ganesh A, Roy J, et al. The relationship between tumor cell differentiation and age at diagnosis in retinoblastoma. *J Pediatr Ophthalmol Strabismus* 2008;45:22–25.

Mullaney J. Retinoblastomas with DNA precipitation. *Arch Ophthalmol* 1969;82:454–456.

Nork TM, Millecchia LL, de Venecia GB, et al. Immunocytochemical features of retinoblastoma in an adult. *Arch Ophthalmol* 1996;114:1402–1406.

Nork TM, Schwartz TL, Doshi HM, et al. Retinoblastoma. Cell of origin. *Arch Ophthalmol* 1995;113:791–802.

Pe'er J, Neufeld M, Baras M, et al. Rubeosis iridis in retinoblastoma. Histologic findings and the possible role of vascular endothelial growth factor in its induction. *Ophthalmology* 1997;104:1251–1258.

Popoff NA, Ellsworth RM. The fine structure of retinoblastoma. In vivo and in vitro observations. *Lab Invest* 1971;25:389–402.

Spaulding G. Rubeosis iridis and retinoblastoma and pseudoglioma. *Trans Am Ophthalmol Soc* 1978;76:584–609.

Stowe GCd, Zakov ZN, Albert DM, et al. Vascular basophilia in ocular and orbital tumors. *Invest Ophthalmol Vis Sci* 1979;18:1068–1075.

Ts'o MO, Fine BS, Zimmerman LE. The Flexner-Wintersteiner rosettes in retinoblastoma. *Arch Pathol* 1969;88:664–671.

Ts'o MO, Fine BS, Zimmerman LE. The nature of retinoblastoma. II. Photoreceptor differentiation: an electron microscopic study. *Am J Ophthalmol* 1970;69:350–359.

Ts'o MO, Zimmerman LE, Fine BS, et al. A cause of radioresistance in retinoblastoma: photoreceptor differentiation. *Trans Am Acad Ophthalmol Otolaryngol* 1970;74:959–969.

Ts'o MO, Zimmerman LE, Fine BS, et al. A cause of radioresistance in retinoblastoma: photoreceptor differentiation. *Trans Am Acad Ophthalmol Otolaryngol* 1970;74:959–969.

Ts'o MO, Zimmerman LE, Fine BS. The nature of retinoblastoma. I. Photoreceptor differentiation: a clinical and histopathologic study. *Am J Ophthalmol* 1970;69:339–349.

Tsokos M, Kyritsis AP, Chader GJ, et al. Differentiation of human retinoblastoma in vitro into cell types with characteristics observed in embryonal or mature retina. *Am J Pathol* 1986;123:542–552.

Vrabec T, Arbizo V, Adamus G, et al. Rod cell-specific antigens in retinoblastoma. *Arch Ophthalmol* 1989;107:1061–1063.

Walton DS, Grant WM. Retinoblastoma and iris neovascularization. *Am J Ophthalmol* 1968;65: 598–599.

Yoshizumi MO, Thomas JV, Smith TR. Glaucoma-inducing mechanisms in eyes with retinoblastoma. *Arch Ophthalmol* 1978;96:105–110.

Yuge K, Nakajima M, Uemura Y, et al. Immunohistochemical features of the human retina and retinoblastoma. *Virchows Arch* 1995;426:571–575.

Risk Factors for Metastasis

Biswas J, Das D, Krishnakumar S, et al. Histopathologic analysis of 232 eyes with retinoblastoma conducted in an Indian tertiary-care ophthalmic center. *J Pediatr Ophthalmol Strabismus* 2003;40:265–267.

Carbajal UM. Metastasis in retinoblastoma. *Am J Ophthalmol* 1959;48:47–69.

Chantada GL, Dunkel IJ, de Dávila MT, et al. Retinoblastoma patients with high-risk ocular pathological features: who needs adjuvant therapy? *Br J Ophthalmol* 2004;88:1069–1073.

De Buen S. Retinoblastoma with spread by direct continuity to the contralateral optic nerve: report of a case. *Am J Ophthalmol* 1960;49:815–819.

Eagle RC Jr. High-risk features and tumor differentiation in retinoblastoma: a retrospective histopathologic study. *Arch Pathol Lab Med* 2009;133:1203–1209.

Khelfaoui F, Validire P, Auperin A, et. al. Histopathologic risk factors in retinoblastoma: a retrospective study of 172 patients treated in a single institution. *Cancer* 1996;77:1206–1213.

Kopelman JE, McLean IW, Rosenberg SH. Multivariate analysis of risk factors for metastasis in retinoblastoma treated by enucleation. *Ophthalmology* 1987;94:371–377.

Lennox EL, Draper GJ, Sanders BM. Retinoblastoma: a study of natural history and prognosis of 268 cases. *Br Med J* 1975;3:731–734.

MacKay CJ, Abramson DH, Ellsworth RM. Metastatic patterns of retinoblastoma. *Arch Ophthalmol* 1984;102:391–396.

Magramm I, Abramson DH, Ellsworth RM. Optic nerve involvement in retinoblastoma. *Ophthalmology* 1989;96:217–222.

McLean IW, Rosenberg SH, Messmer EP, et al. Prognostic factors in cases of retinoblastoma: analysis of 974 patients from Germany and the United States treated by enucleation. In: Bornfeld N, Gragoudas ES, Lommatzsch PK, eds. *Tumors of the Eye. Proceedings of the International Symposium on Tumors of the Eye.* Amsterdam, Netherlands: Kugler Publications, 1991:69–72.

Messmer EP, Heinrich T, Hopping W. Risk factors for metastases in patients with retinoblastoma. *Ophthalmology* 1991;98:136–141.

Redler LD, Elllsworth RM. Prognostic importance of choroidal invasion in retinoblastoma. *Arch Ophthalmol* 1973;90:294–296.

Rootman J, Ellsworth RM, Hofbauer J, et al. Orbital extension of retinoblastoma: a clinicopathological study. *Can J Ophthalmol* 1978;13:72–80.

Rootman J, Hofbauer J, Ellsworth RM, et al. Invasion of the optic nerve by retinoblastoma: a clinicopathological study. *Can J Ophthalmol* 1976;11:106–114.

Rubin CM, Robison LL, Cameron JD, et al. Intraocular retinoblastoma group V: an analysis of prognostic factors. *J Clin Oncol* 1985;3:680–685.

Shields CL, Shields JA, Baez KA, et al. Choroidal invasion of retinoblastoma: metastatic potential and clinical risk factors. *Br J Ophthalmol* 1993;77:544–548.

Shields CL, Shields JA, Baez K, et al. Optic nerve invasion of retinoblastoma. Metastatic potential and clinical risk factors. *Cancer* 1994;73:692–698.

Taktikos A. Investigation of retinoblastoma with special reference to histology and prognosis. *Br J Ophthalmol* 1966;50:225–234.

Uusitalo MS, Van Quill KR, Scott IU, et al. Evaluation of chemoprophylaxis in patients with unilateral retinoblastoma with high-risk features on histopathologic examination. *Arch Ophthalmol* 2001;119:41–48.

Wolter JR. Retinoblastoma extension into the choroid. Pathological study of the neoplastic process and thoughts about its prognostic significance. *Ophthalmic Paediatr Genet* 1987;8:151–157.

Retinoma/Retinocytoma and Spontaneous Regression

Aaby AA, Price RL, Zakov ZN. Spontaneously regressing retinoblastomas, retinoma, or retinoblastoma group 0. *Am J Ophthalmol* 1983;96:315–320.

Abramson DH. Retinoma, retinocytoma, and the retinoblastoma gene [editorial]. *Arch Ophthalmol* 1983;101:1517–1518.

Andersen SR, Jensen OA. Retinoblastoma with necrosis of central retinal artery and vein and partial spontaneous regression. *Acta Ophthalmol (Copenh)* 1974;52:183–193.

Balmer A, Munier F, Gailloud C. Retinoma. Case studies. *Ophthalmic Paediatr Genet* 1991;12:131–137.

Boniuk M, Girard LJ. Spontaneous regression of bilateral retinoblastoma. *Trans Am Acad Ophthalmol Otolaryngol* 1969;73:194–198.

Demirci H, Eagle RC Jr, Shields CL, et al. Histopathologic findings in eyes with retinoblastoma treated only with chemoreduction. *Arch Ophthalmol* 2003;121:1125–1131.

Dimaras H, Khetan V, Halliday W, et al. Loss of RB1 induces non-proliferative retinoma: increasing genomic instability correlates with progression to retinoblastoma. *Hum Mol Genet* 2008;15(17):1363–1372.

Dimaras H, Khetan V, Halliday W, et al. Retinoma underlying retinoblastoma revealed after tumor response to 1 cycle of chemotherapy. *Arch Ophthalmol* 2009;127:1066–1068.

Eagle RC Jr, Shields JA, Donoso L, et al. Malignant transformation of spontaneously regressed retinoblastoma,retinoma/retinocytoma variant. *Ophthalmology* 1989;96:1389–1395.

Eagle RC Jr. High-risk features and tumor differentiation in retinoblastoma: a retrospective histopathologic study. *Arch Pathol Lab Med* 2009;133:1203–1209.

Gallie BL, Campbell C, Devlin H, et al. Developmental basis of retinal-specific induction of cancer by RB mutation. *Cancer Res* 1999;59(7 Suppl):1731s–1735s.

Gallie BL, Ellsworth RM, Abramson DH, et al. Retinoma: spontaneous regression of retinoblastoma or benign manifestation of the mutation? *Br J Cancer* 1982;45:513–521.

Gallie BL, Phillips RA, Ellsworth RM, et al. Significance of retinoma and phthisis bulbi for retinoblastoma. *Ophthalmology* 1982;89:1393–1399.

Gangwar DN, Jain IS, Gupta A, et al. Bilateral spontaneous regression of retinoblastoma with dominant transmission. *Ann Ophthalmol* 1982;14:479–480.

Lindley J, Smith S. Histology and spontaneous regression of retinoblastoma. *Trans Ophthalmol Soc U K* 1974;94:953–967.

Margo C, Hidayat A, Kopelman J, et al. Retinocytoma. A benign variant of retinoblastoma. *Arch Ophthalmol* 1983;101:1519–1531.

Singh AD, Santos CM, Shields CL, et al. Observations on 17 patients with retinocytoma. *Arch Ophthalmol* 2000;118:199–205.

Ts'o MO, Fine BS, Zimmerman LE. The nature of retinoblastoma. II. Photoreceptor differentiation: an electron microscopic study. *Am J Ophthalmol* 1970;69:350–359.

Ts'o MO, Zimmerman LE, Fine BS, et al. A cause of radioresistance in retinoblastoma: photoreceptor differentiation. *Trans Am Acad Ophthalmol Otolaryngol* 1970;74:959–969.

Ts'o MO, Zimmerman LE, Fine BS. The nature of retinoblastoma. I. Photoreceptor differentiation: a clinical and histopathologic study. *Am J Ophthalmol* 1970;69:339–349.

The Retinoblastoma Gene and the Genetics of Retinoblastoma

Balaban-Malenbaum G, Gilbert F, Nichols WW, et al. A deleted chromosome no. 13 in human retinoblastoma cells: relevance to tumorigenesis. *Cancer Genet Cytogenet* 1981;3:243–250.

Balaban G, Gilbert F, Nichols W, et al. Abnormalities of chromosome #13 in retinoblastomas from individuals with normal constitutional karyotypes. *Cancer Genet Cytogenet* 1982;6:213–221.

Benedict WF, Murphree AL, Banerjee A, et al. Patient with 13 chromosome deletion: evidence that the retinoblastoma gene is a recessive cancer gene. *Science* 1983;219:973–975.

Bookstein R, Lee WH. Molecular genetics of the retinoblastoma suppressor gene. *Crit Rev Oncog* 1991;2:211–227.

Cavenee WK, Dryja TP, Phillips RA, et al. Expression of recessive alleles by chromosomal mechanisms in retinoblastoma. *Nature* 1983;305:779–784.

Cavenee WK, Hansen MF, Nordenskjold M, et al. Genetic origin of mutations predisposing to retinoblastoma. *Science* 1985;228:501–503.

Cavenee WK, Murphree AL, Shull MM, et al. Prediction of familial predisposition to retinoblastoma. *N Engl J Med* 1986;314:1201–1207.

Dryja TP, Bruns GA, Orkin SH, et al. Isolation of DNA fragments from chromosome 13. *Retina* 1983;3:121–125.

Dryja TP, Cavenee W, White R, et al. Homozygosity of chromosome 13 in retinoblastoma. *N Engl J Med* 1984;310:550–553.

Dryja TP, Rapaport J, McGee TL, et al. Molecular etiology of low-penetrance retinoblastoma in two pedigrees. *Am J Hum Genet* 1993;52:1122–1128.

Dryja TP, Rapaport JM, Weichselbaum R, et al. Chromosome 13 restriction fragment length polymorphisms. *Hum Genet* 1984;65:320–324.

Fitzgerald PH, Stewart J, Suckling RD. Retinoblastoma mutation rate in New Zealand and support for the two-hit model. *Hum Genet* 1983;64:128–130.

Gallie BL, Phillips RA. Retinoblastoma: a model of oncogenesis. *Ophthalmology* 1984;91:666–672.

Godbout R, Dryja TP, Squire J, et al. Somatic inactivation of genes on chromosome 13 is a common event in retinoblastoma. *Nature* 1983;304:451–453.

Gordon H. Family studies in retinoblastoma. *Birth Defects Orig Artic Ser* 1974;10:185–190.

Harbour JW. Overview of RB gene mutations in patients with retinoblastoma. Implications for clinical genetic screening. *Ophthalmology* 1998;105:1442–1447.

Knudson AG Jr, Hethcote HW, Brown BW. Mutation and childhood cancer: a probabilistic model for the incidence of retinoblastoma. *Proc Natl Acad Sci U S A* 1975;72:5116–5120.

Knudson AG Jr. Mutation and cancer: statistical study of retinoblastoma. *Proc Natl Acad Sci U S A* 1971;68:820–823.

Knudson AG Jr. Retinoblastoma: a prototypic hereditary neoplasm. *Semin Oncol* 1978;5:57–60.

Kratzke RA, Otterson GA, Hogg A, et al. Partial inactivation of the RB product in a family with incomplete penetrance of familial retinoblastoma and benign retinal tumors. *Oncogene* 1994;9:1321–1326.

McGee TL, Yandell DW, Dryja TP. Structure and partial genomic sequence of the human retinoblastoma susceptibility gene. *Gene* 1989;80:119–128.

Murphree AL, Benedict WF. Retinoblastoma: clues to human oncogenesis. *Science* 1984;223:1028–1033.

Murphree AL. Molecular genetics of retinoblastoma. *Ophthalmol Clin North Am* 1995;8:155–166.

Nielsen M, Goldschmidt E. Retinoblastoma among offspring of adult survivors in Denmark. *Acta Ophthalmol (Copenh)* 1968;46:736–741.

Otterson GA, Chen W, Coxon AB, et al. Incomplete penetrance of familial retinoblastoma linked to germ-line mutations that result in partial loss of RB function. *Proc Natl Acad Sci U S A* 1997;94:12036–12040.

Shields CL, Shields JA, Donoso LA. Clinical genetics of retinoblastoma. *Int Ophthalmol Clin* 1993;33:67–76.

Weichselbaum RR, Zakov ZN, Albert DM, et al. New findings in the chromosome 13 long-arm deletion syndrome and retinoblastoma. *Ophthalmology* 1979;86:1191–1201.

Weinberg RA. The retinoblastoma gene and gene product. *Cancer Surv* 1992;12:43–57.

Wiggs J, Nordenskjold M, Yandell D, et al. Prediction of the risk of hereditary retinoblastoma, using DNA polymorphisms within the retinoblastoma gene. *N Engl J Med* 1988;318:151–157.

"Trilateral Retinoblastoma" and Other Second Tumors

Abramson DH, Ellsworth RM, Zimmerman LE. Nonocular cancer in retinoblastoma survivors. *Trans Sect Ophthalmol Am Acad Ophthalmol Otolaryngol* 1976;81:454–457.

Abramson DH. Second nonocular cancers in retinoblastoma: a unified hypothesis. The Franceschetti Lecture. *Ophthalmic Genet* 1999;20:193–204.

Bader JL, Meadows AT, Zimmerman LE, et al. Bilateral retinoblastoma with ectopic intracranial retinoblastoma: trilateral retinoblastoma. *Cancer Genet Cytogenet* 1982;5:203–213.

Dunkel IJ, Gerald WL, Rosenfield NS, et al. Outcome of patients with a history of bilateral retinoblastoma treated for a second malignancy: the Memorial Sloan-Kettering experience. *Med Pediatr Oncol* 1998;30:59–62.

Holladay DA, Holladay A, Montebello JF, et al. Clinical presentation, treatment, and outcome of trilateral retinoblastoma. *Cancer* 1991;67:710–715.

Jakobiec FA, Tso MO, Zimmerman LE, et al. Retinoblastoma and intracranial malignancy. *Cancer* 1977;39:2048–2058.

Li FP, Abramson DH, Tarone RE, et al. Hereditary retinoblastoma, lipoma, and second primary cancers. *J Natl Cancer Inst* 1997;89:83–84.

Meadows AT, Leahey AM. More about second cancers after retinoblastoma. *J Natl Cancer Inst* 2008;100:1743–1745.

Mohney BG, Robertson DM, Schomberg PJ, et al. Second nonocular tumors in survivors of heritable retinoblastoma and prior radiation therapy. *Am J Ophthalmol* 1998;126:269–277.

Moll AC, Imhof SM, Bouter LM, et al. Second primary tumors in patients with retinoblastoma. A review of the literature. *Ophthalmic Genet* 1997;18:27–34.

Pesin SR, Shields JA. Seven cases of trilateral retinoblastoma. *Am J Ophthalmol* 1989;107:121–126.

Roarty JD, McLean IW, Zimmerman LE. Incidence of second neoplasms in patients with bilateral retinoblastoma. *Ophthalmology* 1988;95:1583–1587.

Shields JA, Pesin SR, Shields CL. Trilateral retinoblastoma. *J Clin Neuroophthalmol* 1989;9:222–223.

Wong FL, Boice JD Jr, Abramson DH, et al. Cancer incidence after retinoblastoma. radiation dose and sarcoma risk. *JAMA* 1997;278:1262–1267.

Therapy

Baumal CR, Shields CL, Shields JA, et al. Surgical repair of rhegmatogenous retinal detachment after treatment for retinoblastoma. *Ophthalmology* 1998;105:2134–2139.

Demirci H, Eagle RC Jr, Shields CL, et al. Histopathologic findings in eyes with retinoblastoma treated only with chemoreduction. *Arch Ophthalmol* 2003;121:1125–1131.

Demirci H, Shields CL, Meadows AT, et al. Long-term visual outcome following chemoreduction for retinoblastoma. *Arch Ophthalmol* 2005;123:1525–1530.

Doz F, Khelfaoui F, Mosseri V, et al. The role of chemotherapy in orbital involvement of retinoblastoma. The experience of a single institution with 33 patients. *Cancer* 1994;74:722–732.

Doz F, Neuenschwander S, Plantaz D, et al. Etoposide and carboplatin in extraocular retinoblastoma: a study by the Societe Francaise d'Oncologie Pediatrique. *J Clin Oncol* 1995;13: 902–909.

Freire J, Miyamoto C, Brady LW, et al. Retinoblastoma after chemoreduction and irradiation: preliminary results. *Front Radiat Ther Oncol* 1997;30:88–92.

Gunduz K, Shields CL, Shields JA, et al. The outcome of chemoreduction treatment in patients with Reese-Ellsworth group V retinoblastoma. *Arch Ophthalmol* 1998;116:1613–1617.

Hernandez JC, Brady LW, Shields JA, et al. External beam radiation for retinoblastoma: results, patterns of failure, and a proposal for treatment guidelines. *Int J Radiat Oncol Biol Phys* 1996;35: 125–132.

Howarth C, Meyer D, Hustu HO, et al. Stage-related combined modality treatment of retinoblastoma. Results of a prospective study. *Cancer* 1980;45:851–858.

Pratt CB, Fontanesi J, Chenaille P, et al. Chemotherapy for extraocular retinoblastoma. *Pediatr Hematol Oncol* 1994;11:301–309.

Shields CL, De Potter P, Himelstein BP, et al. Chemoreduction in the initial management of intraocular retinoblastoma. *Arch Ophthalmol* 1996;114:1330–1338.

Shields CL, Mashayekhi A, Au AK, et al. The International Classification of Retinoblastoma predicts chemoreduction success. *Ophthalmology* 2006;113:2276–2280.

Shields CL, Mashayekhi A, Cater J, et al. Chemoreduction for retinoblastoma. Analysis of tumor control and risks for recurrence in 457 tumors. *Am J Ophthalmol* 2004;138:329–337.

Shields CL, Mashayekhi A, Sun H, et al. Iodine 125 plaque radiotherapy as salvage treatment for retinoblastoma recurrence after chemoreduction in 84 tumors. *Ophthalmology* 2006;113: 2087–2092.

Shields CL, Meadows AT, Leahey AM, et al. Continuing challenges in the management of retinoblastoma with chemotherapy. *Retina* 2004;24:849–862.

Shields CL, Palamar M, Sharma P, et al. Retinoblastoma regression patterns following chemoreduction and adjuvant therapy in 557 tumors. *Arch Ophthalmol* 2009;127:282–290.

Shields CL, Ramasubramanian A, Thangappan A, et al. Chemoreduction for group E retinoblastoma: comparison of chemoreduction alone versus chemoreduction plus low-dose external radiotherapy in 76 eyes. *Ophthalmology* 2009;116: 544–551 e541.

Shields CL, Shields JA, De Potter P, et al. Plaque radiotherapy in the management of retinoblastoma. Use as a primary and secondary treatment [see comments]. *Ophthalmology* 1993;100: 216–224.

Shields CL, Shields JA, DePotter P, et al. The effect of chemoreduction on retinoblastoma-induced retinal detachment. *J Pediatr Ophthalmol Strabismus* 1997;34:165–169.

Shields CL, Shields JA, Needle M, et al. Combined chemoreduction and adjuvant treatment for intraocular retinoblastoma [see comments]. *Ophthalmology* 1997;104:2101–2111.

Shields CL, Shields JA. Basic understanding of current classification and management of retinoblastoma. *Curr Opin Ophthalmol* 2006;17:228–234.

Shields JA, Shields CL, De Potter P, et al. Bilateral macular retinoblastoma managed by chemoreduction and chemothermotherapy. *Arch Ophthalmol* 1996;114:1426–1427.

Shields JA, Shields CL, De Potter P. Cryotherapy for retinoblastoma. *Int Ophthalmol Clin* 1993;33:101–105.

Shields JA, Shields CL, De Potter P. Enucleation technique for children with retinoblastoma. *J Pediatr Ophthalmol Strabismus* 1992;29:213–215.

Shields JA, Shields CL, De Potter P. Photocoagulation of retinoblastoma. *Int Ophthalmol Clin* 1993;33:95–99.

Shields JA, Shields CL, Meadows AT. Chemoreduction in the management of retinoblastoma. *Am J Ophthalmol* 2005;140:505–506.

Shields JA, Shields CL. Current management of retinoblastoma. *Mayo Clin Proc* 1994;69:50–56.

Tsokos M, Kyritsis AP, Chader GJ, et al. Differentiation of human retinoblastoma in vitro into cell types with characteristics observed in embryonal or mature retina. *Am J Pathol* 1986;123:542–552.

Vrabec T, Arbizo V, Adamus G, et al. Rod cell-specific antigens in retinoblastoma. *Arch Ophthalmol* 1989;107:1061–1063.

The Differential Diagnosis of Retinoblastoma

Francois J. Differential diagnosis of leukokoria in children. *Ann Ophthalmol* 1978;10:1375–1378, 1381–1372.

Howard GM, Ellsworth RM. Differential diagnosis of retinoblastoma. A statistical survey of 500 children. I. Relative frequency of the lesions which simulate retinoblastoma. *Am J Ophthalmol* 1965;60:610–618.

Margo CE, Zimmerman LE. Retinoblastoma: the accuracy of clinical diagnosis in children treated by enucleation. *J Pediatr Ophthalmol Strabismus* 1983;20:227–229.

Robertson DM, Campbell RJ. Analysis of misdiagnosed retinoblastoma in a series of 726 enucleated eyes. *Mod Probl Ophthalmol* 1977;18:156–159.

Shields JA, Parsons HM, Shields CL, et al. Lesions simulating retinoblastoma. *J Pediatr Ophthalmol Strabismus* 1991;28:338–340.

Shields JA, Shields CL, Parsons HM. Differential diagnosis of retinoblastoma. *Retina* 1991;11:232–243.

Smirniotopoulos JG, Bargallo N, Mafee MF. Differential diagnosis of leukokoria: radiologic-pathologic correlation. *Radiographics* 1994;14:1059–1079; quiz 1081–1052.

Toxocariasis

Belmont JB, Irvine A, Benson W, et al. Vitrectomy in ocular toxocariasis. *Arch Ophthalmol* 1982;100:1912–1915.

Benitez del Castillo JM, Herreros G, Guillen JL, et al. Bilateral ocular toxocariasis demonstrated by aqueous humor enzyme- linked immunosorbent assay. *Am J Ophthalmol* 1995;119:514–516.

Dernouchamps JP, Verougstraete C, Demolder E. Ocular toxocariasis: a presumed case of peripheral granuloma. *Int Ophthalmol* 1990;14:383–388.

Ellis GS Jr, Pakalnis VA, Worley G, et al. Toxocara canis infestation. Clinical and epidemiological associations with seropositivity in kindergarten children. *Ophthalmology* 1986;93:1032–1037.

Kayes SG. Human toxocariasis and the visceral larva migrans syndrome: correlative immunopathology. *Chem Immunol* 1997;66:99–124.

Luxenberg MN. An experimental approach to the study of intraocular Toxocara canis. *Trans Am Ophthalmol Soc* 1979;77:542–602.

Maguire AM, Green WR, Michels RG, et al. Recovery of intraocular Toxocara canis by pars plana vitrectomy. *Ophthalmology* 1990;97:675–680.

Rockey JH, Donnelly JJ, Stromberg BE, et al. Immunopathology of *Toxocara canis* and *Ascaris suum* infections of the eye: the role of the eosinophil. *Invest Ophthalmol Vis Sci* 1979;18:1172–1184.

Schantz PM, Weis PE, Pollard ZF, et al. Risk factors for toxocaral ocular larva migrans: a case-control study. *Am J Public Health* 1980;70:1269–1272.

Searl SS, Moazed K, Albert DM, et al. Ocular toxocariasis presenting as leukocoria in a patient with low ELISA titer to *Toxocara canis*. *Ophthalmology* 1981;88:1302–1306.

Shields JA, Shields CL, Eagle RC Jr, et al. Endogenous endophthalmitis simulating retinoblastoma. The 1993 David and Mary Seslen Endowment Lecture. *Retina* 1995;15:213–219.

Shields JA. Ocular toxocariasis. A review. *Surv Ophthalmol* 1984;28:361–381.

Watzke RC. Ocular *Toxocara canis* infection: clinical and experimental features. *Trans New Orleans Acad Ophthalmol* 1983;31:263–271.

Wilder HC. Nematode endophthalmitis. *Trans Am Acad Ophthalmol Otolaryngol* 1950;55:99–109.

Zinkham WH. Visceral larva migrans. A review and reassessment indicating two forms of clinical expression: visceral and ocular. *Am J Dis Child* 1978;132:627–633.

PHPV/PFV

Boeve MH, van der Linde-Sipman JS, Stades FC, et al. Early morphogenesis of persistent hyperplastic tunica vasculosa lentis and primary vitreous. A transmission electron microscopic study. *Invest Ophthalmol Vis Sci* 1990;31:1886–1894.

Cockburn DM, Dwyer PS. Posterior persistent hyperplastic primary vitreous. *Am J Optom Physiol Opt* 1988;65:316–317.

Dawson DG, Gleiser J, Movaghar M, et al. Persistent fetal vasculature. *Arch Ophthalmol* 2003;121:1340–1341.

Dhingra S, Shears DJ, Blake V, et al. Advanced bilateral persistent fetal vasculature associated with a novel mutation in the Norrie gene. *Br J Ophthalmol* 2006;90:1324–1325.

Doro S, Werblin TP, Haas B, et al. Fetal adenoma of the pigmented ciliary epithelium associated with persistent hyperplastic primary vitreous. *Ophthalmology* 1986;93:1343–1350.

Federman JL, Shields JA, Altman B, et al. The surgical and nonsurgical management of persistent hyperplastic primary vitreous. *Ophthalmology* 1982;89:20–24.

Font RL, Yanoff M, Zimmerman LE. Intraocular adipose tissue and persistent hyperplastic primary vitreous. *Arch Ophthalmol* 1969;82:43–50.

Ganesh A, Mitra S, Koul RL, et al. The full spectrum of persistent fetal vasculature in Aicardi syndrome: an integrated interpretation of ocular malformation. *Br J Ophthalmol* 2000;84:227–228.

Goldberg MF. Persistent fetal vasculature (PFV): an integrated interpretation of signs and symptoms associated with persistent hyperplastic primary vitreous (PHPV). LIV Edward Jackson Memorial Lecture. *Am J Ophthalmol* 1997;124:587–626.

Gulati N, Eagle RC Jr, Tasman W. Unoperated eyes with persistent fetal vasculature. *Trans Am Ophthalmol Soc* 2003;101:59–64, discussion 64–55.

Jampol LM. Persistent fetal vasculature. *Arch Ophthalmol* 2007;125:432.

Jensen OA. Persistent hyperplastic primary vitreous. Cases in Denmark 1942–1966. A mainly histopathological study. *Acta Ophthalmol (Copenh)* 1968;46:418–429.

Meisels H, Goldberg M: Vascular anastomoses between the iris and persistent primary vitreous. *Am J Ophthalmol* 1979;88:179–185.

Reese AB. Persistent hyperplastic primary vitreous. *Am J Ophthalmol* 1955;40:317–331.

Robitaille JM, Wallace K, Zheng B, et al. Phenotypic overlap of familial exudative vitreoretinopathy (FEVR) with persistent fetal vasculature (PFV) caused by FZD4 mutations in two distinct pedigrees. *Ophthalmic Genet* 2009;30:23–30.

Spaulding AG, Naumann G. Persistent hyperplastic primary vitreous in an adult. A brief review of the literature and a histopathologic study. *Arch Ophthalmol* 1967;77:666–671.

Spitznas M, Koch F, Pohl S. Ultrastructural pathology of anterior persistent hyperplastic primary vitreous. *Graefes Arch Clin Exp Ophthalmol* 1990;228:487–496.

Witschel H. Ultrastructure of persistent hyperplastic primary vitreous (PHPV). *Graefes Arch Clin Exp Ophthalmol* 1991;229:297.

Coats Disease

Egbert PR, Chan CC, Winter FC. Flat preparations of the retinal vessels in Coats' disease. *J Pediatr Ophthalmol* 1976;13:336–339.

Frayer WC. Coats' disease: a clinical and pathologic study. *AMA Arch Ophthalmol* 1955;54:240–244.

Goel SD, Augsburger JJ. Hemorrhagic retinal macrocysts in advanced Coats disease. *Retina* 1991;11:437–440.

Green WR. Bilateral Coats' disease. Massive gliosis of the retina. *Arch Ophthalmol* 1967;77:378–383.

Jaffe MS, Shields JA, Canny CL, et al. Retinoblastoma simulating Coats' disease: a clinicopathologic report. *Ann Ophthalmol* 1977;9:863–868.

Kremer I, Nissenkorn I, Ben-Sira I. Cytologic and biochemical examination of the subretinal fluid in diagnosis of Coats' disease. *Acta Ophthalmol (Copenh)* 1989;67:342–346.

Lai WW, Edward DP, Weiss RA, et al. Magnetic resonance imaging findings in a case of advanced Coats' disease. *Ophthalmic Surg Lasers* 1996;27:234–238.

Patel HK, Augsburger JJ, Eagle RC Jr. Unusual presentation of advanced Coats' disease. *J Pediatr Ophthalmol Strabismus* 1995;32:120–122.

Pe'er J. Calcifications in Coats' disease. *Am J Ophthalmol* 1988;106:742–743.

Reese AB. Telangiectasis of the retina and Coats' disease. *Am J Ophthalmol* 1956;42:1–8.

Ridley ME, Shields JA, Brown GC, et al. Coats' disease. Evaluation of management. *Ophthalmology* 1982;89:1381–1387.

Shields JA, Eagle RC Jr, Fammartino J, et al. Coats' disease as a cause of anterior chamber cholesterolosis. *Arch Ophthalmol* 1995;113:975–977.

Shields JA, Shields CL, Honavar SG, et al. Classification and management of Coats disease: the 2000 Proctor Lecture. *Am J Ophthalmol* 2001;131:572–583.

Shields JA, Shields CL, Honavar SG, et al. Clinical variations and complications of Coats disease in 150 cases: the 2000 Sanford Gifford Memorial Lecture. *Am J Ophthalmol* 2001;131:561–571.

Shields JA, Shields CL. Differentiation of coats' disease and retinoblastoma. *J Pediatr Ophthalmol Strabismus* 2001;38:262–266.

Shields JA, Shields CL. Review: coats disease: the 2001 LuEsther T. Mertz lecture. *Retina* 2002;22:80–91.

Shields CL, Zahler J, Falk N, et al. Neovascular glaucoma from advanced Coats disease as the initial manifestation of facioscapulohumeral dystrophy in a 2-year-old child. *Arch Ophthalmol* 2007;125:840–842.

Silodor SW, Augsburger JJ, Shields JA, et al. Natural history and management of advanced Coats' disease. *Ophthalmic Surg* 1988;19:89–93.

Tasman W. Coats' disease. *Am Fam Physician* 1977;15:107.

Retinopathy of Prematurity

An international classification of retinopathy of prematurity. II. The classification of retinal detachment. The International Committee for the Classification of the Late Stages of Retinopathy of Prematurity. *Arch Ophthalmol* 1987;105:906–912.

An international classification of retinopathy of prematurity. The Committee for the Classification of Retinopathy of Prematurity. *Arch Ophthalmol* 1984;102:1130–1134.

Ashton N, Cook C. Direct observation of the effect of oxygen on developing vessels: preliminary report. *Br J Ophthalmol* 1954;38:433–440.

Ashton N, Ward B, Serpell G. Effect of oxygen on developing retinal vessels with particular reference to the problem of retrolental fibroplasia. *Br J Ophthalmol* 1954;38:397–432.

Ashton N. Donders lecture, 1967. Some aspects of the comparative pathology of oxygen toxicity in the retina. *Br J Ophthalmol* 1968;52:505–531.

Ashton N. Oxygen and the growth and development of retinal vessels. In vivo and in vitro studies. The XX Francis I. Proctor Lecture. *Am J Ophthalmol* 1966;62:412–435.

Ashton N. The pathogenesis of retrolental fibroplasia. *Ophthalmology* 1979;86:1695–1699.

Ashton N. The story of blindness in premature babies. *Trans Med Soc Lond* 1987;104:114–125.

de Juan E Jr, Machemer R, Flynn JT, et al. Surgical pathoanatomy in stage 5 retinopathy of prematurity. *Birth Defects Orig Artic Ser* 1988;24:281–286.

Faris B, Tolentino FI, Freeman HM, et al. Retrolental fibroplasia in the cicatricial stage. Fundus and vitreous findings. *Arch Ophthalmol* 1971;85:661–668.

Foos RY. Acute retrolental fibroplasia. *Graefes Arch Clin Exp Ophthalmol* 1975;195:87–100.

Foos RY. Chronic retinopathy of prematurity. *Ophthalmology* 1985;92:563–574.

Garner A, Ashton N. Vaso-obliteration and retrolental fibroplasia. *Proc R Soc Med* 1971;64:774–777.

Good WV, Hardy RJ, Dobson V, et al. The incidence and course of retinopathy of prematurity: findings from the early treatment for retinopathy of prematurity study. *Pediatrics* 2005;116:15–23.

Hittner HM, Kretzer FL. Vitamin E and retrolental fibroplasia: ultrastructural mechanism of clinical efficacy. *Ciba Found Symp* 1983;101:165–185.

Hittner HM, Rhodes LM, McPherson AR. Anterior segment abnormalities in cicatricial retinopathy of prematurity. *Ophthalmology* 1979;86:803–816.

Karlsberg RC, Green WR, Patz A. Congenital retrolental fibroplasia. *Arch Ophthalmol* 1973;89:122–123.

Kinsey VE, Arnold HJ, Kalina RE, et al. PaO2 levels and retrolental fibroplasia: a report of the cooperative study. *Pediatrics* 1977;60:655–668.

Kretzer FL, McPherson AR, Hittner HM. An interpretation of retinopathy of prematurity in terms of spindle cells: relationship to vitamin E prophylaxis and cryotherapy. *Graefes Arch Clin Exp Ophthalmol* 1986;224:205–214.

Naiman J, Green WR, Patz A. Retrolental fibroplasia in hypoxic newborn. *Am J Ophthalmol* 1979;88:55–58.

Palmer EA. Implications of the natural course of retinopathy of prematurity. *Pediatrics* 2003;111:885–886.

Patz A. Current status of role of oxygen in retrolental fibroplasia. *Invest Ophthalmol* 1976;15:337–339.

Patz A. The role of oxygen in retrolental fibroplasia. *Sinai Hosp J (Balt)* 1954;3:6–20.

Patz A, Eastham A, Higginbotham DH, et al. Oxygen studies in retrolental fibroplasia. II. The production of the microscopic changes of retrolental fibroplasia in experimental animals. *Am J Ophthalmol* 1953;36:1511–1522.

Reedy EA. The discovery of retrolental fibroplasia and the role of oxygen: a historical review, 1942–1956. *Neonatal Netw* 2004;23:31–38.

Shastry BS, Pendergast SD, Hartzer MK, et al. Identification of missense mutations in the Norrie disease gene associated with advanced retinopathy of prematurity. *Arch Ophthalmol* 1997;115:651–655.

Tasman W. Vitreoretinal changes in cicatricial retrolental fibroplasia. *Trans Am Ophthalmol Soc* 1970;68:548–594.

Tasman W. The natural history of active retinopathy of prematurity. *Ophthalmology* 1984;91:1499–1503.

Tasman W, Brown GC, Naidoff M, et al. Cryotherapy for active retinopathy of prematurity. *Graefes Arch Clin Exp Ophthalmol* 1987;225:3–4.

Tasman W, Patz A, McNamara JA, et al. Retinopathy of prematurity: the life of a lifetime disease. *Am J Ophthalmol* 2006;141:167–174.

The International Classification of Retinopathy of Prematurity revisited. *Arch Ophthalmol* 2005;123:991–999.

Incontinentia Pigmenti

Bell WR, Green WR, Goldberg MF. Histopathologic and trypsin digestion studies of the retina in incontinentia pigmenti. *Ophthalmology* 2008;115:893–897.

Berlin AL, Paller AS, Chan LS. Incontinentia pigmenti: a review and update on the molecular basis of pathophysiology. *J Am Acad Dermatol* 2002;47:169–187, quiz 188–190.

Brown CA. Incontinentia pigmenti: the development of pseudoglioma. *Br J Ophthalmol* 1988;72:452–455.

Fowell SM, Greenwald MJ, Prendiville JS, et al. Ocular findings of incontinentia pigmenti in a male infant with Klinefelter syndrome. *J Pediatr Ophthalmol Strabismus* 1992;29:180–184.

Goldberg MF. The blinding mechanisms of incontinentia pigmenti. *Trans Am Ophthalmol Soc* 1994;92:167–176, discussion 176–169.

Goldberg MF. Macular vasculopathy and its evolution in incontinentia pigmenti. *Trans Am Ophthalmol Soc* 1998;96:55–65, discussion 65–72.

Goldberg MF. The skin is not the predominant problem in incontinentia pigmenti. *Arch Dermatol* 2004;140:748–750.

Goldberg MF, Custis PH. Retinal and other manifestations of incontinentia pigmenti (Bloch-Sulzberger syndrome). *Ophthalmology* 1993;100:1645–1654.

Heathcote JG, Schoales BA, Willis NR. Incontinentia pigmenti (Bloch-Sulzberger syndrome): a case report and review of the ocular pathological features. *Can J Ophthalmol* 1991;26:229–237.

Mensheha-Manhart O, Rodrigues MM, Shields JA, et al. Retinal pigment epithelium in incontinentia pigmenti. *Am J Ophthalmol* 1975;79:571–577.

Nelson DL. NEMO, NFkappaB signaling and incontinentia pigmenti. *Curr Opin Genet Dev* 2006;16:282–288.

Pacheco TR, Levy M, Collyer JC, et al. Incontinentia pigmenti in male patients. *J Am Acad Dermatol* 2006;55:251–255.

Shields CL, Eagle RC Jr, Shah RM, et al. Multifocal hypopigmented retinal pigment epithelial lesions in incontinentia pigmenti. *Retina* 2006;26:328–333.

Norrie Disease

Apple DJ, Fishman GA, Goldberg MF. Ocular histopathology of Norrie's disease. *Am J Ophthalmol* 1974;78:196–203.

Caballero M, Veske A, Rodriguez JJ, et al. Two novel mutations in the Norrie disease gene associated with the classical ocular phenotype. *Ophthalmic Genet* 1996;17:187–191.

Chen ZY, Battinelli EM, Fielder A, et al. A mutation in the Norrie disease gene (NDP) associated with X-linked familial exudative vitreoretinopathy. *Nat Genet* 1993;5:180–183.

Chynn EW, Walton DS, Hahn LB, et al. Norrie disease. Diagnosis of a simplex case by DNA analysis. *Arch Ophthalmol* 1996;114:1136–1138.

Dickinson JL, Sale MM, Passmore A, et al. Mutations in the NDP gene: contribution to Norrie disease, familial exudative vitreoretinopathy and retinopathy of prematurity. *Clin Experiment Ophthalmol* 2006;34:682–688.

Drenser KA, Fecko A, Dailey W, et al. A characteristic phenotypic retinal appearance in Norrie disease. *Retina* 2007;27:243–246.

Enyedi LB, de Juan E Jr, Gaitan A. Ultrastructural study of Norrie's disease. *Am J Ophthalmol* 1991;111:439–445.

Holmes LB. Norrie's disease: an X-linked syndrome of retinal malformation, mental retardation, and deafness. *J Pediatr* 1971;79:89–92.

Hutcheson KA, Paluru PC, Bernstein SL, et al. Norrie disease gene sequence variants in an ethnically diverse population with retinopathy of prematurity. *Mol Vis* 2005;11:501–508.

Johnson K, Mintz-Hittner HA, Conley YP, et al. X-linked exudative vitreoretinopathy caused by an arginine to leucine substitution (R121L) in the Norrie disease protein. *Clin Genet* 1996;50:113–115.

Kellner U, Fuchs S, Bornfeld N, et al. Ocular phenotypes associated with two mutations (R121W, C126X) in the Norrie disease gene. *Ophthalmic Genet* 1996;17:67–74.

Luhmann UF, Lin J, Acar N, et al. Role of the Norrie disease pseudoglioma gene in sprouting angiogenesis during development of the retinal vasculature. *Invest Ophthalmol Vis Sci* 2005;46:3372–3382.

Mintz-Hittner HA, Ferrell RE, Sims KB, et al. Peripheral retinopathy in offspring of carriers of Norrie disease gene mutations. Possible transplacental effect of abnormal Norrin. *Ophthalmology* 1996;103:2128–2134.

Parsons MA, Curtis D, Blank CE, et al. The ocular pathology of Norrie disease in a fetus of 11 weeks' gestational age. *Graefes Arch Clin Exp Ophthalmol* 1992;230:248–251.

Perez-Vilar J, Hill RL. Norrie disease protein (norrin) forms disulfide-linked oligomers associated with the extracellular matrix. *J Biol Chem* 1997;272:33410–33415.

Riveiro-Alvarez R, Cantalapiedra D, Vallespin E, et al. Gene symbol: NDP. Disease: Norrie disease. *Hum Genet* 2008;124:308.

Schroeder B, Hesse L, Bruck W, et al. Histopathological and immunohistochemical findings associated with a null mutation in the Norrie disease gene. *Ophthalmic Genet* 1997;18:71–77.

Shastry BS, Pendergast SD, Hartzer MK, et al. Identification of missense mutations in the Norrie disease gene associated with advanced retinopathy of prematurity. *Arch Ophthalmol* 1997;115:651–655.

Smallwood PM, Williams J, Xu Q, et al. Mutational analysis of Norrin-Frizzled4 recognition. *J Biol Chem* 2007;282:4057–4068.

Townes PL, Roca PD. Norrie's disease (hereditary oculo-acoustic-cerebral degeneration). Report of a United States family. *Am J Ophthalmol* 1973;76:797–803.

Warburg M. Norrie's disease. *Trans Ophthalmol Soc U K* 1965;85:391–408.

Warburg M. Norrie's disease–differential diagnosis and treatment. *Acta Ophthalmol (Copenh)* 1975;53:217–236.

Warden SM, Andreoli CM, Mukai S. The Wnt signaling pathway in familial exudative vitreoretinopathy and Norrie disease. *Semin Ophthalmol* 2007;22:211–217.

Wolff G, Mayerova A, Wienker TF, et al. Clinical reinvestigation and linkage analysis in the family with Episkopi blindness (Norrie disease). *J Med Genet* 1992;29:816–819.

Wu WC, Drenser K, Trese M, et al. Retinal phenotype-genotype correlation of pediatric patients expressing mutations in the Norrie disease gene. *Arch Ophthalmol* 2007;125:225–230.

Xu Q, Wang Y, Dabdoub A, et al. Vascular development in the retina and inner ear: control by Norrin and Frizzled-4, a high-affinity ligand-receptor pair. *Cell* 2004;116:883–895.

Ye X, Wang Y, Cahill H, et al. Norrin, frizzled-4, and Lrp5 signaling in endothelial cells controls a genetic program for retinal vascularization. *Cell* 2009;139:285–298.

Retinal Dysplasia

Chan A, Lakshminrusimha S, Heffner R, et al. Histogenesis of retinal dysplasia in trisomy 13. *Diagn Pathol* 2007;2:48.

Godel V, Nemet P, Lazar M. Retinal dysplasia. *Doc Ophthalmol* 1981;51:277–288.

Green WR, Iliff WJ, Trotter RR. Malignant teratoid medulloepithelioma of the optic nerve. *Arch Ophthalmol* 1974;91:451–454.

Hoepner J, Yanoff M. Ocular anomalies in trisomy 13–15: an analysis of 13 eyes with two new findings. *Am J Ophthalmol* 1972;74:729–737.

Lahav M, Albert DM, Wyand S. Clinical and histopathologic classification of retinal dysplasia. *Am J Ophthalmol* 1973;75:648–667.

Lloyd IC, Colley A, Tullo AB, et al. Dominantly inherited unilateral retinal dysplasia. *Br J Ophthalmol* 1993;77:378–380.

Mullaney J. Primary malignant medulloepithelioma of the retinal stalk. *Am J Ophthalmol* 1974;77:499–504.

Reese AB, Straatsma BR. Retinal dysplasia. *Am J Ophthalmol* 1958;45:199–211.

Silverstein AM, Osburn BI, Prendergast RA. The pathogenesis of retinal dysplasia. *Am J Ophthalmol* 1971;72:13–21.

Medulloepithelioma

Broughton WL, Zimmerman LE. A clinicopathologic study of 56 cases of intraocular medulloepitheliomas. *Am J Ophthalmol* 1978;85:407–418.

Brownstein S, Barsoum-Homsy M, Conway VH, et al. Nonteratoid medulloepithelioma of the ciliary body. *Ophthalmology* 1984;91:1118–1122.

Canning CR, McCartney AC, Hungerford J. Medulloepithelioma (diktyoma). *Br J Ophthalmol* 1988;72:764–767.

Eagle RC Jr, Font RL, Swerczek TW. Malignant medulloepithelioma of the optic nerve in a horse. *Vet Pathol* 1978;15:488–494.

Font RL, Rishi K. Diffuse retinal involvement in malignant nonteratoid medulloepithelioma of ciliary body in an adult. *Arch Ophthalmol* 2005;123:1136–1138.

Jakobiec FA, Howard GM, Ellsworth RM, et al. Electron microscopic diagnosis of medulloepithelioma. *Am J Ophthalmol* 1975;79:321–329.

Kivela T, Kauniskangas L, Miettinen P, et al. Glioneuroma associated with colobomatous dysplasia of the anterior uvea and retina. A case simulating medulloepithelioma. *Ophthalmology* 1989;96:1799–1808.

Kivela T, Tarkkanen A. Recurrent medulloepithelioma of the ciliary body. Immunohistochemical characteristics. *Ophthalmology* 1988;95:1565–1575.

Lloyd WC III, O'Hara M. Malignant teratoid medulloepithelioma: clinical-echographic-histopathologic correlation. *J AAPOS* 2001;5:395–397.

O'Keefe M, Fulcher T, Kelly P, et al. Medulloepithelioma of the optic nerve head. *Arch Ophthalmol* 1997;115:1325–1327.

Shields JA, Eagle RC Jr, Shields CL, et al. Congenital neoplasms of the nonpigmented ciliary epithelium (medulloepithelioma). *Ophthalmology* 1996;103:1998–2006.

Shields JA, Eagle RC Jr, Shields CL, et al. Pigmented medulloepithelioma of the ciliary body. *Arch Ophthalmol* 2002;120:207–210.

Wilson ME, McClatchey SK, Zimmerman LE: Rhabdomyosarcoma of the ciliary body. *Ophthalmology* 1990;97:1484–1488.

Astrocytic Hamartomas and Astrocytomas

Bornfeld N, Messmer EP, Theodossiadis G, et al. Giant cell astrocytoma of the retina. Clinicopathologic report of a case not associated with Bourneville's disease. *Retina* 1987;7:183–189.

Cleasby GW, Fung WE, Shekter WB. Astrocytoma of the retina. Report of two cases. *Am J Ophthalmol* 1967;(64 Suppl):633–637.

de Juan E Jr, Green WR, Gupta PK, et al. Vitreous seeding by retinal astrocytic hamartoma in a patient with tuberous sclerosis. *Retina* 1984;4:100–102.

Eagle RC Jr, Shields JA, Shields CL, et al. Hamartomas of the iris and ciliary epithelium in tuberous sclerosis complex. *Arch Ophthalmol* 2000;118:711–715.

Gunduz K, Eagle RC Jr, Shields CL, et al. Invasive giant cell astrocytoma of the retina in a patient with tuberous sclerosis. *Ophthalmology* 1999;106:639–642.

Jakobiec FA, Brodie SE, Haik B, et al. Giant cell astrocytoma of the retina. A tumor of possible Mueller cell origin. *Ophthalmology* 1983;90:1565–1576.

Nyboer JH, Robertson DM, Gomez MR. Retinal lesions in tuberous sclerosis. *Arch Ophthalmol* 1976;94:1277–1280.

Robertson DM. Ophthalmic manifestations of tuberous sclerosis. *Ann N Y Acad Sci* 1991;615:17–25.

Shields JA, Eagle RC Jr, Shields CL, et al. Aggressive retinal astrocytomas in four patients with tuberous sclerosis complex. *Trans Am Ophthalmol Soc* 2004;102:139–147, discussion 147–138.

Shields CL, Shields JA, Eagle RC Jr, et al. Progressive enlargement of acquired retinal astrocytoma in 2 cases. *Ophthalmology* 2004;111:363–368.

Shields JA, Shields CL, Ehya H, et al. Atypical retinal astrocytic hamartoma diagnosed by fine-needle biopsy. *Ophthalmology* 1996;103:949–952.

Shields CL, Thangappan A, Hartzell K, et al. Combined hamartoma of the retina and retinal pigment epithelium in 77 consecutive patients visual outcome based on macular versus extramacular tumor location. *Ophthalmology* 2008;115:2246–2252 e2243.

Tay A, Scheithauer BW, Cameron JD, et al. Retinal ependymoma: an immunohistologic and ultrastructural study. *Hum Pathol* 2009;40:578–583.

Ulbright TM, Fulling KH, Helveston EM. Astrocytic tumors of the retina. Differentiation of sporadic tumors from phakomatosis-associated tumors. *Arch Pathol Lab Med* 1984;108:160–163.

Zimmer-Galler IE, Robertson DM. Long-term observation of retinal lesions in tuberous sclerosis. *Am J Ophthalmol* 1995;119:318–324.

Hematopoietic Lesions

Chang MW, Frieden IJ, Good W. The risk intraocular juvenile xanthogranuloma: survey of current practices and assessment of risk. *J Am Acad Dermatol* 1996;34:445–449.

Cho AS, Holland GN, Glasgow BJ, et al. Ocular involvement in patients with posttransplant lymphoproliferative disorder. *Arch Ophthalmol* 2001;119:183–189.

Coupland SE, Foss HD, Bechrakis NE, et al. Secondary ocular involvement in systemic "memory" B-cell lymphocytic leukemia. *Ophthalmology* 2001;108:1289–1295.

Kincaid MC, Green WR. Ocular and orbital involvement in leukemia. *Surv Ophthalmol* 1983;27:211–232.

Leonardy NJ, Rupani M, Dent G, et al. Analysis of 135 autopsy eyes for ocular involvement in leukemia. *Am J Ophthalmol* 1990;109:436–444.

O'Hara M, Lloyd WC III, Scribbick FW, et al. Latent intracellular Epstein-Barr Virus DNA demonstrated in ocular posttransplant lymphoproliferative disorder mimicking granulomatous uveitis with iris nodules in a child. *J Aapos* 2001;5:62–63.

Sanders TE. Intraocular juvenile xanthogranuloma (nevoxanthogranuloma): a survey of 20 cases. *Trans Am Ophthalmol Soc* 1960;58:59–74.

Shields JA, Eagle RC Jr, Shields CL, et al. Iris juvenile xanthogranuloma studied by immunohistochemistry and flow cytometry. *Ophthalmic Surg Lasers* 1997;28:140–144.

Zimmerman LE. Ocular lesions of juvenile xanthogranuloma. Nevoxanthoedothelioma. *Am J Ophthalmol* 1965;60:1011–1035.

Lacrimal Gland Choristomas

Freitag SK, Eagle RC Jr, Shields JA, et al. Melanogenic neuroectodermal tumor of the retina (primary malignant melanoma of the retina). *Arch Ophthalmol* 1997;115:1581–1584.

Ghadially FN, Chisholm IA, Lalonde JM. Ultrastructure of an intraocular lacrimal gland choristoma. *J Submicrosc Cytol* 1986;18:189–198.

Kobrin EG, Shields CL, Danzig CJ, et al. Intraocular lacrimal gland choristoma diagnosed by fine-needle aspiration biopsy. *Cornea* 2007;26:753–755.

Kobrin EG, Shields CL, Danzig CJ, et al. Intraocular lacrimal gland choristoma diagnosed by fine-needle aspiration biopsy. *Cornea* 2007;26:753–755.

Shields JA, Eagle RC Jr, Shields CL, et al. Natural course and histopathologic findings of lacrimal gland choristoma of the iris and ciliary body. *Am J Ophthalmol* 1995;119:219–224.

Shields JA, Hogan RN, Shields CL, et al. Intraocular lacrimal gland choristoma involving iris and ciliary body. *Am J Ophthalmol* 2000;129:673–675.

Other Rare Neoplasms

Kivela T, Kauniskangas L, Miettinen P, et al. Glioneuroma associated with colobomatous dysplasia of the anterior uvea and retina. A case simulating medulloepithelioma. *Ophthalmology* 1989;96:1799–1808.

Patel S, Dondey J, Chan HS. et. al. Leukocoria caused by intraocular heterotopic brain tissue. *Arch Ophthalmol* 2004;122:390–393.

Paysse EA, Coats D, Chevez-Barrios P. An unusual case of leukocoria: heterotopic brain arising from the retina. *Arch Ophthalmol* 2003;121:119–122.

Spencer WH, Jesberg DO. Glioneuroma (choristomatous malformation of the optic cup margin). *Arch Ophthalmol* 1973;89:387–391.

Tiberti A, Damato B, Hiscott P, et al. Iris ectopic thyroid tissue: report of a case. *Arch Ophthalmol* 2006;124:1497–1500.

Miscellaneous Lesions

Brown GC, Shields JA, Oglesby RB. Anterior polar cataracts associated with bilateral retinoblastoma. *Am J Ophthalmol* 1979;87:276.

Friendly DS, Parks MM. Concurrence of hereditary congenital cataracts and hereditary retinoblastoma. *Arch Ophthalmol* 1970;84:525–527.

Mouriaux F, Leroy-Rattier MP, Maurage CA. et. al. Congenital duplication of the anterior segment with central hamartomatous plaque. *Arch Ophthalmol* 2002;120:1377–1379.

13 The Eyelid and Lacrimal Drainage System

INTRODUCTION

The eyelids are flaps of skin with highly modified epidermal appendages that cover and protect the eye. The structure of the eyelids is discussed in Chapter 1 and illustrated in (Fig. 13-1). The eyelids form a moist chamber lined by mucous membrane (conjunctiva) that is absolutely essential for the maintenance of corneal transparency. The importance of the eyelids in the maintenance of corneal health and transparency becomes evident when facial paralysis or stupor prevent normal eyelid closure and produce corneal exposure or lagophthalmos (rabbit eye). If congenital defects in the eyelid called colobomas (coloboma—"a defect") are not corrected expeditiously, corneal ulceration and/or opacification caused by epidermalization invariably result. The corneal epithelium literally turns to skin if it is not continuously moistened.

The external surface of the eyelid is covered by one of the thinnest and most delicate layers of skin in the body (Fig. 13-1D). The epidermis of the eyelid skin is generally only five or six cells in thickness and is covered by a thin layer of surface keratinization. Unlike skin elsewhere, eyelid epidermis lacks rete ridges. The basal cell or germinative layer of the epidermis, where cellular division normally occurs, rests on a delicate basement membrane. Compared to the squamous cells of the overlying epidermis, the basal cells have relatively little cytoplasm. Hence, lesions composed of basal cells such as basal cell carcinoma appear blue or basophilic on low power microscopy. Most of the epidermis is composed of the prickle cells of the stratum spinosum or Malpighian layer. These cells are polygonal in shape and are joined by bundles of tonofilaments evident in light microscopy as intercellular bridges. Squamous cell lesions appear pink or eosinophilic under low power microscopy because the cells have abundant eosinophilic cytoplasm.

TERMS USED IN SKIN PATHOLOGY

Thickening of the prickle cell layer is termed acanthosis (from Gk, *akantha*, thorn) (Fig. 13-2A). As basal cells mature and approach the surface of the skin, they become flattened and squamoid. The nuclei undergo apoptosis as the cells near the surface, releasing intensely basophilic granules of nucleoprotein that form the granular cell layer. The dead, desiccated, anucleate cellular remnants form a thin horny layer of keratin called the stratum corneum (from Latin, *cornu*, a horn). Abnormal thickening of this normally thin surface layer of keratin is called hyperkeratosis (Fig. 13-2A).

Hyperkeratosis is commonly found on the surface of benign squamous papillomas and is responsible for the greasy or scaly character of seborrheic keratoses. Colonies of yeast or bacteria frequently are found in the thick layer of keratin.

Retention of nuclei in the stratum corneum is termed parakeratosis (Fig. 13-2B). Parakeratosis generally occurs in pathologic states when the epidermis is rapidly proliferating. When parakeratosis is present, there is no granular cell layer in the underlying epidermis. Parakeratosis is relatively rare and should alert one that he/she may be dealing with a premalignant lesion such as actinic keratosis.

Dyskeratosis refers to the keratinization of single cells within the prickle cell layer. Dyskeratotic cells are round and intensely eosinophilic and have pyknotic nuclei. Dyskeratosis is particularly striking in the conjunctival lesions of hereditary benign intraepithelial dyskeratosis.

Congenital and Developmental Lesions

Developmental anomalies of the eyelid include ablepharon, cryptophthalmos, colobomas, microblepharon, ankyloblepharon, euryblepharon, blepharophimosis, congenital ectropion, epicanthal folds, and dystopia canthorum. An intact sheet of skin covers the eye in cryptophthalmos. Affected patients may have Fraser syndrome, which also includes syndactyly, renal agenesis, and aural and genital malformations. Colobomas are partial or full-thickness defects in the lid that affect the lid margin. Lid colobomas are common in Goldenhar syndrome and mandibulofacial dysostosis. Isolated strands of skin bridge the palpebral fissure in ankyloblepharon filiforme adnatum. These are related to the fusion of the upper and lower lids that normally occurs *in utero*. Dystopia canthorum, iris heterochromia, a white forelock, synophrys, and deafness comprise Waardenburg syndrome. An accessory row of eyelashes arises from the meibomian glands in distichiasis. Phakomatous choristoma or Zimmerman tumor is a rare congenital neoplasm that involves the lower medial eyelid or anterior orbit. The ultimate choristoma, Zimmerman tumor is composed of extraocular eye lens tissue including lens epithelium, neoplastic lens capsule, and bladder cells like those found in posterior subcapsular cataract (Fig. 13-3).

AGING CHANGES

Aging produces atrophy and laxity of eyelid skin (dermatochalasis), loss of orbital fat and subcutaneous tissue, and relaxation of eyelid ligaments. Folds of redundant skin overhang the upper lid margin, and the orbital fat protrudes

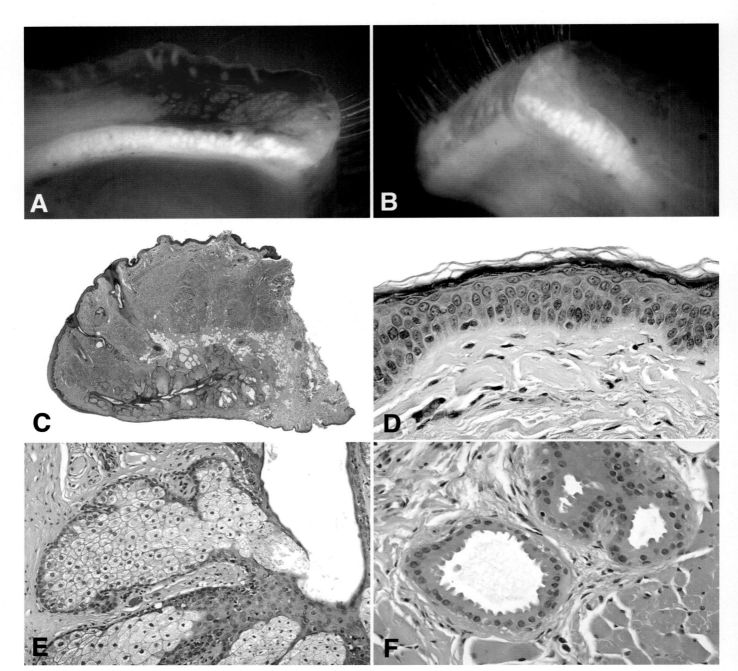

Fig. 13-1. A. Upper eyelid. The upper eyelid is roughly rectangular compared to the lower lid, which is much shorter and triangular in shape. The anterior surface of the lid is covered by skin. A row of cilia (eyelashes) arises near the lid margin (at right) and curves away from the globe. The white foci seen below are the lobules of a Meibomian gland in the tarsal plate, the eyelid's fibrous skeleton. The palpebral conjunctiva is tightly adherent to the back surface of the tarsal plate. **B. Lower eyelid.** The lower eyelid is roughly triangular and has a much shorter tarsal plate and fewer meibomian glands. **C. Histology, lower eyelid.** The anterior surface of the eyelid is covered by a delicate layer of skin. The posterior surface is covered by the palpebral conjunctiva, which is firmly adherent to the tarsal plate. The tarsal plate contains large sebaceous glands called the Meibomian glands. Eosinophilic bundles of orbicularis muscle are seen in cross section in the connective tissue anterior to the tarsus. The tarsal plate of the lower lid is much shorter. The lower lid is roughly triangular in shape. **D. Eyelid skin.** The skin of the eyelid is extremely delicate and lacks rete pegs. The layers of the epidermis include the basal cell layer, the malpighian or prickle cell layer, the granular cell layer, and the superficial keratin layer. **E. Meibomian gland lobule, eyelid.** Each Meibomian gland is composed of multiple sebaceous gland lobules arranged along a central duct, which is oriented perpendicular to the lid margin. Sebaceous glands are holocrine glands; lipidized cells shed into the duct comprise the secretory product. Cellular division occurs in the basal cell layer in the periphery of the lobules. The nuclei become increasingly pyknotic as the cells mature and become lipidized. A flaplike valve of ductal epithelium covers the opening of this lobule. **F. Glands of Moll.** The dilated lumina of these apocrine sweat glands are lined by tall eosinophilic cells capped with the apical snouts that characterize apocrine decapitation secretion. (**C.** H&E ×10, **D.** H&E ×50, **E.** H&E ×50, **F.** H&E ×100)

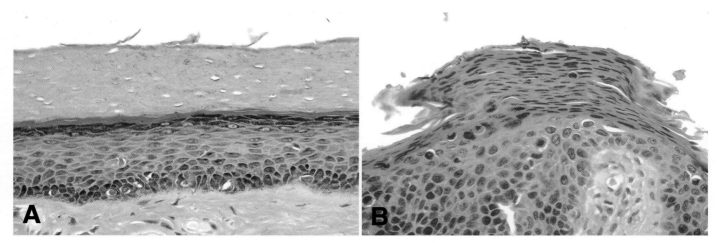

Fig. 13-2. A. Hyperkeratosis. The superficial layer of eosinophilic keratin is markedly thickened. The dead cells comprising the mass of keratin lack nuclei. A granular cell layer is present beneath the keratin. The epidermis in this specimen is mildly thickened. **B. Parakeratosis, actinic keratosis.** The keratin layer retains flattened nuclei, and no granular cell layer is present. Parakeratosis is typically found in actinic keratosis. In this example, the epidermis is composed of mildly atypical squamous cells. (**A.** H&E ×50, **B.** H&E ×100)

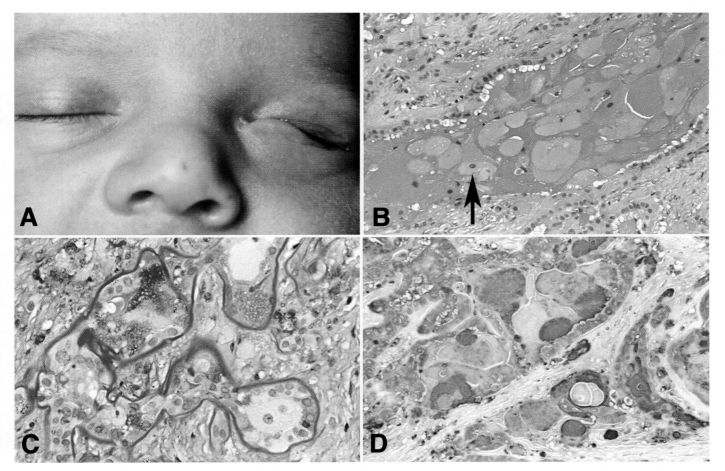

Fig. 13-3. Zimmerman tumor (phakomatous choristoma). A. Phakomatous choristoma is a rare congenital tumor of lenticular anlage that always occurs in the lower medial eyelid or anterior orbit. **B.** The tumor is composed of neoplastic lens epithelial cells. *Arrow* denotes cell resembling bladder or Wedl cell found in posterior subcapsular cataract. **C.** Lens epithelial cells rest on thick PAS-positive basement membrane that mimics lens capsule. **D.** Cells are immunoreactive for lens crystallin. (**B.** H&E ×50, **C.** PAS ×250, **D.** IHC for beta crystalline ×100)

through the attenuated orbital septum, producing bags under the eyes. Chronic light damage (senile or actinic elastosis) is evident histologically as basophilic degeneration of dermal collagen.

Laxity of eyelid tissues predispose to senile entropion or ectropion. Entropion occurs when the preseptal part of the orbicularis muscle overrides the pretarsal part. The lateral canthal tendon is lax in senile ectropion, and the exposed conjunctiva becomes inflamed and undergoes epidermalization. The floppy eyelid syndrome occurs in obese men who have eyelids with a rubbery tarsus that are easily everted. Spontaneous eversion of the eyelids or loss of eyelid contact occurs during sleep, causing chronic papillary conjunctivitis. Patients with floppy eyelid syndrome should be evaluated for obstructive sleep apnea, a potentially fatal condition.

COMMON INFLAMMATORY LESIONS OF THE EYELID

Hordeolums or styes and chalazia are common inflammatory lesions of the eyelid. Hordeolums are acute infections of eyelash follicles (external hordeolums) or meibomian glands (internal hordeolums) that usually are caused by staphylococci. Internal hordeolums are more painful because the inflammation is localized within a confined space. Hordeolums usually respond to conservative therapy, for example, hot compresses, and therefore are rarely examined histopathologically.

Chalazion

Chalazia typically appear as mildly tender nodules, or areas of localized nodular thickening on the eyelid (Fig. 13-4A).

Inflammatory signs such as pain and redness are not especially prominent because chalazia are chronic inflammatory lesions. Chalazia are chronic lipogranulomas, that is, "endogenous foreign body reactions" to the lipid-rich secretions of the meibomian and Zeis glands. When sebum escapes from its normal confines in these sebaceous glands, it is extremely irritating and stimulates chronic granulomatous inflammation. Histopathology discloses epithelioid histiocytes and inflammatory giant cells that typically surround empty spaces (lipid vacuoles) (Fig. 13-4B). *In vivo* the vacuoles contained lipid. During tissue processing solvents such as alcohol and xylene, dissolve out the lipid. Other chronic inflammatory cells such as lymphocytes and plasma cells contribute to the chronic inflammatory infiltrate in chalazion specimens. If the chalazion has ruptured spontaneously, or if prior incision and drainage has been performed, granulation tissue is often found. Although granulation tissue typically is nongranulomatous, the granulation tissue associated with chalazion may contain epithelioid cells or giant cells, which are residua of the lipogranulomatous response. Chalazion curettings often include fragments of tarsal plate.

Sebaceous carcinoma, which also arises in Zeis and meibomian glands, can be confused with chronic chalazia clinically. It is imperative that recurrent or atypical chalazia be submitted for histopathologic examination to exclude the possibility of this potentially fatal eyelid malignancy. The author personally has seen several cases of sebaceous carcinoma that were initially misdiagnosed as chalazia. These lesions were treated with incision and drainage and were not examined histopathologically. When the correct diagnosis was finally made, extensive pagetoid involvement of the conjunctiva by tumor cells necessitated orbital exenteration. Other unusual neoplasms such as sweat gland carcinomas, Merkel cell

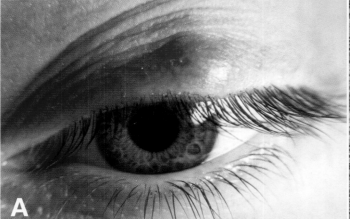
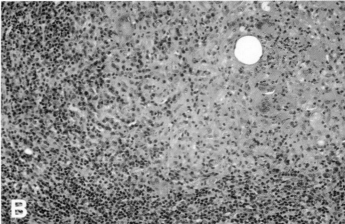

Fig. 13-4. Chalazion. A. The focal area of nodular thickening in the upper eyelid represents a chronic granulomatous inflammatory response to irritating lipid material that has escaped from its normal compartment in the lid. Chalazia usually are only mildly tender and inflamed. Recurrent or atypical "chalazia" should be examined pathologically to exclude simulating lesions such as sebaceous carcinoma. **B.** Pink epithelioid histiocytes and giant cells indicative of chronic granulomatous inflammation surround an empty lipid vacuole. The lipid was dissolved by fat solvents during processing. Empty lipid vacuoles are required for the diagnosis of lipogranulomatous inflammation. The inflammatory infiltrate also contains many plasma cells and lymphocytes. (**B.** H&E ×100)

tumors, and carcinoma metastatic to the eyelid have been misdiagnosed clinically as chalazia.

VIRAL LESIONS

Verruca Vulgaris

Verruca vulgaris, a benign papillomatous skin lesion caused by human papillomavirus type 2 (HPV-2), a DNA papovavirus, occasionally occurs on the eyelid. These viral papillomas are distinguished by elongated spire-shaped papillary fronds and rete ridges that bend inwardly toward the center of the lesion (Fig. 13-5A). Vertical tiers of parakeratosis occur on the crests of papillomatous elevations and overlie foci of vacuolated cells that contain eosinophilic intranuclear and intracytoplasmic viral inclusions (Fig. 13-5B). The viral inclusions, which are necessary for definitive diagnosis, are only found in early lesions. Verruca vulgaris is diagnosed infrequently in the ophthalmic pathology laboratory.

Molluscum Contagiosum

Molluscum contagiosum is a fairly common viral tumor with a distinctive histopathologic appearance (Fig. 13-6). Caused by a pox virus, molluscum contagiosum often is associated with poor hygiene, and lesions may occur in crops on the face and eyelids of children as the result of autoinoculation. Massive involvement of eyelids and adnexal skin has been reported in patients with AIDS. Clinically, molluscum contagiosum appears as either an elevated smooth nodule with a central umbilication, or a larger pore enclosing multiple flattened papillae. Histopathologically, molluscum contagiosum typically has an elevated cup- or crateriform configuration and is composed of lobules of

markedly acanthotic benign epithelium (Fig. 13-6A). The epithelial cells contain large intracytoplasmic inclusion bodies called Henderson Patterson corpuscles (Fig. 13-6B). The inclusions are eosinophilic near the base of the epithelium where they form, and they become denser and more basophilic as they mature and migrate toward the surface where they discharge virus particles. The individual virus particles are quite large and can be resolved with the oil immersion objective of the light microscope in one micron thick plastic-embedded sections. Molluscum contagiosum on the eyelid margin can incite unilateral chronic follicular conjunctivitis by dispersing viral particles into the conjunctival sac. The lids of any patient who has chronic follicular conjunctivitis should be inspected carefully for molluscum contagiosum (or the presence of pubic or "crab" lice whose waste can incite a similar reaction).

Molluscum contagiosum is one of three cup-shaped or crateriform lesions commonly found on eyelid skin. Basal cell carcinoma and keratoacanthoma also are often umbilicated or have a central area of ulceration. Both tend to be larger than molluscum contagiosum.

Other viral lesions that affect eyelid skin include the vesicular eruptions caused by the herpes simplex and varicella-zoster viruses. Herpes simplex infection causes fluid-filled intraepidermal vesicles marked by profound epidermal degeneration and acantholysis (Fig. 13-5C,D). Round acantholytic balloon cells and multinucleated giant cells that contain eosinophilic intranuclear viral inclusions are found.

Benign Cystic Lesions

Eyelid cysts are commonly accessioned by ocular pathology laboratories. Most are epidermal inclusion cysts or sweat ductal cysts.

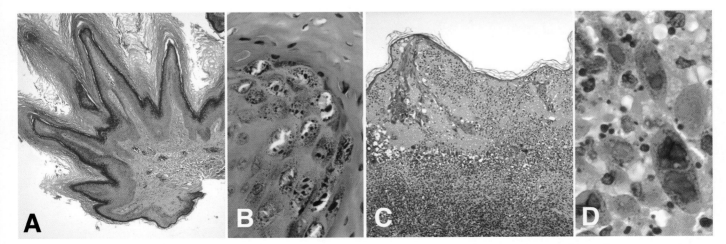

Fig. 13-5. Viral lesions. A. Verruca vulgaris. Viral papilloma is composed of spire-shaped fronds of hyperkeratotic epidermis. **B.** Parakeratosis and vacuolated cells containing viral inclusions are seen on crest of frond. **C. Herpes simplex infection of the skin.** Serous fluid and inflammatory cells fill herpetic vesicle that has formed within the acantholytic epidermis. The underlying dermis is intensely inflamed. **D.** Multinucleated giant cells with Cowdry type A intranuclear inclusions are present. (**A.** H&E ×25, **B.** H&E ×250, **C.** H&E ×25, **D.** H&E ×250)

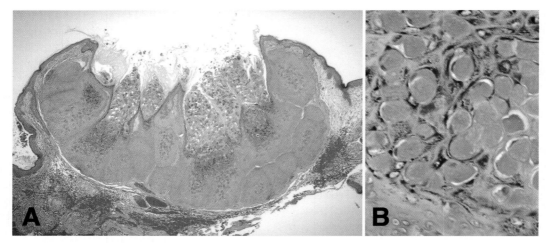

Fig. 13-6. Molluscum contagiosum. A. This viral tumor has a typical crateriform configuration. Inclusions of pox virus shed by the infected acanthotic epithelium fill the crater. **B. Henderson-Patterson corpuscles.** The pox virus infection causes lobular acanthosis of the epidermis. The thickened epidermis contains large oval intracytoplasmic viral inclusions called Henderson-Patterson corpuscles. The inclusions become increasingly basophilic as they mature. (**A.** H&E ×10, **B.** H&E ×100)

Epidermal inclusion cysts are round or oval and unilocular (have a single lumen) and are filled with cheesy, foul-smelling keratin debris. They are lined by keratinizing stratified squamous epithelium that resembles normal epidermis (Fig. 13-7). By definition, the epithelial lining has no epidermal appendages such as pilosebaceous units or sweat glands. (If epidermal appendages are present, and hair shafts are found mixed with the keratin filling the lumen, the cyst probably should be classified as a cystic dermoid, a developmental lesion caused by entrapment of epidermis in bony sutures.) Many epidermal inclusion cysts are caused by the cystic dilatation of hair follicles by keratin debris. Essentially, they result from the cystic dilatation of a single epidermal appendage. *Follicular cyst, infundibular* type is the dermatopathologic term applied to this type of cyst. In such cases, the lining of the cyst may communicate with the skin through a pore. Clinically, epidermal inclusion cysts are called sebaceous cysts, an inappropriate term since they have nothing to do with sebaceous glands or sebum.

Sweat ductal cysts, sudoriferous cysts, or hidrocystomas are caused by the blockage of a sweat duct. These cysts are soft, smooth, and fluctuant and are filled with watery fluid. Some are transparent or translucent, and they readily transilluminate. Some patients have multiple cysts that often involve that skin of both medial or lateral canthi (Fig. 13-8).

Histopathologically, sweat ductal cysts are often multilocular, and their lumens appear empty or contain scant amounts of granular eosinophilic material consistent with serous fluid. The epithelial lining, which is often attenuated, is composed of a dual layer of cells that resembles the normal lining of an eccrine sweat duct (Fig. 13-8B). Although

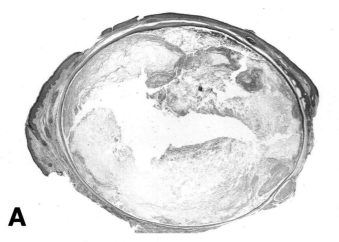

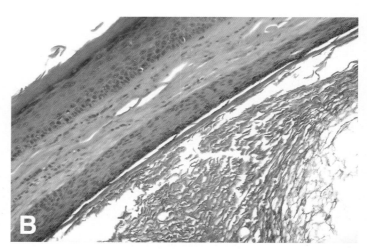

Fig. 13-7. Epidermal inclusion cyst. A. Epidermal inclusion cysts typically are round or oval and unilocular. The lumen of the cyst contains laminated eosinophilic keratin, which had a cheesy appearance grossly. The cyst is lined by keratinized squamous epithelium that resembles skin but lacks epidermal appendages. **B.** The surface of the skin is seen at top left. The cyst is lined by keratinized stratified squamous epithelium resembling epidermis. Laminated keratin fills lumen. (**A.** H&E ×5, **B.** H&E ×50)

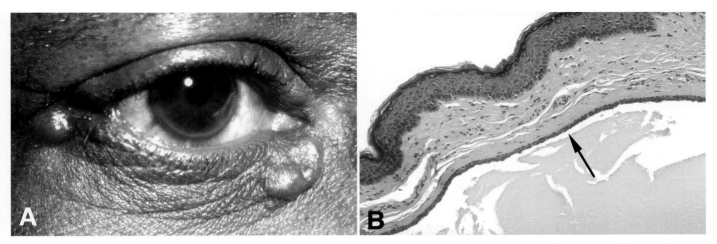

Fig. 13-8. Eccrine hidrocystoma. A. Cysts caused by the blockage of eccrine sweat glands often involve the canthal skin. Multiple cysts occur in some patients. They are filled with watery fluid. Eccrine hidrocystomas also are called sweat ductal or sudoriferous cysts. **B.** The eccrine hidrocystoma is lined by a dual layer of epithelial cells (*arrow*) resembling the epithelium of an eccrine sweat gland duct. The lumen is filled with eosinophilic granular debris consistent with serous fluid. The lumen is often branching and multilocular. (**B.** H&E ×100)

most sudoriferous cysts are eccrine hidrocystomas, the epithelial lining occasionally shows apocrine differentiation. **Apocrine hidrocystomas** (Fig. 13-9) are recognized by their epithelial lining, which is composed of tall cells with eosinophilic cytoplasm and apical snouts of decapitation secretion (Fig. 13-9D). The cytoplasm of the apocrine cells may contain golden-brown granules of lipofuscin pigment that are periodic acid-Schiff-positive. Apocrine hidrocystomas often contain brown fluid stained by this pigment and may be misdiagnosed preoperatively as primary melanocytic lesions (Fig. 13-9A,B).

Benign Epidermal Lesions

Benign tumors that arise from the epidermis generally are located anterior to the plane of the surrounding normal skin because they are composed of cells that are unable to invade or infiltrate the dermis or deeper structures of the lid as malignant lesions can. The redundant epidermis formed by the proliferation of these benign cells typically forms a branching tree-shaped lesion composed of fronds or fingerlike projections that have cores of fibrovascular tissue analogous to dermis. A lesion that exhibits this growth pattern is called a papilloma (Fig. 13-10). Papillomas can be elevated and exophytic or relatively squat and sessile. A variety of lesions show a papillomatous growth pattern including some malignant tumors, for example, papillary squamous cell carcinoma of the conjunctiva.

Benign papillomatous lesions of eyelid skin such as seborrheic keratoses and squamous cell papillomas frequently are submitted for histopathologic evaluation.

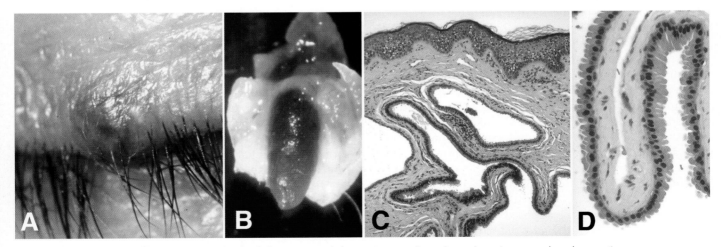

Fig. 13-9. Apocrine hidrocystoma. A. Bluish lesion near lid margin was thought to be pigmented melanocytic nevus preoperatively. **B.** Macrophoto of another case shows brownish fluid filling lumen of cyst. **C.** Branching lumen of multilocular Moll gland cyst appears empty. **D.** The cells comprising the epithelial lining are tall and show apical snouts of decapitation secretion indicative of apocrine differentiation. (**C.** H&E ×25, **D.** H&E ×100)

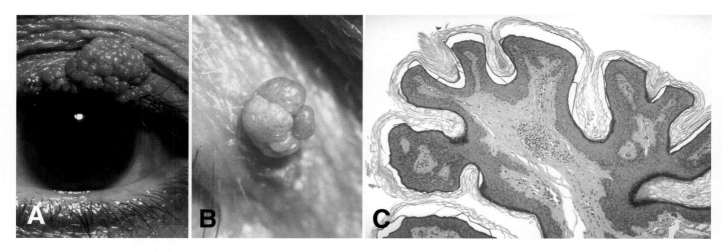

Fig. 13-10. Squamous papillomas. A. Squamous papillomas are very common benign epidermal tumors of the eyelid. They are branching tree-shaped lesions composed of multiple fronds of benign epidermis. A large papilloma is present on upper eyelid. **B.** Smaller pedunculated papillomas are called skin tags, acrochordons, or fibroepithelial polyps. **C.** Multiple fronds or fingerlike projections of epidermis comprise the benign epidermal tumor. The epidermal fronds contain a central core of fibrovascular tissue. Hyperkeratosis is present on the surface of this lesion. (**C.** H&E ×25)

In most instances, the correct diagnosis is suspected preoperatively, and cosmesis is a major indication for excisional biopsy.

Seborrheic Keratosis

Seborrheic keratoses usually occur in elderly patients. They are sharply demarcated, superficial lesions that sit anterior to the plane of surrounding epidermis like a button on the surface of the skin (Fig. 13-11). They typically have a greasy or scaly appearance caused by hyperkeratosis and are often pigmented. Approximately one third of black adults have multiple, small, pigmented seborrheic keratoses on their facial skin, a condition called dermatosis papulosa nigra (Fig. 13-11A).

Seborrheic keratoses are an upward papillomatous proliferation of basaloid cells that resemble normal epidermal basal cells. Therefore, under low magnification, seborrheic keratoses often appear "blue" and are situated "above" the plane of the surrounding skin (signifying a benign lesion of basal cells) (Fig. 13-11B). In contrast to "garden variety" squamous papillomas, acrochordons, or skin tags, which are often exophytic and pedunculated (Fig. 13-10A,B), seborrheic keratoses are often sessile. A thick surface layer of keratin usually is present, and circular spaces filled with keratin called "horn cysts" or "pseudo-horn cysts" are found within the acanthotic epithelium. Most probably represent invaginations of surface keratin (Fig. 13-11B–D).

Interweaving bands composed of benign cells are found in the dermis in the adenoid variant of seborrheic keratosis (Fig. 13-11D), which should not be confused with the highly infiltrative morpheaform variant of basal cell carcinoma. Inverted follicular keratosis (IFK) is considered by some to be an irritated form of seborrheic keratosis. IFK typically has an inverted cup-shaped configuration

and surface invaginations that have been interpreted as hair follicles (Fig. 13-12). Other characteristic histopathologic features include acantholysis (widening of intercellular spaces between squamous cells) and small foci of squamous differentiation called squamous eddies.

Many benign eyelid papillomas do not fulfill all of the diagnostic criteria for seborrheic keratosis. Such lesions tend to be small and pedunculated, and their epidermal component is not particularly basaloid and resembles normal or only slightly acanthotic skin with minimal hyperkeratosis (Fig. 13-10C). The dermal component often contains a sparse to moderate infiltrate of chronic inflammatory cells. Such lesions usually are diagnosed as squamous papillomas and are also called skin tags or acrochordons. Some may be viral in origin.

Keratoacanthoma

Keratoacanthoma is a crater-shaped squamous cell lesion that classically arises rapidly in elderly patients and then undergoes spontaneous involution (Fig. 13-13A). Although keratoacanthoma was classified as a benign pseudoepitheliomatous hyperplasia in the past, some authorities now believe that it actually may be a "deficient squamous cell carcinoma" that tends to involute spontaneously. Rare cases invade deeply like squamous cell carcinomas.

Histopathology discloses a central crater filled with a mass of keratin that is enclosed by markedly acanthotic squamous epithelium that typically extends like a lip or buttress over the side of the crater (Fig. 13-13B). The base of a well-developed lesion appears regular and well demarcated, and the margin is relatively smooth and "pushing " rather than infiltrative. A intense band of inflammation usually is present in the underlying dermis. The overall configuration of the lesion is quite important

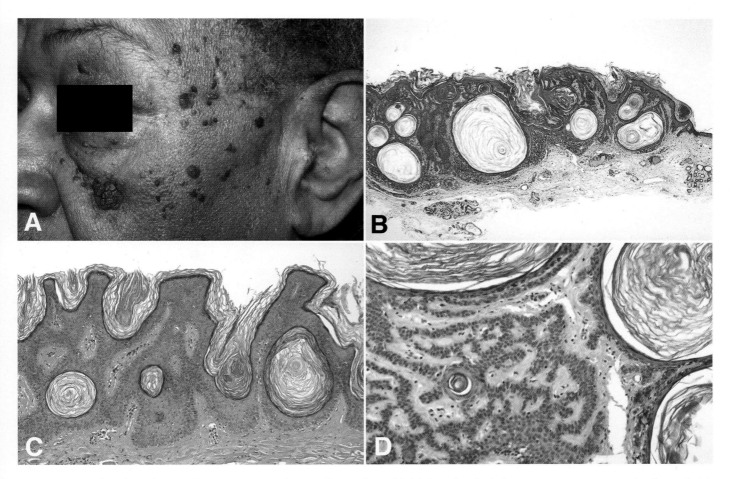

Fig. 13-11. Seborrheic keratosis. A. Dermatosis papulosa nigra. Multiple seborrheic keratoses are seen on the face of this elderly African American woman. **B.** Benign sessile papilloma is situated anterior to the plane of the surrounding skin. Lesion contains many characteristic pseudohorn cysts. **C.** Thick layer of hyperkeratosis covers sessile papilloma. Characteristic pseudohorn cysts filled with keratin are present. **D. Seborrheic keratosis, adenoid type.** The dermis contains interweaving bands of benign epithelial cells. Several keratin-filled pseudohorn cysts are present. (**B.** H&E ×10, **C.** H&E ×25, **D.** H&E ×50)

from a diagnostic standpoint. It is usually impossible to differentiate keratoacanthoma from squamous cell carcinoma in a small incisional biopsy because keratoacan-

thoma frequently harbors atypical cells and mitotic figures. Keratoacanthomas should be totally excised with frozen section control of margins.

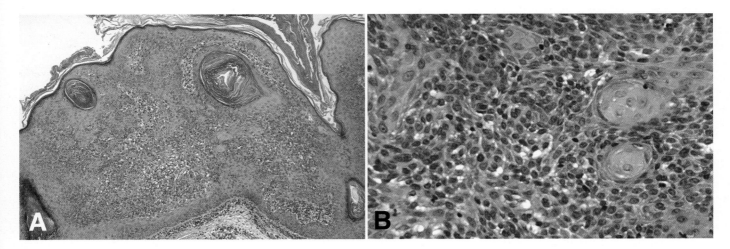

Fig. 13-12. Inverted follicular keratosis. A. IFK is thought to be an irritated variant of seborrheic keratosis. Acantholysis and circular foci of squamous cells (squamous eddies) are characteristic histologic features. **B.** Several oval foci of squamous differentiation called squamous cells are seen at right. The smaller basaloid cells show mild acantholysis. (**A.** H&E ×25, **B.** H&E ×100)

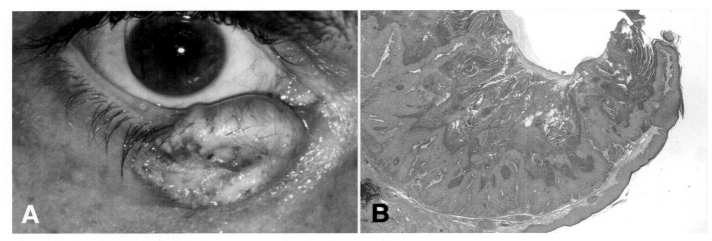

Fig. 13-13. Keratoacanthoma. A. Keratin fills irregular crater in large biopsy-confirmed keratoacanthoma of the lower eyelid. The tumor developed rapidly. Some authorities now believe that keratoacanthoma is a "deficient squamous cell carcinoma" that tends to involute spontaneously. **B.** A mass of keratin fills the crater-shaped tumor, which is composed of squamous cells with eosinophilic cytoplasm. A lateral buttress of normal skin is seen at right. The base of the lesion has a smooth "pushing" margin. The general configuration of the lesion is important in histopathologic diagnosis. It usually is impossible to distinguish keratoacanthoma from squamous cell carcinoma in a small incisional biopsy. (**B.** H&E ×5)

MALIGNANT TUMORS OF THE EYELID

Basal Cell Carcinoma

Basal cell carcinoma is the most common malignant tumor affecting the periocular skin. Basal cell carcinomas tend to affect fair skinned adults but can occur in younger persons. They arise in sun-exposed skin and are thought to be caused by actinic damage.

Several variants of basal cell carcinoma are recognized clinically. Nodulo-ulcerative basal cell carcinomas are firm, elevated, pearly nodules whose surface initially may be marked by telangiectatic vessels (Fig. 13-14A). Ulceration often develops centrally as the nodules increase in size. More advanced lesions appear as a slowly enlarging ulcers with prominent rolled pearly borders. Nodulo-ulcerative basal cell carcinomas usually have relatively distinct margins.

In contrast, the sclerosing or morpheaform variant of basal cell carcinoma frequently has relatively indistinct margins and does not tend to ulcerate until late. (The term morpheaform alludes to the lesion's similarity to morphea, a circumscribed type of scleroderma.) Widespread superficial multicentric involvement occurs in some patients. Extensive areas of ulceration called "rodent ulcers" are found in neglected cases. Patients who are cancerphobic, are afraid of doctors, or manifest excessive denial may present late in the course of the disease with ghastly disfiguring facial destruction (Fig. 13-15A).

Basal cell carcinoma occurs 15 to 40 times more often than squamous cell carcinoma on the eyelids. The tumor arises most frequently in the lower eyelid, followed by the inner canthus, upper lid, and outer canthus. Considering its frequency, it is fortunate that basal cell carcinoma rarely metastasizes. The unusual cases that do metastasize usually are of the metatypical or basosquamous type. Rare fatalities can result, however, when deeply infiltrative, ulcerative lesions invade the orbital bones and meninges and cause secondary meningitis.

Basal cell carcinoma appears "blue" and "below" on low power light microscopy. The neoplastic basaloid cells of basal cell carcinoma typically form large masses or fields, or smaller nests, islands, or cords (Figs. 13-15 and 13-16). Peripheral palisading of nuclei and retraction artifact are seen at the periphery of the tumor lobules (Figs. 13-15D and 13-16A). Peripheral palisading refers to an arrangement of peripheral nuclei perpendicular to the margin of a tumor lobule, which has been likened to a row of logs comprising a wooden fort or palisade. Shrinkage of the mucin-rich stroma during processing causes retraction artifact, an empty space or cleft between the tumor lobule and the surrounding stroma. The fibrous stroma that separates the lobules of neoplastic epithelial cells in basal cell carcinoma is generally more fibrotic and much denser than the adjacent normal dermis. The stimulation of fibrosis by the tumor is called desmoplasia.

Several histopathologic variants of basal cell carcinoma are recognized. In these variants, the tumor appears to be undergoing differentiation toward various epidermal appendages. Mucin production is evident as intralobular pools of foamy, lucent, slightly basophilic material in the adenoid variant of basal cell carcinoma. Keratotic basal cell carcinomas contain small keratinized horn cysts that may represent abortive pilar differentiation. Sebaceous differentiation is quite rare and should raise concern about an internal malignancy (see Muir–Torre syndrome below). Pigmented basal cell carcinomas contain melanin pigment

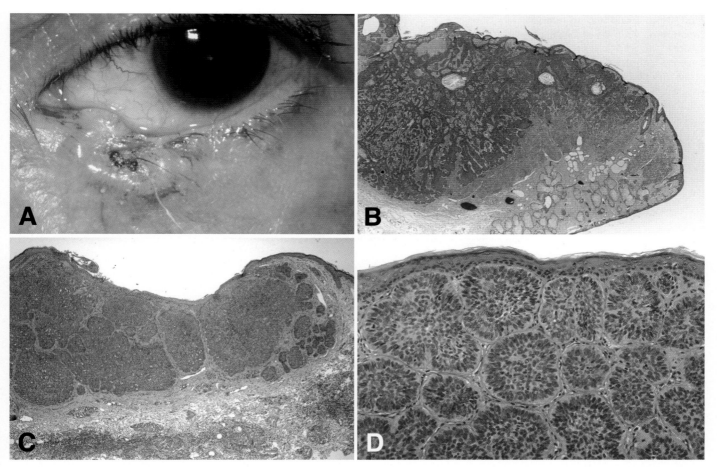

Fig. 13-14. Basal cell carcinoma. A. Nodulo-ulcerative basal cell carcinoma of lower lid has pearly elevated margins. **B.** Basal cell carcinoma of lower eyelid appears "blue and below." Its cells are basophilic and are located deep to the plane of the epidermis. **C.** The surface of this tumor is ulcerated. Basophilic lobules invade dermis. **D.** Well-differentiated basal cell carcinoma is composed of nests of basaloid cells that show peripheral palisading of nuclei. Retraction artifact is not present. No connection with epidermis is evident in this field. (**D.** H&E ×100)

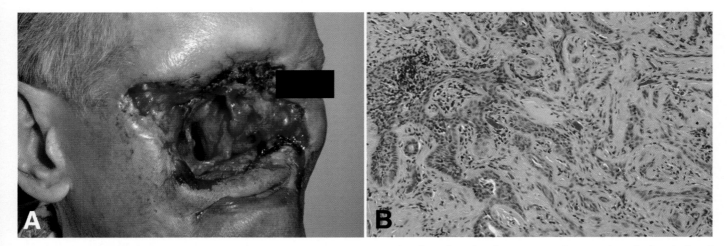

Fig. 13-15. Morpheaform basal cell carcinoma. A. Neglected morpheaform basal cell carcinoma has produced ghastly facial disfigurement. **B.** Morpheaform basal cell carcinoma is a poorly differentiated variant of basal cell carcinoma that is composed of slender infiltrating tendrils of tumor cells similar to those found in scirrhous breast carcinoma. The margins of morpheaform basal cell carcinoma are often indistinct clinically, and the tumor tends to infiltrate deeply. (**B.** H&E ×25)

Fig. 13-16. Basal and squamous cell carcinoma. A. Invasive basal cell carcinoma (*at left*) appears basophilic because tumor cells have scant cytoplasm. Peripheral palisading and retraction artifact are present. **B.** Invasive squamous cell carcinoma is composed of cells with eosinophilic cytoplasm. The surface is keratinized. (**A.** H&E ×25, **B.** H&E ×50)

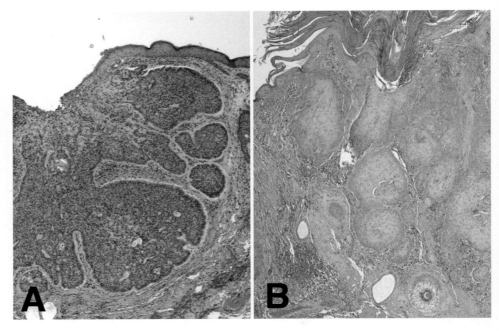

and may be confused clinically with malignant melanomas or nevi. Pseudocystic basal cell carcinomas are formed by necrobiosis in the center of a large mass of tumor cells, which is somewhat analogous to holocrine secretion. Morpheaform basal cell carcinomas are composed of slender cords or tendrils of tumor cells embedded in a densely fibrotic stroma (Fig. 13-15B). Morpheaform tumors can widely and deeply infiltrate the tissues of the eyelid and orbit, and have indistinct margins. Excision may be incomplete unless frozen section control of margins or MOHS surgery are performed.

Optimally, basal cell carcinomas of the eyelid and periocular skin should be excised with frozen section control of surgical margins. Frozen sections probably are unnecessary for some smaller nodulo-ulcerative lesions that have clinically distinct margins. The time-consuming modified MOHS technique is best suited for extensive and deeply infiltrative lesions arising in areas like the inner canthus where the danger of orbital invasion is great. Basal cell carcinoma does not invariably recur after incomplete excision. We frequently find no residual basal cell carcinoma histopathologically when tumors that were reported as having been incompletely removed are re-excised. The initial trauma of surgery or postoperative inflammation may destroy the residual tumor in such cases.

In approximately 0.7% of cases, multiple basal cell carcinomas occur on the face and body of young patients who inherit an autosomal dominantly inherited syndrome that includes a predisposition to the tumor. Patients with the basal cell nevus or Gorlin-Goltz syndrome also have odontogenic keratocysts of the jaw, skeletal anomalies such as bifid ribs, neurologic abnormalities, and endocrine disorders. Basal cell carcinomas from patients with the basal cell nevus syndrome may contain spicules of bone.

Actinic Keratosis and Squamous Cell Carcinoma

Actinic keratosis is a premalignant lesion of squamous cells that develops on the sun-exposed skin of fair-skinned middle-aged individuals. Clinically, these keratoses appear as scaly, keratotic, flat-topped lesions, or erythematous nodules. Microscopy reveals thickened epidermis that is partially replaced by atypical squamous cells (Fig. 13-17). Parakeratosis usually is present, and the granular cell layer is absent. Irregular buds of atypical keratinocytes extend into the papillary dermis at the base of some lesions. The disease spares the openings of the pilosebaceous units. The underlying dermis characteristically shows solar elastosis (elastotic degeneration) similar to that seen in pinguecula and pterygium. The elastotic degeneration stains positively with the Verhoeff–van Gieson stain for elastic tissue. If severe atypia is present but invasion is not present, the diagnosis of squamous cell carcinoma in situ is warranted.

Squamous cell carcinoma of the eyelid is relatively rare compared to basal cell carcinoma. Squamous cell carcinoma typically affects elderly, fair-skinned individuals. Although the lower lid margin is typically involved, squamous cell carcinoma is said to be more common than basal cell carcinoma in the upper lid and outer canthus.

Histopathologically, squamous cell carcinomas are composed of nests, cords, and islands of malignant squamous cells that have abundant eosinophilic cytoplasm and appear "pink" under low power (Figs. 13-16B and 13-18). Reflecting the tumor's invasive malignant potential, tumor cells are seen deep to the plane of the epidermis. More differentiated tumors produce keratin. Squamous cell carcinomas of the eyelid rarely metastasize. Metastatic disease is particularly uncommon if the squamous cell carcinoma has arisen from a preexisting actinic keratosis (Fig. 13-17B).

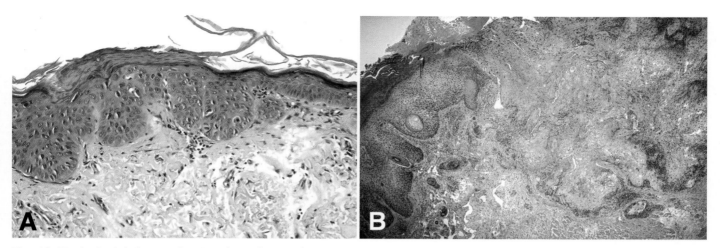

Fig. 13-17. A. Actinic keratosis. A surface plaque of parakeratosis covers a thickened segment of epidermis that is replaced by atypical squamous cells. Irregular buds of atypical keratinocytes extend into the papillary dermis at the base of some lesions. The dermis shows actinic elastosis. Normal epidermis is seen at **right. B. Squamous cell carcinoma arising from actinic keratosis.** Atypical squamous cells remain confined by the basement membrane of the markedly acanthotic epithelium at **left**. Eosinophilic squamous cell carcinoma invades the dermis at **right**. The tumor has incited a chronic inflammatory response. (**A.** H&E ×100, **B.** H&E ×10)

Approximately 12% of patients who had actinic keratosis in one series developed a nonaggressive form of squamous cell carcinoma that had an excellent prognosis compared to squamous cell carcinoma that arose de novo. The incidence of metastatic disease was only 0.5%. A larger study from Australia found a much lower incidence (0.1%) of progression to squamous cell carcinoma. Many actinic keratoses in that series underwent spontaneous regression.

Sebaceous Carcinoma and Other Sebaceous Tumors

Sebaceous carcinoma or **Sebaceous gland carcinoma** is about as common as squamous cell carcinoma of the eyelid. Rarely encountered before age 40, sebaceous carcinoma typically occurs in elderly patients and is also more common in women and Asians. Sebaceous carcinoma has a definite predilection for the sebaceous glands of the eyelid but is quite rare elsewhere in the body. It can arise from the meibomian glands, the glands of Zeis, or rarely the sebaceous glands in the caruncle.

Sebaceous carcinoma is an important tumor that can confound both ophthalmologists and pathologists. Lesions that arise deep in the substance of the lid, for example, meibomian carcinomas, typically cause no abnormalities in the overlying skin until late in the course of the disease. Meibomian gland carcinomas can be confused with chalazia, which typically arise within the tarsal plate. Recurrent or atypical chalazia should be submitted for histopathologic examination.

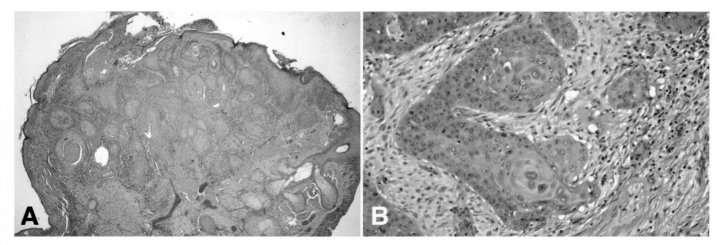

Fig. 13-18. Squamous cell carcinoma. A. Eosinophilic nests of squamous cell carcinoma infiltrate the eyelid margin. A thick layer of surface keratinization is present. **B.** Infiltrating nests of squamous cell carcinoma are composed of neoplastic squamous cells with abundant eosinophilic cytoplasm. (**A.** H&E ×10, **B.** H&E ×100)

Rarely, sebaceous carcinoma presents as a chronic unilateral keratoconjunctivitis that is unresponsive to therapy. This "masquerade syndrome" is caused by the intraepithelial spread of tumor that has replaced the conjunctival epithelium in a pagetoid or bowenoid fashion. Any elderly patient who has unilateral chronic keratoconjunctivitis that does not respond to treatment should be biopsied.

Two thirds of sebaceous carcinomas arise in the upper eyelid, undoubtedly reflecting the greater mass of meibomian gland tissue in the upper lid (Fig. 13-19A). Sebaceous carcinoma grows forming lobules and sheets whose size and shape are somewhat reminiscent of normal sebaceous glands (Fig. 13-19B). Meibomian glands in the tarsus are often completely replaced by tumor. The tumor lobules lack peripheral palisading, and the nuclei of the cells tend to be larger, and more pleomorphic, hyperchromatic, and atypical than those in basal cell carcinoma. Mitotic figures are common and may be abnormal. In well-differentiated cases, the cytoplasm of the tumor cells has a frothy or foamy appearance caused by lipid vacuoles.

Large lobules of sebaceous carcinoma frequently are necrotic centrally, a feature called the comedocarcinoma pattern, which recapitulates the necrobiosis that occurs during normal holocrine secretion (Fig. 13-19C). Another characteristic and extremely important feature of sebaceous carcinoma is the tumor's ability to invade and replace eyelid skin and conjunctival epithelium in a pagetoid fashion (Fig. 13-19D). The term pagetoid derives from the similarity of this process to Paget disease of the nipple, which is marked by replacement of the epidermis by breast carcinoma cells. The observation of pagetoid involvement of the skin or conjunctiva helps to confirm the diagnosis of sebaceous carcinoma. The ability to invade and replace the conjunctival epithelium is one of the tumor's most insidious features. A relatively small eyelid tumor can give rise to extensive intraepithelial spread. Histopathologically, the affected segments of conjunctival epithelium are thickened and often are totally replaced by tumor cells (Fig. 13-19F,G). The infiltrated epithelium is often poorly adherent and may be lost or desquamated leading to nondiagnostic biopsies.

Fat stains such as oil red O can help to confirm the diagnosis by demonstrating the presence of intracytoplasmic lipid. They must be performed on frozen sections, however, because the solvents used in normal tissue processing and paraffin embedding dissolve fat (Fig. 13-19C). In practice, experienced ocular pathologists perform fat stains infrequently, reserving it for exceptional cases with equivocal sebaceous differentiation. However, pathologists who are less familiar with the tumor may wish to confirm the presence of lipid. Surgeons who suspect sebaceous carcinoma clinically should always inform the pathologist, so wet tissue can be reserved for possible fat stains.

Immunohistochemical techniques for diagnosing sebaceous carcinoma are not particularly satisfactory as they tend to work best on well-differentiated cases that are easily diagnosed using routine sections. One protocol recommends the use of epithelial membrane antigen (EMA), CAM 5.2 and breast marker BRST-1. Sebaceous carcinoma often stains with EMA and shows focal immunoreactivity with BRST-1. P-16 readily highlights pagetoid cells within the epidermis and conjunctival epithelium.

Sebaceous carcinoma can spread by direct extension and can metastasize to regional lymph nodes and distant sites such as lung, liver, brain, and skull. Tumor mortality was estimated to be about 15% in a large series by Rao et al. from the Armed Forces Institute of Pathology that included many advanced lesions. Factors associated with poor prognosis include origin from the upper eyelid, tumor diameter >10 mm, origin from meibomian glands, duration of symptoms before diagnosis >6 months, an infiltrative growth pattern, poor sebaceous differentiation, extensive pagetoid invasion, and invasion of lymphatics, vessels, and the orbit.

Early diagnosis and treatment are important. No fatal tumors were reported in recent series, reflecting increased awareness of sebaceous carcinoma by ophthalmologists. Wide local excision with frozen section control of surgical margins should be performed. Radiation should be reserved only for palliation of advanced cases that refuse or cannot tolerate radical surgery. Orbital exenteration is performed in many institutions if there is orbital invasion or extensive pagetoid replacement of the conjunctiva. Some have questioned whether exenteration is excessive therapy for the latter, which essentially is an *in situ* disease process. Cryotherapy of conjunctival disease has been advocated to treat this diffuse, yet relatively localized form of the disease. Topical chemotherapy with mitomycin C has been used to treat intraepithelial sebaceous carcinoma in some instances.

Senile sebaceous gland hyperplasia and sebaceous adenoma are other sebaceous lesions that occur on facial and eyelid skin. Relatively common, senile sebaceous gland hyperplasia appears as a nodule that may be umbilicated and often is misdiagnosed as basal cell carcinoma. Histopathology shows mature sebaceous gland lobules surrounding a central dilated duct (Fig. 13-20A).

Sebaceous adenoma is a rare tumor composed of irregular lobules of incompletely differentiated sebaceous glands composed of foamy sebaceous cells, nonlipidized germinative cells, and intermediate cells (Fig. 13-20B). The lobules are not arranged around a duct. Multiple sebaceous gland neoplasms, especially sebaceous adenomas, are associated with visceral cancer, especially colon carcinoma, in the Muir-Torre syndrome, which is caused by inherited defects in DNA mismatch repair genes MSH2 and MLH1.

Melanocytic Lesions

Melanocytic nevi are relatively common eyelid lesions. They are often misdiagnosed preoperatively when they are amelanotic or papillary in configuration. Nevi are classified as junctional, intradermal, or compound. Junctional

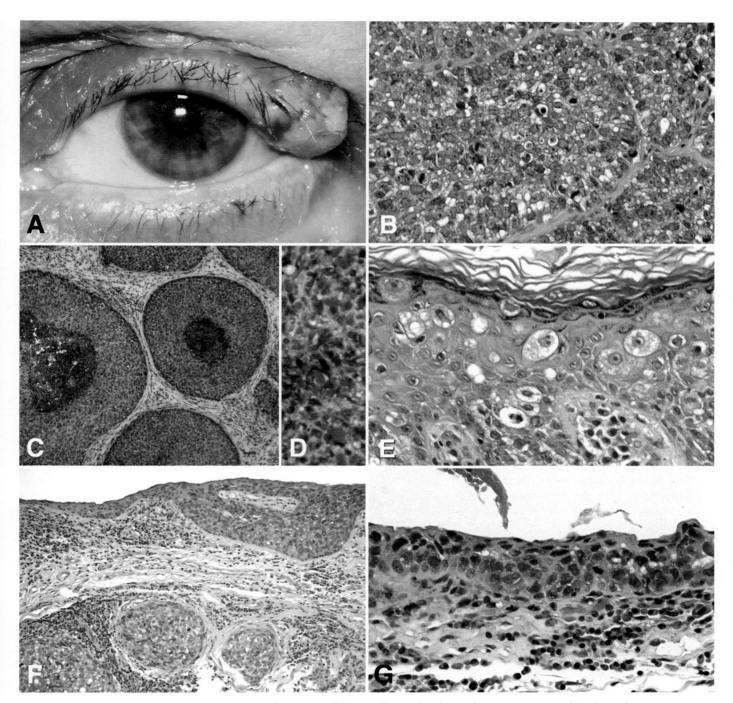

Fig. 13-19. Sebaceous carcinoma. A. Tumor of upper eyelid has yellow color that indicates presence of lipid. Madarosis is present. **B.** Tumor is composed of lobules of cells with foamy vacuolated cytoplasm. Numerous mitoses are present. Peripheral palisading is not seen. **C.** Large lobules of sebaceous carcinoma show central necrosis (comedocarcinoma pattern) mimicking holocrine secretion. **D.** Oil red O stain performed on frozen sectioned material confirms the presence of lipid in cytoplasmic vacuoles. **E. Pagetoid invasion of eyelid skin by sebaceous carcinoma.** Individual tumor cells with vacuolated cytoplasm from an underlying sebaceous carcinoma infiltrate the epidermis in a fashion analogous to Paget disease of the breast. **F.** Tarsal conjunctiva shows intraepithelial sebaceous carcinoma. Lobules of tumor are present in tarsal plate. **G.** Intraepithelial sebaceous carcinoma, conjunctiva. Atypical cells with large, hyperchromatic nuclei and cytoplasmic vacuoles replace basal half of conjunctival epithelium. (**B.** H&E ×100, **C.** Oil red O ×50, **D.** Oil red O ×250, **E.** H&E ×100, **F.** H&E ×50, **G.** H&E ×100)

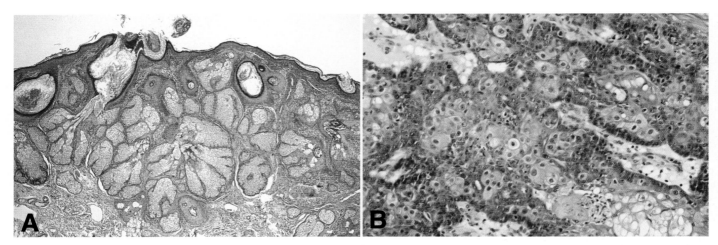

Fig. 13-20. A. Senile sebaceous gland hyperplasia. Lobules of mature benign hyperplastic sebaceous glands form a nodule in the dermis. These show typical arrangement around central duct. The nodule was misdiagnosed as basal cell carcinoma preoperatively. **B. Sebaceous adenoma.** Incompletely lipidized cells comprising low-grade sebaceous neoplasm form disorderly lobules. Differential diagnosis included sebaceous adenoma or low-grade sebaceous carcinoma. Sebaceous adenomas serve as a clinical marker for systemic malignancy in patients with the Muir-Torre syndrome. (**A.** H&E ×10, **B.** H&E ×100)

nevi are flat, pigmented, and relatively rare. The nevus cells in junctional nevi are confined to the junction between the epidermis and the dermis. Junctional activity is much more common in younger patients. As we age, nevus cells tend to leave the epidermal-dermal junction and migrate into the underlying dermis. Most nevi submitted to ophthalmic pathology laboratories are intradermal (or dermal) nevi (Fig. 13-21A). They are often papillomatous, pedunculated, or dome-shaped; bear hairs; and are frequently amelanotic or only slightly pigmented. Because a junctional component is absent, malignant transformation almost never occurs. Microscopy shows infiltration of the dermis by nevus cells arranged in nests. A cell-free collagenous grenz zone (*grenz*, German for border) separates the nevus cells in the dermis from the epidermis. The nevus

cells in intradermal nevi typically show polarity, that is, the cellular morphology changes with location. Large type A nevus cells are found in the upper dermis. Type B cells found in the mid-dermis are smaller and are often lymphocytoid (i.e., they superficially resemble lymphocytes). Type C cells in the lower dermis have little or no melanin and tend to appear fibroblastic with spindled nuclei. In elderly individuals, the deeper cells may have a distinctly neural appearance. Benign nevi can infiltrate the deeper structures in the lid and occasionally may contain multinucleated giant cells. If one observes mitotic figures, atypical cells with prominent nucleoli, or an intense infiltrate of inflammatory cells in a nevus, or finds "junctional activity" or epithelial involvement in an older patient, the diagnosis may be malignant melanoma.

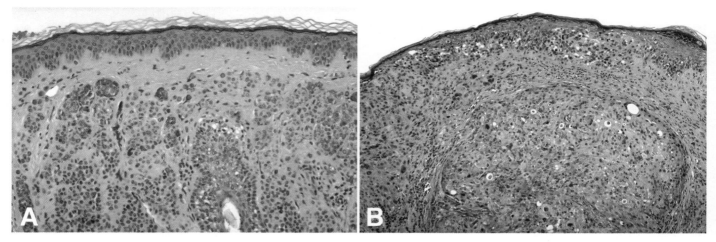

Fig. 13-21. A. Intradermal nevus. Nests of benign nevus cells infiltrate the dermis. An acellular "grenz" zone separates the nevus cells from the epidermis. No junctional activity persists. Some of the cells are lightly pigmented. **B. Malignant melanoma, eyelid.** Lobules of frankly malignant melanocytes including epithelioid cells invade the dermis. The basal half of the overlying epidermis is replaced by atypical melanocytic hyperplasia. (**A.** H&E ×25, **B.** H&E ×50)

Compound nevi usually are slightly elevated, papillomatous, and pigmented. The term compound indicates that nevus cells occur both at the junction and in the dermis. Other forms of nevi occasionally are encountered. Blue nevi are composed of heavily pigmented spindled or dendritic melanocytes that are located in the deeper tissues. The gray blue skin pigmentation in the Nevus of Ota (congenital oculodermal melanocytosis) is caused by an extensive blue nevus. Cellular blue nevi can undergo malignant transformation into melanoma.

Malignant melanomas of eyelid skin (Fig. 13-21B) are relatively rare tumors that constitute <1% of eyelid malignancies. The prognosis of skin melanoma depends on the type of tumor, its thickness, and depth of invasion. Lentigo maligna melanoma has the best prognosis. It develops in elderly individuals who have lentigo maligna or Hutchinson malignant freckle. Patients with nodular melanoma tend to do poorly, while the prognosis of superficial spreading melanoma is intermediate.

Adnexal Tumors

A variety of eyelid neoplasms are derived from adnexal structures such as sweat glands and hair follicles. Most are quite rare. Syringomas are relatively common benign tumors of eccrine sweat glands that occur as multiple flesh-colored nodules on the faces of young women. Histopathology discloses small cysts and/or comma or tadpole-shaped ductules lined by a dual layer of eccrine ductal epithelium embedded in a dense fibrous stroma (Fig. 13-22). Primary malignant sweat gland tumors also occur on the eyelid. Primary mucous secreting adenocarcinoma of sweat gland origin, which is probably the fifth most common primary malignant eyelid tumor, has a relatively high incidence (38%) of distant metastasis (Fig. 13-23B). Some eccrine adenocarcinomas are composed of signet ring

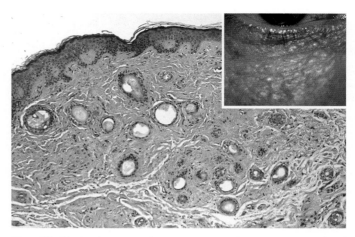

Fig. 13-22. Syringoma. Syringomas are benign sweat gland tumors. Oval and comma or tadpole-shaped epithelial ductules are found amidst dense fibrous stroma. The ducts mimic the straight dermal duct of eccrine sweat glands. Syringomas often occur as multiple elevated papules on the facial skin of young women (**inset**) (H&E ×50)

cells. A malignant variant of syringoma called microcystic carcinoma can present with enophthalmos, like scirrhous breast carcinoma. Microcystic carcinoma has little metastatic potential, but it deeply infiltrates the lid and orbit, causing stromal desmoplasia. Apocrine tumors of the eyelid include syringocystadenoma papilliferum (Fig. 13-23A) and rare adenomas and adenocarcinomas of the glands of Moll.

Tumors of hair follicle origin include trichofolliculomas, trichoadenomas, trichoepitheliomas, trichilemmomas, and pilomatrixomas. Most of these "tricky" tumors are rare and are a diagnostic challenge to dermatopathologists. Pilomatrixoma (or pilomatricoma), which often presents as a reddish nodule on the upper lid or brow

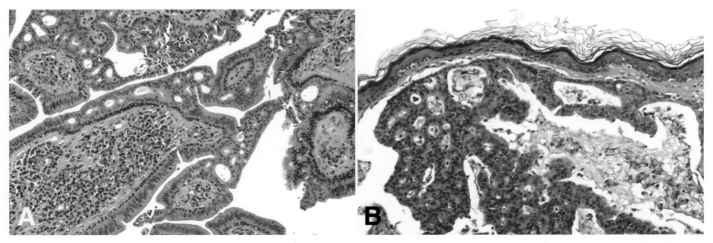

Fig. 13-23. A. Syringocystadenoma papilliferum. A papillary proliferation of benign apocrine sweat glandular epithelium lines and partially fills cystic spaces in the dermis. Plasma cells infiltrate the stroma. The overlying epidermis was acanthotic. **B. Primary mucous-secreting sweat gland carcinoma.** Pools of mucous surround cords of malignant sweat gland epithelium. Primary sweat gland carcinomas can metastasize but fortunately are quite rare. A metastasis to the lid from a distant primary carcinoma must be excluded clinically. (**A.** H&E ×50, **B.** H&E ×50)

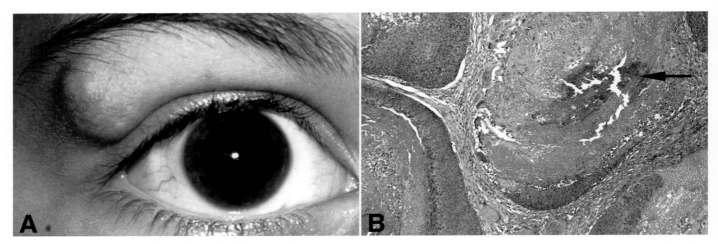

Fig. 13-24. Pilomatrixoma (calcifying epithelioma of Malherbe). A. Tumor beneath brow in child appears clinically as slightly erythematous subepidermal nodule. **B.** Tumor is composed of viable hair matrix cells, which are basophilic, and sheets of nonviable eosinophilic shadow cells. *Arrow* denotes focus of dystrophic calcification in necrotic area. (**B.** H&E ×50)

of young patients, is relatively common (Fig. 13-24). Both its eponymic designation (the calcifying epithelioma of Malherbe) and its histopathologic features are memorable. Pilomatrixoma contains sheets of bland, uniform, basophilic cells (hair matrix cells) that readily undergo necrosis forming eosinophilic shadow cells with ghostly nuclei. Dystrophic calcification characteristically develops in the necrotic areas, and a prominent foreign body giant cell response to the sheets of dead cells typically is observed.

Other Lesions

Xanthelasmas are soft, flat or slightly elevated, yellowish plaques that typically occur near the inner canthi (Fig. 13-25A). Cosmesis often is an indication for removal. Xanthelasmas are predominantly dermal lesions. Histopathologic examination reveals sheets of foamy, lipid-laden histiocytes (xanthoma cells) that tend to aggregate around vessels in the dermis (Fig. 13-25B). The epidermis is normal. Although xanthelasmas occasionally signify hyperlipidemia, two thirds of patients have normal lipids. Indurated, atypical xanthelasma-like lesions are eyelid markers for several xanthogranulomatous disorders including Erdheim-Chester disease, necrobiotic xanthogranuloma, and orbital xanthogranuloma with adult onset asthma. The xanthogranulomatous infiltrates in the latter disorders are deeper and more extensive than that seen in xanthelasma and typically contain Touton giant cells. Bilateral orbital infiltration, retroperitoneal fibrosis, and characteristic bone lesions occur in Erdheim-Chester disease, a rare and potentially fatal systemic disorder. The xanthogranulomatous infiltrate in patients with adult onset asthma usually contains foci of follicular lymphoid hyperplasia (Fig. 13-26).

Multiple waxy nodules located along the eyelid margins that contain acellular eosinophilic hyaline material of unknown composition are found in autosomal recessively inherited lipoid proteinosis or Urbach-Wiethe disease.

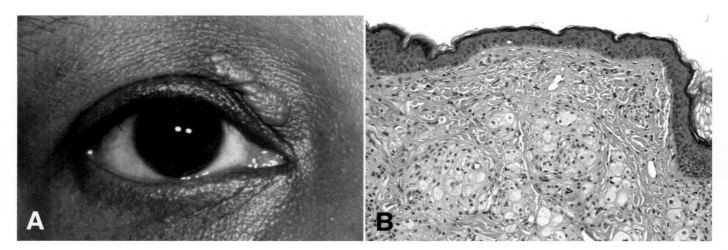

Fig. 13-25. Xanthelasma. A. Elevated yellowish plaque involves inner canthal skin of upper lid. **B.** The dermis contains an infiltrate of xanthoma cells (lipid-laden histiocytes). The epidermis is normal. (**B.** H&E ×50)

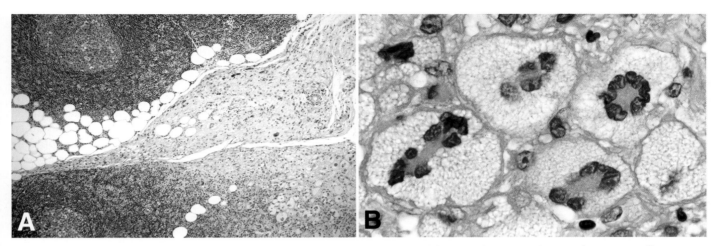

Fig. 13-26. Orbital xanthogranuloma with adult-onset asthma. A. Orbital biopsy shows xanthogranulomatous inflammation with Touton giant cells and benign follicular lymphoid hyperplasia with germinal centers. **B.** Higher magnification of Touton giant cells. (**A.** H&E ×25, **B.** H&E ×250)

Patients who have primary systemic amyloidosis may develop multiple confluent waxy purpuric papules on the eyelid skin that hemorrhage spontaneously or after minor trauma. The AI amyloid deposits are composed of immunoglobulin light chains. Slightly elevated or umbilicated papules, which may be partially depigmented in blacks, are an eyelid manifestation of sarcoidosis. Histopathology shows noncaseating granulomas. Multiple eyelid nodules and severe mutilating arthritis occur in patients with multicentric reticulohistiocytosis.

Eyelid Markers for Systemic Malignancy

Rare eyelid tumors serve as clinical markers for internal malignancy in patients with several hereditary syndromes. Trichilemmomas of the eyelid have been reported in Cowden multiple hamartoma-neoplasia syndrome, which predisposes to the development of breast cancer in one third of affected women. Sebaceous adenomas, other sebaceous neoplasms and keratoacanthomas occur in Muir-Torre syndrome, a variant of the Lynch or hereditary nonpolyposis colorectal cancer syndrome (Fig. 13-20B). Myxomas of the eyelid (Fig. 13-27A,B) and spotty lentiginous pigmentation of the lids and conjunctiva, which often involves the caruncle and semilunar fold, are ocular markers for cardiac myxomas, endocrine abnormalities, and rare testicular tumors in autosomal dominantly inherited Carney complex, caused by mutations in the PRKAR1A gene on chromosome 17q. Atypical xanthelasma-like lesions that contain xanthoma

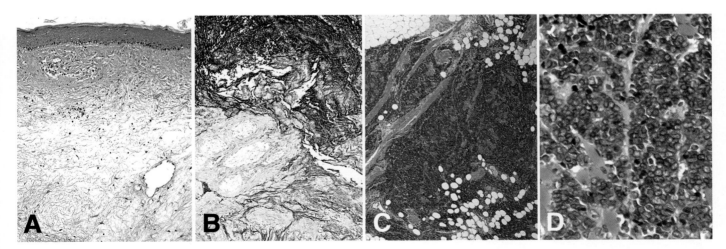

Fig. 13-27. Eyelid myxoma, Carney complex. A. Lucent pools of relatively acellular mucin are present deep in the dermis. **B.** The alcian blue stain confirms the presence of acid mucopolysaccharide. The patient had Carney syndrome, an autosomal dominantly inherited syndrome that includes multiple myxomas, spotty mucocutaneous pigmentation, and endocrine abnormalities. **C. Merkel cell tumor.** Primary neuroendocrine tumor of eyelid skin infiltrates orbicularis muscle. **D.** Lobules of poorly differentiated basophilic cells lack peripheral palisading. Tumor was immunoreactive for keratin, neuron specific enolase, and chromogranin. (**A.** H&E ×50, **B.** alcian blue ×100, **C.** H&E ×25, **D.** H&E ×100)

cells, Touton giant cells, cholesterol clefts, and foci of necrobiosis are found in patients with necrobiotic xanthogranuloma who may have systemic monoclonal gammopathies and plasma cell dyscrasias. Patients with the Brooke-Spiegler syndrome develop multiple skin appendage tumors of the head and neck including cylindromas, trichoepitheliomas, and spiradenomas.

Other rare malignant eyelid tumors include metastases from distant primary cancers and the trabecular carcinoma or Merkel cell tumor (Fig. 13-27C,D). A cutaneous APUDoma, the Merkel cell tumor typically presents as a violaceous or reddish-blue nodule. The tumor is a neuroendocrine neoplasm of the skin that has a carcinoid-like histology. Electron microscopy shows dense core neurosecretory granules and immunohistochemistry typically shows the dual expression of epithelial markers and neural markers chromogranin and neuron specific enolase. Dotlike staining for cytokeratin 20 (CK 20) distinguishes Merkel cell tumor from metastatic small cell carcinoma. The fatality rate is 20%. Merkel cell tumor should be locally resected with frozen section control of surgical margins.

Lacrimal Drainage System

Tears are drained into the nose through the nasolacrimal drainage system, which is located nasally and is composed of the puncta, canaliculi, lacrimal sac, and nasolacrimal duct. The puncta are the openings of the canaliculi. They are located in upper and lower eyelids near the inner canthus. The canaliculi are small tubules lined with epithelium that run from the puncta to the lacrimal sac. The lacrimal sac is located the lacrimal fossa in anteromedial wall of the orbit. A downward extension of the lacrimal sac called the nasolacrimal duct enters the nasal cavity on the lateral wall of the inferior nasal meatus. The nasolacrimal duct is enclosed in a bony canal about 12 mm long.

Congenital obstruction of the nasal lacrimal duct is a relatively common cause of tearing (epiphora) in infants. This usually is caused by incomplete canalization of the duct near its lower end. Chronic dacryocystitis is the most common cause of nasolacrimal duct obstruction or stenosis in adults. Surgical specimens obtained at dacryocystorhinostomy typically contain an infiltrate of lymphocytes and plasma cells in the wall of the lacrimal sac (Fig. 13-28A). Concretions or casts occasionally are found within the lumina of the canaliculi or sac. These include masses of the Gram-positive filamentous fungus Actinomyces (Fig. 13-28B) and dacryoliths composed of laminated inspissated protein that may contain fungal elements. Chronic nasolacrimal duct obstruction can predispose to acute bacterial infection of the lacrimal sac (acute dacryocystitis).

Neoplasms of the lacrimal sac are a rare cause of nasolacrimal duct obstruction and recurrent dacryocystitis. In addition to tearing, patients present with a mass in the inner canthal region that is situated below the medial canthal tendon. Hemorrhage (bloody discharge or epistaxis) and pain are signs suggestive of a malignant neoplasm.

Most lacrimal sac tumors are papillomatous neoplasms that arise from the epithelial lining of the sac (Fig. 13-29). They include exophytic and inverted papillomas composed of squamous cells, transitional cells, or a mixture of both. The papillomas may be benign, show focal atypia, or progress to invasive carcinoma. Invasive carcinoma typically arises from papillomas that have an inverted growth pattern. Less than one third of lacrimal gland tumors are nonepithelial. Lymphomas, malignant melanomas, fibrous histiocytomas, hemangiopericytomas, neurilemmomas, and angiosarcomas occasionally occur in this site.

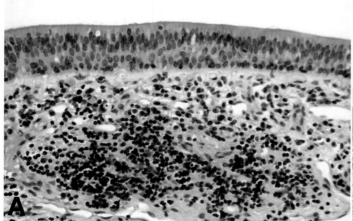
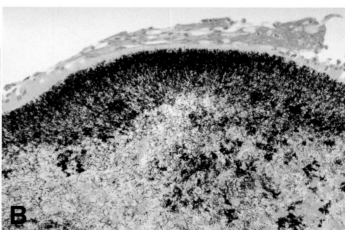

Fig. 13-28. A. Chronic nongranulomatous dacryocystitis. Infiltrate of lymphocytes and plasma cells is present in stroma beneath respiratory epithelial lining of lacrimal sac. **B. Actinomycotic lacrimal cast.** Mass of Gram-positive filamentous fungi removed from canaliculus has laminated appearance. (**A.** H&E ×100, **B.** Gram stain ×100)

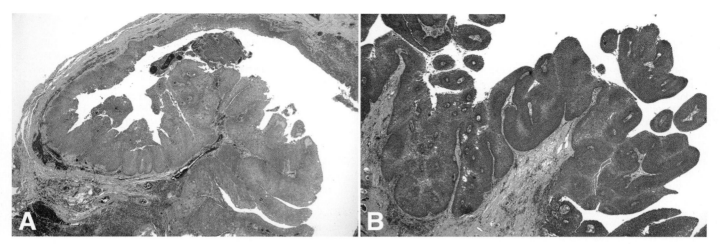

Fig. 13-29. A. Papillary squamous carcinoma, lacrimal sac. Exophytic papillary epithelial tumor partially fills lumen of the lacrimal sac. Foci of squamous differentiation are present. **B. Inverted papilloma, lacrimal sac.** Acanthotic fronds of transitional epithelium invade stroma. Most lacrimal gland carcinomas arise from inverted papillomas. (**A.** H&E ×10, **B.** H&E ×25)

BIBLIOGRAPHY

General References

Eagle RC Jr. Specimen handling in the ophthalmic pathology laboratory. In: Grossniklaus HE, Margo CE, eds. *Advances in Ophthalmic Pathology. Ophthalmol Clin North Am* 1995;8:1–15.

Font RL. Eyelids and lacrimal drainage system. In: Spencer W, ed. *Ophthalmic Pathology: An Atlas and Textbook*, 4th ed, vol. 2. Philadelphia, PA: WB Saunders, 1996:2218–2437.

Lever WF, Schaumburg-Lever G. *Histopathology of the Skin*, 7th ed. Philadelphia, PA: JB Lippincott, 1990.

Developmental Lesions

Boyd PA, Keeling JW, Lindenbaum RH. Fraser syndrome (cryptophthalmos-syndactyly syndrome): a review of eleven cases with postmortem findings. *Am J Med Genet* 1988;31:159–168.

Culbertson WW, Ostler HB. The floppy eyelid syndrome. *Am J Ophthalmol* 1981;92:568–575.

Ellis FJ, Eagle RC Jr, Shields JA. Phakomatous choristoma (Zimmerman's tumor): immunohistochemical confirmation of lens-specific proteins. *Ophthalmology* 1993;100:955–960.

Kidwell ED, Tenzel RR. Repair of congenital colobomas of the lids. *Arch Ophthalmol* 1979;97:1931–1932.

Mansour AM, Wang F, Henkind P, et al. Ocular findings in the facio-auriculovertebral sequence (Goldenhar-Gorlin syndrome). *Am J Ophthalmol* 1985;100:555–559.

Pe'er J, BenEzra D, Sela M, et al. Cryptophthalmos syndrome. Clinical and histopathological findings. *Ophthalmic Paediatr Genet* 1987;8:177–182.

Schauer GM, Dunn LK, Godmilow L, et al. Prenatal diagnosis of Fraser syndrome at 18.5 weeks gestation, with autopsy findings at 19 weeks. *Am J Med Genet* 1990;37:583–591.

Schwartz LK, Gelender H, Forster RK. Chronic conjunctivitis associated with 'floppy eyelids'. *Arch Ophthalmol* 1983;101:1884–1888.

Stefanyszyn MA, Hidayat AA, Flanagan JC. The histopathology of involutional ectropion. *Ophthalmology* 1985;92:120–127.

Waardenburg P. A new syndrome combining developmental anomalies of the eyelids, eyebrows and nose root with pigmentary defects of the iris and headhair with congenital deafness. *Am J Hum Genet* 1951;3:195–253.

Whitaker LA, Katowitz JA, Jacobs WE. Ocular adnexal problems in craniofacial deformities. *J Maxillofac Surg* 1979;7:55–60.

Benign Lesions

Al-Hazzaa SA, Hidayat AA. Molluscum contagiosum of the eyelid and infraorbital margin—a clinicopathologic study with light and electron microscopic observations. *J Pediatr Ophthalmol Strabismus* 1993;30:58–59.

Averbuch D, Jaouni T, Pe'er J, et al. Confluent molluscum contagiosum covering the eyelids of an HIV-positive child. *Clin Experiment Ophthalmol* 2009;37:525–527.

Boniuk M, Zimmerman LE. Eyelid tumors with reference to lesions confused with squamous cell carcinoma. II. Inverted follicular keratosis. *Arch Ophthalmol* 1963;69:698–707.

Henderer JD, Tanenbaum M. Excision of multiple eyelid apocrine hidrocystomas via an en-bloc lower eyelid blepharoplasty incision. *Ophthalmic Surg Lasers* 2000;31:157–161.

Kwitko ML, Boniuk M, Zimmerman LE. Eyelid tumors with reference to lesions confused with squamous cell carcinoma. I. Incidence and errors in diagnosis. *Arch Ophthalmol* 1963;69:693–697.

Leahey AB, Shane JJ, Listhaus A, et al. Molluscum contagiosum eyelid lesions as the initial manifestation of acquired immunodeficiency syndrome. *Am J Ophthalmol* 1997;124:240–241.

Luque Aranda R, Baquero Aranda I, Salido Hidalgo C, et al. Molluscum contagiosum in a patient with no risk factors. *Eur J Ophthalmol* 2006;16:621–623.

Mencia-Gutierrez E, Gutierrez-Diaz E, Redondo-Marcos I, et al. Cutaneous horns of the eyelid: a clinicopathological study of 48 cases. *J Cutan Pathol* 2004;31:539–543.

Mulugeta A. Giant molluscum contagiosum presenting as a tumour in an HIV-infected patient: case report. *Ethiop Med J* 2000;38:125–130.

Perez-Blazquez E, Villafruela I, Madero S. Eyelid molluscum contagiosum in patients with human immunodeficiency virus infection. *Orbit* 1999;18:75–81.

Robinson MR, Udell IJ, Garber PF, et al. Molluscum contagiosum of the eyelids in patients with acquired immune deficiency syndrome. *Ophthalmology* 1992;99:1745–1747.

Sassani JW, Yanoff M. Inverted follicular keratosis. *Am J Ophthalmol* 1979;87:810–813.

Shields JA, Eagle RC Jr, Shields CL, et al. Apocrine hidrocystoma of the eyelid. *Arch Ophthalmol* 1993;111:866–867.

Keratoacanthoma

Boniuk M, Zimmerman LE. Eyelid tumors with reference to lesions confused with squamous cell carcinoma. III. Keratoacanthoma. *Arch Ophthalmol* 1967;77:29–40.

Cribier B. Keratoacanthoma? Better to say "squamous cell carcinoma, keratoacanthoma type". *Ann Dermatol Venereol* 2008;135:541–546.

Grossniklaus HE, Wojno TH, Yanoff M, et al. Invasive keratoacanthoma of the eyelid and ocular adnexa. *Ophthalmology* 1996;103:937–941.

Hodak E, Jones RE, Ackerman AB. Solitary keratoacanthoma is a squamous-cell carcinoma: three examples with metastases. *Am J Dermatopathol* 1993;15:332–342.

Mandrell JC, Santa Cruz D. Keratoacanthoma: hyperplasia, benign neoplasm, or a type of squamous cell carcinoma? *Semin Diagn Pathol* 2009;26:150–163.

Requena L, Romero E, Sanchez M, et al. Aggressive keratoacanthoma of the eyelid: "malignant" keratoacanthoma or squamous cell carcinoma? *J Dermatol Surg Oncol* 1990;16:564–568.

Tan KB, Lee YS. Immunoexpression of Bcl-x in squamous cell carcinoma and keratoacanthoma: differences in pattern and correlation with pathobiology. *Histopathology* 2009;55: 338–345.

Basal Cell Carcinoma

Doxanas MT, Green WR, Iliff CE. Factors in the successful surgical management of basal cell carcinoma of the eyelid. *Am J Ophthalmol* 1981;91:726–736.

Einaugler RB, Henkind P. Basal cell carcinoma of the eyelid: apparent incomplete removal. *Am J Ophthalmol* 1969;67:413–417.

Honavar SG, Shields JA, Shields CL, et al. Basal cell carcinoma of the eyelid associated with Gorlin-Goltz syndrome. *Ophthalmology* 2001;108:1115–1123.

Jakobiec FA, Hanna E, Townsend DJ. Basal cell carcinoma of the eyelid with exceptional histomorphologic expressions. *Ophthal Plast Reconstr Surg* 2009;25:232–234.

Kimonis VE, Goldstein AM, Pastakia B, et al. Clinical manifestations in 105 persons with nevoid basal cell carcinoma syndrome. *Am J Med Genet* 1997;69:299–308.

Kimonis VE, Mehta SG, Digiovanna JJ, et al. Radiological features in 82 patients with nevoid basal cell carcinoma (NBCC or Gorlin) syndrome. *Genet Med* 2004;6:495–502.

Margo CE, Waltz K. Basal cell carcinoma of the eyelid and periocular skin. *Surv Ophthalmol* 1993;38:169–192.

Shields CL. Basal cell carcinoma of the eyelids. *Int Ophthalmol Clin* 1993;33:1–4.

Squamous Cell Carcinoma and Predisposing Lesions

Caya JG, Hidayat AA, Weiner JM. A clinicopathologic study of 21 cases of adenoid squamous cell carcinoma of the eyelid and periorbital region. *Am J Ophthalmol* 1985;99:291–297.

Dailey JR, Kennedy RH, Flaharty PM, et al. Squamous cell carcinoma of the eyelid. *Ophthal Plast Reconstr Surg* 1994;10:153–159.

Faustina M, Diba R, Ahmadi MA, et al. Patterns of regional and distant metastasis in patients with eyelid and periocular squamous cell carcinoma. *Ophthalmology* 2004;111:1930–1932.

Gaasterland DE, Rodrigues MM, Moshell AN. Ocular involvement in xeroderma pigmentosa. *Ophthalmology* 1982;89:980–986.

Hadi U, Tohmeh H, Maalouf R. Squamous cell carcinoma of the lower lid in a 19-month-old girl with xeroderma pigmentosum. *Eur Arch Otorhinolaryngol* 2000;257:77–79.

Lopez-Tizon E, Mencia-Gutierrez E, Garrido-Ruiz M, et al. Clinicopathological study of 21 cases of eyelid actinic keratosis. *Int Ophthalmol* 2009;29:379–384.

Lund HZ. How often does squamous cell carcinoma of the eyelid metastasize. *Arch Dermatol* 1965;92:635–637.

Marks R, Foley P, Goodman G, et al. Spontaneous remission of solar keratoses: the case for conservative management. *Br J Dermatol* 1986;115:649–655.

Proia AD, Selim MA, Reutter JC, et al. Basal cell-signet-ring squamous cell carcinoma of the eyelid. *Arch Pathol Lab Med* 2006;130:393–396.

Reifler DM, Hornblass A. Squamous cell carcinoma of the eyelid. *Surv Ophthalmol* 1986;30:349–365.

Scott KR, Kronish JW. Premalignant lesions and squamous cell carcinoma. In: Albert DM, Jakobiec FA, eds. *Principles and Practice of Ophthalmology: Clinical Practice*, vol. 3. Philadelphia, PA: WB Saunders, 1994:1733–1744.

Sullivan TJ. Squamous cell carcinoma of eyelid, periocular, and periorbital skin. *Int Ophthalmol Clin* 2009;49:17–24.

Sullivan TJ, Boulton JE, Whitehead KJ. Intraepidermal carcinoma of the eyelid. *Clin Experiment Ophthalmol* 2002;30:23–27.

Sebaceous Tumors

Abbas O, Mahalingam M. Cutaneous sebaceous neoplasms as markers of Muir-Torre syndrome: a diagnostic algorithm. *J Cutan Pathol* 2009;36:613–619.

Demirci H, Nelson CC, Shields CL, et al. Eyelid sebaceous carcinoma associated with Muir-Torre syndrome in two cases. *Ophthal Plast Reconstr Surg* 2007;23:77–79.

Dores GM, Curtis RE, Toro JR, et al. Incidence of cutaneous sebaceous carcinoma and risk of associated neoplasms: insight into Muir-Torre syndrome. *Cancer* 2008;113:3372–3381.

Doxanas MT, Green WR. Sebaceous gland carcinoma. Review of 40 cases. *Arch Ophthalmol* 1984;102:245–249.

Font RL, Rishi K. Sebaceous gland adenoma of the tarsal conjunctiva in a patient with Muir-Torre syndrome. *Ophthalmology* 2003;110:1833–1836.

Hidayat AA, Font RL. Sebaceous carcinoma of the eyelids and caruncle of eyelid and eyebrow: a clinicopathologic study of 31 cases. *Arch Ophthalmol* 1980;98: 844–847.

Honavar SG, Shields CL, Maus M, et al. Primary intraepithelial sebaceous gland carcinoma of the palpebral conjunctiva. *Arch Ophthalmol* 2001;119:764–767.

Jakobiec FA, Zimmerman LE, La Piana F, et al. Unusual eyelid tumors with sebaceous differentiation in the Muir-Torre syndrome. Rapid clinical regrowth and frank squamous transformation after biopsy. *Ophthalmology* 1988;95:1543–1548.

Jakobiec FA. Sebaceous adenoma of the eyelid and visceral malignancy. *Am J Ophthalmol* 1974;78:952–960.

Jakobiec FA. Sebaceous tumors of the ocular adnexa. In: Albert DM, Jakobiec FA, eds. *Principles and Practice of Ophthalmology: Clinical Practice*, vol. 3. Philadelphia, PA: WB Saunders, 1994:1745–1770.

Margo CE, Grossniklaus HE. Intraepithelial sebaceous neoplasia without underlying invasive carcinoma. *Surv Ophthalmol* 1995;39:293–301.

Pettey AA, Walsh JS. Muir-Torre syndrome: a case report and review of the literature. *Cutis* 2005;75:149–155.

Rao NA, Hidayat AA, McLean IW, et al. Sebaceous gland carcinoma of the ocular adnexa: a clinicopathologic study of 104 cases with five year follow-up data. *Hum Pathol* 1982;13:113–122.

Rishi K, Font RL. Sebaceous gland tumors of the eyelids and conjunctiva in the Muir-Torre syndrome: a clinicopathologic study of five cases and literature review. *Ophthal Plast Reconstr Surg* 2004;20:31–36.

Shields JA, Demirci H, Marr BP, et al. Conjunctival epithelial involvement by eyelid sebaceous carcinoma. The 2003 J. Howard Stokes lecture. *Ophthal Plast Reconstr Surg* 2005;21:92–96.

Shields JA, Demirci H, Marr BP, et al. Sebaceous carcinoma of the eyelids: personal experience with 60 cases. *Ophthalmology* 2004;111:2151–2157.

Shields JA, Demirci H, Marr BP, et al. Sebaceous carcinoma of the ocular region: a review. *Surv Ophthalmol* 2005;50:103–122.

Sinard JH. Immunohistochemical distinction of ocular sebaceous carcinoma from basal cell and squamous cell carcinoma. *Arch Ophthalmol* 1999;117:776–783.

Singh AD, Mudhar HS, Bhola R, et al. Sebaceous adenoma of the eyelid in Muir-Torre syndrome. *Arch Ophthalmol* 2005;123: 562–565.

Wolfe JT III, Yeatts RP, Wick MR, et al. Sebaceous carcinoma of the eyelid: errors in clinical and pathological diagnosis. *Am J Surg Pathol* 1984;8:597–606.

Melanocytic Lesions

Chan FM, O'Donnell BA, Whitehead K, et al. Treatment and outcomes of malignant melanoma of the eyelid: a review of 29 cases in Australia. *Ophthalmology* 2007;114:187–92.

Esmaeli B, Youssef A, Naderi A, et al. Margins of excision for cutaneous melanoma of the eyelid skin: the Collaborative Eyelid Skin Melanoma Group Report. *Ophthal Plast Reconstr Surg* 2003;19: 96–101.

Margo C. Pigmented lesions of the eyelid. In: Albert DM, Jakobiec FA, eds. *Principles and Practice of Ophthalmology: Clinical Practice*, vol. 3. Philadelphia, PA: WB Saunders, 1994:1797–1812.

Naidoff MA, Bernardino VB Jr, Clark WH. Melanocytic lesions of the eyelid skin. *Am J Ophthalmol* 1976;82: 371–382.

Putterman AM. Intradermal nevi of the eyelid. *Ophthalmic Surg* 1980;11:584–587.

Rodriguez-Sains RS, Jakobiec FA, Iwamoto T. Lentigo maligna of the lateral canthal skin. *Ophthalmology* 1981;88:1186–92.

Sanchez R, Ivan D, Esmaeli B. Eyelid and periorbital cutaneous malignant melanoma. *Int Ophthalmol Clin* 2009;49:25–43.

Tahery DP, Goldberg R, Moy RL. Malignant melanoma of the eyelid. A report of eight cases and a review of the literature. *J Am Acad Dermatol* 1992;27:17–21.

Vaziri M, Buffam FV, Martinka M, et al. Clinicopathologic features and behavior of cutaneous eyelid melanoma. *Ophthalmology* 2002;109:901–908.

Wang Q, Prieto V, Esmaeli B, et al. Cellular blue nevi of the eyelid: a possible diagnostic pitfall. *J Am Acad Dermatol* 2008;58:257–260.

Adnexal Tumors

Aurora AL, Luxenberg MN. Case report of adenocarcinoma of the glands of Moll. *Am J Ophthalmol* 1970;70:984–990.

Auw-Haedrich C, Boehm N, Weissenberger C. Signet ring carcinoma of the eccrine sweat gland in the eyelid, treated by radiotherapy alone. *Br J Ophthalmol* 2001;85:112–113.

Barker-Griffith AE, Streeten BW, Charles NC. Moll gland neoplasms of the eyelid: a clinical and pathological spectrum in 5 cases. *Arch Ophthalmol* 2006;124:1645–1649.

Buchi ER, Peng Y, Eng AM, et al. Eccrine acrospiroma of the eyelid with oncocytic, apocrine and sebaceous differentiation. Further evidence for pluripotentiality of the adnexal epithelia. *Eur J Ophthalmol* 1991;1:187–193.

Hidayat AA, Font RL. Trichilemmoma of eyelid and eyebrow. A clinicopathologic study of 31 cases. *Arch Ophthalmol* 1980;98: 844–847.

Katowitz WR, Shields CL, Shields JA, et al. Pilomatrixoma of the eyelid simulating a chalazion. *J Pediatr Ophthalmol Strabismus* 2003;40:247–248.

Khalil M, Brownstein S, Codere F, et al. Eccrine sweat gland carcinoma of the eyelid with orbital involvement. *Arch Ophthalmol* 1980;98:2210–2214.

Kramer TR, Grossniklaus HE, McLean IW, et al. Histocytoid variant of eccrine sweat gland carcinoma of the eyelid and orbit: report of five cases. *Ophthalmology* 2002;109:553–559.

Lahav M, Albert DM, Bahr R, et al. Eyelid tumors of sweat gland origin. *Graefes Arch Klin Ophthalmol* 1981;216:301–311.

Levy J, Ilsar M, Deckel Y, et al. Eyelid pilomatrixoma: a description of 16 cases and a review of the literature. *Surv Ophthalmol* 2008;53:526–535.

Mehta S, Thiagalingam S, Zembowicz A, et al. Endocrine mucin-producing sweat gland carcinoma of the eyelid. *Ophthal Plast Reconstr Surg* 2008;24:164–165.

Netland PA, Townsend DJ, Albert DM, et al. Hidradenoma papilliferum of the upper eyelid arising from the apocrine gland of Moll. *Ophthalmology* 1990;97:1593–1598.

Perez RC, Nicholson DH. Malherbe's calcifying epithelioma (pilomatrixoma) of the eyelid. Clinical features. *Arch Ophthalmol* 1979;97:314–315.

Shields JA, Shields CL, Eagle RC Jr, et al. Pilomatrixoma of the eyelid. *J Pediatr Ophthalmol Strabismus* 1995;32:260–261.

Shintaku M, Tsuta K, Yoshida H, et al. Apocrine adenocarcinoma of the eyelid with aggressive biological behavior: report of a case. *Pathol Int* 2002;52:169–173.

Shuster AR, Maskin SL, Leone CR Jr. Primary mucinous sweat gland carcinoma of the eyelid. *Ophthalmic Surg* 1989;20:808–810.

Thomas JW, Fu YS, Levine MR. Primary mucinous sweat gland carcinoma of the eyelid simulating metastatic carcinoma. *Am J Ophthalmol* 1979;87:29–33.

Tong JT, Flanagan JC, Eagle RC Jr, et al. Benign mixed tumor arising from an accessory lacrimal gland of Wolfring. *Ophthal Plast Reconstr Surg* 1995;11:136–368.

Topping NC, Chakrabarty A, Edrich C, et al. Desmoplastic trichilemmoma of the upper eyelid. *Eye (Lond)* 1999;13 (Pt 4):593–594.

Wright JD, Font RL. Mucinous sweat gland carcinoma of the eyelid. A clinicopathologic study of 21 cases with histochemical and electron microscopic observations. *Cancer* 1979;44:1757–1768.

Yap EY, Hohberger GG, Bartley GB. Pilomatrixoma of the eyelids and eyebrows in children and adolescents. *Ophthal Plast Reconstr Surg* 1999;15:185–189.

Eyelid Markers for Systemic Disease

Bardenstein DS, McLean IW, Nerney J, et al. Cowden's disease. *Ophthalmology* 1988;95:1038–1041.

Bianciotto C, Demirci H, Shields CL, et al. Metastatic tumors to the eyelid: report of 20 cases and review of the literature. *Arch Ophthalmol* 2009;127:999–1005.

Bianciotto CG, Demirci HY, Shields CL, et al. Simultaneous eyelid and choroidal metastases 36 years after diagnosis of medullary thyroid carcinoma. *Ophthal Plast Reconstr Surg* 2008;24:62–63.

Carney JA. Carney complex: the complex of myxomas, spotty pigmentation, endocrine overactivity, and schwannomas. *Semin Dermatol* 1995;14:90–98.

Jonsson A. Sigfusson N. Significance of xanthelasma palpebrarum in the normal population. *Lancet* 1976;1(7955):372.

Kennedy RH, Flanagan JC, Eagle RC Jr, et al. The Carney complex with ocular signs suggestive of cardiac myxoma. *Am J Ophthalmol* 1991;111:699–702.

Mansour AH, Hidayat AA. Metastatic eyelid disease. *Ophthalmology* 1987;94: 667–670.

Ozdol S, Sahin S, Tokgozoglu L. Xanthelasma palpebrarum and its relation to atherosclerotic risk factors and lipoprotein (a). *Int J Dermatol* 2008;47:785–789.

Robertson DM, Winkelmann RK. Ophthalmic features of necrobiotic xanthogranuloma with paraproteinemia. *Am J Ophthalmol* 1984;97:173–183.

Rohrich RJ, Janis JE, Pownell PH. Xanthelasma palpebrarum: a review and current management principles. *Plast Reconstr Surg* 2002;110:1310–1314.

Shields JA, Eagle RC Jr, Gausas RE, et al. Retrograde metastasis of cutaneous melanoma to conjunctival lymphatics. *Arch Ophthalmol* 2009;127:1222–1224.

Tsilou ET, Chan CC, Sandrini F, et al. Eyelid myxoma in Carney complex without PRKAR1A allelic loss. *Am J Med Genet A* 2004;130A:395–397.

Merkel Cell Carcinoma

Chan JK, Suster S, Wenig BM, et al. Cytokeratin 20 immunoreactivity distinguishes Merkel cell (primary cutaneous neuroendocrine) carcinomas and salivary gland small cell carcinomas from small cell carcinomas of various sites. *Am J Surg Pathol* 1997;21: 226–234.

Cummings HL, Green WR. Merkel cell carcinoma of the eyelid: a report of two new cases and a review of the literature. *Md Med J* 1992;41:149–153.

D'Agostino M, Cinelli C, Willard R, et al. Epidermotropic Merkel cell carcinoma: a case series with histopathologic examination. *J Am Acad Dermatol* 2010;62:463–468.

Kivela T, Tarkkanen A. The Merkel cell and associated neoplasms in the eyelids and periocular region. *Surv Ophthalmol* 1990;35: 171–187.

Rubsamen PE, Tanenbaum M, Grove AS, et al. Merkel cell carcinoma of the eyelid and periocular tissues. *Am J Ophthalmol* 1992;113:674–680.

Miscellaneous Lesions

Alper MG, Zimmerman LE, LaPiana FG. Orbital manifestations of Erdheim-Chester disease. *Trans Am Ophthalmol Soc* 1983;81:64–85.

Eagle RC Jr, Penne RA, Hneleski IS Jr. Eyelid involvement in multicentric reticulohistiocytosis. *Ophthalmology* 1995;102: 426–430.

Feiler-Ofry V, Lewy A, Regenbogen L, et al. Lipoid proteinosis (Urbach-Wiethe syndrome). *Br J Ophthalmol* 1979;63:694–698.

Ferry AP. Subcutaneous granuloma annulare ("pseudorheumatoid nodule") of the eyebrow. *J Pediatr Ophthalmol* 1977;14: 154–157.

Floyd BB, Brown B, Isaacs H, et al. Pseudorheumatoid nodule involving the orbit. *Arch Ophthalmol* 1982;100:1478–1480.

Game JA, Davies R. Mycosis fungoides causing severe lower eyelid ulceration. *Clin Experiment Ophthalmol* 2002;30:369–371.

Girard C, Johnson WC, Graham JH. Cutaneous angiosarcomas. *Cancer* 1970;26:868–883.

Rosenthal G, Lifshitz T, Monos T, et al. Carbon dioxide laser treatment for lipoid proteinosis (Urbach-Wiethe syndrome) involving the eyelids [letter]. *Br J Ophthalmol* 1997;81:253.

Sanka RK, Eagle R Jr, Wojno TH, et al. Spectrum of CD30+ lymphoid proliferations in the eyelid lymphomatoid papulosis, cutaneous anaplastic large cell lymphoma, and anaplastic large cell lymphoma. *Ophthalmology* 2009;117:343–351.

Scupham RK, Fretzin DF. Necrobiotic xanthogranuloma with paraproteinemia. *Arch Pathol Lab Med* 1989;113:1389–1391.

Valentine EA, Friedman HD, Zamkoff KW, et al. Necrobiotic xanthogranuloma with IgA multiple myeloma: a case report and literature review. *Am J Hematol* 1990;35:283–285.

Lacrimal Sac

Pe'er JJ. Stefanyszyn M, Hidayat AA. Nonepithelial tumors of the lacrimal sac. *Am J Ophthalmol* 1994;118:650–658.

Ryan SJ, Font RL. Primary epithelial neoplasms of the lacrimal sac. *Am J Ophthalmol* 1973;76: 73–88.

Stefanyszyn MA. Hidayat AA. Pe'er JJ. Flanagan JC. Lacrimal sac tumors. *Ophthal Plastic Reconstr Surg* 1994;10:169–184.

14 Orbit

INTRODUCTION

Orbital disease is relatively uncommon but quite diverse in nature. Inflammatory diseases, such as infectious cellulitis, and immunological disorders, such as thyroid ophthalmopathy and idiopathic orbital inflammation or "pseudotumor," are encountered most often in general clinical practice. However, the soft tissues of the orbit occasionally give rise to a relatively broad spectrum of primary neoplasms, and the orbit can be involved secondarily by systemic lymphoma, metastases from distant primary cancers, or by tumors that arise in neighboring tissues such as conjunctiva, eyelid, paranasal sinuses, or even the intracranial cavity (Fig. 14-1).

The essential clinical manifestation of orbital disease is ocular proptosis or exophthalmos (Fig. 14-2A). The eye usually is pushed forward because the orbit is a semi-confined space bounded by bony walls, and most orbital diseases are space-occupying. The proptotic eye may be pushed directly forward (axial proptosis) or in other directions (e.g., down and in) that are determined by, and serve to indicate the location of, the orbital lesion. For example, tumors of the lacrimal gland, which is located in the superotemporal orbit, typically push the eye inferomedially as well as forward, while mucoceles of the ethmoid sinus in the medial orbital wall cause lateral displacement. Retraction of the eye or enophthalmos occurs occasionally. Causes of enophthalmos include traumatic blow-out fractures of the orbital floor and sclerosing tumors such as metastatic scirrhous breast carcinoma. Other symptoms and signs of orbital disease include pain, loss of vision, and ocular motility disturbances, which may or may not be conspicuous

depending on the underlying cause; some orbital tumors, for example, lymphomas, tend to be well-tolerated. Others, such as metastatic carcinoma, are more likely to be symptomatic.

ORBITAL INFLAMMATORY DISEASE

Most orbital diseases encountered by ophthalmologists in general practice are inflammatory in nature. The most common inflammatory diseases of the orbit include infectious orbital cellulitides, noninfectious idiopathic orbital inflammation (inflammatory orbital pseudotumor), and Graves disease or thyroid orbitopathy.

Orbital Cellulitis

Orbital cellulitis usually is caused by the extension of a primary sinus infection into adjacent soft tissues of the orbit (Fig. 14-3). Abscesses can form beneath the periosteum (subperiosteal abscess) or in the orbital soft tissues. Patients with orbital cellulitis have signs of acute inflammation including erythema and pain as well as proptosis. Although most orbital cellulitis is caused by bacteria, fungi such as *Aspergillus* or *Mucor* occasionally invade the orbit from primary foci in the sinuses. *Haemophilus influenzae* is an important cause of orbital cellulitis in children but is becoming rare due to immunization. Rarely, a clinical picture resembling orbital cellulitis may be caused by an extensively necrotic intraocular retinoblastoma or melanoma. Orbital involvement has been reported in allergic fungal sinusitis (Fig. 14-4).

MUCORMYCOSIS

Mucormycosis (zygomycosis) is a potentially lethal opportunistic infection by saprophytic fungi that usually occurs in acidotic persons such as poorly controlled diabetics. The fungus is vasotropic and invades orbital vessels causing thrombosis and necrosis (Fig. 14-5). Histopathology shows both acute and chronic granulomatous inflammation and necrotic tissue. The hyphae are large and nonseptate and are easily identified in standard hematoxylin and eosin-stained sections. Lives occasionally can be saved if an expedient diagnosis is made and antifungal therapy is instituted.

THYROID EYE DISEASE

Thyroid eye disease (thyroid ophthalmopathy, Graves orbitopathy) is the most common cause of unilateral or bilateral exophthalmos (Fig. 14-2). Affected patients have an

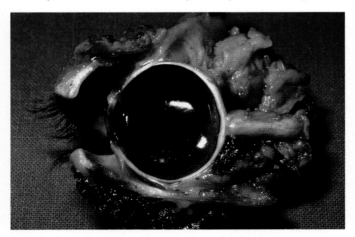

Fig. 14-1. A. Orbital contents. The orbital contents include the eye, optic nerve, smooth and striated muscle, vessels, nerves, fatty and fibrous connective tissue, and the lacrimal gland. They are delimited anteriorly by a fibrous tissue septum and protected by the eyelids.

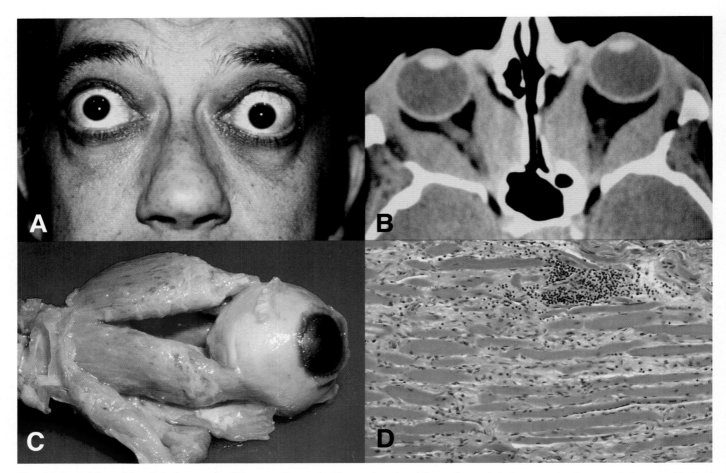

Fig. 14-2. A. Thyroid ophthalmopathy (Graves disease). The patient has bilateral exophthalmos and a characteristic stare. Vertical extraocular muscle imbalance (left hypotropia) reflects fibrosis of left inferior rectus muscle. **B.** CT shows massive enlargement of extraocular muscles. **C.** Postmortem exenteration specimen from patient with thyroid optic neuropathy shows massive enlargement of extraocular muscles. **D.** Extraocular muscle from case seen grossly in Figure C contains patchy foci of chronic inflammatory cells composed largely of lymphocytes. The myofibers are separated by fibrosis. The inflammation in Graves disease characteristically spares the tendons of the extraocular muscles and the orbital fat, features that serve to distinguish the disorder histopathologically from idiopathic orbital inflammatory pseudotumor. (**C.** Photo by the author. [From Hufnagel TJ, Hickey WF, Cobbs WH, et al. *Ophthalmology* 1984;91:1411. Courtesy of Ophthalmology.], **D.** H&E ×50)

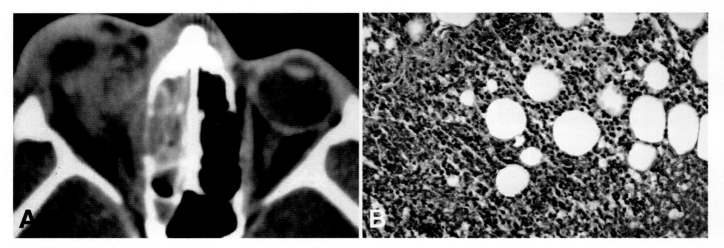

Fig. 14-3. Orbital cellulitis. A. CT scan of patient with orbital cellulitis shows opacification of adjacent infected sinus. Orbital cellulitis often is caused by extension of a primary sinus infection into orbital soft tissues. **B. Orbital abscess.** An abscess is a focal collection of polymorphonuclear leukocytes. Many of the polys infiltrating the orbital fat are degenerated. Basophilia reflects necrosis. (**A.** Photo courtesy of Jurij Bilyk, MD, Wills Eye Institute, **B.** H&E ×100)

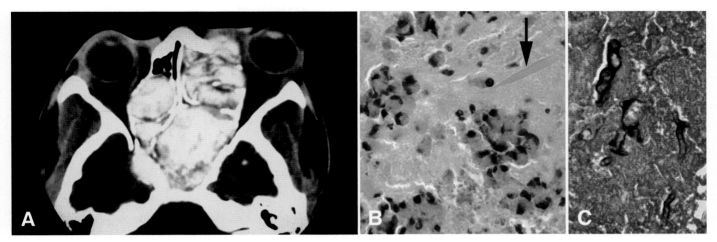

Fig. 14-4. Allergic fungal sinusitis. A. CT scan shows massive involvement and expansion of sinuses by allergic mucin. **B.** Allergic mucin contains clumps of eosinophils and Charcot-Leyden crystals (*arrow*). **C.** Gomori methenamine silver (GMS) stain discloses hyphae of noninvasive fungus within mucin. (**B.** H&E ×250, **C.** GMS ×250)

underlying immunological disorder, which is complex and still poorly understood, that affects both the thyroid gland and orbital structures, especially the extraocular muscles. The exophthalmos is caused by enlargement of the extraocular muscles (Fig. 14-2B,C). The enlarged muscles contain foci of chronic nongranulomatous inflammation and increased quantities of glycosaminoglycans and show endomysial fibrosis (Fig. 14-2D). The tendon of the extraocular muscle and the orbital fat characteristically are noninflamed, a feature that serves to differentiate thyroid ophthalmopathy from idiopathic orbital inflammation (pseudotumor). Visual loss due to compressive optic neuropathy occurs in some patients when the swollen muscle bellies press on the optic nerve in the crowded orbital apex. Corneal complications caused by exposure can also cause visual loss. Graves ophthalmopathy can occur in patients whose thyroid function tests are high, low, or even normal. Most cases are readily diagnosed by the demonstration of enlarged extraocular muscles on computed tomography (CT) or magnetic resonance imaging (MRI) scans. Very few cases are biopsied.

IDIOPATHIC ORBITAL INFLAMMATION

Idiopathic orbital inflammation or pseudotumor is relatively common. Although orbital pseudotumor undoubtedly is an immunological disorder, the details of its immunopathology and the identity of the antigens responsible for inciting the inflammation are still unclear. Idiopathic orbital inflammatory pseudotumor is a diagnosis of exclusion, from both the clinical and histopathologic standpoint. The presence of fungi, bacteria and acid fast organisms, foreign substances, and other specific inflammatory diseases such as Wegener granulomatosis or sarcoidosis must be excluded with special stains or appropriate tests.

Idiopathic orbital inflammation can affect both adults and children who may have either unilateral or bilateral disease. Although occasional cases are relatively asymptomatic and indolent in their course, idiopathic orbital inflammation classically presents explosively with the acute onset of pain, ocular proptosis, muscle paresis, and sometimes visual

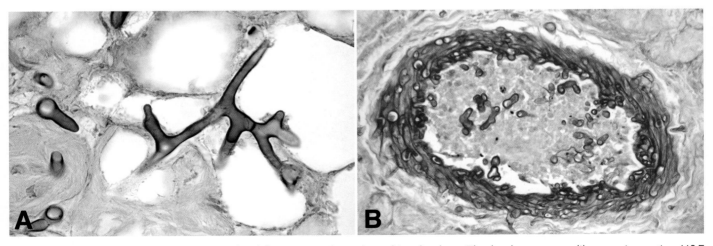

Fig. 14-5. Mucormycosis. A. Necrotic orbital fat contains large branching hyphae. The hyphae are readily seen in routine H&E sections. **B.** Fungus infiltrates wall and lumen of thrombosed vessel. (**A.** H&E ×250, **B.** H&E ×100)

loss. The inflammation may be localized to single orbital structures such as the extraocular muscles (orbital myositis), the lacrimal gland (chronic dacryoadenitis), or the sclera or episclera (scleritis or episcleritis). A diagnostic trial of systemic corticosteroids may be administered to patients suspected of having idiopathic orbital inflammation, because the disorder is exquisitely sensitive to steroids.

Biopsy is often performed on patients with orbital inflammatory pseudotumor. Microscopy typically discloses a polymorphous infiltrate of inflammatory cells that may contain lymphocytes, plasma cells, eosinophils, macrophages, and occasionally epithelioid histiocytes (Fig. 14-6A,B). Although vessels ringed or cuffed by chronic inflammation can be seen, this reflects diapedesis of lymphocytes, not true vasculitis. Lymphoid follicles and germinal centers occur in some cases, and fibrosis is often extensive. If the lacrimal gland is involved, its acini are destroyed by the inflammatory process and fibrosis replaces the parenchyma. The fibrosis is responsible for the typically eosinophilic appearance of specimens under low magnification light microscopy. This eosinophilia usually distinguishes "pseudotumor" from lymphoid tumors, which are composed of sheets of basophilic cells. Fibrosis is particularly marked in the sclerosing type of pseudotumor, which may be a subset of IgG4-related sclerosing disorders. Follicular lymphoid hyperplasia is considered to be an orbital lymphoid tumor by ophthalmic pathologists; it should not be called an inflammatory pseudotumor.

Lacrimal gland biopsy typically discloses discrete noncaseating granulomas composed of epithelioid histiocytes and giant cells in sarcoidosis, which is another diagnosis of exclusion (Fig. 14-6C). Lacrimal gland biopsy occasionally is performed to confirm the diagnosis of sarcoidosis histopathologically.

If true vasculitis, granulomatous inflammation, and focal necrosis are observed, the patient may have Wegener granulomatosis. About one third of patients with Wegener granulomatosis have ophthalmic manifestations during

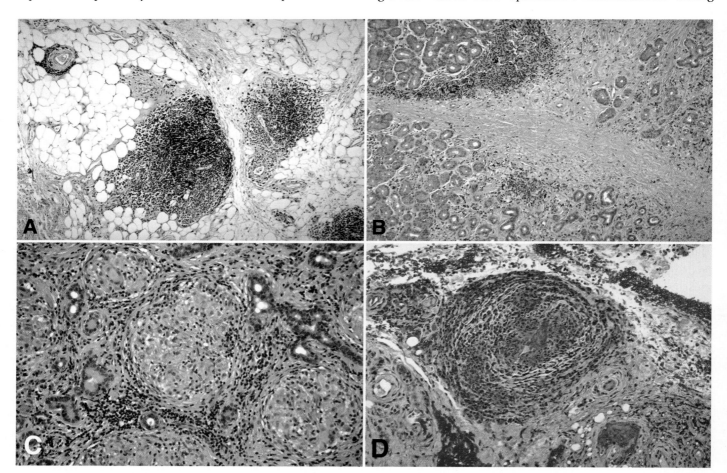

Fig. 14-6. A. **Idiopathic orbital inflammation, orbital fat (idiopathic inflammatory pseudotumor).** The orbital fat contains patchy foci of chronic inflammatory cells. The polymorphous inflammatory infiltrate was composed largely of lymphocytes and plasma cells. B. **Idiopathic orbital inflammation with fibrosis, lacrimal gland (sclerosing idiopathic inflammatory pseudotumor).** A few residual ductules persist in the eosinophilic, chronically inflamed scar tissue that has replaced the lacrimal gland. Patchy foci of chronic inflammatory cells are present. Higher magnification disclosed a polymorphous inflammatory infiltrate composed largely of lymphocytes and plasma cells. C. **Sarcoidosis.** Atrophic parenchyma of lacrimal glands contains multiple discrete noncaseating granuloma consistent with sarcoidosis. D. **Wegener granulomatosis.** Granulomatous vasculitis involves orbital vessel. Foci of necrosis were present. (**A.** H&E ×25, **B.** H&E ×25, **C.** H&E ×50, **D.** H&E ×50)

the course of their disease, and they may present with ocular findings such as orbital infiltration or peripheral corneal ulceration. Clinical suspicion is important because the classic histopathologic features of Wegener granulomatosis are found in few orbital biopsies (Fig. 14-6D). Most patients have concurrent sinus disease. The cytoplasmic antineutrophilic cytoplasmic antibody (c-ANCA) test is a helpful diagnostic adjunct but may be negative in the early stages of the disease.

ORBITAL TUMORS

A wide variety of benign and malignant primary neoplasms are spawned by the tissues of the orbit. Most of these tumors are relatively rare. Secondary involvement of the orbit by blood-borne metastases, systemic lymphoproliferative disorders, or direct invasion from contiguous structures also occurs. Children and adults are affected by different spectra of orbital tumors.

Orbital Tumors in Adults

Primary orbital tumors that are encountered fairly often in adults include cavernous hemangioma, schwannoma, fibrous histiocytoma (FH) or solitary fibrous tumor (SFT), hemangiopericytoma, epithelial tumors of the lacrimal gland, and lymphoid tumors. Cavernous hemangioma and lymphoid tumors are encountered most often.

LYMPHOID TUMORS

Orbital lymphoid tumors comprise a spectrum that includes polyclonal reactive lymphoid hyperplasias and malignant lymphomas composed of clonal proliferations of lymphoid cells (Figs. 14-7 and 14-8). Immunophenotypic analysis has shown that most lesions previously classified light microscopically as atypical lymphoid hyperplasias are low-grade lymphomas. Lymphoma is also discussed in Chapter 5.

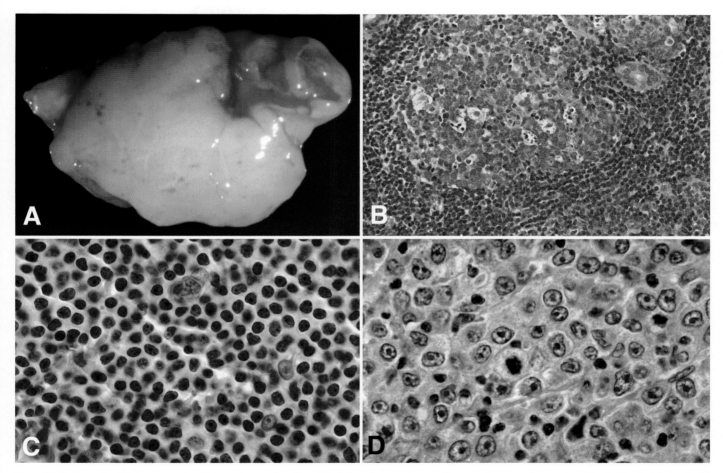

Fig. 14-7. Lymphoid tumors. A. Cut surface of soft orbital lymphoma has uniform salmon-yellow-color. **B. Follicular lymphoid hyperplasia.** Small well-differentiated lymphocytes surround a germinal center. The lighter cells in the germinal center are tingible body macrophages, which are antigen presenting cells. Mitoses normally are found in germinal centers. The germinal center and adjacent mantle zone are composed largely of B lymphocytes. **C. Diffuse non-Hodgkin lymphoma, well-differentiated lymphocytic type.** Infiltrate is composed of monotonous monomorphic sheet of small well-differentiated lymphocytes. Immunophenotypic studies disclosed a monoclonal population of B lymphocytes. **D. Diffuse large cell lymphoma**. This obviously malignant tumor is composed of large, atypical immunoblastic B cells that have prominent nucleoli. Apoptotic cells and mitoses are present. (**B.** H&E ×100, **C.** H&E ×250, **D.** H&E ×250)

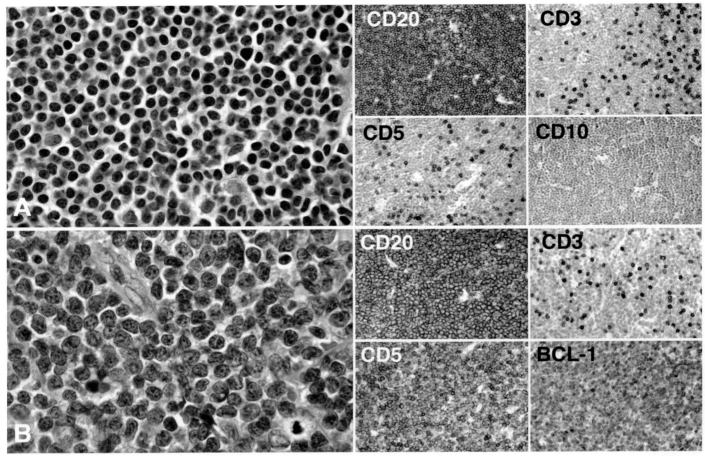

Fig. 14-8. A. Extranodal marginal zone lymphoma of mucosa-associated lymphoid tissue (MALT lymphoma). Lymphoma is composed of diffuse infiltrate of small, well-differentiated B lymphocytes. IHC panel at right shows that neoplastic B cells express B cell marker CD20 but are negative for CD3, CD5, and CD10. More than half of ocular adnexal lymphomas are MALT lymphomas. **B. Mantle cell lymphoma.** The neoplastic B cells comprising mantle cell lymphoma usually have irregular cleaved nuclei. The CD20-positive B cells coexpress T cell marker CD5 but are negative for CD3. Positive immunoreactivity for BCL-1 (cyclin D1) confirms the diagnosis. Mantle cell lymphoma has a poor prognosis. (**A. main figure**, H&E ×250; **insets**, IHC for CD20, CD3, CD5, and D10, all ×100; **B. main figure**, H&E ×250; **insets**, IHC for CD20, CD3, CD5 and bcl-1, all ×100)

Orbital lymphoma usually is a disorder of older patients that is diagnosed on average at age 60 years. The onset of orbital lymphoma is usually insidious. Orbital lymphoid tumors typically present with painless, well-tolerated proptosis, because the tumor has no fibrous stroma, is soft and pliable, and molds to the globe and other orbital structures. Some patients may present with a conjunctival mass or patch of salmon-colored tissue on the epibulbar surface or fornix (Fig. 5-29). The tumor's characteristic salmon hue reflects the presence of many fine capillaries (Fig. 14-7A). The lymphoid infiltrate is often delimited sharply by tissue planes. The latter are evident on imaging studies as linear margins. Lymphomas diffusely infiltrate and thicken the lacrimal gland, which drapes around the globe assuming an appearance that Jakobiec has facetiously termed a "pregnant pancake." The latter contrasts with epithelial neoplasms of the lacrimal gland, which typically are rounded. Ninety percent of orbital lymphomas involve the superior part of the orbit behind the orbital septum. More than 40% involve

the lacrimal gland and often affect its palpebral lobe. Bone destruction is very rare except in multiple myeloma. When extraocular muscles are involved, usually a single muscle is affected. Motility remains normal because the lymphoma does not stimulate fibrosis.

Ocular lymphomas are extranodal by definition because the orbit lacks lymphatics and lymph nodes, and most are diffuse, as well. About two thirds of ocular adnexal lymphoid tumors are malignant non-Hodgkin lymphomas (NHLs) composed of a monoclonal proliferation of B lymphocytes, and most of the these are low grade lesions composed of well-differentiated lymphocytes. In recent years, pathologists have used the WHO classification to classify lymphomas. Types of NHL in the WHO classification that typically affect the ocular adnexa include extranodal marginal zone lymphoma of mucosa-associated lymphoid tissue (often called MALT lymphoma), follicular lymphoma, mantle cell lymphoma, diffuse large cell lymphoma, and small lymphocytic lymphoma.

More than half of ocular adnexal lymphomas are MALT lymphomas (Fig. 14-8A). About 23% are follicular lymphomas, 5% mantle cell, and 4% small lymphocytic lymphoma (SLL/CLL). These four entities are very difficult to differentiate using routine light microscopy alone, but distinguishing them is important clinically because they differ greatly in prognosis and the proper choice of therapy requires accurate classification. The cells of extranodal marginal zone or MALT lymphoma are CD20 positive but are negative for CD3, CD5, and CD10 (Fig. 14-8A). Mantle cell lymphoma (Fig. 14-8B) is usually widely disseminated on presentation and has a poor prognosis. Its CD20-positive B cells co-express T cell marker CD5 and bcl-1 (also called cyclin D1). The cells comprising the neoplastic follicles of follicular lymphoma stain with CD20, CD10, and bcl-2. About one third of patients who have orbital lymphomas have, have a history of, or will develop systemic lymphoma. All patients with ocular adnexal lymphoid tumors need to be evaluated by a hematologist-oncologist. Some patients with polyclonal lymphoid proliferations are a risk for systemic lymphoma.

Lymphoid tumors of the orbit and ocular adnexa are treated with external beam radiotherapy with appropriate eye shielding if there is no evidence of systemic disease. Chemotherapy or immunotherapy should be used if extraocular systemic lymphoma is present. This may be supplemented with adjuvant radiotherapy if ocular regression is subtotal.

VASCULAR LESIONS

Cavernous Hemangioma

Cavernous hemangioma is probably the most common primary orbital neoplasm. This benign vascular tumor typically occurs in middle-aged women. Cavernous hemangiomas cause low-grade proptosis and usually are well-tolerated, sparing vision and ocular motility. Some cases are discovered incidentally when imaging is performed for headache or other indications (Fig. 14-9A). These benign vascular tumors are well-circumscribed, encapsulated lesions with

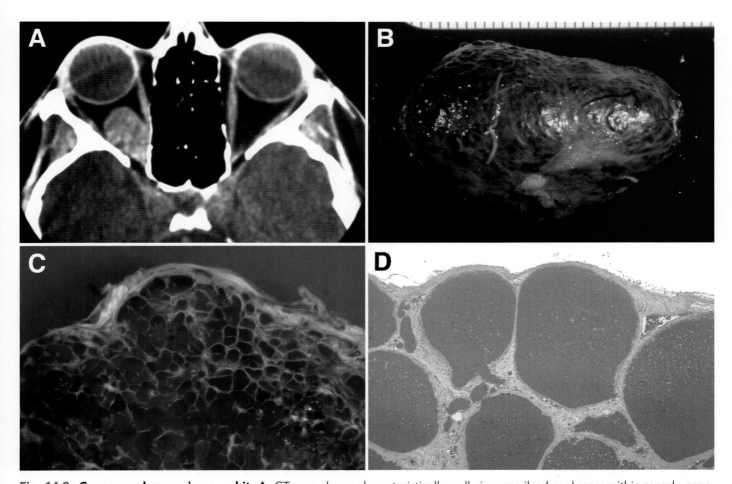

Fig. 14-9. Cavernous hemangioma, orbit. A. CT scan shows characteristically well-circumscribed oval mass within muscle cone. The differential diagnosis of a well-circumscribed orbital tumor also includes schwannoma, hemangiopericytoma and SFT. **B.** After fixation, the well-circumscribed, encapsulated tumor appears bluish-purple in color and has a pebbly surface. **C.** The benign encapsulated tumor is composed of large blood-filled vascular channels separated by fibrous septa that are evident grossly. **D.** The large vascular channels comprising the benign vascular tumor are lined by a single layer of endothelial cells. The fibrous septa separating the vessels often contain smooth muscle. (**D.** H&E ×25)

a pebbly surface that appear dusky-red or purplish-blue grossly (Fig. 14-9B). They are composed of large round or oval vascular spaces lined by endothelium, which are separated by thick septa of fibrous tissue that may contain smooth muscle (Fig. 14-9C,D). Cavernous hemangiomas show little contrast enhancement on imaging studies because their circulation is relatively stagnant. This feature helps to distinguish them from the much rarer encapsulated vascular tumor hemangiopericytoma, which enhances vividly.

Hemangiopericytoma

Hemangiopericytomas is a relatively rare orbital lesion. Hemangiopericytoma was originally thought to be a soft tissue tumor that arose from pericytes in the walls of capillaries. Large branching sinusoidal vessels with a "stag-horn" configuration are a classic histopathologic feature, and the reticulin stain shows that its constituent cells are totally enveloped by basement membrane (Fig. 14-10). About 15% of patients who were diagnosed as having orbital hemangiopericytoma at the Armed Forces Institute of Pathology developed distant metastases. The histologic appearance of the tumor did not always predict metastatic potential, as metastatic disease occasionally developed in patients with benign-appearing tumors. In recent years, authorities have stressed that many other neoplasms may show a branching staghorn hemangiopericytomatous vascular pattern. It is now believed that many tumors diagnosed as hemangiopericytomas in the past probably would now be classified as solitary fibrous tumors (SFTs) (Fig. 14-13).

Lymphangioma

Lymphangiomas and capillary hemangiomas (hemangioma of infancy) and are the most common vascular tumors of the orbit in children (Fig. 14-11). Lymphangiomas are poorly circumscribed choristomatous lesions composed of large endothelial-lined channels filled with lymph or serosanguineous fluid (Fig. 14-11A,B). Focal lymphoid infiltrates in the contiguous stroma, which may contain germinal centers, serve to differentiate lymphangioma from cavernous hemangioma, particularly in cases where there has been secondary hemorrhage into the lymphatic vessels. Acute enlargement of lymphangioma is often caused by intralesional hemorrhage, which can produce a blood-filled "chocolate cyst" (Fig. 14-11A). Lymphangiomas also may enlarge during upper respiratory infections, presumably because their lymphoid component undergoes hyperplasia. Lymphangiomas are usually quite infiltrative in their growth pattern, and they do not undergo spontaneous involution. Surgical removal may be quite difficult. Orbital lymphangiomas stain positively with the D2-40 immunohistochemical (IHC) stain for lymphatic endothelial cells.

Capillary (Infantile) Hemangioma

Involvement of eyelid skin by a capillary hemangioma is readily apparent as a bright red strawberry nevus. Infantile hemangiomas confined to the orbit are more subtle and may present with proptosis and bluish discoloration of the skin. Poorly circumscribed and unencapsulated, these benign vascular tumors are composed of lobules of capillary-caliber vessels or sheets of capillary endothelial cells (Fig. 14-11C). Hemangiomas in very young infants tend to be quite cellular; capillary lumens appear and enlarge as the lesions mature. Although infantile hemangiomas eventually involute spontaneously, they may be a major cosmetic blemish and often produce potentially reversible visual loss (amblyopia) by causing corneal astigmatism or by occluding the pupil. Nonsurgical therapy includes intralesional injection of steroids, interferon α-2a and systemic propranolol.

Other vascular lesions that affect the orbit include varices and arteriovenous malformations. Patients with orbital varices often show variable proptosis that depends on head position and is increased by a Valsalva maneuver. Histopathology

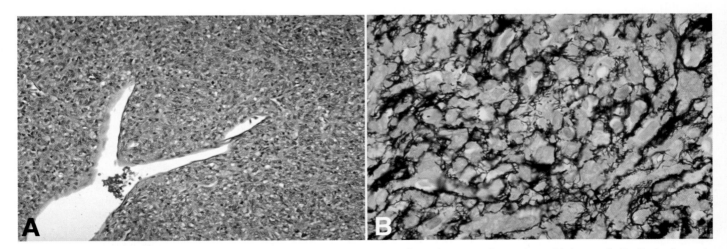

Fig. 14-10. Hemangiopericytoma. A. Highly cellular tumor contains branching staghorn sinusoidal vessel. **B.** Reticulin stain highlights basement membrane encompassing neoplastic pericytes. (**A.** H&E ×50, **B.** Wilder reticulin ×250)

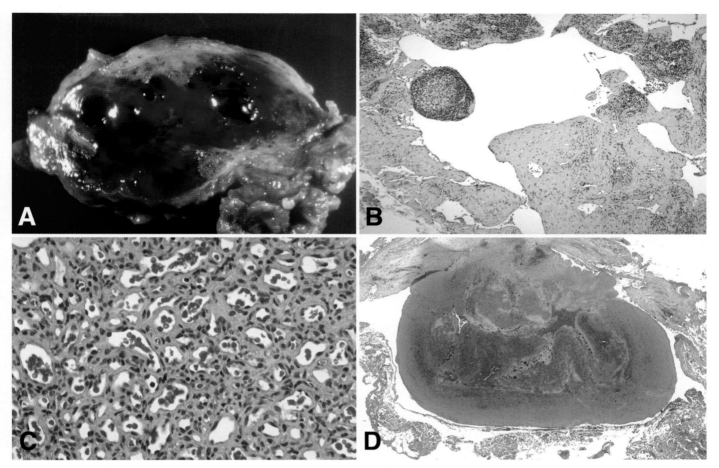

Fig. 14-11. Vascular lesions. A. Lymphangioma with secondary hemorrhage. Blood-filled chocolate cysts caused by secondary hemorrhage into lymphangioma are evident in this gross specimen. Many lymphangiomas contain blood. Lymphangiomas typically are unencapsulated and show an infiltrative growth pattern. **B. Lymphangioma, orbit.** Lymphoid channels comprising lymphangioma vary markedly in size and shape. They appear empty or contain serous fluid if intralesional hemorrhage has not occurred. Lymphoid foci in intervascular septa help to differentiate a lymphangioma with secondary hemorrhage from a cavernous hemangioma. Lymphangiomas typically are unencapsulated and have an infiltrative growth pattern. **C. Capillary hemangioma.** Mature capillary hemangioma is composed of a plexus of capillary caliber vessels. Early lesions often are composed predominantly of a solid sheet of endothelial cells. Vascular lumina develop and become progressively ectatic at the lesion matures. **D. Thrombosed varix, orbit.** A varix is a dilated or ectatic vein. An organized thrombus adheres to the wall of this orbital varix. (**B.** H&E ×10, **C.** H&E ×100, **D.** H&E ×5)

shows a markedly dilated vein that may contain a thrombus (Fig. 14-11D). Intravascular papillary endothelial hyperplasia may develop in the thrombosed varix.

Neurogenic Tumors

Neurogenic tumors of the orbit include schwannomas, neurofibromas, amputation neuromas, and malignant peripheral nerve sheath tumors.

Schwannoma

Schwannoma or neurilemmoma is a well-circumscribed, encapsulated orbital tumor of adults composed of a neoplastic proliferation of Schwann cells, the perineural cells that form the myelin sheaths around axons in peripheral nerves (Fig. 14-12A). Many orbital schwannomas arise from sensory branches of the ophthalmic division of the trigeminal nerve,

and may be painful. Histopathology shows an encapsulated spindle cell neoplasm composed of cells with eosinophilic cytoplasm that have indistinct cellular borders and bland elongated oval nuclei. Two growth patterns are recognized. Tumors with the solid Antoni A pattern show bands of nuclear palisading and structures called Verocay bodies (Fig. 14-12B). The Antoni B pattern is marked by a loose myxomatous background. Schwannomas are immunoreactive with neural markers such as S-100 protein and CD57.

Neurofibroma

Isolated neurofibromas cause diffuse enlargement of the affected nerve and contain axons. They are pseudoencapsulated. Schwannomas and neurofibromas are often grouped together under the designation peripheral nerve sheath tumor. Schwannomas and isolated neurofibromas are more prevalent in patients who have neurofibromatosis.

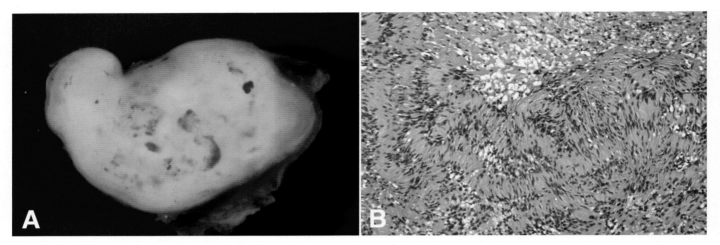

Fig. 14-12. Schwannoma (neurilemoma). A. Cut surface of well-circumscribed schwannoma is yellow-tan in color. **B.** Antoni A portion of benign peripheral nerve sheath tumor (below) is composed of highly regimented fascicles of bland spindle cells that show nuclear palisading and enclose tangles of fibrillary processes called Verocay bodies. Small focus of looser myxoid tumor (Antoni B pattern) is seen above. Schwannomas are well-circumscribed, encapsulated tumors that are associated with a peripheral nerve. (**B.** H&E ×100)

Plexiform neurofibromas and diffuse neurofibromas are characterstic manifestations of NF-1. Malignant peripheral nerve sheath tumors are encountered rarely.

Mesenchymal Tumors

A variety of rare mesenchymal tumors of fibrous, fibro-osseous, smooth muscle, adipose tissue, or cartilaginous derivation occur in the orbit. Other extremely rare primary orbital tumors include endodermal sinus tumor, alveolar soft part sarcoma, granular cell tumor, paraganglioma, primary orbital carcinoid, primary orbital melanoma, retinal anlage tumor, neuroepithelioma, ectomesenchymal tumor, malignant rhabdoid tumor, and primitive neuroectodermal tumor.

Fibrous Histiocytoma and Solitary Fibrous Tumor

FH is said to be the most common mesenchymal tumor of the orbit in adults. Typically well-circumscribed but non-encapsulated, FH is composed of spindle cells arranged in a characteristic whirling, pinwheel or storiform pattern. Benign, locally aggressive and rare malignant variants of FH are recognized. Although benign and locally aggressive FH cannot metastasize, total excision is recommended to prevent recurrence. Many tumors that were diagnosed as FH in the past probably would be classified today as solitary fibrous tumors (SFTs), a newly recognized orbital spindle cell neoplasm that shares many features with FH (Fig. 14-13). The cells in SFT are arranged in a "patternless pattern" and are immunoreactive for CD-34, CD99, and bcl-2.

Fibro-osseous Lesions

Common fibro-osseous lesions of the orbital bones include fibrous dysplasia, juvenile psammomatoid ossifying fibroma, and ivory osteoma. Ivory osteoma is the most common bony lesion in adults. Fibrous dysplasia generally occurs in the first two decades and may spread across suture lines to involve multiple orbital bones. The affected bones have a "ground

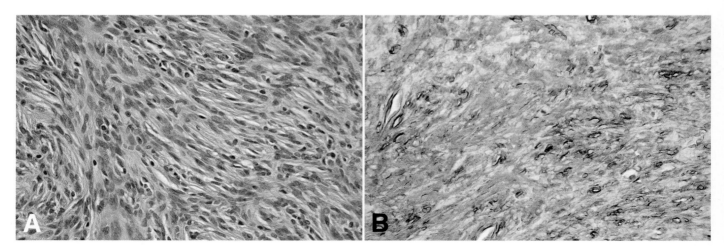

Fig. 14-13. Solitary fibrous tumor, orbit. A. Spindle cells comprising SFT are arranged in a "paternless pattern." **B.** Tumor cells are immunoreactive for CD34 (shown here), CD99 and bcl-2. (**A.** H&E ×100, **B.** IHC for CD34 ×100)

glass" appearance in CT bone windows (Fig. 14-14A–D). Fibrous dysplasia is composed of irregular trabeculae of immature woven bone surrounded by fibrous stroma. The bony trabeculae are not rimmed by osteoblasts and are often shaped like Chinese characters.

Juvenile ossifying fibroma is a more aggressive expansile lesion that usually is restricted to a single bone. Radiographically, it has a sclerotic margin and a less radiodense center. The cellular fibrous stroma of the psammomatoid variant of juvenile ossifying fibroma contains bony spicules that can be confused with psammoma bodies and lead to the misdiagnosis of meningioma (Fig. 14-14E).

The orbital bones occasionally are affected by a perplexing group of rare osseous lesions that contain giant cells including aneurysmal bone cyst, giant cell reparative granuloma, giant cell tumor, the brown tumor of hyperparathyroidism, and eosinophilic granuloma (see below).

Osteogenic sarcoma and other soft tissue sarcomas can arise after radiotherapy for retinoblastoma.

Lacrimal Gland Lesions

The lacrimal gland is a minor salivary gland that is located in a bony fossa behind the superotemporal orbital rim (Fig. 14-15). Lacrimal gland tumors constitute only 10% to 15% of orbital lesions. Most lacrimal gland lesions encountered in nonreferral clinical practice are inflammatory or lymphoid tumors, which are at least five times more prevalent than primary epithelial tumors. Epithelial neoplasms of the lacrimal gland are quite rare, but they are important because about half are highly malignant tumors that are potentially lethal.

Granulomatous dacryoadenitis can cause bilateral lacrimal gland enlargement and a characteristic "S"-shaped

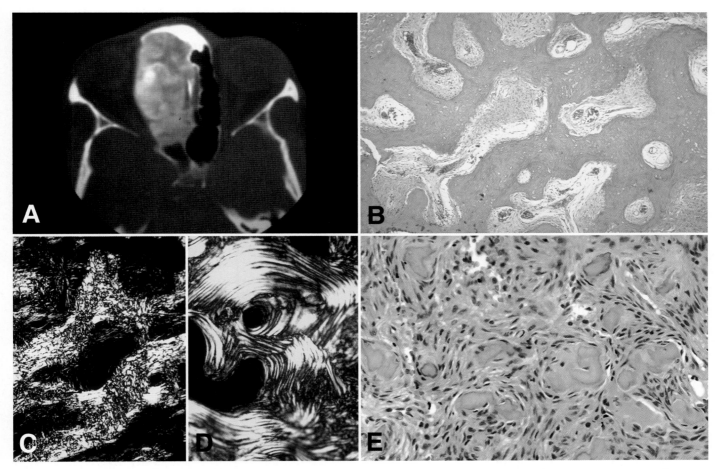

Fig. 14-14. Fibro-osseous lesions. A. Fibrous dysplasia. Lesion of nasal bones has "ground glass" appearance on CT scan. Fibrous dysplasia may spread across suture lines to involve multiple orbital bones. **B. Fibrous dysplasia.** Fibrous stroma contains irregular trabeculae of immature woven bone, which are not rimmed by osteoclasts. Fibrous dysplasia represents an arrest in the maturation of bone. **C.** Polarization microscopy of fibrous dysplasia discloses an irregular interweaving pattern of collagenous matrix that resembles the fibers in woven cloth. **D.** In contrast, collagen fibers disclosed by polarization in mature lamellar bone form highly regular, parallel lamellae. **E. Psammomatoid ossifying fibroma.** The cellular stroma contains spindle cells and small spicules of bone called ossicles that can be confused with the psammoma bodies of meningioma. This benign lesion found in young individuals has an expansile growth pattern and behaves more aggressively than fibrous dysplasia. It usually does not cross suture lines and is restricted to a single orbital bone. (**B.** H&E ×25, **C.** H&E with crossed polarizers ×50, **D.** H&E with crossed polarizers ×50, **E.** H&E ×100)

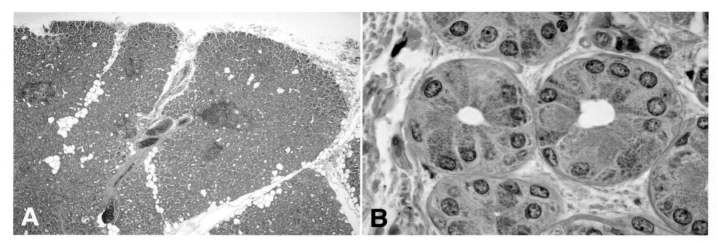

Fig. 14-15. Lacrimal gland. A. Fibrofatty stroma separates multiple lobules composed of glandular acini. Patchy foci of chronic inflammation are present. **B. Lacrimal gland, acini.** Inner layer of tall columnar secretory cells and a relatively inconspicuous discontinuous outer layer of contractile myoepithelial cells comprise acini of lacrimal gland. Large intensely eosinophilic secretory granules called zymogen granules are found in the apical cytoplasm of the secretory cells. (**A.** H&E ×10, **B.** H&E ×250)

lid fissure in patients with sarcoidosis (Fig. 14-6C). Kerato conjunctivitis sicca develops in patients with Sjögren syndrome when intense lymphocytic infiltration replaces the parenchyma of the lacrimal gland. Damaged ducts and epimyoepithelial islands persist in the resultant benign lymphoepithelial lesion, and patients are at risk for lymphoma. Cystic dilation of lacrimal gland ducts (dacryops) may simulate a primary lacrimal gland tumor. Concretions or stones (dacryolithiasis) occasionally form in the ducts of the lacrimal gland.

Epithelial Tumors of the Lacrimal Gland

Compared to other salivary glands, the lacrimal gland gives rise to a relatively limited spectrum of primary epithelial neoplasms. About one half of epithelial tumors of the lacrimal gland are pleomorphic adenomas or benign mixed tumors and half are malignant. Lacrimal gland malignancies include adenoid cystic carcinomas, malignant mixed tumors derived from pleomorphic adenomas, and a variety of rare adenocarcinoma that have arisen de novo. Mucoepidermoid carcinoma is quite rare in the lacrimal gland and acinic cell and Warthin tumors are almost nonexistent. The lacrimal gland gives rise to a greater proportion of malignant tumors than the parotid gland.

Epithelial tumors of the lacrimal gland typically arise in relatively young individuals whose average age at diagnosis is about age forty. Several signs and symptoms are very important in the clinical evaluation of patients with lacrimal gland tumors. These include the duration of symptoms, the presence of pain, and the status of the orbital bones on imaging studies. A tumor is probably malignant if it is has been present for <6 months, the patient complains of pain, and there is radiographic evidence of bony erosion. Benign pleomorphic adenomas produce a regular, well-corticated fossa in the bone, not bone erosion.

Pleomorphic Adenoma (Benign Mixed Tumor)

Pleomorphic adenoma or benign mixed tumor has a slight male predominance. The patient typically presents with painless proptosis that has been present for a year or more (Fig. 14-16). The eye is displaced inferonasally. Imaging studies disclose a rounded or oval mass that usually involves the gland's orbital lobe. As noted above, the pressure of the slowly enlarging lesion does not destroy bone; rather, it accentuates the lacrimal fossa (Fig. 14-16A). Macroscopically, the tumor is well-circumscribed and pseudoencapsulated, and its surface is marked by convex bosselations (Fig. 14-16B). Sectioning may disclose mucinous or myxomatous areas and hemorrhage. The term *mixed tumor* reflects the biphasic mixture of epithelial and mesenchymal elements seen histopathologically (Fig. 14-16C,D). The epithelial components include ducts composed of an inner layer of cuboidal or columnar cells and an outer layer of flattened or spindled myoepithelial cells. The myoepithelial cells typically spindle-off into the stroma where they may maintain a spindled configuration, or undergo metaplasia forming the mesenchymal part of the tumor including myxoid tissue, cartilage, or rarely fat or bone. Electron microscopic studies suggest that pleomorphic adenomas probably are derived from the duct cells of the lacrimal gland.

If pleomorphic adenoma of the lacrimal gland is suspected clinically, the tumor should be totally excised within an intact capsule. Benign mixed tumors should never be biopsied. An orbital recurrence will develop in about one third of patients after incisional biopsy is performed. Recurrent benign mixed tumor can infiltrate orbital soft tissues and even bone and brain, and the recurrences also are prone to malignant degeneration. The rate of malignant degeneration in recurrent benign mixed tumor is 10% and 20%, respectively, at 20 and 30 years.

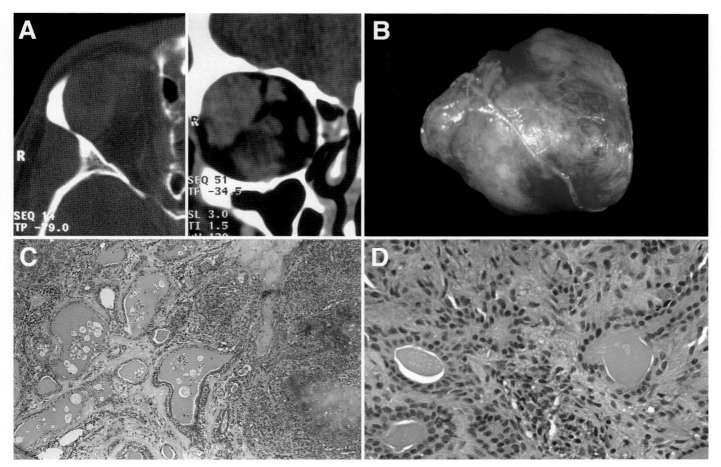

Fig. 14-16. Pleomorphic adenoma (benign mixed tumor), lacrimal gland. A. Sagittal and coronal CT scans of right orbit disclose well-circumscribed tumor in superotemporal orbit that has produced accentuation of lacrimal fossa. **B.** Convex bosselations are present on surface of well-circumscribed, pseudoencapsulated tumor. **C.** Tumor is composed of neoplastic ductules of epithelial cells set in a fibromyxoid stroma. The term *mixed tumor* refers to this mixture of epithelial and mesenchymal elements. **D.** The epithelial ductules are composed of two layers of cells. Myoepithelial cells from the outer layer spindle-off into the surrounding stroma where they may undergo metaplasia into myxoid tissue, cartilage, or rarely bone. (**C.** H&E ×25, **D.** H&E ×100)

Adenoid Cystic Carcinoma

Adenoid cystic carcinoma (Fig. 14-17) is the second most common epithelial neoplasm of the lacrimal gland, constituting 25% to 30% of cases. About 60% of cases occur in women. Although the average age at presentation is 40 years, adenoid cystic carcinoma has a biphasic age distribution, and tumors occasionally develop in children. Patients with adenoid cystic carcinoma typically have had symptoms for a relatively short period of time. The tumor has a propensity for perineural invasion (Fig. 14-17C) and can present with pain and/or numbness, blepharoptosis, and ocular motility deficits. Unfortunately, it may have already extended out of the orbit via nerves before becoming symptomatic.

Adenoid cystic carcinoma tends to be rounded or globular in imaging studies like pleomorphic adenoma, but the margin of the tumor is often irregular or serrated, and it may extend into the medial or posterior orbit (Fig. 14-17A). Bone destruction is seen in 80% of cases. Five histologic patterns of adenoid cystic carcinoma are recognized: the cribriform

or "Swiss cheese," the basaloid or solid pattern, a sclerosing pattern, a tubular pattern with true duct formation, and a comedocarcinoma pattern marked by tumor lobules with central necrosis. A thick basement membrane surrounds the epithelial elements in the cylindromatous variant. The cribriform pattern is characterized by smoothly rounded biomorphic sheets of deceptively bland appearing basaloid cells that contain round pools of mucin that mimic glands (Fig. 14-17B). The term adenoid means "gland-like."

The prognosis of adenoid cystic carcinoma of the lacrimal gland is dismal; only 20% of patients survive 10 years. Many fatal tumors invade the middle cranial fossa through the superior orbital fissure. Late pulmonary metastases also occur. Survival correlates with tumor histology; the poorly differentiated basaloid pattern is particularly ominous (Fig. 14-17D). If foci of basaloid tumor are found, the 5-year survival is 21% and the median survival is 3 years. If no basaloid tumor is found, the 5-year survival increases to 71% and the median survival to 8 years.

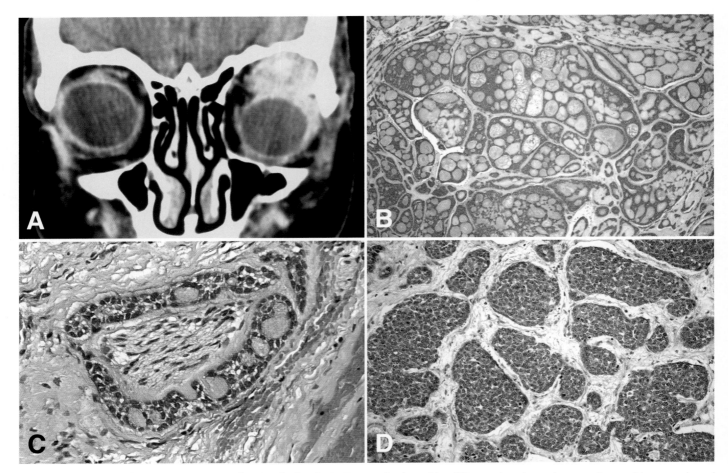

Fig. 14-17. Adenoid cystic carcinoma, lacrimal gland. A. Tumor disclosed by CT scan has irregular margins and has produced scalloped fossa in orbital bone. The tumor developed rapidly and was painful. **B. Adenoid cystic carcinoma, lacrimal gland (cribriform pattern).** Multiple pools of mucin impart a "Swiss cheese" appearance to the basophilic lobules of cells comprising the cribriform pattern of adenoid cystic carcinoma. The tumor cells are relatively uniform and have a deceptively bland appearance. Adenoid cystic carcinoma has a dismal prognosis. **C. Adenoid cystic carcinoma, lacrimal gland, perineural invasion.** Infiltrative adenoid cystic carcinoma surrounds a large orbital nerve. This highly malignant tumor has a propensity for neural and perineural invasion. Patients may present with pain. **D. Adenoid cystic carcinoma, lacrimal gland (basaloid pattern).** Poorly differentiated tumor is composed of solid lobules of deeply basophilic cells with scanty cytoplasm. Absence of peripheral palisading serves to differentiate basaloid adenoid cystic carcinoma from invasive basal cell carcinoma. Adenoid cystic carcinoma with a basaloid component has a poor prognosis. (**B.** H&E ×25, **C.** H&E ×150, **D.** H&E ×100)

The management of adenoid cystic carcinoma of the lacrimal gland is controversial. An incisional biopsy should be performed if the diagnosis is suspected on clinical grounds. Orbital exenteration should be performed after the diagnosis is confirmed by a review of permanent sections. The decision to perform a mutilating operation such as orbital exenteration should never be based on frozen section diagnosis. Some authorities recommend en bloc resection of the tumor and contiguous bone or radical orbitectomy including the roof and lateral walls of the orbit.

Other Malignant Tumors of the Lacrimal Gland

Other malignant neoplasms of the lacrimal gland include malignant mixed tumor (pleomorphic adenocarcinoma), mucoepidermoid carcinoma, acinic cell carcinoma, and a variety of other rare adenocarcinomas such as ductal

carcinoma (Fig. 14-18). Malignant mixed tumor (pleomorphic adenocarcinoma) usually results from the malignant transformation of benign mixed tumor (Fig. 14-18B). Patients with malignant mixed tumors generally are older than patients who have benign mixed tumors. In most cases, the tumor contains a clone of poorly differentiated adenocarcinoma that may show squamous, acinar, or sebaceous differentiation. Patients usually succumb within 3 years with lung and lymphatic node metastases. The prognosis of adenocarcinoma de novo is equally poor. Most of these poorly differentiated tumors occur in older men. Mucoepidermoid carcinoma of the lacrimal gland has a better prognosis than other epithelial malignancies but is quite rare. Histopathologically, the tumor contains paving stonelike squamous elements and mucous-secreting goblet cells (Fig. 14-18A). Treatment includes exenteration or wide local excision. Rare examples of primary ductal adenocarcinoma, basal cell

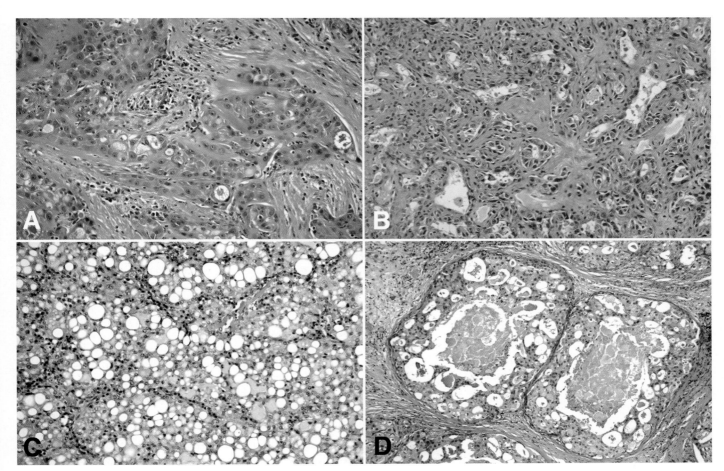

Fig. 14-18. Rare malignant tumors of lacrimal gland. A. Mucoepidermoid carcinoma, lacrimal gland. Tumor is composed of sheets of eosinophilic squamous cells with a "paving stone" arrangement and mucus-producing goblet cells. Mucoepidermoid carcinoma is an extremely rare lacrimal gland tumor that behaves less aggressively than other lacrimal gland malignancies. **B. Malignant mixed tumor, lacrimal gland.** The epithelial tubules comprising this field are composed of frankly malignant cells. Most malignant mixed tumors result from the malignant degeneration of a benign mixed tumor. **C. Acinic cell carcinoma, lacrimal gland.** Acinic cell carcinomas of the lacrimal gland are very rare. **D. Ductal adenocarcinoma, lacrimal gland.** Malignant cells within ducts are arranged in cribriform pattern. This rare variant of lacrimal gland adenocarcinoma resembles ductal carcinoma of the breast. (**A.** H&E ×100, **B.** H&E ×50, **C.** H&E ×50, **D.** H&E ×25)

adenocarcinoma, lymphoepithelial carcinoma, epithelial-myoepithelial carcinoma, and cystadenocarcinoma have been reported in the lacrimal gland.

Secondary Orbital Tumors

Secondary orbital neoplasms in adults include metastases from distant primary tumors and tumors that have invaded the orbit from contiguous structures. Breast carcinoma metastasizes to the orbit most frequently, constituting 42% of 195 orbital metastases in a combined series (Fig. 14-19A). Other common sources of orbital metastases include lung (12.8%), prostate (6.7%), and gastrointestinal carcinomas (4.1%). The primary tumor was unknown in 11.3% of cases.

Tumors that directly invade the orbit include basal cell, squamous cell, and sebaceous gland carcinomas of the eyelid and malignant melanomas and squamous cell and mucoepidermoid carcinomas of the conjunctiva.

Secondary orbital tumors also result from the extraocular extension of intraocular tumors, most notably retinoblastoma and uveal melanoma. In underdeveloped countries, retinoblastoma frequently presents as an orbital tumor that requires exenteration. Sinus carcinomas and lacrimal sac tumors can also invade the orbit. Benign cystic lesions lined by respiratory epithelium called mucoceles occasionally erode through orbital bones and impinge on the orbital contents (Fig. 14-19B). Most occur in patients who have chronic sinusitis. Secondary orbital invasion by intracranial meningioma actually is more common than primary optic nerve meningioma.

Pediatric Orbital Tumors

Pediatric vascular tumors of the orbit are discussed above.

Congenital teratomas of the orbit may present at birth with hideously deforming proptosis (Fig. 14-20A).

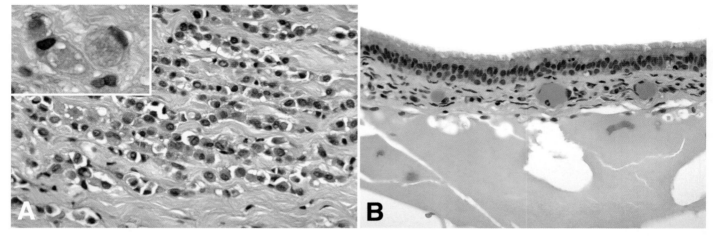

Fig. 14-19. Secondary orbital lesions. A. Metastatic breast carcinoma, orbit. The carcinoma cells are arranged in a linear "Indian file" fashion. Inset shows signet ring cells with prominent cytoplasmic vacuoles of mucin. **B. Mucocele**. The mucocele is lined by ciliated respiratory epithelium. It arose in the ethmoid sinus. (**A.** H&E ×100; **inset** H&E ×250, **B.** H&E ×100)

Dermoid Cyst

The dermoid cyst or cystic dermoid is the most common orbital lesion found in infants and children. Caused by entrapment of surface ectoderm in bony sutures during development, these choristomatous lesions typically are located in the superotemporal quadrant. Cystic dermoids resemble epidermal inclusion cysts histopathologically, but the keratinized stratified squamous epithelial lining also has epidermal appendages such as pilosebaceous units and sweat glands (Fig. 14-21). Hairs are often found mixed with the cheesy, keratinous material filling the lumen. Polarization microscopy helps to highlight the hair shafts during examination. The epithelial lining of a dermoid cyst may be partially replaced by a layer of foreign body giant cells. A rare variant of dermoid cyst, which has been termed a "conjunctivoid," occasionally is found in the nasal orbit. These unusual dermoids

are lined by nonkeratinized epithelium with goblet cells that resembles conjunctiva but has epidermal appendages.

Childhood neural tumors include plexiform neurofibroma found in von Recklinghausen neurofibromatosis type I (Fig. 2-8) and juvenile pilocytic astrocytoma (optic nerve glioma) (Fig. 15-7), which also complicates neurofibromatosis. Plexiform neurofibroma feels like a "bag of worms" when palpated because the malformation is composed of an interweaving plexus of nerves that are markedly enlarged by a proliferation of Schwann cells and mucoid material. The upper eyelid fissure often has an "S" configuration on the side of the plexiform neurofibroma.

Rhabdomyosarcoma

Rhabdomyosarcoma (Fig. 14-22) is the most common malignant orbital tumor of childhood. The tumor presents on

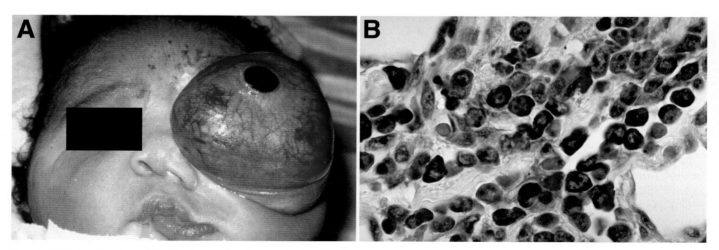

Fig. 14-20. Pediatric orbital lesions. A. Congenital orbital teratoma. Congenital orbital tumor produces hideous proptosis. (Case presented by Dr. Harry Brown, 1993 meeting of the Verhoeff Society, Coral Gables, Florida.) **B. Granulocytic (myeloid) sarcoma**. Positive (red) Leder naphthol AS-D chloroacetate esterase stain confirms the presence of granulocytic differentiation. This use of this stain has largely been supplanted by more specific IHC stains. Granulocytic or myeloid sarcoma must be excluded when an apparent "lymphoma" is encountered in the orbit of a child. (**B.** Leder stain, ×250)

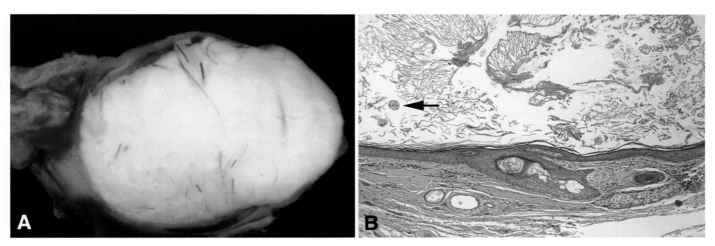

Fig. 14-21. Dermoid cyst. A. Cheesy keratin debris with hair shafts fills lumen of sectioned cyst. **B.** The cyst is filled with laminated keratin. It is lined with keratinized stratified squamous epithelium that resembles skin and has pilosebaceous units and other epidermal appendages. A few hair shafts are mixed with the keratin (*arrow*). (**B.** H&E ×50)

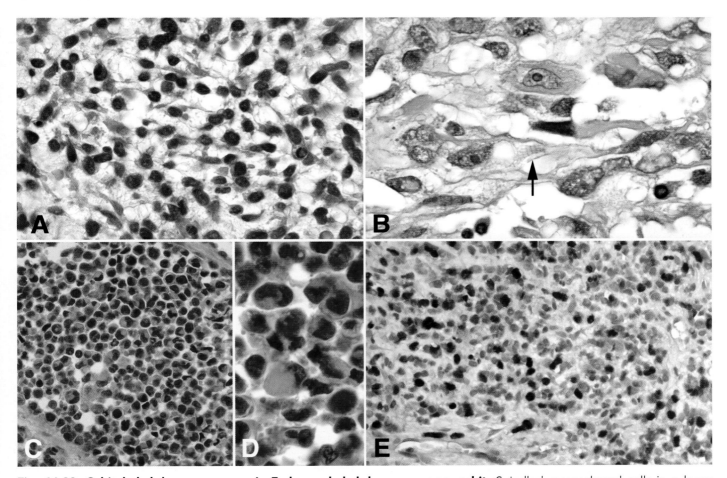

Fig. 14-22. Orbital rhabdomyosarcoma. A. Embryonal rhabdomyosarcoma, orbit. Spindled mesenchymal cells in a loose myxoid stroma constitute poorly differentiated embryonal tumor. Most orbital rhabdomyosarcomas are classified as embryonal. **B. Orbital rhabdomyosarcoma with cross striations and rhabdomyoblasts.** *Arrow* points to eosinophilic strap cell with cross striations. Rhabdomyoblast above has eosinophilic cytoplasm. Many embryonal rhabdomyosarcomas lack cross striations. Immunohistochemistry is used to demonstrate striated muscle differentiation. **C. Alveolar rhabdomyosarcoma.** Round, poorly cohesive tumor cells are compartmentalized by fibrous septa that resemble pulmonary alveoli. **D. Inset** shows large polygonal tumor cells with eosinophilic cytoplasm. **E. Rhabdomyosarcoma, immunohistochemical diagnosis.** Cells in embryonal tumor show positive nuclear staining for myogenin, a transcription factor specific for striated muscle. The tumor was also immunoreactive for MyoD, desmin, and muscle specific actin. (**A.** H&E ×150, **B.** H&E ×250, **C.** H&E ×50, **D.** H&E ×250, **E.** IHC for myogenin ×100)

average at age 7 and is more common in boys. The possibility of rhabdomyosarcoma should be considered in any child with orbital disease. Orbital rhabdomyosarcoma often grows rapidly and can cause fulminant proptosis. Occasionally, progression is so rapid that the tumor can be confused with inflammatory disease. Orbital rhabdomyosarcoma affects the superior orbit most commonly and may appear deceptively well circumscribed on imaging studies. About 60% of cases erode through the ethmoidal lamina papyracea in the medial orbital wall. Infrequently, rhabdomyosarcoma arises in the paranasal sinuses and invades the orbit secondarily. Macroscopically, fresh tumor usually is fleshy or yellow in color and may be focally hemorrhagic.

Histologically, rhabdomyosarcoma is nonencapsulated, and its growth pattern is usually infiltrative, although "pushing" margins occasionally are encountered. Several histologic variants of orbital rhabdomyosarcoma are recognized. Most orbital tumors are embryonal rhabdomyosarcomas, which are poorly differentiated neoplasms composed of spindle and strap cells arranged haphazardly in a loose, myxomatous stroma (Fig. 14-22A). Cross striations (Fig. 14-22B) are found in <60% of cases, but rhabdomyoblasts, which appear as globoid cells, with abundant eosinophilic cytoplasm may be present. Immunohistochemistry is used to confirm the diagnosis in most cases (see below). In some instances, special studies including immunohistochemistry or electron microscopy fail to reveal evidence of striated muscle differentiation. Such tumors are called embryonic sarcomas. Botryoid rhabdomyosarcoma is a variant of embryonal rhabdomyosarcoma that is associated with a mucous membrane like the conjunctiva. Botryoid rhabdomyosarcomas have a multinodular grapelike appearance clinically.

Alveolar rhabdomyosarcoma is less common, tends to arise in the inferior orbit, and tends to have a poorer prognosis. Approximately 75% of alveolar rhabdomyosarcomas have characteristic chromosomal translocations t(2;13) or t(1;13) that result in fusion of the PAX3 or PAX7 genes with the FKHR or FOXO1A gene on chromosome 13. The latter can be detected with molecular genetic techniques. The tumor cells in alveolar rhabdomyosarcoma are enclosed by fibrous tissue septa that resemble alveoli in the lungs (Fig. 14-22C,D). The large polygonal tumor cells have abundant eosinophilic cytoplasm. Pleomorphic or differentiated rhabdomyosarcomas are rare in the orbit and occur in adults.

Orbital rhabdomyosarcomas probably arise from pluripotential mesenchymal cells and are not derived from the dedifferentiation of an extraocular muscle. The diagnosis can be rapidly confirmed by immunohistochemistry that shows the presence of myogenesis-associated proteins such as desmin, myogenin, and MyoD (Fig. 14-22E). Diagnostic transmission electron microscopy can also disclose sarcomeric units and 150 Å myosin filaments but is rarely performed. After orbital rhabdomyosarcoma is diagnosed by expedient biopsy, the tumor usually is treated with a combination of radiation and adjuvant chemotherapy. Orbital exenteration is rarely necessary. The prognosis of orbital rhabdomyosarcoma is relatively good. The Intergroup Rhabdomyosarcoma Study-IV found that the 3-year failure free survival rate was 91%.

Hematopoietic Lesions

Lymphomas are rare in childhood. If an apparent "lymphoma" is encountered in the orbit of a child, an infiltrate of leukemic cells called a granulocytic or myeloid

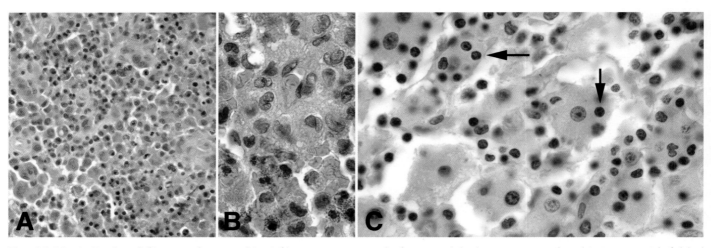

Fig. 14-23. A. Eosinophilic granuloma, orbit. Infiltrate is composed of eosinophils, large mononuclear histiocytes with folded nuclei, and small round osteoclast-like giant cells. **B.** Higher magnification shows folds in histiocytic nuclei. Eosinophilic granuloma is a localized form of Langerhans cell histiocytosis that characteristically forms a lytic lesion in the superotemporal orbital bone. The cells stain positively for CD-1A and S-100 protein and contain racket-shaped Birbeck granules disclosed by electron microscopy. **C. Sinus histiocytosis with massive lymphadenopathy (Rosai-Dorfman disease).** Large histiocytes in orbital infiltrate have phagocytized lymphocytes (*arrows*), a process called emperipolesis. The histiocytes are S-100 positive. (**A.** H&E ×100, **B.** H&E ×250, **C.** H&E ×250)

sarcoma must be excluded. In the past, the Leder esterase stain (Fig. 14-20B) was used to confirm granulocytic differentiation, but this has largely been supplanted by IHC stains for antigens including myeloperoxidase, lysozyme, and CD43. In the past, granulocytic sarcomas were called chloromas, reflecting a greenish hue caused by myeloperoxidase in some tumors. Infiltration of the orbital tissues by leukemic cells may antedate peripheral leukemia or even bone marrow involvement by several months.

Orbital involvement can occur in Langerhans cell histiocytosis (Histiocytosis X), especially the eosinophilic granuloma variant, which typically causes a cystic or erosive lesion in the superotemporal orbital bone. Biopsy shows a mixture of histiocytes with folded nuclei, eosinophils, and small round osteoclast-like giant cells (Fig. 14-23A). The histiocytes stain positively for Langerhans cell marker CD1a and S-100 protein. Electron microscopy shows rod or tennis racket–shaped Birbeck granules in the cytoplasm of the Langerhans cells.

Sinus histiocytosis with massive lymphadenopathy (Rosai-Dorfman disease) can involve the orbit. The histiocytes are S-100 protein positive and show emperipolesis (Fig. 14-23B).

Most orbital metastases in children stem from neuroblastoma or Ewing Sarcoma. Metastatic orbital neuroblastoma occurs in the late stages of the disease in children who are known to have the tumor. Metastases from neuroblastoma are often hemorrhagic and cause periocular ecchymoses, an appearance termed "raccoon eyes."

BIBLIOGRAPHY

General References

Henderson JW. (in Collaboration with Campbell RJ, Farrow GM and Garrity JA). *Orbital Tumors*, 3rd ed. New York, NY: Raven Press, 1994.

Jakobiec FA, Bilyk JR, Font RL. Orbit. In: Spencer W, ed. *Ophthalmic Pathology: An Atlas and Textbook*, 4th ed., vol. 2, Philadelphia, PA: WB Saunders, 1996:2438–2933.

Rootman J. *Diseases of the Orbit*. Philadelphia, PA: JB Lipincott, 1988.

Shields JA. *Diagnosis and Management of Orbital Tumors*. Philadelphia, PA: WB Saunders, 1989.

Shields JA, Shields CL, Scartozzi R. Survey of 1264 patients with orbital tumors and simulating lesions: the 2002 Montgomery Lecture, part 1. *Ophthalmology* 2004;111:997–1008.

Orbital Cellulitis

Bilyk JR. Periocular infection. *Curr Opin Ophthalmol* 2007;18:414–423.

Hornblass A, Herschorn BJ, Stern K, et al. Orbital abscess. *Surv Ophthalmol* 1984;29:169–179.

Macy HI, Mandelbaum SH, Minckler DA. Orbital cellulitis. *Ophthalmology* 1980;87:1309–1314.

Shields JA, Shields CL, Suvarnamani C, et al. Retinoblastoma manifesting as orbital cellulitis. *Am J Ophthalmol* 1991;112:442–449.

Watters EC, Wallar PH, Hiles DA, et al. Acute orbital cellulitis. *Arch Ophthalmol* 1976;94:785–788.

Weiss A, Friendly D, Eglin K, et al. Bacterial periorbital and orbital cellulitis in childhood. *Ophthalmology* 1983;90:195–203.

Youssef OH, Stefanyszyn MA, Bilyk JR. Odontogenic orbital cellulitis. *Ophthal Plast Reconstr Surg* 2008;24:29–35.

Fungal Infection

Chang WJ, Shields CL, Shields JA, et al. Bilateral orbital involvement with massive allergic fungal sinusitis [letter]. *Arch Ophthalmol* 1996;114:767–768.

DeJuan E, Green WR, Iliff NT. Allergic periorbital mucopyocele in children. *Am J Ophthalmol* 1983;96:299–303.

Ferry AP, Abedi S. Diagnosis and management of rhino-orbitocerebral mucormycosis (phycomycosis). *Ophthalmology* 1983;90:1096–1104.

Green WR, Font RL, Zimmerman LE. Aspergillosis of the orbit: report of ten cases and review of the literature. *Arch Ophthalmol* 1969;82: 302–312.

Houle T, Ellis P. Aspergillosis of the orbit with immunosuppressive therapy. *Surv Ophthalmol* 1975;20:35–41.

Klapper SR, Lee AG, Patrinely JR, et al. Orbital involvement in allergic fungal sinusitis. *Ophthalmology* 1997;104:2094–2100.

Yohai RA, Bullock JD, Aziz AA, et al. Survival factors in rhino-orbital-cerebral mucormycosis. *Surv Ophthalmol* 1994;39:3–22.

Thyroid Ophthalmology

Bahn RS. Clinical review 157: pathophysiology of Graves' ophthalmopathy: the cycle of disease. *J Clin Endocrinol Metab* 2003;88:1939–1946.

Char DH. The ophthalmopathy of Graves' disease. *Med Clin North Am* 1991;70:97–119.

Goldstein SM, Katowitz WR, Moshang T, et al. Pediatric thyroid-associated orbitopathy: the Children's Hospital of Philadelphia experience and literature review. *Thyroid* 2008;18:997–999.

Heufelder AE. Involvement of the orbital fibroblast and TSH receptor in the pathogenesis of Graves' ophthalmopathy. *Thyroid* 1995;5:331–340.

Hufnagel TJ, Hickey WF, Cobbs WH, et al. Immunohistochemical and ultrastructural studies on the exenterated orbital tissues of a patient with Graves' disease. *Ophthalmology* 1984;91:1411–1419.

Netland PA, Dallow RL. Thyroid ophthalmology. In: Albert DM, Jakobiec FA, eds. *Principles and Practice of Ophthalmology: Clinical Practice*, vol. 5. Philadelphia, PA: WB Saunders, 1994:2937–2955.

Sergott RC, Glaser JS. Graves' ophthalmopathy. A clinical and immunologic review. *Surv Ophthalmol* 1981;26:1–21.

van der Gaag R, Vernimmen R, Fiebelkorn N, et al. Graves' ophthalmopathy: what is the evidence for extraocular muscle specific autoantibodies. *Int Ophthalmol* 1990;14:25–30.

Wall JR, Bernard N, Boucher A, et al. Pathogenesis of thyroid-associated ophthalmopathy: an autoimmune disorder of the eye muscle associated with Graves' hyperthyroidism and Hashimoto's thyroiditis. *Clin Immunol Immunopathol* 1993;68:1–8.

Weetman AP, McGregor AM, Hall R. Ocular manifestations of Graves' disease: a review. *J R Soc Med* 1984;77:936–942.

Werner WC. Modification of the classification of the eye changes of Graves' disease. *Am J Ophthalmol* 1977;83:725–727.

Idiopathic Orbital Inflammation (Pseudotumor)

Abramovitz JN, Kasdon DL, Satala F, et al. Sclerosing orbital pseudotumor. *Neurosurgery* 1983;12:463–468.

Brannan PA. A review of sclerosing idiopathic orbital inflammation. *Curr Opin Ophthalmol* 2007;18:402–404.

Chavis RM, Garner A, Wright JE. Inflammatory orbital pseudotumor. A clinicopathologic study. *Arch Ophthalmol* 1978;96: 1817–1822.

Gordon LK. Orbital inflammatory disease: a diagnostic and therapeutic challenge. *Eye (Lond)* 2006;20:1196–1206.

Hara Y, Ohnishi Y. Orbital inflammatory pseudotumor: clinico-pathologic study of 22 cases. *Jpn J Ophthalmol* 1983;27:80–89.

Kennerdell JS, Dresner SC. The nonspecific orbital inflammatory syndromes. *Surv Ophthalmol* 1984;29:93–103.

McCarthy JM, White VA, Harris G, et al. Idiopathic sclerosing inflammation of the orbit: immunohistologic analysis and comparison with retroperitoneal fibrosis. *Mod Pathol* 1993;6:581–587.

Mehta M, Frederick Jakobiec FA, Fay A. Idiopathic fibroinflammatory disease of the face, eyelids, and periorbital membrane with immunoglobulin G4–positive plasma cells. *Arch Pathol Lab Med* 2009;133:1251–1255.

Mombaerts I, Goldschmeding R, Schlingemann RO, et al. What is orbital pseudotumor? *Surv Ophthalmol* 1996;41:66–78.

Mottow-Lippa L, Jakobiec FA. Idiopathic inflammatory orbital pseudotumor in childhood. *Arch Ophthalmol* 1978;96:1410–1417.

Rootman J, McCarthy M, White V, et al. Idiopathic sclerosing inflammation of the orbit. A distinct clinicopathologic entity. *Ophthalmology* 1994;101:570–584.

Uy HS, Nguyen QD, Arbour J, et al. Sclerosing inflammatory pseudotumor of the eye. *Arch Ophthalmol* 2001;119:603–607.

Wegener's Granulomatosis

Bullen CL, Liesegang TJ, McDonald TJ. Ocular complications of Wegener's granulomatosis. *Ophthalmology* 1983;90:279–290.

Kalina PH, Lie JT, Campbell RJ, et al. Diagnostic value and limitations of orbital biopsy in Wegener's granulomatosis. *Ophthalmology* 1994;99:120–124.

Koyama T, Matsuo N, Watanabe Y, et al. Wegener's granulomatosis with destructive ocular manifestations. *Am J Ophthalmol* 1984;98:736–740.

Perry SR, Rootman J, White VA. The clinical and pathologic constellation of Wegener granulomatosis of the orbit. *Ophthalmology* 1997;104:683–694.

Trocme SD, Bartley GB, Campbell RJ, et al. Eosinophil and neutrophil degranulation in ophthalmic lesions of Wegener's granulomatosis. *Arch Ophthalmol* 1991;109:1585–1589.

Orbital Xanthogranuloma

Hammond MD, Niemi EW, Ward TP, et al. Adult orbital xanthogranuloma with associated adult-onset asthma. *Ophthal Plast Reconstr Surg* 2004;20:329–332.

Karcioglu ZA, Sharara N, Boles TL, et al. Orbital xanthogranuloma: clinical and morphologic features in eight patients. *Ophthal Plast Reconstr Surg* 2003;19:372–381.

Miszkiel KA, Sohaib SA, Rose GE, et al. Radiological and clinicopathological features of orbital xanthogranuloma. *Br J Ophthalmol* 2000;84:251–258.

Sheu SY, Wenzel RR, Kersting C, et al. Erdheim-Chester disease: case report with multisystemic manifestations including testes, thyroid, and lymph nodes, and a review of literature. *J Clin Pathol* 2004;57:1225–1228.

Sivak-Callcott JA, Rootman J, Rasmussen SL, et al. Adult xanthogranulomatous disease of the orbit and ocular adnexa: new immunohistochemical findings and clinical review. *Br J Ophthalmol* 2006;90:602–608.

Lymphoid Tumors

Adkins JW, Shields JA, Shields CL, et al. Plasmacytoma of the eye and orbit. *Int Ophthalmol* 1996;20:339–343.

Chan JK. The new World Health Organization classification of lymphomas: the past, the present and the future. *Hematol Oncol* 2001;19:129–150.

Coupland SE, Damato B. Lymphomas involving the eye and the ocular adnexa. *Curr Opin Ophthalmol* 2006;17:523–531.

Coupland SE, Hummel M, Stein H. Ocular adnexal lymphomas: five case presentations and a review of the literature. *Surv Ophthalmol* 2002;47:470–490.

Coupland SE, Krause L, Delecluse HJ, et al. Lymphoproliferative lesions of the ocular adnexa. Analysis of 112 cases. *Ophthalmology* 1998;105:1430–1441.

Craig FE. Flow cytometric evaluation of B-cell lymphoid neoplasms. *Clin Lab Med* 2007;27:487–512.

Demirci H, Shields CL, Karatza EC, et al. Orbital lymphoproliferative tumors: analysis of clinical features and systemic involvement in 160 cases. *Ophthalmology* 2008;115:1626–1631.

Ferry JA, Fung CY, Zukerberg L, et al. Lymphoma of the ocular adnexa: a study of 353 cases. *Am J Surg Pathol* 2007;31:170–184.

Kaleem Z. Flow cytometric analysis of lymphomas: current status and usefulness. *Arch Pathol Lab Med* 2006;130:1850–1858.

Knowles DM, Jakobiec FA, McNally L, et al. Lymphoid hyperplasia and malignant lymphoma occurring in the ocular adnexa (orbit, conjunctiva, and eyelids): a prospective multiparametric analysis of 108 case during 1977 to 1987. *Hum Pathol* 1990;21:959–973.

Looi A, Gascoyne RD, Chhanabhai M, et al. Mantle cell lymphoma in the ocular adnexal region. *Ophthalmology* 2005;112:114–119.

Margo CE. Orbital and ocular adnexal lymphoma: evolving concepts. In: Grossniklaus HE, Margo CE, eds. *Advances in Ophthalmic Pathology. Ophthalmol Clin North Am* 1995;8:167–177.

Medeiros LJ, Harris NL. Immunuhistologic analysis of small lymphocytic infiltrates of the orbit and conjunctiva. *Hum Pathol* 1990;21:1126–1131.

Swerdlow SH, Campo E, Harris NL, et al., eds. *WHO Classification of Tumours of Haemopoietic and Lymphoid Tissues*, 4th ed. Geneva, Switzerland: World Health Organization, 2008.

White WL, Ferry JA, Harris NL, et al. Ocular adnexal lymphoma. A clinicopathologic study with identification of lymphomas of mucosa-associated lymphoid tissue type. *Ophthalmology* 1995;102:1994–2006.

Vascular Tumors

Croxatto JO, Font RL. Hemangiopericytoma of the orbit: a clinicopathologic study of 30 cases. *Hum Pathol* 1982;13:210–218.

Font RL, Wheeler TM, Boniuk M. Intravascular papillary endothelial hyperplasia of the orbit and ocular adnexa. A report of five cases. *Arch Ophthalmol* 1983;101:1731–1736.

Harris GJ, Jakobiec FA. Cavernous hemangioma of the orbit: an analysis of 66 cases. *J Neurosurg* 1979;51:219–228.

Henderson JW, Farrow GM. Primary orbital hemangiopericytoma: an aggressive and potentially malignant neoplasm. *Arch Ophthalmol* 1978;96:666–673.

Iwamoto T, Jakobiec FA. Ultrastructural comparison of capillary and cavernous hemangiomas of the orbit. *Arch Ophthalmol* 1979;97:1144–1153.

Ruchman MC, Flanagan J. Cavernous hemangiomas of the orbit. *Ophthalmology* 1983;90:1328–1336.

Shields JA, Shields CL, Eagle RC Jr. Cavernous hemangioma of the orbit. *Arch Ophthalmol* 1987;105:853.

Werner MS, Hornblass A, Reifler DM, et al. Intravascular papillary endothelial hyperplasia: collection of four cases and a review of the literature. *Ophthal Plast Reconstr Surg* 1997;13:48–56.

Neural Tumors

Blodi FC. Amputation neuroma in the orbit. *Am J Ophthalmol* 1949;32:929–932.

Coleman DJ, Jack RL, Franzen LA. Neurogenic tumors of the orbit. *Arch Ophthalmol* 1972;88:380–384.

Krohel GB, Rosenberg MD, Wright JE Jr, et al. Localized orbital neurofibromas. *Am J Ophthalmol* 1985;100:458–464.

Rootman J, Goldberg C, Robertson W. Primary orbital schwannomas. *Br J Ophthalmol* 1982;66:194–204.

Mesenchymal Tumors

Bartley GB, Yeatts RP, Garrity JA, et al. Spindle cell lipoma of the orbit. *Am J Ophthalmol* 1985;100:605–609.

Dorfman DM, To K, Dickersin GR, et al. Solitary fibrous tumor of the orbit. *Am J Surg Pathol* 1994;18:281–287.

Folberg R, Cleasby G, Flanagan JA, et al. Orbital leiomyosarcoma after radiation therapy for bilateral retinoblastoma. *Arch Ophthalmol* 1983;101:1562–1565.

Font RL, Hidayat AA. Fibrous histiocytoma of the orbit: a clinicopathologic study of 150 cases. *Hum Pathol* 1982;13:199–209.

Font RL, Jurco S III, Brechner RJ: Postradiation leiomyosarcoma of the orbit complicating bilateral retinoblastoma. *Arch Ophthalmol* 1983;101:1557–1561.

Goldsmith JD, van de Rijn M, Syed N. Orbital hemangiopericytoma and solitary fibrous tumor: a morphologic continuum. *Int J Surg Pathol* 2001;9:295–302.

Guccion J, Font RL, Enzinger FM, et al. Extraskeletal mesenchymal chondrosarcoma. *Arch Pathol* 1973;95:336–340.

Hidayat AA, Font RL. Juvenile fibromatosis of the periorbital region and eyelid. A clinicopathologic study of six cases. *Arch Ophthalmol* 1980;98:280–285.

Holland MG, Allen JH, Ichinose H. Chondrosarcoma of the orbit. *Trans Am Acad Ophthalmol Otolaryngol* 1961;65:898–905.

Jakobiec FA, Rini F, Char D, et al. Primary liposarcoma of the orbit. Problems in the diagnosis and management of five cases. *Ophthalmology* 1989;96:180–191.

Krishnakumar S, Subramanian N, Mohan ER, et al. Solitary fibrous tumor of the orbit: a clinicopathologic study of six cases with review of the literature. *Surv Ophthalmol* 2003;48:544–554.

Sanborn GE, Valenzuela RE, Green WR. Leiomyoma of the orbit. *Am J Ophthalmol* 1979;87:371–375.

Weiner JM, Hidayat AA. Juvenile fibrosarcoma of the orbit and eyelid. *Arch Ophthalmol* 1983;101:253–259.

Rare Orbital Tumors

Folpe AL, Goldblum JR, Rubin BP, et al. Morphologic and immunophenotypic diversity in Ewing family tumors: a study of 66 genetically confirmed cases. *Am J Surg Pathol* 2005;29:1025–1033.

Font RL, Jurco S III, Zimmerman LE. Alveolar soft-part sarcoma of the orbit. *Hum Pathol* 1982;13:569–579.

Goldstein BG, Font RL, Alper MG. Granular cell tumor of the orbit: a case report including electron microscopic observation. *Ann Ophthalmol* 1982;14:231–238.

Gunduz K, Shields JA, Eagle RC Jr, et al. Malignant rhabdoid tumor of the orbit. *Arch Ophthalmol* 1998;116:243–246.

Jakobiec FA, Ellsworth R, Tannenbaum M. Primary orbital melanoma. *Am J Ophthalmol* 1974;78:24–39.

Lamping KA, Albert DM, Lack E, et al. Melanotic neuroectodermal tumor of infancy (retinal anlage tumor). *Ophthalmology* 1985;92:143–147.

Margo CE, Folberg R, Zimmerman LE, et al. Endodermal sinus tumor (yolk sac tumor) of the orbit. *Ophthalmology* 1983;90:1426–1432.

Rootman J, DamJi KF, Dimmick JE. Malignant rhabdoid tumor of the orbit. *Ophthalmology* 1989;96:1650–1604.

Singh AD, Husson M, Shields CL, et al. Primitive neuroectodermal tumor of the orbit. *Arch Ophthalmol* 1994;112:217–221.

Tellada M, Specht CS, McLean IW, et al. Primary orbital melanomas. *Ophthalmology* 1996;103:929–932.

Zimmerman LE, Stangl R, Riddle PJ. Primary carcinoid tumor of the orbit. *Arch Ophthalmol* 1983;101:1395–1398.

Osseous and Fibro-osseous Lesions

Blodi FC. Pathology of orbital bones. *Am J Ophthalmol* 1976;81:1–26.

Fu YS, Perzin KH. Non-epithelial tumors of the nasal cavity, paranasal sinuses, and nasopharynx: a clinicopathological study. II. Osseous and fibro-osseous lesions, including osteoma, fibrous dysplasia, ossifying fibroma, osteoblastoma, giant cell tumor and osteosarcoma. *Cancer* 1974;33:1289–1305.

Hoopes PC, Anderson RL, Blodi FC. Giant cell (reparative) granuloma of the orbit. *Ophthalmology* 1981;88:1361–1366.

Klepach GL, Ho REM, Kelly JK. Aneurysmal bone cyst of the orbit. *J Clin Neuro-Ophthalmol* 1984;4:49–52.

Margo CE, Ragsdale B, Purman K, et al. Psammomatoid (juvenile) ossifying fibroma of the orbit. *Ophthalmology* 1985;92:150–159.

Moore AT, Buncic R. Fibrous dysplasia of the orbit in childhood: clinical features and management. *Ophthalmology* 1985;92:12–20.

Naiman J, Green WR, D'Heurle D, et al. Brown tumor of the orbit associated with primary hyperparathyroidism. *Am J Ophthalmol* 1980;90:565–571.

Spraul CW, Wojno TH, Grossniklaus HE, et al. Reparative giant cell granuloma with orbital involvement. *Klin Monatsbl Augenheilkd* 1997;211:133–134.

Lacrimal Gland Tumors

Ahmad SM, Esmaeli B, Williams M, et al. American Joint Committee on Cancer classification predicts outcome of patients with lacrimal gland adenoid cystic carcinoma. *Ophthalmology* 2009;116:1210–1215.

Bartley GB, Harris GJ. Adenoid cystic carcinoma of the lacrimal gland: is there a cure…yet? *Ophthal Plast Reconstr Surg* 2002;18:315–318.

Biggs SL, Font RL. Oncocytic lesions of the lacrimal gland. *Arch Ophthalmol* 1977;95:474–478.

Bonavolonta G, Tranfa F, Staibano S, et al. Warthin tumor of the lacrimal gland. *Am J Ophthalmol* 1997;124:857–858.

Briscoe D, Mahmood S, Bonshek R, et al. Primary sebaceous carcinoma of the lacrimal gland. *Br J Ophthalmol* 2001;85:625–626.

Brownstein S, Belin MW, Krohel GB, et al. Orbital dacryops. *Ophthalmology* 1984;91:1424–1428.

Chan WM, Liu DT, Lam LY, et al. Primary epithelial-myoepithelial carcinoma of the lacrimal gland. *Arch Ophthalmol* 2004;122:1714–1717.

Chang CJ, Lin TK, Wei LC, et al. Carcinoma ex pleomorphic adenoma of the lacrimal gland: a case report. *Ann Ophthalmol (Skokie)* 2006;38:141–144.

Cunningham RD. Lacrimal gland tumors. In: Fraunfelder FT, Roy FH, eds. *Current Ocular Therapy 4*. Philadelphia, PA: WB Saunders, 1995:693–695.

Eviatar JA, Hornblass A. Mucoepidermoid carcinoma of the lacrimal gland: 25 cases and a review and update of the literature. *Ophthal Plast Reconstr Surg* 1993;9:170–181.

Fenton S, Srinivasan S, Harnett A, et al. Primary squamous cell carcinoma of the lacrimal gland. *Eye (Lond)* 2003;17:424–425.

Font RL, Gamel JW. Adenoid cystic carcinoma of the lacrimal gland: a clinicopathological study of 79 cases. In: Nicholson DH, ed. *Ocular Pathology Update*. New York, NY: Masson Publishing USA, 1980:277–283.

Font RL, Gamel JW. Epithelial tumors of the lacrimal gland: an analysis of 256 cases. In: Jakobiec FA, ed. *Ocular and Adnexal Tumors*. Birmingham, AL: Aesculapius, 1978:787–805.

Font RL, Yanoff M, Zimmerman LE. Benign lymphoepithelial lesion of the lacrimal gland and its relationship to Sjogren's syndrome. *Am J Clin Pathol* 1967;48:365–376.

Gamel JW, Font RL. Adenoid cystic carcinoma of the lacrimal gland: the clinical significance of a basaloid histologic pattern. *Hum Pathol* 1982;13:219–225.

Gibson A, Mavrikakis I, Rootman J, et al. Lacrimal gland pleomorphic adenomas with low-density zones resembling cystic change on computed tomography. *Ophthal Plast Reconstr Surg* 2007;23:234–235.

Grossniklaus HE, Wojno TH, Wilson MW, et al. Myoepithelioma of the lacrimal gland. *Arch Ophthalmol* 1997;115:1588–1590.

Henderson JW. Adenoid cystic carcinoma of the lacrimal gland, is there a cure? *Trans Am Ophthalmol Soc* 1987;85:312–319.

Hotta K, Arisawa T, Mito H, et al. Primary squamous cell carcinoma of the lacrimal gland. *Clin Experiment Ophthalmol* 2005;33:534–536.

Ishida M, Hotta M, Kushima R, et al. Case of ductal adenocarcinoma ex pleomorphic adenoma of the lacrimal gland. *Rinsho Byori* 2009;57:746–751.

Iwamota T, Jakobiec FA. A comparative ultrastructural study of the normal lacrimal gland and its epithelial tumors. *Hum Pathol* 1982;13:236–262.

Jang J, Kie JH, Lee SY, et al. Acinic cell carcinoma of the lacrimal gland with intracranial extension: a case report. *Ophthal Plast Reconstr Surg* 2001;17:454–457.

Katz SE, Rootman J, Dolman PJ, et al. Primary ductal adenocarcinoma of the lacrimal gland. *Ophthalmology* 1996;103:157–162.

Khalil M, Arthurs B. Basal cell adenocarcinoma of the lacrimal gland. *Ophthalmology* 2000;107:164–168.

Lee DA, Campbell RJ, Waller RR, et al. A clinicopathologic study of primary adenoid cystic carcinoma of the lacrimal gland. *Ophthalmology* 1985;92:128–134.

Lee YJ, Oh YH. Primary ductal adenocarcinoma of the lacrimal gland. *Jpn J Ophthalmol* 2009;53:268–270.

Lin SC, Kau HC, Yang CF, et al. Adenoid cystic carcinoma arising in the inferior orbit without evidence of lacrimal gland involvement. *Ophthal Plast Reconstr Surg* 2008;24:74–76.

Malhotra GS, Paul SD, Batra DV. Mucoepidermoid carcinoma of the lacrimal gland. *Ophthalmologica* 1967;153:184–190.

Milman T, Shields JA, Husson M, et al. Primary ductal adenocarcinoma of the lacrimal gland. *Ophthalmology* 2005;112:2048–2051.

Ostrowski ML, Font RL, Halpern J, et al. Clear cell epithelial-myoepithelial carcinoma arising in pleomorphic adenoma of the lacrimal gland. *Ophthalmology* 1994;101:925–930.

Perzin K, Jakobiec FA, LiVolsi V, et al. Malignant mixed tumors of the lacrimal gland. *Cancer* 1980;45:2593–606.

Rao NA, Kaiser E, Quiros PA, et al. Lymphoepithelial carcinoma of the lacrimal gland. *Arch Ophthalmol* 2002;120:1745–1748.

Rootman J, White VA. Changes in the 7th edition of the AJCC TNM classification and recommendations for pathologic analysis of lacrimal gland tumors. *Arch Pathol Lab Med* 2009;133:1268–1271.

Rose GE, Wright JE. Pleomorphic adenoma of the lacrimal gland. *Br J Ophthalmol* 1992;76:395–400.

Rosenbaum PS, Mahadevia PS, Goodman LA, et al. Acinic cell carcinoma of the lacrimal gland. *Arch Ophthalmol* 1995;113:781–785.

Selva D, Davis GJ, Dodd T, et al. Polymorphous low-grade adenocarcinoma of the lacrimal gland. *Arch Ophthalmol* 2004;122:915–917.

Shields CL, Shields JA, Eagle RC. Rathmell JP. Clinicopathologic review of 142 cases of lacrimal gland lesions. *Ophthalmology* 1989;96:431–435.

Shields JA, Shields CL, Eagle RC Jr, et al. Adenoid cystic carcinoma developing in the nasal orbit. *Am J Ophthalmol* 1997;123:398–389.

Shields JA, Shields CL, Epstein JA, et al. Review: primary epithelial malignancies of the lacrimal gland: the 2003 Ramon L. Font lecture. *Ophthal Plast Reconstr Surg* 2004;20:10–21.

Sofinski SJ, Brown BZ, Rao N, et al. Mucoepidermoid carcinoma of the lacrimal gland. Case report and review of the literature. *Ophthal Plast Reconstr Surg* 1986;2:147–151.

Su GW, Patipa M, Font RL. Primary squamous cell carcinoma arising from an epithelium-lined cyst of the lacrimal gland. *Ophthal Plast Reconstr Surg* 2005;21:383–385.

Takahira M, Minato H, Takahashi M, et al. Cystic carcinoma ex pleomorphic adenoma of the lacrimal gland. *Ophthal Plast Reconstr Surg* 2007;23:407–409.

Tellado MV, McLean IW, Specht CS, et al. Adenoid cystic carcinomas of the lacrimal gland in childhood and adolescence. *Ophthalmology* 1997;104:1622–1625.

Vangveeravong S, Katz SE, Rootman J, et al. Tumors arising in the palpebral lobe of the lacrimal gland. *Ophthalmology* 1996;103:1606–1612.

Wagoner MD, Chuo N, Gonder JR. Mucoepidermoid carcinoma of the lacrimal gland. *Ann Ophthalmol* 1982;14:383–386.

Weis E, Rootman J, Joly TJ, et al. Epithelial lacrimal gland tumors: pathologic classification and current understanding. *Arch Ophthalmol* 2009;127:1016–1028.

Wiwatwongwana D, Berean KW, Dolman PJ, et al. Unusual carcinomas of the lacrimal gland: epithelial-myoepithelial carcinoma and myoepithelial carcinoma. *Arch Ophthalmol* 2009;127:1054–1056.

Wright JE, Rose GE, Garner A. Primary malignant neoplasms of the lacrimal gland. *Br J Ophthalmol* 1992;76:401–407.

Yamamoto N, Mizoe JE, Hasegawa A, et al. Primary sebaceous carcinoma of the lacrimal gland treated by carbon ion radiotherapy. *Int J Clin Oncol* 2003;8:386–390.

Orbital Metastasis

Ahmad SM, Esmaeli B. Metastatic tumors of the orbit and ocular adnexa. *Curr Opin Ophthalmol* 2007;18:405–413.

Cline RA, Rootman J. Enophthalmos: a clinical review. *Ophthalmology* 1984;91:229–237.

Font RL, Ferry AP. Carcinoma metastatic to the eye and orbit. III. A clinicopathologic study of 28 cases metastatic to the orbit. *Cancer* 1976;38:1326–1335.

Goldberg RA, Rootman J, Cline RA. Tumors metastatic to the orbit: a changing picture. *Surv Ophthalmol* 1990;35:1–24.

Holland D, Maune S, Kovacs G, et al. Metastatic tumors of the orbit: a retrospective study. *Orbit* 2003;22:15–24.

Sabatini P, Ducic Y. Bilateral lacrimal gland masses: unusual case of metastatic renal cell carcinoma. *J Otolaryngol Head Neck Surg* 2009;38:E1–E2.

Shields CL, Shields JA, Peggs M. Tumors metastatic to the orbit. *Ophthal Plast Reconstr Surg* 1988;4:73–80.

Shields JA, Shields CL, Brotman HK, et al. Cancer metastatic to the orbit: the 2000 Robert M. Curts Lecture. *Ophthal Plast Reconstr Surg* 2001;17:346–354.

Watkins LM, Rubin PA. Metastatic tumors of the eye and orbit. *Int Ophthalmol Clin* 1998;38:117–128.

Zografos L, Ducrey N, Beati D, et al. Metastatic melanoma in the eye and orbit. *Ophthalmology* 2003;110:2245–2256.

Mucocele

Alberti PWRM, Marshall HF, Black HIM. Frontoethmoidal mucocoele as a cause of unilateral proptosis. *Br J Ophthalmol* 1968;52:833–838.

Avery G, Tang RA, Close LG. Ophthalmic manifestations of mucoceles. *Ann Ophthalmol* 1983;15:734–737.

Iliff CE. Mucoceles in the orbit. *Arch Ophthalmol* 1973;89:392–395.

Dermoid Cysts

Dutton JJ, Fowler AM, Proia AD. Dermoid cyst of conjunctival origin. *Ophthal Plast Reconstr Surg* 2006;22:137–139.

Emerick GT, Shields CL, Shields JA, et al. Chewing-induced visual impairment from a dumbbell dermoid cyst. *Ophthal Plast Reconstr Surg* 1997;13:57–61.

Jakobiec FA, Bonanno PA. Conjunctival adnexal cysts and dermoids. *Arch Ophthalmol* 1978;96:1040–1049.

Shields JA, Kaden IH, Eagle RC Jr, et al. Orbital dermoid cysts: clinicopathologic correlations, classification and management. The 1997 Josephine E. Schueler Lecture. *Ophthal Plast Reconstr Surg* 1997;13:265–276.

Rhabdomyosarcoma

Abramson DH, Ellsworth RM, Tretter P, et al. The treatment of orbital rhabdomyosarcoma with irradiation and chemotherapy. *Ophthalmology* 1979;86:1330–1335.

Ashton N. Embryonal sarcoma and embryonal rhabdomyosarcoma of the orbit. *J Clin Pathol* 1965;18:699–714.

Crist WM, Anderson JR, Meza JL, et al. Intergroup rhabdomyosarcoma study-IV: results for patients with nonmetastatic disease. *J Clin Oncol* 2001;19:3091–3102.

Donaldson SS, Meza J, Breneman JC, et al. Results from the IRS-IV randomized trial of hyperfractionated radiotherapy in children with rhabdomyosarcoma—a report from the IRSG. *Int J Radiat Oncol Biol Phys* 2001;51:718–728.

Jakobiec FA, Font RL. Ocular and orbital tumors. In: Johanessen JV, ed. *The Nervous System, Sensory Organs and Respiratory Tract. Electron Microscopy in Human Diseases*, vol. VI. New York, NY: McGraw-Hill Book Co., 1979:346–368.

Karcioglu ZA, Hadjistilianou D, Rozans M, et al. Orbital rhabdomyosarcoma. *Cancer Control* 2004;11:328–333.

Knowles DM II, Jakobiec FA, Potter G, et al. Ophthalmic striated muscle neoplasms. *Surv Ophthalmol* 1976;21:219–261.

Newton WA, Soule EH, Hamoudi AB, et al. Histopathology of childhood sarcomas, intergroup rhabdomyosarcoma studies I and II: clinicopathologic correlation. *J Clin Oncol* 1988;6:67–75.

Porterfield JF, Zimmerman LE. Rhabdomyosarcoma of the orbit: a clinicopathologic study of 55 cases. *Virchows Arch [A]* 1962;335:329–344.

Raney RB, Anderson JR, Barr FG, et al. Rhabdomyosarcoma and undifferentiated sarcoma in the first two decades of life: a selective review of intergroup rhabdomyosarcoma study group experience and rationale for Intergroup Rhabdomyosarcoma Study V. *J Pediatr Hematol Oncol* 2001;23:215–220.

Raney RB, Anderson JR, Kollath J, et al. Late effects of therapy in 94 patients with localized rhabdomyosarcoma of the orbit: report from the Intergroup Rhabdomyosarcoma Study (IRS)-III, 1984–1991. *Med Pediatr Oncol* 2000;34:413–420.

Raney RB, Maurer HM, Anderson JR, et al. The Intergroup Rhabdomyosarcoma Study Group (IRSG): major lessons from the IRS-I through IRS-IV studies as background for the current IRS-V treatment protocols. *Sarcoma* 2001;5:9–15.

Shields CL, Shields JA, Honavar SG, et al. Clinical spectrum of primary ophthalmic rhabdomyosarcoma. *Ophthalmology* 2001;108:2284–2292.

Shields CL, Shields JA, Honavar SG, et al. Primary ophthalmic rhabdomyosarcoma in 33 patients. *Trans Am Ophthalmol Soc* 2001;99:133–142, discussion 142–133.

Shields JA, Shields CL. Rhabdomyosarcoma: review for the ophthalmologist. *Surv Ophthalmol* 2003;48:39–57.

Other Pediatric Orbital Tumors

Barnes CM, Christison-Lagay EA, Folkman J. The placenta theory and the origin of infantile hemangioma. *Lymphat Res Biol* 2007;5:245–255.

Barnes CM, Huang S, Kaipainen A, et al. Evidence by molecular profiling for a placental origin of infantile hemangioma. *Proc Natl Acad Sci U S A* 2005;102:19097–19102.

Ellis FJ, Eagle RC Jr, Shields JA. Phakomatous choristoma (Zimmerman's tumor): immunohistochemical confirmation of lens-specific proteins. *Ophthalmology* 1993;100:955–960.

Fay A, Nguyen J, Jakobiec FA, et al. Propranolol for isolated orbital infantile hemangioma. *Arch Ophthalmol* 2010;128:256–258.

Ferry AP, Font AP. The phakomatoses. *Int Ophthalmol Clin* 1972;12:1–50.

Folpe AL, Goldblum JR, Rubin BP, et al. Morphologic and immuno-phenotypic diversity in Ewing family tumors: a study of 66 genetically confirmed cases. *Am J Surg Pathol* 2005;29:1025–1033.

Galambos C, Nodit L. Identification of lymphatic endothelium in pediatric vascular tumors and malformations. *Pediatr Dev Pathol* 2005;8:181–189.

Gausas RE, Daly T, Fogt F. D2-40 expression demonstrates lymphatic vessel characteristics in the dural portion of the optic nerve sheath. *Ophthal Plast Reconstr Surg* 2007;Jan-Feb(23):32–36.

Haik BG, Karcioglu ZA, Gordon RA, et al. Capillary hemangioma (infantile periocular hemangioma). *Surv Ophthalmol* 1994;38:399–426.

Hidayat AA, Cameron JD, Font RL, et al. Angiolymphoid hyperplasia with eosinophilia (Kimura's disease) of the orbit and ocular adnexa. *Am J Ophthalmol* 1983;96:176–189.

Illif WJ, Green WR. Orbital lymphangiomas. *Ophthalmology* 1979;86:914–929.

Kivela T, Tarkkanen A. Orbital germ cell tumors revisted: a clinicopathological approach to classification. *Surv Ophthalmol* 1994;38:541–554.

Kobrin JL, Blodi FC, Weingeist TA. Ocular and orbital manifestations of neurofibromatosis. *Surv Ophthalmol* 1979;24:45–51.

Leaute-Labreze C, Dumas de la Roque E, Hubiche T, et al. Propranolol for severe hemangiomas of infancy. *N Engl J Med* 2008;358(24):2649–2651.

Lo K, Mihm M, Fay A. Current theories on the pathogenesis of infantile hemangioma. *Semin Ophthalmol* 2009;24:172–177.

McEachren TM, Brownstein S, Jordan DR, et al. Epithelioid hemangioma of the orbit. *Ophthalmology* 2000;107:806–810.

Ramchandani PL, Sabesan T, Hussein K. Angiolymphoid hyperplasia with eosinophilia masquerading as Kimura disease. *Br J Oral Maxillofac Surg* 2005;43:249–252.

Sartelet H, Grossi L, Pasquier D, et al. Detection of N-myc amplification by FISH in immature areas of fixed neuroblastomas: more efficient than Southern blot/PCR. *J Pathol* 2002;198:83–91.

Shields JA, Bakewell B, Augsburger JJ, et al. Space-occupying orbital masses in children: a review of 250 consecutive biopsies. *Ophthalmology* 1986;93:379–384.

Singh AD, Husson M, Shields CL, et al. Primitive neuroectodermal tumor of the orbit. *Arch Ophthalmol* 1994;112:217–221.

Sun ZY, Yi CG, Zhao H, et al. Infantile hemangioma is originated from placental trophoblast, fact or fiction? *Med Hypotheses* 2008;71:444–448.

Tajiri T, Shono K, Fujii Y, et al. Highly sensitive analysis for N-myc amplification in neuroblastoma based on fluorescence in situ hybridization. *J Pediatr Surg* 1999;34:1615–1619.

Wilson DJ, Dailey RA, Griffeth MT, et al. Primary Ewing sarcoma of the orbit. *Ophthal Plast Reconstr Surg* 2001;17:300–303.

Woog JJ, Albert DM, Solt LC, et al. Neurofibromatosis of the eyeball and orbit. *Int Ophthalmol Clin* 1982;22:157–187.

Leukemic and Histiocytic Disorders

Davis JL, Parke DW II, Font RL. Granulocytic sarcoma of the orbit: a clinicopathologic study. *Ophthalmology* 1985;92:1758–1762.

Emile JF, Wechsler J, Brousse N, et al. Langerhans' cell histiocytosis. Definitive diagnosis with the use of monoclonal antibody O10 on routinely paraffin-embedded samples. *Am J Surg Pathol* 1995;19:636–641.

Feldman RB, Moore DM, Hood CI, et al. Solitary eosinophilic granuloma of the lateral orbital wall. *Am J Ophthalmol* 1985;100:318–323.

Foucar E, Rosai J, Dorfman RF. The ophthalmologic manifestations of sinus histiocytosis with massive lymphadenopathy. *Am J Ophthalmol* 1979;87:354–367.

Friendly DS, Font RL, Rao NA. Orbital involvement in "sinus" histiocytosis: a report of four cases. *Arch Ophthalmol* 1977;95:2006–2011.

Gunduz K, Palamar M, Parmak N, et al. Eosinophilic granuloma of the orbit: report of two cases. *J AAPOS* 2007;11:506–508.

Hidayat AA, Mafee MF, Laver NV, et al. Langerhans' cell histiocytosis and juvenile xanthogranuloma of the orbit. Clinicopathologic, CT, and MR imaging features. *Radiol Clin North Am* 1998;36:1229–1240.

Khan R, Moriarty P, Kennedy S. Rosai Dorfman disease or sinus histiocytosis with massive lymphadenopathy of the orbit. *Br J Ophthalmol* 2003;87:1054.

Kincaid MC, Green WR. Ocular and orbital involvement in leukemia. *Surv Ophthalmol* 1983;27:211–232.

Kramer TR, Noecker RJ, Miller JM, et al. Langerhans cell histiocytosis with orbital involvement. *Am J Ophthalmol* 1997;124: 814–824.

Paulli M, Rosso R, Kindl S, et al. Immunophenotypic characterization of the cell infiltrate in five cases of sinus histiocytosis with massive lymphadenopathy (Rosai-Dorfman disease). *Hum Pathol* 1992;23:647–654.

Puri P, Grover AK. Granulocytic sarcoma of orbit preceding acute myeloid leukaemia: a case report. *Eur J Cancer Care (Engl)* 1999;8:113–115.

Vemuganti GK, Naik MN, Honavar SG. Rosai dorfman disease of the orbit. *J Hematol Oncol* 2008;1:7.

Willman CL, Busque L, Griffith BB, et al. Langerhans'-cell histiocytosis (histiocytosis X)—a clonal proliferative disease. *N Engl J Med* 1994;331:191–193.

15 Optic Nerve

DEVELOPMENTAL ANOMALIES

Developmental anomalies of the optic nerve include optic nerve aplasia and hypoplasia, optic pits, optic nerve colobomas, and the morning glory syndrome. Bilateral hypoplasia is often associated with congenital syndromes such as de Morsier syndrome of septo-optic dysplasia, which includes bilateral hypoplastic nerves, absent septum pellucidum, and hemiplegia, and Aicardi syndrome, which affects only women and includes peripapillary chorioretinal lacunae, ectopic retinal pigment epithelium (RPE), agenesis of the corpus callosum, infantile spasms, and mental retardation.

Colobomas of the optic nerve (Fig. 15-1) are caused by incomplete closure of the posterior portion of the fetal fissure. Eyes with extensive optic nerve colobomas may be microophthalmic and have a cystic out-pouching of the posterior sclera (microphthalmos with cyst) (Fig. 2-2). The cyst typically is lined by dysplastic neuroectodermal tissue, which communicates with the retina via the coloboma. Optic nerve colobomas occasionally are associated with choristomatous malformations that contain smooth muscle and heterotopic fat.

Optic pits are small craterlike holes that usually occur unilaterally at the temporal margin of the optic disc. Pathogenesis probably is related to anomalous closure of the superior margin of the embryonic fissure. Optic pits frequently are complicated by serous detachment of the macula, complicated by schisis of its inner layers. The subretinal fluid may be derived from the vitreous.

The morning glory syndrome is an optic nerve anomaly characterized by a funnel-shaped optic nerve head, which appears to contain a central dot of connective tissue believed to be residual Bergmeister papilla. The retinal vessels emerge from the margin of the disc, which is surrounded by an elevated annulus of disturbed chorioretinal pigment. Bilateral cases occasionally have been associated with midline neurologic and craniofacial anomalies.

OPTIC DISC DRUSEN

Optic disc drusen are globular aggregates of concentrically laminated, calcified material that are located deep in the substance of the optic nerve head anterior to the lamina cribrosa within the scleral ring (Fig. 15-2). Optic disc drusen appear ophthalmoscopically as tan, yellow, or straw-colored glistening or refractile spheric structures. They typically are found in a small, crowded optic disc that has a small or absent cup. Optic disc drusen are unrelated to drusen of the RPE or the heavily calcified epipapillary astrocytomas called giant drusen of the optic disc that occur in some patients with tuberous sclerosis complex. Optic disc drusen are important clinically because they may be misdiagnosed as papilledema and prompt an unnecessary neurologic evaluation. The pathogenesis of optic disc drusen may be related to blockage of axoplasmic flow in ganglion cell axons within a narrow crowded scleral canal. Calcified mitochondria dispersed from prelaminar corpora amylacea may provide a nidus for further calcium deposition. Optic disc drusen occur sporadically or may be inherited as an irregular autosomal dominant trait. Disc drusen also occur in some patients with retinitis pigmentosa or pseudoxanthoma elasticum with angioid streaks.

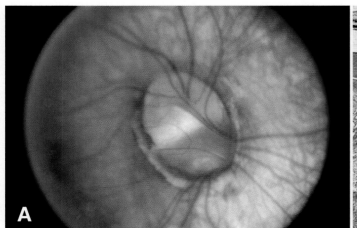
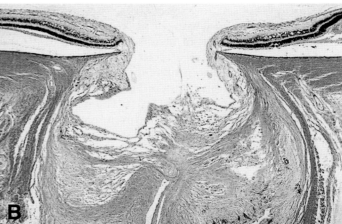

Fig. 15-1. A, B. Optic nerve coloboma. Optic nerve colobomas are caused by incomplete closure of the fetal fissure. (**B.** H&E ×10)

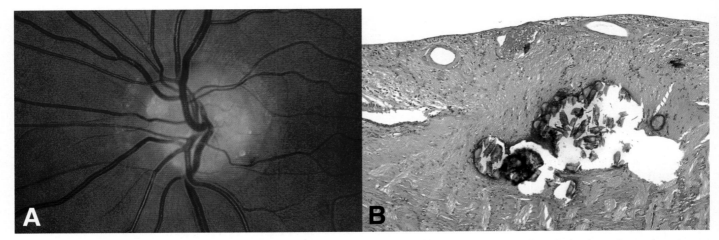

Fig. 15-2. Optic disc drusen. A. Anterior substance of optic disc contains yellow spherical refractile bodies. Optic disc drusen may be misdiagnosed clinically as papilledema. **B.** A conglomeration of calcareous deposits is present in the optic nerve anterior to the lamina cribrosa. The drusen have fractured during sectioning. They were unsuspected, and the specimen was not decalcified. (**A.** Photo courtesy of Dr. Peter Savino, **B.** H&E ×25)

OPTIC DISC EDEMA

Although optic disc edema (papilledema) classically is associated with elevated intracranial pressure and space-occupying intracranial lesions, swollen optic discs also occur in eyes with acute glaucoma, ocular hypotony, central retinal vein occlusion, juxtapapillary tumors, and severe hypertensive retinopathy (Fig. 15-3). Optic disc edema does not result from an accumulation of fluid in the extracellular spaces of the disc. Rather, the increase in the volume of the nerve head reflects the intracytoplasmic swelling and thickening of ganglion cell axons caused by blockage of axoplasmic flow in the distorted lamina cribrosa. The pores of the lamina cribrosa are distorted by a pressure gradient between the intraocular pressure and pressure in the retrolaminar optic nerve. A pressure gradient can form if the intracranial pressure is elevated (classic papilledema), the intraocular pressure is low (hypotony), or the intraocular pressure is acutely elevated (acute glaucoma).

Histopathologically, the nerve head is swollen and the physiological cup is narrowed (Fig. 15-3B–C). The increase in the volume of nerve head tissue displaces the photoreceptors laterally from the margin of the disc. This lateral displacement of photoreceptors and an accompanying shallow peripapillary collection of serous subretinal fluid are responsible for enlargement of the blind spot on visual field testing. Folds are also found in the outer retinal layers (Paton folds). Extensive gliosis and axonal loss occur in chronic papilledema.

OPTIC ATROPHY

Optic nerve atrophy is characterized pathologically by shrinkage of the parenchyma of the optic nerve caused by loss of ganglion cell axons (Fig. 15-4). The subarachnoid space around the shrunken nerve becomes widened, and the dura may appear redundant and folded. Light microscopy discloses loss of axons and thickening of the

pia mater and pial septa. Gliosis may or may not become prominent depending on the cause of the atrophy.

By convention, the terms primary or descending optic atrophy are applied to atrophy of the nerve caused by lesions in the central nervous system or orbit. Primary optic atrophy generally is not associated with an ophthalmoscopically visible glial or mesenchymal reaction. Causes of primary optic atrophy include optic nerve trauma, compression by neoplasms or enlarged extraocular muscles in thyroid ophthalmopathy, neurosyphilis, demyelinating diseases including multiple sclerosis, heritable leukodystrophies, and toxic and nutritional optic neuropathies.

Inflammatory, neoplastic, or vascular lesions located in the retina or the vicinity of the optic disc cause secondary or ascending optic atrophy, which is often marked by pronounced alterations in the glial and mesenchymal tissues of the nerve head. Common retinal causes of optic atrophy include chorioretinitis, retinitis pigmentosa, and trauma.

Leber hereditary optic neuropathy is caused by several point mutations in genes encoding complex I subunits of the mitochondrial respiratory chain. The subunit 4 gene of mitochondrial DNA encoding NADH dehydrogenase is mutated most often. Mitochondrial DNA is maternally inherited. Leber hereditary optic atrophy usually presents with subacute progressive bilateral central visual loss in men between 18 and 30 years of age. Some patients have disc swelling and telangiectatic peripapillary vessels.

Although retinal ganglion cells and axons are lost in both primary and glaucomatous optic atrophy, cupping of the disc generally occurs in glaucomatous optic atrophy and is not prominent in primary optic atrophy. Schnabel's cavernous optic atrophy is a relatively rare type of optic atrophy characterized by the presence of large spaces filled with hyaluronic acid in the retrolaminar part of the nerve (Fig. 15-5). Schnabel's cavernous optic atrophy classically was associated with an acute elevation of intraocular pressure, but a large postmortem study found many cases in elderly women with systemic vascular disease who had

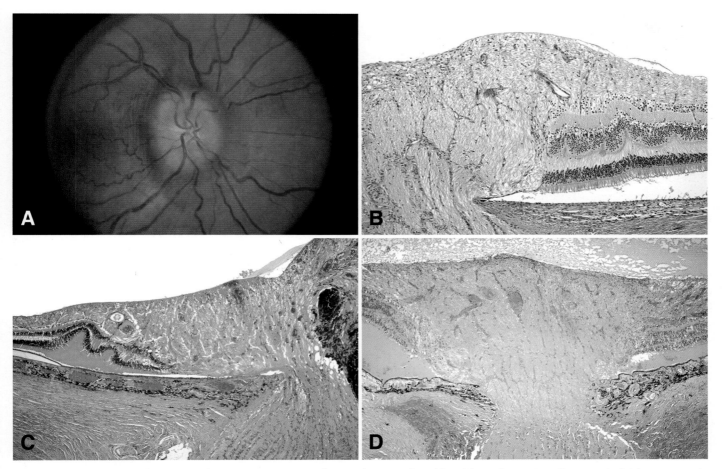

Fig. 15-3. Optic disc edema. A. The optic nerve is swollen and injected and has blurred margins. Concentric folds are seen in the adjacent retina. **B.** The nerve head is swollen. The photoreceptors are displaced laterally. **C.** Optic disc edema, secondary to juxtapapillary melanoma. The optic nerve head is compressed by an infiltrating juxtapapillary tumor, causing blockage of axoplasmic flow. The photoreceptors of the swollen optic nerve are displaced laterally and the peripapillary retina is detached by serous fluid. Folds are noted in the outer retina. **D.** Optic disc edema, hypotony. The optic disc is massively swollen. The photoreceptors are displaced laterally, and a shallow exudative retinal detachment is present. Severe hypotony caused by uveitis was the cause of the disc edema. (**B.** H&E ×50, **C.** H&E ×25, **D.** H&E ×25)

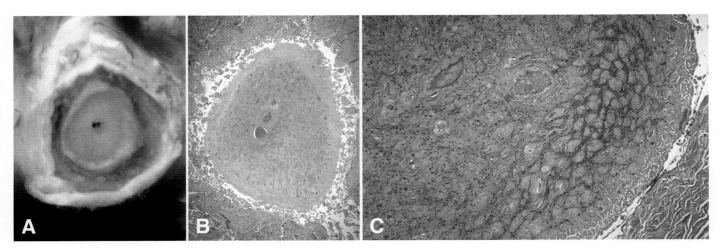

Fig. 15-4. Optic atrophy. A. The optic nerve is atrophic, and the subarachnoid space is widened. The severity of the optic atrophy makes the meninges appear redundant. **B.** The pia and pial septa are markedly thickened, and the substance of the nerve is severely atrophic. **C.** Transverse section shows that most of the parenchyma of the severely atrophic optic nerve has been replaced by blue-staining collagenous connective tissue. The pia and pial septa are markedly widened. (**B.** H&E ×10, **C.** Masson trichrome ×25)

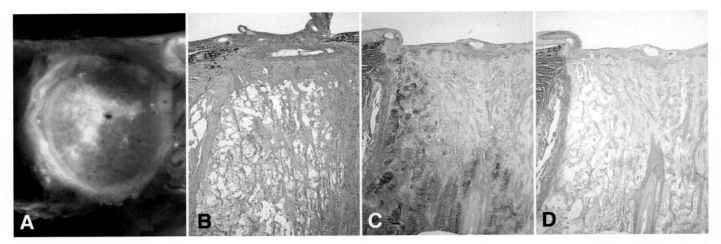

Fig. 15-5. Schnabel's cavernous optic atrophy. A. Diameter of transversely sectioned optic nerve is markedly widening. Small cystoid spaces replace myelinated parenchyma. **B.** Retrolaminar optic nerve contains pools of clear mucoid material. **C.** Clear spaces in retrolaminar optic nerve stain intensely for acid mucopolysaccharide (AMP). **D.** Positive staining is abolished by pretreatment with hyaluronidase indicating that the substance is hyaluronic acid. (**B.** H&E ×10, **C.** Colloidal iron for AMP ×10, **D.** colloidal iron after hyaluronidase digestion ×10)

no evidence of glaucoma. Hypothetical sources of the mucopolysaccharide include the vitreous in glaucomatous eyes or *in situ* production within areas of optic nerve infarction. No gliosis or histiocytic reaction typically is seen. Intraocular silicone oil can infiltrate the optic nerve producing pseudo-Schnabel's cavernous degeneration. In rare instances, the oil can migrate to the brain.

OPTIC NEURITIS

The term optic neuritis refers to involvement of any part of the optic nerve by an inflammatory disease process. The process is called retrobulbar neuritis clinically when the inflammation involves the retrobulbar part of the optic nerve, and ophthalmoscopy initially reveals no abnormalities. Multiple sclerosis is a relatively common cause of retrobulbar neuritis. The term papillitis is used when the optic disc is affected, and the process is called neuroretinitis if the peripapillary retina is involved by edema, hemorrhage, and inflammation. Optic neuritis is classified topographically as perineuritis, periaxial neuritis, axial neuritis, and transverse neuritis. It can be caused by bacterial, mycobacterial, viral, mycotic, and parasitic infection as well as by granulomatous disorders such as sarcoidosis and Wegener granulomatosis (Fig. 15-6). Large granulomas occur on the surface of the optic disc in some patients with sarcoidosis.

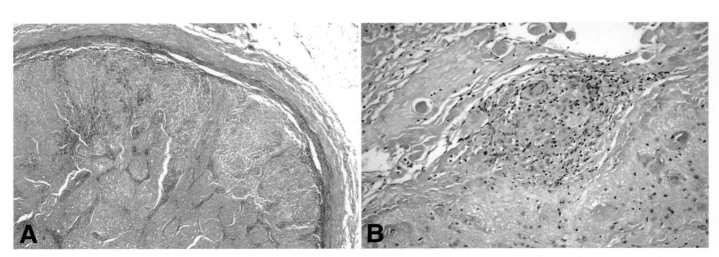

Fig. 15-6. Sarcoid optic neuropathy. A. The parenchyma of the nerve contains a prominent focus of chronic granulomatous inflammation composed of pale-staining epithelioid histiocytes and lymphocytes. The inflammation is concentrated in the periphery of the nerve. **B.** Discrete noncaseating granuloma in nerve is composed of epithelioid histiocytes. (**A.** H&E ×25, **B.** H&E ×100)

NEOPLASMS OF THE OPTIC NERVE

Most primary tumors of the optic nerve are optic nerve gliomas and meningiomas. Although melanocytoma (magnocellular nevus) can occur anywhere in the uveal tract, it typically affects the optic nerve head (Fig. 11-3). Large epipapillary astrocytomas occur in some patients with tuberous sclerosis, and the optic nerve head can be affected by hemangioblastoma in von Hippel–Lindau syndrome. Rare medulloepitheliomas of the optic nerve have been reported. Combined hamartoma of the RPE and retina may affect the optic disc and may be associated with neurofibromatosis type 2.

OPTIC NERVE GLIOMA

Optic nerve glioma (pilocytic astrocytoma) usually presents between 2 and 6 years of age with unilateral visual loss and axial proptosis. Ophthalmoscopy may disclose either optic atrophy or papilledema. Strabismus, an afferent pupillary defect, and enlargement of the ipsilateral optic canal may be present. There is a strong association with neurofibromatosis type I (10%–50%). Optic nerve gliomas cause a fusiform swelling of the optic nerve (Fig. 15-7A–C). The tumor does not invade the orbital tissues because it typically remains confined by the intact dura (Fig. 15-7B). Optic nerve gliomas in children are grade I astrocytomas, which are composed of spindly cells that have long, delicate, hairlike processes (Fig. 15-7E). The term *pilocytic* astrocytoma reflects that feature. Eosinophilic clumps of fibrils called Rosenthal fibers are a prominent finding in some tumors (Fig. 15-7F). Optic nerve gliomas associated with neurofibromatosis often break through the pia and proliferate in the subarachnoid space within the intact dura (arachnoidal gliomatosis) (Fig. 15-7D). In such cases, the central remnant of the optic nerve may be evident on imaging studies. Arachnoidal gliomatosis may be confused with meningioma in a superficial biopsy. Presently, many optic nerve gliomas are followed conservatively. Surgical excision, usually sparing the eye, may be indicated for high degrees of cosmetically unacceptable proptosis, or when the tumor threatens to extend intracranially and involves the chiasm. The use of radiotherapy and chemotherapy is

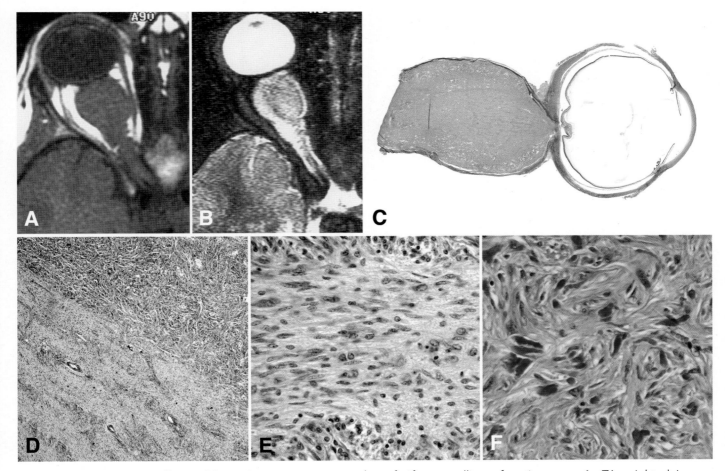

Fig. 15-7. Optic nerve glioma. Magnetic resonance scans show fusiform swelling of optic nerve. **A.** T1-weighted image. **B.** T2-weighted image. **C.** Meninges of markedly swollen nerve are intact. **D.** Glial cells infiltrate arachnoid above (arachnoid gliomatosis). **E.** Cells comprising low-grade pilocytic astrocytoma of optic nerve have bland nuclei and slender cellular processes. **F.** This tumor contains many periodic acid-Schiff (PAS)-positive Rosenthal fibers. (**C.** Case presented by J. Douglas Cameron, MD at the 2010 meeting of the Verhoeff-Zimmerman Society—H&E ×1.5, **D.** H&E ×25, **E.** H&E ×100, **F.** PAS ×100)

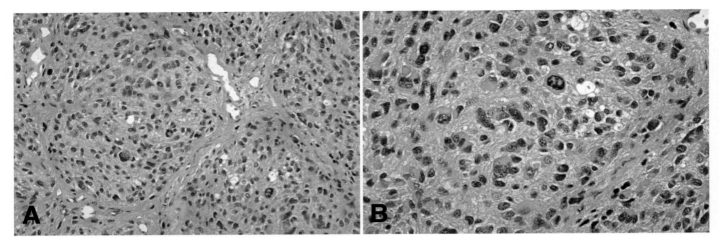

Fig. 15-8. Malignant glioma, optic nerve. Hypercellular tumor is composed of highly atypical glial cells with hyperchromatic pleomorphic nuclei. Malignant gliomas of the optic nerve are quite rare and have a poor prognosis. (**A.** H&E ×100, **B.** H&E ×250)

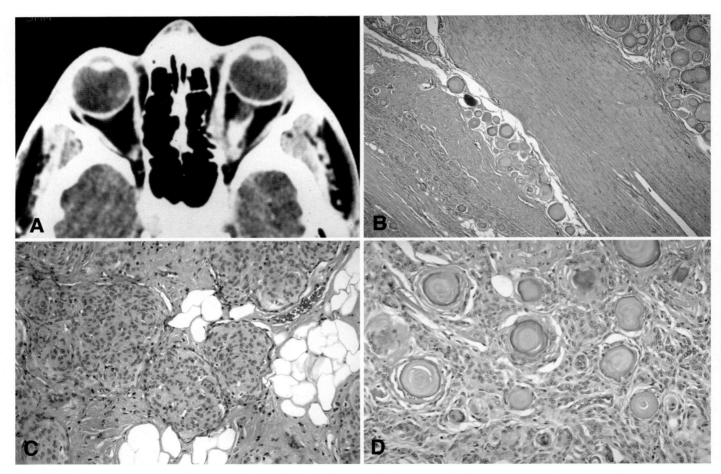

Fig. 15-9. Meningioma of optic nerve. A. Involved optic nerve is thickened. **B.** Tumor compressing the optic nerve contains many psammoma bodies. The patient had neurofibromatosis. **C.** Meningothelial meningioma, optic nerve. Whorls of bland meningothelial cells comprise this tumor. Psammoma bodies are not present. **D.** Meningothelial meningioma with psammoma bodies. Most meningiomas cannot metastasize but are locally infiltrative. Orbital meningiomas arise primarily from the optic nerve sheath or invade the orbit secondarily from the intracranial meninges. Rare ectopic meningiomas derived from extradural meningothelial rests have been reported. (**B.** H&E ×10, **C.** H&E ×100, **D.** H&E ×100)

controversial. High grade malignant gliomas of chiasm or optic nerve occur rarely in adults and have a dismal prognosis (Fig. 15-8).

OPTIC NERVE MENINGIOMA

Primary meningiomas of the optic nerve can occur in either adults or children. They may behave aggressively in children. Clinically, optic nerve meningiomas compress the optic nerve causing optic atrophy and visual loss (Fig. 15-9). Ophthalmoscopy may reveal opticociliary (retinochoroidal) venous shunt vessels on the optic disc. Primary orbital meningiomas arise from the meninges of the optic nerve or rarely from ectopic rests of arachnoidal tissue. Primary intracranial meningiomas also invade the orbit secondarily. Most primary meningiomas of the orbit are either meningothelial or transitional. The tumor cells typically are arranged in whorls or paving stone clusters and may have intranuclear vacuoles of herniated cytoplasm (Fig. 15-9C). Calcified psammomma bodies may be present (Fig. 15-9B,D). Meningiomas typically stain for vimentin, epithelial membrane antigen (EMA) and cytokeratin. Unlike optic nerve gliomas, optic nerve meningiomas frequently erode through the meninges and invade the soft tissue of the orbit. Fractionated external beam radiotherapy improves or stabilizes visual acuity in many patients and has been recommended as initial therapy.

BIBLIOGRAPHY

Developmental Lesions

Brockhurst RJ. Optic pits and posterior retinal detachment. *Trans Am Ophthalmol Soc* 1975;73:264–291.
Brown GC, Shields JA, Patty BE, et al. Congenital pits of the optic nerve head. I. Experimental studies in collie dogs. *Arch Ophthalmol* 1979;97:1341–1344.
Eustis HS, Sanders MR, Zimmerman T. Morning glory syndrome in children: Association with endocrine and central nervous system anomalies. *Arch Ophthalmol* 1994;112:204–207.
Font RL, Zimmerman LE. Intrascleral smooth muscle in coloboma of the optic disc: Electron microscopic verification. *Am J Ophthalmol* 1971;72:452–457.
Gass JDM. Serous detachment of the macula secondary to congenital pit of the optic nerve head. *Am J Ophthalmol* 1969;67:821–841.
Hoyt CS, Billson FA, Ouvrier R, et al. Ocular features of Aicardi's syndrome. *Arch Ophthalmol* 1978;96:291–295.
Jensen PE, Kalina RE. Congenital anomalies of the optic disk. *Am J Ophthalmol* 1976;82:27–31.
Kindler P. Morning glory syndrome: unusual congenital optic disk anomaly. *Am J Ophthalmol* 1970;69:376–384.
Lieb W, Rochels R, Gronemeyer U. Microphthalmos with colobomatous orbital cyst: clinical, histological, immunohistological, and electronmicroscopic findings. *Br J Ophthalmol* 1990;74:59–62.
Mafee MF, Jampol LM, Langer BG, et al. Computed tomography of optic nerve colobomas, morning glory anomaly, and colobomatous cyst. *Radiol Clin North Am* 1987;25:693–699.
Pagon RA. Ocular coloboma. *Surv Ophthalmol* 1981;25:223–223.
Pollock S. The morning glory disc anomaly: contractile movement, classification, and embryogenesis. *Doc Ophthalmol* 1987;65:439–460.

Slamovits TL, Kimball GP, Friberg TR, et al. Bilateral optic disc colobomas with orbital cysts and hypoplastic optic nerves and chiasm. *J Clin Neuroophthalmol* 1989;9:172–177.
Waring GO, Roth AM, Rodrigues MM. Clinicopathologic correlation of microphthalmos with cyst. *Am J Ophthalmol* 1976;82:714–721.
Weiss A, Martinez C, Greenwald M. Microphthalmos with cyst: clinical presentations and computed tomographic findings. *J Pediatr Ophthalmol Strabismus* 1985;22:6–12.
Wiggins RE, von Noorden GK, Boniuk M. Optic nerve coloboma with cyst: a case report and review. *J Pediatr Ophthalmol Strabismus* 1991;28:274–277.
Zeki SM, Dutton GN. Optic nerve hypoplasia in children: Mini review. *Br J Ophthalmol* 1990;74:300–304.

Optic Disk Drusen

Spencer WH. Drusen of the optic nerve (XXXIV Edward Jackson Memorial Lecture). *Am J Ophthalmol* 1978;85:1–12.
Tso MOM. Pathology and pathogenesis of drusen of the optic nerve head. *Ophthalmology* 1981;188:1066–1080.

Optic Disk Edema

Galbraith JEK, Sullivan JH. Decompression of the perioptic meninges for relief of papilledema. *Am J Ophthalmol* 1973;76:687–692.
Tso MOM, Fine BS. Electron microscopic study of papilledema in man. *Am J Ophthalmol* 1976;82:424–434.
Tso MOM, Hayreh SS. Optic disc edema in raised intracranial pressure. III. A pathologic study of experimental papilledema. *Arch Ophthalmol* 1977;95:1458–1462.

Optic Atrophy

Andersen DR. Ascending and descending optic atrophy produced experimentally in squirrel monkeys. *Am J Ophthalmol* 1973;76:693–711.
Brown MD, Voljavec AS, Lott MT, et al. Leber's hereditary optic neuropathy: a model for mitochondrial neurodegenerative diseases. *Faseb J* 1992;6:2791–2799.
Howell N. Leber hereditary optic neuropathy: how do mitochondrial DNA mutations cause degeneration of the optic nerve? *J Bioenerg Biomembr* 1997;29:165–173.
Kerrison JB, Newman NJ. Clinical spectrum of Leber's hereditary optic neuropathy. *Clin Neurosci* 1997;4:295–301.
Morris MA. Mitochondrial mutations in neuro-ophthalmological diseases. A review. *J Clin Neuroophthalmol* 1990;10:159–166.
Phillips CI, Gosden CM. Leber's hereditary optic neuropathy and Kearns-Sayre syndrome: mitochondrial DNA mutations. *Surv Ophthalmol* 1991;35:463–472.
Riordan-Eva P, Wood NW. Mitochondrial disorders in neuro-ophthalmology. *Curr Opin Neurol* 1996;9:1–4.

Glaucomatous Optic Atrophy

Gong H, Ye W, Freddo TF, et al. Hyaluronic acid in the normal and glaucomatous optic nerve. *Exp Eye Res* 1997;64:587–595.
Kalvin NH, Hamasaki DI, Gass JDM. Experimental glaucoma in monkeys. I. Relationship between intraocular pressure and cupping of the optic disc and cavernous atrophy of the optic nerve. *Arch Ophthalmol* 1966;76:82–93.
Shields CL, Eagle RC Jr. Pseudo-Schnabel's cavernous degeneration of the optic nerve secondary to intraocular silicone oil. *Arch Ophthalmol* 1989;107:714–717.
Zimmerman LE, deVenecia G, Hamasaki DI. Pathology of the optic nerve in experimental acute glaucoma. *Invest Ophthalmol* 1967;6:109–125.

Optic Neuritis

Warner J, Lessell S. Neuro-ophthalmology of multiple sclerosis. *Clin Neurosci* 1994;2:180–188.
Newman NJ. Neuro-ophthalmology: the afferent visual system. *Curr Opin Neurol* 1993;6:738–746.
Newman NJ. Optic neuropathy. *Neurology* 1996;46:315–322.

Laties AM, Scheie HG. Sarcoid granuloma of the optic disk: evolution of multiple small tumors. *Trans Am Ophthalmol Soc* 1970;689:219–233.

Miller NR. The optic nerve. *Curr Opin Neurol* 1996;9:5–15.

Optic Nerve Gliomas

Borit A, Richardson EP Jr. The biological and clinical behavior of pilocytic astrocytomas of the optic pathways. *Brain* 1982;105:161–187.

Cummings TJ, Provenzale JM, Hunter SB, et al. Gliomas of the optic nerve: histological, immunohistochemical (MIB-1 and p53), and MRI analysis. *Acta Neuropathol* 2000;99:563–570.

Dutton JJ. Gliomas of the anterior visual pathway. *Surv Ophthalmol* 1994;38:427–452.

Lewis RA, Gerson LP, Axelson KA, et al. Von Recklinghausen's neurofibromatosis. II. Incidence of optic gliomata. *Ophthalmology* 1984;91:929–935.

Miller NR, Illif WJ, Green WR. Evaluation and management of gliomas of the anterior visual pathways. *Brain* 1974;97:743–754.

Rush JA, Younge BR, Campbell RJ, et al. Optic glioma. Long-term follow-up of 85 histopathologically verified cases. *Ophthalmology* 1982;89:1213–1219.

Spoor TC, Kennerdell JS, Martinez AJ, et al. Malignant gliomas of the optic nerve pathways. *Am J Ophthalmol* 1980;89:284–292.

Stern J, Jakobiec FA, Housepian E. The architecture of optic nerve gliomas with and without neurofibromatosis. *Arch Ophthalmol* 1980;98:505–511.

Tibbetts KM, Emnett RJ, Gao F, et al. Histopathologic predictors of pilocytic astrocytoma event-free survival. *Acta Neuropathol* 2009;117:657–665.

Weiss L, Sagerman RH, King GA, et al. Controversy in the management of optic nerve glioma. *Cancer* 1987;59:1000–1004.

Optic Nerve Meningiomas

Dutton JJ. Optic nerve gliomas and meningiomas. *Neurol Clin* 1991;9:163–77.

Dutton JJ. Optic nerve sheath meningiomas. *Surv Ophthalmol* 1992;37:167–183.

Karp LA, Zimmerman LE, Borit A, et al. Primary intraorbital meningiomas. *Arch Ophthalmol* 1974;91:24–28.

Marquardt MD, Zimmerman LE. Histopathology of meningiomas and gliomas of the optic nerve. *Hum Pathol* 1982;13:226–235.

Pravdenkova S, Al-Mefty O, Sawyer J, et al. Progesterone and estrogen receptors: opposing prognostic indicators in meningiomas. *J Neurosurg* 2006;105:163–173.

16 Laboratory Techniques, Special Stains and Immunohistochemistry

SPECIMEN HANDLING IN THE OPHTHALMIC PATHOLOGY LABORATORY

This chapter discusses the basic principles of practical ocular histopathology and summarizes techniques used in the handling, gross dissection, and submission of enucleated eyes and other ocular specimens for routine histopathologic examination. Special histochemical and immunohistochemical stains also are discussed.

Fixation

Routinely, unopened enucleated eyes are fixed for at least 24 hours by total immersion in a relatively large volume (50–100 mL) of 10% neutral buffered formalin. The large volume of fixative is necessary because the solution must penetrate through the sclera. Bouin solution (bright yellow in color) should not be used because it hardens the sclera, making eyes extremely difficult to section. Newer alcohol-based fixatives are also unsatisfactory because they precipitate protein in the vitreous and interfere with gross examination. Enucleated eyeballs should be briefly rinsed in running tap water to remove excess fixative prior to handling.

Specimen Orientation

Determination of laterality (right or left eye) is a prerequisite for proper specimen orientation (Fig. 16-1). The laterality of an eye is determined by identifying key anatomic landmarks. These include the long posterior ciliary vessels, which appear as blue lines on the posterior sclera on either side of the optic nerve in the horizontal plane; the cornea, whose horizontal diameter is usually a millimeter longer than its vertical diameter; and the insertions of the superior and inferior oblique muscles. The inferior oblique muscle lacks a tendon; its fibers insert directly into the sclera in the inferotemporal quadrant. The nasal end of the muscular inferior oblique insertion lies close to the fovea. The shiny tendinous insertion of the superior oblique muscle is located superiorly and temporally and is an excellent landmark for the superior pole of the eye. After the horizontal meridian and the superior pole have been located, the nasal and temporal sides of the eye are readily identified. It is important to remember that both oblique muscles insert on the temporal side of the eye and their fibers run nasally. The temporal arc of the posterior sclera is longer than the nasal arc because the optic nerve enters the eye 15 degrees nasal to the posterior pole. The angulation of the optic nerve stump cannot be relied upon to determine laterality, however, because it often bends temporally after fixation.

Measurement

The oriented eye is measured using calipers or a millimeter ruler. Standard measurements include the anteroposterior (AP), horizontal, and vertical diameters of the eye; the length of the optic nerve segment attached; the horizontal and vertical diameters of the cornea; and the size of the pupil (Fig. 16-2A). Measurements should be made and

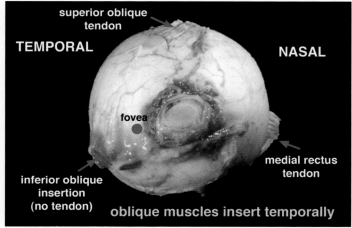
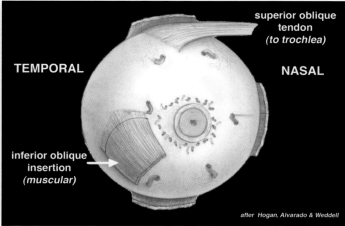

Fig. 16-1. Orientation of globe, posterior landmarks. The temporal insertions of the oblique muscles are helpful landmarks. The inferior oblique lacks a tendon and its muscular fibers insert inferonasally near the fovea. The tendinous insertion of the superior oblique muscle is located superotemporally. The long posterior ciliary vessels are often evident as blue lines on either side of the optic nerve in the horizontal plane.

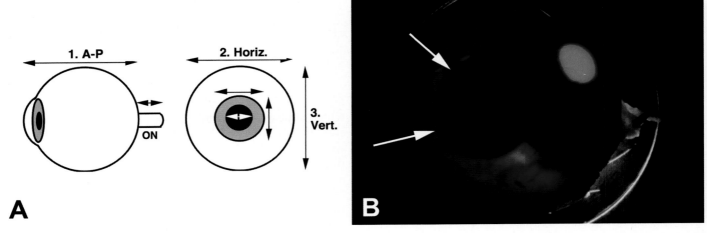

Fig. 16-2. A. Ocular measurements. Standard measurements include the AP, horizontal, and vertical diameters of the eye; the length of the optic nerve segment; the horizontal and vertical diameters of the cornea; and the size of the pupil. **B. Transillumination of globe.** Transillumination is used to localize ciliochoroidal melanoma in enucleated eye. *Arrows* point to round shadow cast by choroidal part of pigmented tumor. The pupil glows brightly.

recorded in a standardized sequence, that is, AP, horizontal, and vertical. Important pathologic features such as wounds, lacerations, and tumors should also be measured and their location noted. Most normal human eyes are slightly less than 1 inch in diameter (24–25 mm), and the normal cornea is approximately 1 cm in diameter (11 × 10 mm).

It is easier to section an eye if the optic nerve is removed first. The nerve should be sectioned a millimeter or two posterior to the sclera to avoid "buttonholing" a deeply cupped nerve head. A transverse section of the optic nerve should always be submitted if the nerve has not been cut flush with the globe. The surgical margin should be marked with India ink or an indelible colored pencil before the nerve is removed. The optic nerve segment should always be removed before the globe is opened to preclude potential contamination of the surgical margin with intraocular tumor. This is especially important if the eye contains retinoblastoma, which tends to invade the optic nerve. Surgeons occasionally submit the optic nerve in a separate container. In such specimens, blood staining and crushing serve to identify the true surgical margin.

INSPECTION AND DESCRIPTION

The general consistency and character of the eye are noted. Descriptive terms that are commonly used include normal, soft, collapsed, ruptured, lacerated, hard, rubbery, phthisic, etc. Before it is opened, the external surface of the eye should be carefully and systematically examined with a dissecting microscope, starting anteriorly. The cornea is usually slightly hazy in fixed or postmortem specimens. The presence of corneal opacities, scars, vascularization, ulcers, band keratopathy, wounds, and incisions should be described and measured when appropriate. The shape and size of the pupil, the color of the iris, and the presence

and location of iridectomies and surgical iris colobomas should be recorded. If the cornea is hazy, iris defects are readily disclosed by transillumination.

The rest of the globe should be carefully inspected looking for signs of surgical or nonsurgical trauma or extraocular tumor extension. The presence, type, location, and size of wounds, scars, vitrectomy ports, sutures, and prosthetic devices such as retinal implants, explants, and encircling bands and tube shunts should be precisely noted. The use of "clock hours," for example, "between 1 and 3 o'clock," is helpful in the description of wounds and other important lesions.

Drawing a diagram of the findings on the pathology protocol facilitates description and permits reconstruction of the gross description if the dictation is lost.

TRANSILLUMINATION

Eyes are transilluminated before they are opened to disclose occult pathology that may not be evident on external examination. Transillumination is performed by holding the eye directly on the surface of a bright light in a darkened chamber. Transillumination is especially helpful during the orientation of eyes that contain intraocular tumors, particularly uveal malignant melanomas (Fig. 16-2B). Pigmented melanomas usually cast a dark shadow on the sclera, which should be localized and measured. When clinical data are absent, transillumination may disclose signs of previous surgery, for example, an iridectomy, that may be an indication for vertical sectioning. Eyes that are filled with blood or contain dense gelatinous exudate often transmit light poorly, as do specimens from heavily pigmented individuals. Staphylomas and cyclodestructive procedures cause increased light transmission.

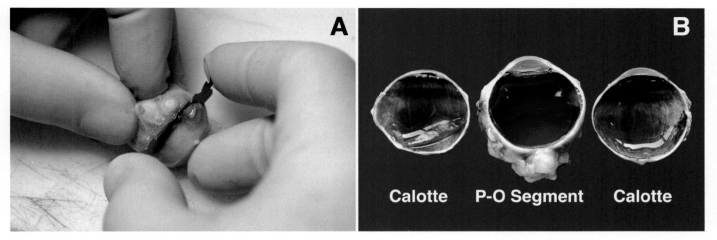

Fig. 16-3. **A. Sectioning technique for globe.** Globe is sectioned cornea down with a razor blade. **B. P-O segment and calottes.** The central P-O segment, which is submitted for sectioning includes the pupil and optic nerve.

DISSECTION

Microscopic sections are cut from a paraffin block that contains a short cylindrical segment of the eyeball called the pupil-optic nerve or P-O segment. The P-O segment includes most of the cornea, iris, and pupil anteriorly and the optic nerve posteriorly (Fig. 16-3B).

When tissue is submitted for histopathologic examination, care must be taken to ensure that the microscopic sections will include important lesions such as tumors, lacerations, or incisions. The presence and location of the ocular pathology determine how the eye is opened. It is routine practice to open eyes horizontally if they do not contain wounds or other focal lesions. Horizontal P-O sections include the macula as well as the pupil and optic nerve.

Eyes that have had prior surgery may be opened vertically to include a superior limbal surgical wound in the microscopic sections. This category includes eyes that have had cataract surgery or filtering procedures for glaucoma. If an eye with a small superior incision is opened horizontally, the microscopic sections will not include the wound, and the pathologist will be unable to document its presence.

Traumatic lacerations and intraocular tumors can occur anywhere. Such eyes are opened along the meridian that includes the main part of the lesion. The localization of intraocular tumors by transillumination greatly aids sectioning.

SECTIONING TECHNIQUE

I currently section eyes using one half of a standard double-edged razor blade that has been snapped in half within its protective wrapper. The two ends of the blade are held between the apposed surfaces of the thumb and forefinger, and a gentle sawing and pushing motion is used. During the initial cut, the eye is steadied with the nondominant hand and held cornea side down on the cutting block (Fig. 16-3A). Guidelines drawn on the eye with colored pencil facilitate sectioning and assure that the eye maintains proper orientation. The first cut is begun just external to the dural sheath of the optic nerve and should enter the periphery of the anterior chamber anteriorly. The two dome-shaped caps of tissue that are removed are called calottes (French for visor-less cap). The first calotte should include about one fourth or one fifth of the peripheral anterior chamber. Ideally, the central P-O segment should be about 8- to 10-mm thick. The globe is placed cut surface down on the cutting board during removal of the second calotte. Eye protection (glasses, goggles, or face shield) should be worn during the initial cut to protect against occasional squirts or splashes of fixative and intraocular contents that can occur if the intraocular pressure is high.

Any material that flows from the eye during sectioning (blood, crystals, pigment-tinged fluid, or silicone oil) should be described. Gritty, hard, or even impenetrable intraocular material may be encountered. When this happens, possibilities include intraocular bone, a calcified cataractous lens, or a prosthetic intraocular lens. Intraocular bone is an extremely common finding in phthisical eyes. Eyes that contain bone must be decalcified before they are submitted. In some instances, decalcification is a prerequisite for initial dissection.

Every specimen should be examined carefully and systematically with the dissecting microscope, and macrophotography performed if indicated. Disturbing light reflexes are minimized during gross examination and macrophotography by immersing the specimen in a flat-bottomed cylindrical dish filled with 60% "grossing" alcohol. Placing the flat-bottomed cylindrical dish on a plate of dark blue Plexiglas provides an aesthetic background for the gross photographs, which is enhanced if the bottom of the dish is coupled to the plastic with a thin layer of alcohol. The calottes are retained in alcohol as "wet tissue" and may be retrieved if additional sections or studies are necessary.

ROUTINE HISTOPATHOLOGY: DEHYDRATION, EMBEDDING, AND MICROTOMY

The P-O segment is embedded in a block of paraffin wax to facilitate the cutting of microscopic sections. Because water and wax are not miscible, the aqueous fixative and the water in the tissue must be removed before the specimen can be embedded. This process is called dehydration. Tissue is dehydrated by passing it through increasing concentrations of ethanol until absolute ethanol is reached. The dehydrated tissue is then transferred to xylene, which is miscible with both absolute alcohol and paraffin, and then infiltrated with molten paraffin under vacuum. After infiltration, the specimen is placed in a plastic mold that is filled with molten paraffin. The paraffin is cooled and hardens into a block, which fits into the chuck of a rotary microtome. The support provided by the surrounding paraffin matrix allows the tissue to be sectioned thinly (6–8 m). The thin slices of paraffin and tissue are then floated onto the surface of a bath of heated water, which causes the paraffin to expand. The tissue sections are then mounted on glass slides, which are heated in an oven to promote tissue adherence.

STAINING

Most human tissues are relatively transparent unless they contain endogenous pigment (Fig. 16-4A). To facilitate examination, microscopic slides are stained with dyes such as **hematoxylin and eosin** (H&E) that color certain tissue components. Because aqueous solutions of these stains usually are used, the tissue sections must be deparaffinized and rehydrated before they can be stained. This is done by immersing the slides in successive baths of xylene and absolute alcohol and then decreasing the concentrations of alcohol and water. After staining, the tissue subsequently is dehydrated and coverslipped.

In most laboratories, routine histopathologic sections are stained with H&E (Fig. 16-4D). Hematoxylin is a basic

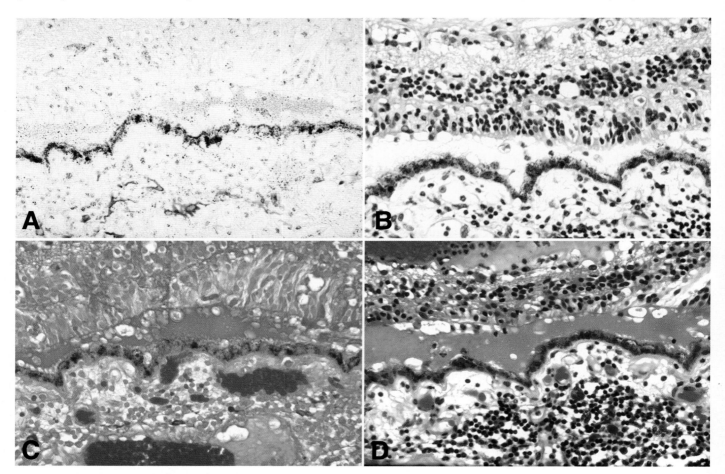

Fig. 16-4. Staining, Hematoxylin and eosin stain. A. Unstained section. Presence of endogenous pigment allows identification of retinal pigment epithelium and choroidal melanocytes. **B. Hematoxylin-stained section** (same area as that in Fig. 16-4A). Basic dye stains DNA in cellular nuclei, highlighting retinal nuclear layers and inflammatory cells in choroid. **C. Eosin-stained section** (same area as that in Fig. 16-4A). Acidic dye stains cytoplasm, erythrocytes in choroidal vessels, and proteinaceous subretinal fluid. **D. Hematoxylin and eosin-stained section** (same area as that in Fig. 16-4A). A shallow retinal detachment and chronic nongranulomatous choroiditis are present. Photoreceptor atrophy denotes chronic process. (**A.** Unstained section ×100, **B.** Hematoxylin ×100, **C.** Eosin ×100, **D.** Hematoxylin and eosin ×100)

dye that binds to acidic materials including the DNA in the nuclei of cells (Fig. 16-4B). Eosin (tetrabromofluorescein) is acidic and stains basic substances such as proteins pink (Fig. 16-4C).

H&E staining provides helpful diagnostic color cues. Lesions composed of cells with scanty cytoplasm tend to look blue or basophilic during microscopy. Examples of basophilic lesions include inflammatory infiltrates, lymphoid tumors, retinoblastoma, and basal cell carcinoma. Necrosis, calcification, and DNA deposition in eyes with retinoblastoma also appear blue. In contrast, cells that have abundant cytoplasm (e.g., squamous cells or epithelioid histiocytes) appear pink. Squamous cell carcinomas usually are eosinophilic. Normal ocular structures composed largely of connective tissue such as the cornea and sclera appear pink in H&E sections. Protein-rich subretinal fluid, lens material, amyloid, and exfoliation material also are eosinophilic.

The **periodic acid-Schiff (PAS) stain** is used routinely in most ophthalmic pathology laboratories because it vividly highlights the thick basement membranes of the eye (lens capsule and Descemet membrane). PAS stains materials that contain unsubstituted vicinal glycol groups (CHOH-CHOH). The vicinal glycol groups are oxidized to dialdehydes (CHO-CHO) by periodic acid, and the Schiff reagent (leucofuchsin) reacts with the dialdehydes forming complexes that range in color from red to magenta. In addition to basement membranes and aggregates of basement membrane material such as guttae and cuticular drusen, PAS stains glycogen, some mucins (e.g., conjunctival goblet cells), and many but not all fungal hyphae.

SPECIAL HISTOCHEMICAL STAINS

A variety of special histochemical stains occasionally are ordered in the ophthalmic pathology laboratory to demonstrate the presence of microorganisms and highlight special structures and materials in histologic sections. Standard histochemical stains rely on chemical reactions to demonstrate the presence of substances. All special stains must be used in conjunction with positive control slides that contain the sought-for organisms or materials. These control slides confirm that the special stains are working. In some instances, the use of histochemical stains has been replaced by immunohistochemical stains, which are more specific.

Special stains for microorganisms are ordered most often. These include modifications of the Gram stain for bacteria called the Brown and Hopps and the Brown and Brenn stains (Fig. 16-5A), several acid fast stains for mycobacteria (Fig. 16-5B), and the Gomori methenamine silver (GMS) stain for fungi (Fig. 16-5C). The nonspecific fluorochrome stain calcofluor white can be used to detect fungi and acanthamoeba cysts, but requires an ultraviolet microscope (Fig. 16-5D). The Dieterle and Warthin-Starry silver impregnation techniques for spirochetes, *Bartonella*, and *Legionella* occasionally are ordered (Fig. 5-9). Fungi and yeast are impregnated with silver and appear black against a green counterstain when stained with the GMS stain (Fig. 16-5C). The Ziehl-Neelson and Fite-Firaco acid fast stains are used to demonstrate the acid fast organisms that cause tuberculosis, leprosy, nocardiosis, and atypical mycobacterial infections (Fig. 16-5B). The organisms appear red ("red snappers") against a blue background.

Several histochemical stains are used to demonstrate the presence of metals in tissue. These include the Perls Prussian blue reaction for iron and the von Kossa and Alizarin red stains for calcium. The iron stain is used to demonstrate the deposition of iron in ocular epithelial structures in hemosiderosis and siderosis (Figs. 4-7 and 4-11) and in corneal iron lines (Fig. 6-17F,G). The iron deposits are blue. The von Kossa stain for calcium actually stains the anionic material that binds with calcium. This silver stain stains calcium deposits black (Fig. 12-6D). The Alizarin red stain forms complexes with calcium, which appear red against a green counterstain. The ruthenium red stain and rhodanine stains for copper are relatively nonspecific and are used infrequently.

The Masson trichrome stain stains collagen blue and cellular tissue red and is used to demonstrate the presence of fibrosis (Fig. 9-10B). Masson trichrome is the histochemical stain of choice for granular corneal dystrophy (Fig. 6-21D). Stains for acid mucopolysaccharides (AMP) include Alcian blue, Hale's colloidal iron, and mucicarmine. The first two stain mucin blue because the histochemical reaction is based partially on the iron stain. AMP stains are used to demonstrate mucin production in tumors (Fig. 11-19E) and to assess corneal dystrophies. They are the stains of choice for macular corneal dystrophy (Fig. 6-23). The Verhoeff-van Gieson stain for elastic tissue demonstrates the internal elastic lamina in arteries (e.g., temporal artery biopsies) and the excessive production of elastic components (elastotic degeneration) in pterygium, pinguecula, and chronic actinic keratopathy (Figs. 5-14 and 6-13). In the latter, the elastotic degeneration stains black, but the reaction is not quenched by pretreatment with elastase. The reticulin stain occasionally is used in the assessment of certain neoplasms such as hemangiopericytoma and lymphomas (Fig. 14-10).

Although amyloid can be stained with the metachromatic stain crystal violet and the fluorescent stain thioflavine T, the Congo red stain is generally used in clinical practice (Figs. 5-15C,D, 6-20C,D, and 11-7B). The amyloid deposits stain light orange and show apple green birefrigence and dichroism during polarization microscopy. Congo red is the stain of choice for lattice corneal dystrophy (Fig. 6-22).

Other histochemical stains that are occasionally ordered include the Fontana-Masson stain for melanin, the luxol fast blue stain for myelin, the Bodian stain for axons, and the Oil red O (ORO) stain for lipid (Fig. 13-19C). ORO must be used on frozen-sectioned tissue because fat is dissolved during normal tissue processing.

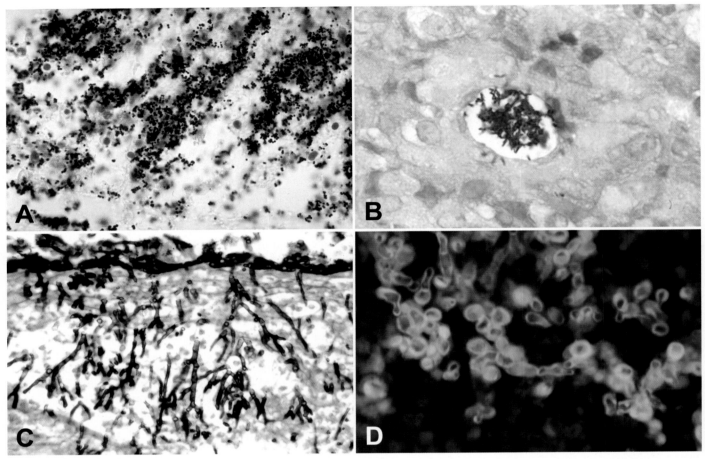

Fig. 16-5. Special stains for microorganisms. A. Tissue Gram stain. Tissue Gram stain discloses myriad Gram-positive cocci in exudate from eye with endophthalmitis. **B. Acid fast stain.** Stain discloses large colony of atypical mycobacteria within vacuole in granulomatous inflammation. Patient developed infection after blepharoplasty. **C. GMS stain for fungus.** Branching septate Aspergillus hyphae in choroid of patient with endogeneous endophthalmitis are stained black by silver impregnation. **D. Calcofluor white.** Yeast stained with nonspecific fluorochrome stain calcofluor white fluoresces vividly during ultraviolet microscopy. (**A.** Brown and Hopps ×250, **B.** Ziehl-Neelson ×250, **C.** GMS ×250, **D.** Calcofluor white ×400)

IMMUNOHISTOCHEMISTRY

Immunohistochemistry (IHC) is a powerful technique that has revolutionized histopathologic diagnosis in the past several decades. IHC employs antibodies to identify antigens or epitopes whose expression is limited to certain types of cells. This technique has markedly improved diagnostic accuracy. Using IHC, pathologists are now able to diagnose many poorly differentiated neoplasms that were unclassifiable by routine light microscopy in the past. Carcinomas, amelanotic melanomas, and high-grade lymphomas are identified by the expression of characteristic antigens that serve as cellular markers. These include cytokeratins and other epithelial markers that are expressed by and serve to identify carcinomas; melanocytic markers such as S-100, HMB-45, Melan-A, and MITF expressed by melanoma; and leukocyte common antigen CD45 expressed by most neoplastic B and T lymphocytes.

Many antibodies employed in diagnostic IHC work well in sections prepared from routinely processed, paraffin-embedded tissue. Tissue sections for IHC are cut, placed on polylysine-coated "plus" slides which promote tissue adherence, and deparaffinized and hydrated. A battery of primary antibodies that are directed against a series of potential antigens are then applied and allowed to react with the tissue (Fig. 16-6A). The choice of antibodies depends on the histopathologic differential diagnosis.

A second antibody of a different class (made in another species), which is directed against the first class of antibody, is then applied (Fig. 16-6B). Binding of the second antibody occurs if the primary antibody has reacted with its complementary antigen. Although techniques and reagents vary, the second, or occasionally third, antibody is labeled with an enzyme (usually peroxidase) that reacts with a substrate called chromogen to produce a colored reaction product (Fig. 16-6C). Often brown, the reaction product is deposited in the tissue and serves as a permanent marker for the presence and location of the antigen. Appropriate negative and positive controls are mandatory to ensure that results are accurate and meaningful.

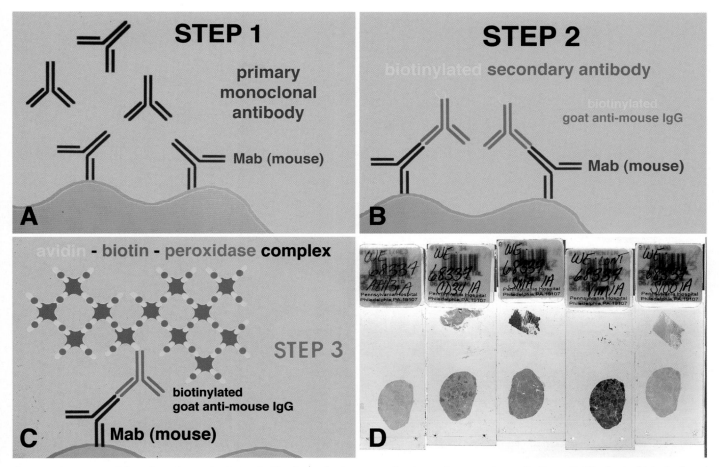

Fig. 16-6. Immunohistochemistry. A. Step 1. Binding of primary antibody to tissue antigen. **B. Step 2.** Binding of biotinylated secondary antibody to primary antibody. **C. Step 3.** Avidin-biotin—peroxidase complex and chromogen form colored reaction product that permanently marks the site of antigen. **D. Solitary fibrous tumor stained with a battery of immunohistochemical stains.** Sectioned tumor in microslides shows positive brown staining for CD34, vimentin, and smooth muscle actin, and negative staining for S-100 and cytokeratin AE1/AE3.

The prudent practice of diagnostic IHC employs a battery of antibodies directed against a number of potential tissue markers, not a single stain or two. The final diagnosis is based on the tumor's pattern of positive and negative immunoreactivity (Fig. 16-6D). For example, both malignant melanoma and schwannoma typically stain for S-100 protein, but only the melanoma should react with more specific melanocytic markers such as HMB-45, Melan-A, or MITF. In addition, a melanoma should not stain for neural markers, neurofilament protein, or CD57. In contrast, a schwannoma should be positive for neural markers and negative for melanocytic markers.

In addition to facilitating diagnosis, IHC increasingly is being used to assess prognosis and guide therapy. For example, metastatic breast carcinoma typically is evaluated for the presence of estrogen and progesterone receptors and the expression of HER2/neu (Fig. 16-7). Estrogen receptor-positive breast cancers are treated with *selective estrogen receptor modulator*

drugs such as tamoxifen or aromatase inhibitors that decrease estrogen production by the adrenal glands in postmenopausal women. About 15% to 20% of breast carcinomas overexpress HER2/neu, which is targeted by the therapeutic monoclonal antibody trastuzumab (Herceptin).

In the ophthalmic pathology laboratory at the Wills Eye Institute, IHC is frequently used to classify lymphoid lesions, assess melanocytic lesions of the conjunctiva, and investigate tumors that have metastasized to the uvea or orbit. These uses have been discussed in Chapters 5, 11, and 14. In some instances, IHC can identify the nature of an occult primary tumor that spawned an ocular metastasis (Fig. 11-20). IHC is also invaluable in the classification of many spindle cell and the so-called small round blue cell tumors of the orbit.

Immunohistochemical markers that are commonly used in the diagnostic ophthalmic pathology laboratory are listed in Table 16-1. Immunoprofiles of various ocular lesions are shown in Table 16-2.

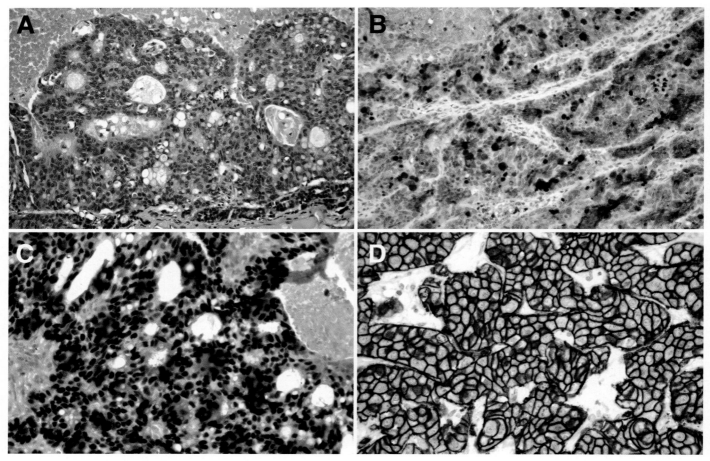

Fig. 16-7. Immunohistochemistry in breast carcinoma. A. Choroidal metastasis found in woman with remote history of breast carcinoma. **B.** Positive immunoreactivity with BRST-2 confirms that the tumor is breast carcinoma. **C. Estrogen receptors.** Black staining of tumor cell nuclei indicates the presence of estrogen receptors. **D. HER2/neu-positive breast carcinoma.** Tumor cells show intense continuous immunostaining of cell membranes for HER2/neu protein, indicating that the patient is a candidate for trastuzumab therapy. (**A.** H&E ×100, **B.** IHC for BRST-2, **C.** IHC for estrogen receptors ×150, **D.** IHC for HER2/neu ×200)

Other Ocular Specimens

Other tissue specimens processed by ophthalmic pathology laboratories include eyelid, conjunctival, and orbital biopsies; corneal specimens; ocular evisceration and orbital exenteration specimens; intraocular biopsies including intraocular tumors that have been locally resected; fine needle aspiration biopsies (FNABs); and vitreous fluid and particulates from diagnostic vitrectomies.

Unoriented biopsies of soft tissue with no obvious epithelial lining are measured and described. The description should include the color and consistency of the tissue, and any distinguishing characteristics. Larger specimens should be sectioned before submitting, typically by "bread-loafing."

Skin lesions and other specimens with an epithelium must be embedded on their side so that the resultant sections include a cross section of the epithelium. Benign skin lesions (papillomas, cysts) usually are excised with a surrounding ellipse of skin. Larger ellipses should be bisected, and the two new cut surfaces marked with India ink or a blue pencil as a guide for embedding. If the specimen has been oriented by the surgeon (using sutures and/or diagrams), the margins should be examined. This usually is done by submitting a number of designated tissue segments in separate cassettes.

Full-thickness eyelid resection usually is performed to remove malignant tumors such as basal cell, squamous, or sebaceous carcinomas. Separate nasal and temporal margins are submitted to determine if the tumor has been totally excised (Fig. 16-8A). The true surgical margin is marked with ink or a colored pencil before the specimen is dissected. The central part of the resection (main specimen) is sectioned perpendicular to the lid margin in a bread-loaf fashion and totally submitted. The nasal and temporal margins of an eyelid resection are readily determined if the laterality (OD vs. OS) and location (upper or lower lid) of the specimen are known. The upper eyelid can be distinguished by the length of the tarsal plate and its roughly rectangular configuration. The lower lid is roughly triangular in shape.

Many malignant tumors of the eyelid are excised with frozen section control of surgical margins. After the frozen sections are prepared, the marginal tissue samples are fixed

TABLE 16-1	Immunohistochemical Markers Commonly Used in Ophthalmic Pathology

Abbreviation or CD Designation	Name	Antigenic Target	Major Use in Eye Pathology	Abbreviation or CD Designation	Name	Antigenic Target	Major Use in Eye Pathology
CD1a		Langerhans cells	Langerhans cell histiocytosis	SMA	Smooth muscle actin	Smooth muscle actin	Leiomyoma, soft tissue tumors, myofibroblasts
CD3	T-cell receptor (TCR) complex	T lymphocytes	Inflammation; T-cell lymphomas	MSA	Muscle-specific actin	Muscle-specific actin	Rhabdomyo-sarcoma
CD5		T lymphocytes	Mantle cell lymphoma; CLL/SLL	CD57	HNK1 (human natural killer 1) or LEU7	Natural killer cells, neuroec-toderm	Schwannoma, neural tumors
CD10	Common acute lymphoblastic leukemia anti-gen (CALLA)	T lymphocytes	Follicular lymphoma, renal carcinoma	NFL	Neurofilaments	Cytoskeleton in axons and dendrites	Optic nerve, neural tumors
CD15		Reed-Sternberg cells	Hodgkin disease	CAM 5.2	Low MW cytokeratin cocktail	Cytokeratins 8, 18, and 19	Epithelial marker, carcinoma
CD20		B lymphocytes	Most ocular adnexal non-Hodgkin lymphomas	AE1/AE3	Pankeratin cocktail	Cytokeratins 1–8, 10, 14–16, and 19	Epithelial marker, carcinoma, PPMD, epithelial downgrowth
CD23		Follicular den-dritic cells	Evaluation of lymphoid lesions				
CD30		Reed-Sternberg cells, etc.	Hodgkin disease, anaplastic large cell lymphoma	CK7	Cytokeratin 7	Low molecular weight cytokeratin 7	Evaluation of metastatic carcinoma
CD45	Leukocyte common antigen	All hemopoietic cells except erythrocytes	Assessment of poorly differentiated neoplasms	CK20	Cytokeratin 20	Low molecular weight cytok-eratin 20	Evaluation of metastatic carcinoma
CD68	KP1, macrosialin	Histiocytes	Histiocytic lesions, juvenile xanthogranu-loma	EMA	Epithelial membrane antigen, CD227	Mucin glycoprotein–glandular epithelium	Epithelial marker, meningioma
CD79a	Pan–B-cell marker	All B cells and plasma cells	B cells, plasma cells	DES	Desmin	Intermediate filament in stri-ated muscle	Rhabdomyo-sarcoma
CD138	Syndecan-1	Plasma cells	Plasma cells, myeloma	MYO D1	Myogenic dif-ferentiaton 1	Myogenic transcriptional regulatory protein	Rhabdomyo-sarcoma
Bcl-1	Cyclin D1, B-cell leukemia/lymphoma 1	Protein that phosphorylates Rb protein	Mantle cell lymphoma	MYOG	Myogenin (myogenic factor 4)	Myogenic transcriptional regulatory protein	Rhabdomyo-sarcoma
Bcl-2	B-cell lym-phoma No. 2	Protein that blocks apop-tosis	Follicular lymphoma, lymphoma diagnosis	CD99	MIC2	Surface glycoprotein primitive neu-roectodermal cells	Ewing Sarcoma/PNET
VIM	Vimentin	Mesenchymal cells	Mesenchy-mal tumors, adequacy of tissue for IHC	HMB45	Melanoma-specific antigen	Melanosomal protein	Melanoma marker
S-100	S-100 protein	Neural crest derivatives	Melanocytic and neural tumors, etc.	Melan-A (Mart-1)		Melanoma cells and nevus cells	Melanocytic lesions

(Continued)

| TABLE 16-1 | | Immunohistochemical Markers Commonly Used in Ophthalmic Pathology *(continued)* |

Abbreviation or CD Designation	Name	Antigenic Target	Major Use in Eye Pathology
MITF	Microphthalmia transcription factor	melanocytes	Melanocytic lesions
NSE	Neuron-specific enolase	Neuroendocrine cells and tumors	Neuroectodermal and Neuroendocrine tumors
GCDFP-15 (BRST-2)	Gross cystic disease fluid protein	Breast, apocrine epithelium	Breast carcinoma, apocrine lid tumors
ER	Estrogen receptors	Estrogen receptors	Treatment of breast carcinoma
PR	Progesterone receptors	Progesterone receptors	Breast carcinoma, meningioma
Thyroglobulin	Thyroglobulin	Thyroid hormone	Thyroid carcinoma
TTF-1	Thyroid transcription factor 1	Lung and thyroid cells	Lung and thyroid carcinoma, negative in Merkel cell tumor
CEA (CD66e)	Carcinoembryonic antigen	Adenocarcinoma cells	Colorectal carcinoma, other adenocarcinomas
Calcitonin		Polypeptide hormone of thyroid C cells	Medullary thyroid carcinoma, MEN2B
RCC	Renal cell carcinoma marker	Renal tubular cells	Renal cell carcinoma
PSA	Prostate-specific antigen	Prostatic tissue	Prostate carcinoma

Abbreviation or CD Designation	Name	Antigenic Target	Major Use in Eye Pathology
PAP	Prostatic acid phosphatase	Enzyme produced by prostatic tissue	Prostate carcinoma
CHR	Chromogranin A	Neurosecretory granules	Neuroendocrine tumors
Ki-67 (MIB-1)		Cells in G1, S, G2, and M phases of cell cycle	Cycling cells, proliferation index, melanoma vs nevus
GFAP	Glial fibrillary acidic protein	Intermediate filament of glial cells	Glial tumors, gliosis
CD31	Platelet endothelial cell adhesion molecule	Vascular endothelial cells	Vascular tumors, highlight vessels
Factor VIII	Coagulation factor VIII	Vascular endothelial cells	Vascular tumors, highlight vessels
CD34		Vascular endothelial cells, dendritic interstitial cells	Vascular tumors, solitary fibrous tumor
D2-40	Lymphatic endothelial marker	Lymphatic endothelial cells	Lymphangioma, lymphatics
HSV	Herpes simplex virus	Herpes simplex virus	Keratitis, viral retinitis
CMV	Cytomegalovirus	Cytomegalovirus	Viral retinitis
HHV8	Human herpesvirus 8	Human herpesvirus 8	Kaposi sarcoma
HER2/neu (ErbB-2)	Human epidermal growth factor receptor 2	Human epidermal growth factor receptor 2	Prognostic assessment of breast cancer

CLL/SLL, small lymphocytic lymphoma; IHC, immunohistochemistry; JXG, juvenile xanthogranuloma; MEN2B, multiple endocrine neoplasia syndrome 2B; PNET, primitive neuroectodermal tumor; PPMD, posterior polymorphous dystrophy.
From Eagle RC Jr. Immunohistochemistry in diagnostic ophthalmic pathology: a review. *Clin Experiment Ophthalmol* 2008;36:675–688.

in formaldehyde and submitted for permanent control sections. It is unnecessary to re-examine the margins of the main fixed tissue specimen because the true surgical margins already have been examined using the frozen sections.

Corneal buttons obtained at penetrating keratoplasty usually are bisected before submission. The halves are wrapped in tissue to avoid specimen loss. Specimens from lamellar keratoplasty procedures also are commonly accessioned. These include thick lamellas of anterior cornea from deep anterior lamellar keratoplasty procedures, diaphanous sheets of Descemet membrane from Descemet-stripping endothelial keratoplasty (DSEK) procedures, and thin lamellas of posterior stroma and Descemet membrane from "failed" DSEK procedures. Our laboratory currently examines the stripped sheets of Descemet membrane from DSEK procedures as flat mounts.

Conjunctival biopsies tend to roll or ballup in fixative, making assessment of margins nearly impossible. Conjunctival biopsies should be gently spread out stromal side down on heavy paper or the thin cardboard used

TABLE 16-2	Immunoprofiles of Various Ocular Lesions
Merkel cell tumor	CAM5.2 (+), NSE (+), CK20 (+), CK7 (−), TTF-1 (−), S-100 (−)
Langerhans cell histiocytosis	CD1a (+), S-100 (+), CD68 (+) histiocytes
Rosai-Dorfman Disease	S-100 (+) , CD68 (+), CD1A (−) histiocytes
Sebaceous carcinoma	EMA (+), BRST-1 (+), CAM5.2 (+)
Squamous cell carcinoma	EMA (+), BRST-1 (−), CAM5.2 (−)
Basal cell carcinoma	EMA (−), BRST-1 (−), CAM5.2 (+)
Lymphangioma	D2-40 (+)
Mesectodermal leiomyoma	SMA (+), S100 (−), Melan A (−)
Peripheral nerve sheath tumor	SMA (−), S100 (+), Melan A (−), CD57 (+)
Uveal melanoma	SMA (−), S100 (+), Melan A (+), HMB45 (+), MITF (+), CD57 (−)
Meningioma	EMA (+), VIM (+), S-100 (+), SMA (+/−)
Retinoblastoma	NSE (+)
Metastatic carcinoma	CK (+), S-100 (−), CD45 (−)
Breast carcinoma	CK7 (+). CK20 (−), BRST-2 (+), ER (+/−), PR (+/−), HER2/neu (+/−)
Lung carcinoma	CK7 (−). CK20 (+), TTF-1 (+)
Colorectal carcinoma	CK7 (−). CK20 (+), CDX-2 (+)
Solitary fibrous tumor	CD34 (+), bcl-2 (+), CD99 (+)

From Eagle, RC Jr., Immunohistochemistry in diagnostic ophthalmic pathology: a review. *Clin Experiment Ophthalmol.* 2008;36:675-688.

to package sutures before they are immersed in fixative (Fig. 16-8B). If this is done, the specimen is fixed as a flat sheet, which is much easier to manipulate and section.

Ocular evisceration involves excision of the cornea and a rim of surrounding sclera and removal of the intraocular contents including uvea, retina, and vitreous. The scleral shell is left behind in the orbit. Some oculoplastic surgeons prefer to eviscerate eyes because postoperative ocular motility is superior. However, evisceration does not totally prevent the development of sympathetic uveitis, and blind painful eyes occasionally harbor unsuspected malignant neoplasms. A malignant tumor should be excluded with imaging, preferably B-scan ultrasonography, prior to eviscerating a blind painful eye. The large corneoscleral button and the intraocular contents are bisected and entirely submitted.

Orbital exenteration involves removal of the eye and all of the orbital contents. Orbital exenteration usually is performed when the orbit contains an unresectable primary tumor or has been invaded by an eyelid or conjunctival malignancy. Exenteration specimens are large and multiple surgical margins must be submitted. Orientation must be

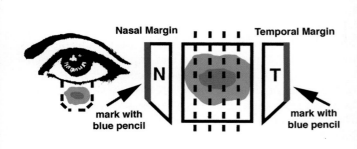

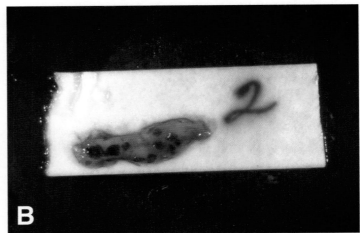

Fig. 16-8. A. Sectioning technique for full-thickness eyelid resection of malignant tumor. **B.** Conjunctival lesions like this nevus should be spread on cardboard prior to fixation to minimize distortion.

maintained during dissection. Before dissection, the surgical margin (external aspect of the specimen) is marked by coating the specimen with India ink. Immersing the ink-coated specimen in Bouin fixative binds the ink to the tissue.

Temporal artery biopsy is performed to rule out giant cell arteritis (Fig. 8-18). To avoid skip lesions, an adequate biopsy should be at least 2 cm long. After fixation, the artery is divided into a series of transverse segments, which are embedded cut-surface down. It much is easier to interpret transverse sections. Arteries that are positive for giant cell arteritis may appear thickened and opacified on gross examination.

Frozen Section Diagnosis

Frozen sections are cut from a block of fresh unfixed tissue that is flash frozen in liquid nitrogen or refrigerated isopentane. The frozen tissue is sectioned with a refrigerated microtome called a cryostat and is stained with a rapid H&E technique. Sections usually are ready for interpretation in 10 minutes or less.

The most common indication for frozen section diagnosis in ophthalmic pathology is the intraoperative assessment of surgical margins during excision of malignant eyelid tumors. In orbital surgery, frozen sections are used to determine if the tissue obtained is representative or adequate for diagnosis. The decision to exenterate an orbit should always be based on examination of the permanent sections.

Rapid diagnosis is the main advantage of frozen section diagnosis, but speed has its price. The technical quality of frozen sections is always substantially inferior to that of routine sections prepared from paraffin-embedded tissue. The quality of frozen sections usually is sufficient to determine if a basal cell carcinoma or some other common eyelid tumor has been totally excised, although sebaceous and melanocytic lesions may be problematic. In many instances, the final diagnosis of orbital lesions must be deferred to permanent sections. One should remember that frozen section diagnosis consumes valuable tissue that might be better utilized if it were fixed in formaldehyde and processed routinely for light microscopy.

Lymphoid Tumors

Lymphoid tumors are discussed in the chapters on conjunctiva and orbit. If lymphoma is suspected clinically, fresh unfixed tissue should be submitted for immunophenotypic assessment by flow cytometry. Flow cytometry is superior to IHC performed on sections of paraffin-embedded tissue, because flow cytometry can determine clonality by assessing immunoglobulin light chains and quantifies the different types of lymphocytes as well. An adequate sample of fresh tissue is necessary for flow cytometry. Optimally, the sample should be at least as large as a pea, which excludes some

conjunctival lesions. Specimens for flow cytometry should be forwarded expeditiously to the laboratory in a closed, moist container that contains a piece of gauze moistened with saline to prevent drying. The specimen should not be immersed in saline.

Other Diagnostic Tools

Transmission (TEM) and scanning electron microscopy (SEM) occasionally are used as adjuncts to routine histology in diagnostic pathology laboratories, and are tools in ocular research. TEM is still used occasionally for the diagnosis of tumors and unusual lesions, but it has been largely supplanted by immunohistochemistry, which is cheaper, faster, and less labor intensive. SEM shows the three-dimensional shape of objects at high magnification and resolution and can reveal patterns of disease that are not immediately obvious in sectioned material (Fig. 9-17A). Specially equipped scanning electron microscopes can rapidly determine the elemental composition of materials such as foreign bodies using energy dispersive x-ray spectroscopy.

As noted above, flow cytometry is primarily used to assess the immunophenotype of adnexal lymphoid lesions in ophthalmic pathology. A suspension of fresh, unfixed cells is prepared and aliquots are reacted with a variety of antibodies directed against selected lymphocytic markers. Suspended in fluid, the cells flow rapidly through a thin tube past detectors that are able to detect and accurately quantify them. Flow cytometry has been used to measure the DNA content of tumor cells and assess the ploidy of neoplasms. This has not proved to be especially beneficial in the evaluation of ocular tumors.

In situ hybridization employs nucleic acid probes whose sequences are complementary to a specific sought-for sequence of DNA or RNA in tissue. *In situ* hybridization is used to detect the presence of pathogens such as bacteria or viruses in tissue sections. Fluorescent *in situ* hybridization is used to detect chromosomal deletions and translocations. Examples include the evaluation of uveal melanoma for monosomy 3 and the assessment of rhabdomyosarcoma for the characteristic translocations found in the alveolar form of the tumor.

The polymerase chain reaction is used to detect the presence of organisms by amplifying species-specific parts of their genetic material. The technique uses two single-stranded DNA primers that are complementary to segments of the target organism's DNA. DNA synthesis is catalyzed by a heat-resistant form of DNA polymerase obtained from *Thermus aquaticus*, bacteria isolated from a hot spring in Yellowstone National Park. Repeated cycles of thermal denaturation, annealing, and synthesis amplify the sought-after segment of DNA a millionfold, producing quantities that are large enough to detect. Southern blot analysis is used to identify the DNA.

Gene expression profiling is a research tool that employs DNA microarray technology to measure the activity of thousands of genes. Microarray analysis of uveal malignant melanoma has identified two classes of tumors that differ markedly in their risk of metastasis.

The Ophthalmologist and the Pathology Laboratory

Effective and accurate communication is the most important element in the relationship between the practicing ophthalmologist and the pathology laboratory. Pathologists are consultants who require accurate clinical data to provide their clinical colleagues with optimum service. Few physicians would refer a patient to a consultant without a clinical summary or letter of introduction, yet specimens constantly arrive in pathology laboratories with little or no clinical data.

Ophthalmologists usually communicate with the pathology laboratory in writing using the pathology slip or transmittal form. Information on the slip should include the age, sex, and race (if pertinent) of the patient; the laterality and location of the lesion; the operation performed; the clinical impression (preoperative diagnosis); the postoperative diagnosis if different; and any other appropriate clinical information. If the specimen is a globe, the visual acuity and intraocular pressure should also be listed. Many surgeons do not realize that satisfactory completion of pathology slips is a requirement of hospital and laboratory accrediting organizations such as the Joint Commission and the College of American Pathologists.

The patient's age and sex should always be listed. Age is an extremely important factor in the interpretation of melanocytic lesions of the conjunctiva. Junctional nevi of the conjunctiva do occur rarely in children, but a "junctional nevus" in a middle-aged or elderly patient is almost always primary acquired melanosis, a precursor of conjunctival malignant melanoma. The sex of the patient is important in the assessment of metastatic disease. Breast carcinoma is the most common source of ocular metastases in women, but is quite rare in men. The patient's race should be noted if it is pertinent and important from a clinical standpoint. Certain tumors such as uveal melanoma occur infrequently in patients of African ancestry, while sarcoidosis is common.

"Lesion" is not a particularly helpful or informative preoperative diagnosis. Always list the diagnosis if you are fairly certain what the "lesion" is, or at least indicate important entities that you would like to rule out. Your clinical impression is important because it may influence how your specimen is processed. For example, if the pathologist knows that you are concerned about sebaceous carcinoma, he or she usually will reserve some "wet tissue" for possible fat stains, which may be necessary to confirm the diagnosis in poorly differentiated cases. Fat stains cannot be done if the entire specimen has been embedded in paraffin because the fat is dissolved out by the solvents used in processing. Although routine tissue processing precludes staining for fat, fixation does not. Fresh unfixed tissue is easier to cut, but frozen sections can still be prepared from formalin-fixed tissue.

Direct personal communication with your pathologist is advised if your case is unusual or important, you are concerned about the diagnosis, or have questions about proper specimen handling. Call your pathologist if you have questions or concerns. Personal contact is the fastest and most efficient (and most confidential) means of conveying important clinical data. Furthermore, it decreases the likelihood that your specimen will be mishandled and may give your pathologist additional insight that can contribute to an accurate diagnosis. Your pathologist is your best guide to laboratory services and may be able to suggest additional tests, techniques, or methods of tissue processing that can facilitate diagnosis. He or she can also inform you about special fixation or processing requirements (e.g., fresh tissue for flow cytometric analysis of lymphoid tumors).

Personal communication is always best if you think your specimen may need special stains or special procedures such as electron microscopy. Ordering the pathologist to do a certain stain on the pathology slip without discussing the case beforehand is tantamount to the pathologist instructing the surgeon what operation to perform and what instruments to use. The pathologist usually knows what stains and procedures are indicated and should be ordered (assuming that he or she is aware of your problem and has been supplied with adequate clinical data). You should also speak to the pathologist directly if you need photographs for presentation or publication. Most cases are not photographed routinely and the cost of photography is not reimbursed. You are asking the pathologist to expend his or her time and resources to do you a favor.

If possible, you should consider personally handdelivering your important specimens to the laboratory. This assures that your specimen will arrive expeditiously and will not be misplaced in the operating room or lost in transit. It also evidences your interest and concern.

Batching and submitting multiple specimens excised from different locations in a single container is dangerous. This occasionally is done by ophthalmologists who believe that they are excising multiple benign cysts or papillomas. If one of the lesions proves to be an unexpected malignancy (e.g., an incompletely excised basal cell carcinoma), its location will be unknown.

All ophthalmologists are encouraged to visit the pathology laboratory and review their cases with the pathologist under the microscope. Always review the histopathology with your pathologist if your clinical impression and the pathologic diagnosis are discordant, and question diagnoses that are unexpected or make no sense. If you remain unsatisfied, request a consultation with an experienced ophthalmic pathologist. Finally, always forward rare or unusual ocular lesions to ophthalmic pathology laboratories that appreciate their significance and have the experience and expertise to process and evaluate them.

BIBLIOGRAPHY

Boenisch T. *Handbook on Immunohistochemical Staining Methods*, 3rd ed. Carpinteria, CA: Dako Corporation, 2001.

DeLellis RA, Resnick M, Frable WJ. General and special techniques in surgical pathology and cytopathology. In: Silverberg SG, DeLellis RA, Frable WJ, et al., eds. *Silverberg's Principles And Practice Of Surgical Pathology And Cytopathology*. Philadelphia, PA: Churchhill Livingstone/Elsevier, 2006:25–54.

Eagle RC Jr. Specimen handling in the ophthalmic pathology laboratory. *Ophthalmol Clin N Am* 1995;8:1–15.

Eagle RC Jr. Photographic tips for the ophthalmic pathology laboratory. In: Wilson R, ed. *The Year Book of Ophthalmology*. Mosby, 1997:341–354.

Eagle RC Jr. Immunohistochemistry in diagnostic ophthalmic pathology: a review. *Clin Experiment Ophthalmol* 2008;36:675–688.

Guesdon Jl, Ternynck T, Avrameas S. The uses of avidin-biotin interaction in immunoenzymatic techniques. *J Histochem Cytochem* 1979;27:1131–1139.

Hsu S-M, Raine L, Fanger H. Use of avidin-biotin-peroxidase complex (abc) in immunoperoxidase techniques: a comparison between abc and unlabeled antibody (pap) procedures. *J Histochem Cytochem* 1981;29:577–580.

Hsu S-M, Raine L. Protein A, avidin and biotin in immunocytochemistry. *J Histochem Cytochem* 1981;29:1349–1353.

Ramos-Vara JA. Technical aspects of immunohistochemistry. *Vet Pathol* 2005;42:405–426.

Shi SR, Key ME, Kalra KL. Antigen retrieval in formalin-fixed, paraffin-embedded tissues: an enhancement method for immunohistochemical staining based on microwave oven heating of tissue sections. *J Histochem Cytochem* 1991;39:741–748.

INDEX

Page numbers in *italics* denote figures; those followed by a "t" denote tables.